Encyclopedia
of
BIOETHICS

Encyclopedia
of
BIOETHICS

WARREN T. REICH, *Editor in Chief*

GEORGETOWN UNIVERSITY

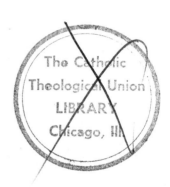

VOLUME **1**

THE FREE PRESS
A Division of Macmillan Publishing Co., Inc.
NEW YORK

Collier Macmillan Publishers
LONDON

THE FREE PRESS
A Division of Macmillan Publishing Co., Inc.
866 Third Avenue, New York, N.Y. 10022

Collier Macmillan Canada, Ltd.

Library of Congress Catalog Card Number: 78–8821

Printed in the United States of America

printing number

2 3 4 5 6 7 8 9 10

Library of Congress Cataloging in Publication Data
Main entry under title:

Encyclopedia of bioethics.

  Includes bibliographies and index.
  1. Bioethics–Dictionaries. 2. Medical ethics–
Dictionaries. I. Reich, Warren T. [DNLM: 1. Bio-
ethics–Encyclopedias. QH302.5 E56]
QH332.E52   174′.2   78-8821
ISBN 0-02-926060-4

The *Encyclopedia of Bioethics* project was made possible by a grant from the National Endowment for the Humanities. In funding the project the Endowment matched gifts from non-federal sources including The Joseph P. Kennedy, Jr. Foundation, the Raskob Foundation, The Commonwealth Fund, The Loyola Foundation, Inc., and The David J. Greene Foundation, Inc. The views expressed in this encyclopedia are not necessarily those of the Endowment or of these foundations.

Contents

Editorial Advisory Board

Preface

When a special encyclopedia—one aiming to be comprehensive in a particular discipline—is the first in its field, its appearance has the potential for marking an important stage in the development of one aspect of human knowledge. Yet its production invariably is attended by unique problems that can be surmounted only by a combination of loyal support, careful planning, and capable personnel. The *Encyclopedia of Bioethics* has been no exception to this rule.

This encyclopedia could not have been developed had it not been for the intellectual vision and continual labors of André E. Hellegers, first director of The Joseph and Rose Kennedy Institute of Ethics at Georgetown University. His constant supportive efforts made possible the launching and sustaining of this project.

Georgetown University provided a stimulating and supportive academic atmosphere in addition to financial assistance for carrying out this project. We are particularly indebted to two Presidents of the University, Robert J. Henle and Timothy S. Healy, for their faith in this project.

The National Endowment for the Humanities, a federal grant-making agency, provided the principal funding for the project by matching gifts from private sources, including The Joseph P. Kennedy, Jr. Foundation, the Raskob Foundation, The Commonwealth Fund, The Loyola Foundation, Inc., and The David J. Greene Foundation, Inc. Ronald Berman, Chairman of the National Endowment for the Humanities during most of this project, and Robert Kingston, Deputy Chairman, showed a strong interest in the project at its inception and gave their consistent support through its final stages. The encyclopedia was completed while Joseph Duffey was Chairman of the Endowment. The *Encyclopedia of Bioethics* is a project of the Endowment's Program of Science, Technology and Human Values. We are grateful to Richard Hedrich, coordinator of that program, for his continuous encouragement and assistance.

The organizations that funded the encyclopedia project, and Georgetown University, were firmly committed to the principle that the editors and contributors would present all views—in an interdisciplinary, intercultural, and international context.

As Senior Research Scholar at The Kennedy Institute during the first year of its existence (1971–1972), I conceived the idea of developing a reference work that would gather together what was known about the scientific state of the art and the full range of ethical views and policy options in matters dealing with the life sciences. After extensive consultation with experts in the organization of knowledge, in the fields bearing on bioethics, in editing, and in publishing, I developed the basic plan for the project and selected the Editorial Advisory Board, the Associate Editors, and the editorial staff. As Editor in Chief, I directed the various phases of the work, commissioned the articles, maintained direct contact with the contributors, and determined the acceptability of the articles and of all other materials in light of the purpose, scope, and desired level of quality of the work.

In the fall of 1972, approximately twenty-two members of the Editorial Advisory Board assembled for two meetings held at Georgetown University to test the feasibility of this encyclopedia and to recommend topics, organizational ideas, and personnel. The sixty members of the Editorial Advisory Board, listed elsewhere in these introductory pages, are from eleven countries and represent all the disciplines converging on bioethics. They reviewed several drafts of the table of contents, made suggestions of topics and contributors, and responded to specific editorial questions that arose in the course of the work. Some of them also reviewed manuscripts. It is a pleasure to thank this distinguished international and interdisciplinary Editorial Advisory Board for their advice and encouragement.

Eight Associate Editors, who played a crucial role in designing and evaluating the contents of the work, were selected on the basis of their outstanding knowledge of the field of bioethics, the diversity of their intellectual and methodological backgrounds, and the special areas in which each of them had excelled. They contributed to this project a level of expertise and dedication that could scarcely have been matched by any other group.

Each Associate Editor submitted descriptions of the intended scope of the articles in a specific area, prepared a list of contributors for each article, judged the quality of the manuscripts, and decided on their acceptability. We integrated the entire plan at several meetings and constantly adapted it as the articles were being prepared.

The Associate Editors and I, working collaboratively, exercised full autonomy in setting editorial policies, selecting contributors, and approving the contents of the work.

A complete editorial staff was hired specifically for this project at The Kennedy Institute. This group included the assistant editors, managing editor, bibliographers, and editorial secretaries. In addition, we hired research assistants, bibliographic assistants, copy editors, proofreaders, an assistant managing editor, computer specialists, and a clerical staff to perform specific tasks as needs arose.

Sandra Hass, the encyclopedia's managing editor, did outstanding work in directing the editorial staff and coordinating contact with the contributors, advisors, reviewers, and publisher. We are indebted to her for her loyalty and her persistence in setting and maintaining high standards of excellence for stylistic editing of the work.

The consulting editor, Philip Wiener, editor of the *Dictionary of the History of Ideas,* gave extensive advice and also made editorial suggestions regarding the articles.

The assistant editors rendered an indispensable service, especially in correcting and evaluating manuscripts at the revision stage. Many phases of the project could not have been brought to successful completion without the competent help of the research and editorial staffs; I would like to thank especially Cheryl Calhoun, Sara Hannum Chase, Ronald S. Gass, Nina Shafran, Mary Ellen Timbol, and Susan White.

The bibliographies are a major component of this encyclopedia. The task of verifying and copy editing all bibliographic listings, as well as occasionally suggesting additional bibliographic items, was carried out with meticulous and professional attention by the bibliographer, William Pitt. He was assisted at various times by a total of twenty-seven persons.

Credit for the quality of the articles must go principally to the contributors. They accommodated themselves to the integrated plan, the scholarly standards, the succinct yet comprehensive style, and the demanding schedule of the encyclopedia. Edited manuscripts were returned to the contributors for their correction and approval; a final copy of the text was mailed to them in the form of printed galleys.

The following standards guided us in the selection of contributors: that each should have highly respected qualifications to write on the topic as well as the ability to write well, and that they should include diverse intellectual backgrounds and appropriate geographical and institutional representation. The names and institutional affiliations of all contributors are listed in the front matter of this encyclopedia, together with the titles of their articles. We are especially grateful to those contributors who prepared excellent articles on extremely short notice as we approached the end of the project.

All manuscripts were thoroughly reviewed for appropriateness of scope, accuracy of content, and clarity of style by at least four editors. In addition, we called on special reviewers to evaluate manuscripts that included material beyond the special expertise of the editors. These special reviewers, whose names are listed elsewhere in the front matter of this encyclopedia, made an important contribution to the accuracy of this work.

My colleagues, the scholars of The Kennedy Institute, have been most generous with their time and advice, and have been a constant and indispensable resource for the development of this project. They include these philosophers, religious ethicists, biologists, physicians, demographers, economists, and lawyers, who have been permanent and visiting scholars of the Institute: Francisco Abel, Robert C. Baumiller, Tom L. Beauchamp, Roy Branson, Frederick Carney, Kenneth Casebeer, James F. Childress, John Connery, Charles E. Curran, H. Tristram Engelhardt, Jr., Murray Gendell, Bernard Häring, Stanley Hauerwas, André E. Hellegers, James Jones, Leon R. Kass, Patricia A. King, Karen Lebacqz, Sid Z. Leiman, Richard A. McCormick, Thomas Merrick, Gene Outka, Seymour Perlin, Ralph B. Potter, Jeanne Clare Ridley, Bruno Schüller, Henry S. Shryock, Joan Sieber, Seymour Siegel, David Smith, Conrad Taeuber, and LeRoy Walters.

In the early planning stages of the encyclopedia project, the editors of several scholarly journals agreed to serve as advisory editors. They were asked to recommend contributors and reviewers and to comment on the topics to be included in the work. Several of them also served as critical reviewers of manuscripts. They are Philip H. Abelson, editor of *Science;* Walter J. Burghardt, editor of *Theological Studies;* Marshall Cohen, editor of *Philosophy & Public Affairs;* T. George Harris, editor in chief of *Psychology Today;* Franz J. Ingelfinger, editor of *The New England Journal of Medicine;* Paul Kurtz, editor of *The Humanist;* Peter J. M. McEwan, editor in chief of *Ethics in Science & Medicine;* Robert H. Moser, editor of *The Journal of the American Medical Association;* Nicholas Rescher, editor of *American Philosophical Quarterly;* Wolfgang Schweitzer, editor of *Zeitschrift für Evangelische Ethik;* and Edward F. Shotter, member of the Editorial Board for the *Journal of Medical Ethics.*

Preparation of the bibliographies, which embrace a wide variety of disciplines and cultures, could not have been accomplished without the resources and personnel of many libraries. We wish to thank the following libraries of Georgetown University: The Center for Bioethics Library, Kennedy Institute of Ethics; Lauinger Library—its Reference, Serials, Government Documents, Acquisitions, Special Collections, Cataloging, and Circulation staffs; Woodstock Theological Center Library; Dahlgren Medical Library; Bloomer Science Library; the Library of the Center for Population Research; and the Dennis Library of the Georgetown University Law Center.

We are also indebted to: The Library of Congress, especially its Reference staff, its Law Library, and its Orientalia Division; the National Library of Medicine, its Reference staff, and its Rare Book staff; the National Institutes of Health Library; the Theology, Philosophy, and Canon Law Library of the Catholic University of America; The George Washington University Library and Burns Law Library; the American University Library; Wesley Theological

Seminary Library; the Howard University Medical-Dental Library; the University of Maryland libraries; and the State Library of Maryland.

There were many university, college, public, and private special libraries in the District of Columbia area that helped us, as well as those librarians who responded to telephone inquiries throughout the United States and Canada. Special reference help came from the United Nations and associated international organizations, as well as from various embassies, notably those of Canada, the United Kingdom, the Federal Republic of Germany, and the Peoples' Republic of China.

Many individuals, too numerous to mention, assisted in the completion of this encyclopedia. We thank all of them, especially David Eggenberger, David Sills, and John Bradley for their advice and encouragement; Dorothy Sawicki for her careful preparation of manuscripts for the printer, her supervision of the proofreading, and her correction of the galley proofs; George Rowland of The Free Press, who served as the publisher's managing editor, for his extraordinary cooperation and steadfast concern for the quality and appearance of this work; William E. May for his astute evaluation and speedy editing of manuscripts in the crucial final stage of the project; Doris Goldstein, Kennedy Institute librarian, for her cooperation in obtaining information and for preparing Additional Resources in Bioethics, which appears at the end of this encyclopedia; David Webster for his helpful legal advice; and the following for their advice on topics and contributors: James Luther Adams, Harry Gordon, James Gustafson, R. M. Hare, Joseph Kitagawa, Frank Reynolds, Daniel Robinson, Lloyd Stevenson, and Owsei Temkin.

A special acknowledgment must be given to The Joseph P. Kennedy, Jr. Foundation for contributing generously to the support of this project and for establishing The Joseph and Rose Kennedy Institute of Ethics, a research center at Georgetown University. This encyclopedia project could not have been completed without the scholarly resources of The Kennedy Institute. It was The Kennedy Foundation's deep interest in the well-being of the mentally retarded and of children—groups so vulnerable to neglect and exploitation—that led the Foundation to create The Kennedy Institute and to support a variety of research and teaching endeavors in the field of bioethics.

Finally, a special expression of gratitude goes to Sargent Shriver, Chairman of The Kennedy Institute's International Advisory Board. He has worked with singular dedication for the support of this project and for the advancement of the discipline of ethics, both basic and applied, in the biomedical and other professions.

WARREN T. REICH
Senior Research Scholar, Center for Bioethics,
*   The Joseph and Rose Kennedy Institute of Ethics*
Associate Professor of Bioethics, School of Medicine
Georgetown University
Washington, D.C.

Introduction

The *Encyclopedia of Bioethics* is the first encyclopedia in its field. Its purpose is to synthesize, analyze, and compare the positions taken on the problems of bioethics, in the past as well as in the present, to indicate which issues require further examination, and to point to anticipated developments in the ethics of the life sciences and health care.

The emergence of bioethics as a field of study is a contemporary phenomenon traceable to several causes. First, the issues of bioethics have captured the contemporary mind because they represent major conflicts in the area of technology and basic human values, those dealing with life, death, and health. Although many bioethical issues have been discussed since ancient times, the introduction of modern biomedical technologies, especially since the 1950s, has intensified some age-old questions and has given rise to perplexing new problems—the prolongation of life, euthanasia, prenatal diagnosis and abortion, human experimentation, genetic interventions and reproductive technologies, behavior control and psychosurgery, the definition of death, the right to privacy, allocation of scarce health resources, and dilemmas in the maintenance of environmental health.

Second, there is an intense and widespread interest in bioethics because it offers a stimulating intellectual and moral challenge. In contrast to earlier eras, when ethical world views were held in common and offered a certain security for dealing with moral dilemmas, today the very tools for coping with these problems are themselves subject of considerable controversy. There is an uncertainty about moral values, ethical principles, and their priorities; the contemporary world is experiencing a philosophical upheaval; and many systems of theological thought are questioning traditional assumptions in religious ethics. Bioethics has already had a significant intellectual impact, for it has precipitated a reexamination of basic moral values and methods of applying them to practical ethical questions.

Third, the rapid growth of the field of bioethics has been facilitated by the openness to multidisciplinary work that characterizes many scholars and academic institutions today, especially in matters dealing with personal and social aspects of human behavior.

Bioethics, like other special fields of learning, has manifested the "explosion of knowledge" characteristic of our era. Courses of study in bioethics have proliferated in universities, professional schools, colleges, and high schools; a number of scholarly journals specially devoted to the field have begun publication; hundreds of journals in disciplines bearing directly on bioethical concerns—such as medicine, law, psychology, philosophy, religious studies, biology, and political sciences—have dramatically increased the amount of space they offer to bioethics articles; monographs and anthologies have multiplied; and research institutes have been established.

The Editors and Editorial Advisory Board of this work were convinced that a reference work was needed that would gather together, as comprehensively yet as succinctly as possible, what is known about the questions of bioethics, the data from which they arise, a full range of responses to them, and the principles and values that account for those responses.

We believe that the articles and accompanying bibliographies in the *Encyclopedia of Bioethics* will be helpful to those who have been seeking a reliable and comprehensive treatment of topics in bioethics. Our prospective readers fall into four groups:

- teachers and their students—in departments or programs of philosophy, religion, biology, medicine, social sciences, psychology, law, health sciences, and other disciplines—who are increasingly involved in education, research, and writing in the field
- nonacademic scholars, journalists, and other writers whose important contributions to bioethics would be greatly strengthened by a reference work in this field
- health professionals who would draw on such a work to inform and enrich their professional lives, e.g., physicians, health administrators, nurses, psychologists, social workers, lawyers, and counselors
- those involved in the formulation and execution of public policy bearing on the life sciences and health care, such as legislators, judges, public officials, health planners, and members of research committees

This encyclopedia was designed, then, not only to meet educational needs, but to serve as a resource for professional decision making, for the development of public policies, and for further research.

Although it is unusual, perhaps unprecedented, for a special encyclopedia to be produced almost simultaneously with the emergence of its field, several reasons persuaded us that this work was not premature. First, many of the issues and methodological roots of bioethics are not new; they were waiting to be gleaned from centuries of literature in the fields of philosophy, medical ethics, history of medicine, and other fields. Second, the plethora of contemporary literature badly needed systematization: Approximately 1,500 significant items are published annually in the English language alone. Third, an encyclopedia could assist the formation of this field of study.

In a field as fast-growing as bioethics, one difficulty is that the encyclopedia might be outdated too quickly. This problem is not unique to bioethics: Most active fields of learning are subject to constant change and development, with the result that most special encyclopedias, and even general encyclopedias, are faced with the need to adapt to a rapid growth in knowledge. An encyclopedia cannot be a vehicle for definitive statements in fixed categories of thought; it must be a tool that reflects and facilitates the development of ideas. The purpose of this encyclopedia, then, was not to freeze knowledge, but to summarize and analyze the historical and current state of knowledge in bioethics in such a way as to facilitate learning what is known in this area and to stimulate further thought and research. Furthermore, we have attempted to minimize the problem of obsolescence by asking the contributors to emphasize major positions and schemes of analysis. Supplements to or revisions of this reference work can serve future needs by reporting new scientific data and summarizing further developments in the field of bioethics.

SCOPE OF THE ENCYCLOPEDIA

The range of subject matter within this encyclopedia was chosen to make the work reasonably self-contained. The scope of topics, discussed in more detail below, can be viewed at several levels: (I) the range of *concrete ethical and legal problems* included within bioethics; (II) the basic *concepts* that clarify bioethical issues and the *principles* appealed to as guides for human behavior in this area; (III) the various *ethical theories* that account for how one knows human values and justifies the norms that should guide human conduct; (IV) the *religious traditions,* which also account for what is good and bad, right and wrong in bioethical matters; (V) *historical perspectives,* particularly in the traditional area of medical ethics which deals specifically with the physician–patient relationship; and (VI) information about *disciplines bearing on bioethics.*

The following outline offers an overview of the contents of the encyclopedia under the six headings mentioned above.

I. **Concrete Ethical and Legal Problems.**   This category of entries deals with specific normative questions—i.e., value questions requiring an answer as to what ought or ought not to be done. These questions may arise, for example, in reference to specific kinds of actions (such as sterilization of the retarded), value aspects of relationships (e.g., What sort of confidentiality should characterize the psychiatrist–patient relationship?), and public policy options and legal structures (e.g., What policy should govern the cessation of medical treatment of the incompetent elderly?). More than any other single factor, the range of these issues defines the scope of bioethics. The following headings represent the broad spectrum of concrete ethical problems in bioethics; under each heading some examples are given representing article titles in the encyclopedia.

The Therapeutic Relationship—e.g., truth-telling, informed consent, confidentiality, medical malpractice, and the patients' rights movement. We have also singled out some dominant health professions as titles of separate articles, trusting that the issues they encounter would serve as models for discussing the ethical problems of the innumerable health professions and specialties. Some of the articles treating individual professions include medicine, nursing, dentistry, surgery, pharmacy, medical social work, public health, and social medicine. The mental health professions are included topically, that is, in articles dealing with such topics as mental health therapies.

Codes of Professional Ethics—articles dealing with the history and ethical analysis of codes of medical ethics. The encyclopedia also includes an Appendix, which is a selective annotated collection of the texts of the most important codes from the earliest to contemporary times. The Appendix is organized under four headings: I. GENERAL CODES FOR THE PRACTICE OF MEDICINE; II. DIRECTIVES FOR HUMAN EXPERIMENTATION; III. PATIENTS' BILLS OF RIGHTS; and IV. CODES OF SPECIALTY HEALTH-CARE ASSOCIATIONS. Highlights of most of these codes are synthesized and analyzed in the Appendix's introductory article on CODES OF THE HEALTH-CARE PROFESSIONS.

Health Care—including such topics as humanization and dehumanization of health care, right to health-care services, rationing of medical treatment, international health, and health policy.

Sociopolitical Problems in Biomedicine—for example, torture and the health professional, biomedical science and war, and racism.

Biomedical and Behavioral Research—including articles on the social and professional control of human experimentation, informed consent in human research, research on children, and research on the mentally handicapped.

Mental Health and Behavioral Issues—embracing such questions as drug use, abuse, and dependence; self-realization therapies; behavior control; psychosurgery; and institutionalization.

Sexuality, Contraception, Sterilization, and Abortion—embracing such topics as sex therapy and sex research; sexual ethics; abortion: historical and contemporary perspectives; and sterilization: ethical and legal aspects.

Genetics—including genetic screening, genetic counseling, gene therapy, eugenics, and genetic aspects of human behavior.

Reproductive Technologies—for example, artificial insemination, in vitro fertilization, sex selection, and asexual human reproduction ("cloning").

Organ and Tissue Transplantation and Artificial Organs—blood transfusion, organ transplantation, heart transplantation, and kidney dialysis and transplantation.

Death and Dying—including such topics as definition and determination of death, euthanasia and sustaining life, suicide, and ethical perspectives on the care of infants.

Population—e.g., history of population policies; compulsory population control programs; and genetic implications of population control.

Environment—e.g., environmental health and human disease, and the problem of growth.

II. **Basic Concepts and Principles.** Also discussed in this encyclopedia are underlying concepts that clarify or give shape to ethical attitudes and positions in bioethics, e.g., health and disease, pain and suffering, life, death in Eastern and Western thought, and paternalism. Principles, i.e., norms of right conduct, are listed under such titles as justice, rights, double effect, and obligations to future generations.

III. **Ethical Theories.** Systematic philosophical methods of viewing the moral life and of accounting for what is good and right in human conduct are explained, for example, in the entry titled ETHICS. This entry—which is intended to be a virtual primer in ethical theory with examples taken from bioethics—contains twelve articles dealing with a broad range of ethical theories, beginning with the introductory article on THE TASK OF ETHICS, and including such titles as UTILITARIANISM, DEONTOLOGICAL THEORIES, RULES AND PRINCIPLES, and THEOLOGICAL ETHICS. The reader would do well to relate these articles and the entries on religious traditions to the entry on BIOETHICS to grasp the ethical underpinnings of the field.

IV. **Religious Traditions.** The great traditions of religious ethics embody beliefs and principles that are applicable to problems in bioethics. The implications of these religious traditions for bioethics have been synthesized —several of them for the first time—in this encyclopedia. They include Buddhism, Confucianism, Eastern Orthodox Christianity, Hinduism, Islam, Judaism, Protestantism, Roman Catholicism, and Taoism. Additionally, some articles deal expressly with the ethical approaches taken by various religious groups to specific issues in bioethics. These are found either as separate titles—e.g., Islamic perspectives on population ethics— or combined with nonreligious views, as in the article on the ethical aspects of sterilization.

V. **Historical Perspectives.** A unique feature of this encyclopedia is the comprehensive 97,000-word entry on the history of medical ethics. Its twenty-nine articles, designed to reward a reading either separately or in sequence, are divided into four sections: PRIMITIVE SOCIETIES; NEAR AND MIDDLE EAST AND AFRICA; SOUTH AND EAST ASIA; and EUROPE AND THE AMERICAS. Each section contains articles in chronological sequence, with such titles as: ANCIENT NEAR EAST; PREREPUBLICAN CHINA; MEDIEVAL EUROPE: FOURTH TO SIXTEENTH CENTURY; NORTH AMERICA: SEVENTEENTH TO NINETEENTH CENTURY; and EASTERN EUROPE IN THE TWENTIETH CENTURY. Other historical articles are situated topically within the encyclopedia, such as those on the history of the therapeutic relationship and the history of human experimentation.

VI. **Disciplines Bearing on Bioethics.** Some entries survey an entire discipline, presenting in succinct fashion an overview of the discipline and its bearing on bioethics. In this category are entries on the philosophy of biology; the anthropology of medicine; the philosophy of medicine; the sociology of medicine; and the sociology of science.

DEFINING THE FIELD OF BIOETHICS

Bioethics is a composite term derived from the Greek words *bios* (life) and *ēthikē* (ethics). It can be defined as the systematic study of human conduct in the area of the life sciences and health care, insofar as this conduct is examined in the light of moral values and principles.

Bioethics is an area of interdisciplinary studies whose focus depends on the kinds of issues it examines and the nature of ethical inquiry. The scope of the field has been outlined earlier in this Introduction under "Scope of the Encyclopedia," especially in the thirteen areas of "Concrete Ethical and Legal Problems." Further explanation may help define more fully the scope of bioethics as presupposed in this encyclopedia and in the interdisciplinary approach we have taken.

Bioethics encompasses medical ethics and extends beyond it. Medical ethics in its traditional meaning deals with value-related problems that arise in the physician–patient relationship. Bioethics is more inclusive in four significant respects:

> It embraces the value-related problems that arise in all health professions, including the "allied" health professions, mental health professions, and so forth.
>
> It extends to biomedical and behavioral research, whether or not that research has a direct bearing on therapy.
>
> It includes a broad range of social issues, such as those associated with public health, occupational health, international health, and the ethics of population control.
>
> It extends beyond human life and health to embrace issues involving animal and plant life, e.g., in the topics dealing with animal experimentation and competing environmental claims.

These four main areas can be accounted for as the cardinal issues of bioethics by two key terms in our definition of bioethics: the *life sciences* and *health care*. Both of these terms have acquired broad connotations in the contemporary world. Health care cannot be restricted to physical health nor confined to the medical profession. A life science may also be defined somewhat broadly as "a branch of science (as biology, medicine, anthropology, or sociology) that deals with living organisms and life processes" (*Webster's New Collegiate Dictionary*, 1973).

The appropriateness of including a broad range of health professions within bioethics is obvious simply because health-care services are rendered by so many professions. Both biomedical and behavioral research can be viewed either as activities of the life sciences or as endeavors inextricably linked with health care or both. Similarly, a broad range of social issues is associated with health care; the competing interests of human, animal, and plant life are deeply enmeshed in the life sciences; and demographic concerns are inseparable from health care and the life sciences.

For example, environmental health and occupational health raise ethical issues at least as important as those encountered on an individual basis in the clinic; and the biological disciplines, so central to the life sciences, embrace not only molecular and cell biology, but organismic biology (including ecology, eugenics, and genetics) and population biology (which has an integral relationship with population ecology, population genetics, and sociology). Furthermore, even the perennial problems of medical ethics, such as the ethics of sterilization and abortion, cannot be adequately discussed except in the context of demographic and environmental perspectives.

Certainly not all scholars would agree on the precise scope of bioethics. The explanation offered here gives a rationale for the broad perspective on the scope of bioethics that is presumed in the structure of this encyclopedia.

Bioethics is further defined by the nature of ethical inquiry and the competence presumed for it.

Contributions are made to bioethics by philosophers, biologists, physicians, theologians, psychologists, lawyers, various health professionals, social scientists, and many others. Some have claimed that the right ethical answers can be known directly from the implications of the biomedical sciences themselves, or simply from sociological studies of human behavior in the area of biomedicine. These claims represent particular theories of moral knowledge; but it is the aim of this encyclopedia to present all significant theories and viewpoints.

The assumption underlying this work is that all the contributing disciplines are concerned with an evaluative endeavor and that each discipline brings a different competence and methodology to such questions as these: What should be done (e.g., in supporting human life)? Who should decide? What policies should guide society in these areas? In assembling the encyclopedia, we have been guided by the special competence of each discipline.

Leading scientists were invited to prepare articles about the biomedical aspects of topics such as sterilization. These scientists were asked to present accurate scientific data on the "state of the art" to the extent necessary for discussing the ethical questions and to give a clear statement of the ethical issues arising in research or practice. The biomedical sciences make further contributions to the delineation of ethical issues by offering conceptual schemes, explaining the consequences of therapeutic actions, and adopting certain notions of professional responsibility.

Articles dealing with social or sociological aspects of bioethical questions explain the behavior of individuals and the policies that guide them, as well as some of the factors that account for behavior and preferred public policies; but the social science contributors were not asked to analyze the ultimate ethical question—what that behavior or policy ought to be. Again, the conceptual schemes offered by the sociologists are helpful in understanding the ethical issues and options, e.g., in the area of human experimentation.

Articles on legal aspects of bioethical questions—for example, the legal aspects of reproductive technologies or of informed consent in the therapeutic relationship—do not offer a mere history of statutory law in the area but are a systematic presentation of the legal principles employed, illustrated by landmark cases. Our assumption has been that the law supplies concepts and principles of action that are useful in arriving at ethical conclusions and in developing better public policies, but that the law itself should be examined from an ethical perspective to test its suitability as public policy.

Articles dealing explicitly and systematically with the ethical aspects of a topic—i.e., with a summary of ethical viewpoints and an explanation of their justifications—were usually prepared by leading ethicists: philosophers and theologians whose special area of expertise is ethics, many of whom have specialized even further in bioethics. They were asked to summarize a variety of ethical views in terms of values and goods, rights and responsibilities, duties and obligations. When these articles were prepared by someone from a discipline other than ethics, such as medicine or law, the contributor was selected particularly because of his or her special competence in ethics.

In some cases, rather than offer two articles, for example, on the medical and ethical aspects of a topic, we achieved a multidisciplinary approach to the subject by arranging for coauthorship or by enlisting a contributor with competence in more than one field.

SPECIAL FEATURES OF THE ENCYCLOPEDIA

The international and interdisciplinary character of the encyclopedia is evident from the fact that the 285 contributors are from fifteen countries and represent many fields of learning including ethics, biology, medicine, the allied health professions, psychology, sexology, philosophy, religion, sociology, anthropology, law, political science, demography, and history.

Contributors were asked to make all topical presentations as international as possible. While they could not be expected to be equally competent in the mores, laws, and ethical systems found in every part of the world, and while some emphasis is placed understandably on the country of origin of this encyclopedia, every effort has been made—both in stating issues and in examples used—to give the work a pronounced international dimension. Articles in the entry MEDICAL ETHICS, HISTORY OF offer an explicit treatment of bioethical themes as they are perceived in many parts of the world.

All of the entries consist of original, signed articles. Contributors were asked to present significant ethical viewpoints from a variety of perspectives, rather than to settle differences of opinion arbitrarily or articulate a purely personal view. They were also asked to compare and contrast various methodologies or approaches, so as to encourage ethical reflection on the part of the reader. A few contributors were asked to write creative essays in areas that have been notably neglected in bioethical studies. A number of the essays will undoubtedly be unique contributions to the literature of bioethics.

All encyclopedias must face the problem of bias, which affects even the most distinguished scholars in all fields of learning. In an encyclopedia dealing exclusively with ethics and values, the presumption is that biases and ideologies might insinuate themselves even more easily. The contributors were asked to give fair representation to a variety of ethical views on a given topic. A number of well-written articles were rejected because they did not meet this requirement. Frequently the perspective of the individual author cannot be entirely concealed: If some ethical, philosophical, or religious perspectives are not fully acknowledged in a given article, we believe this is counterbalanced by the breadth of perspectives offered in related entries.

All articles are directed to the educated person who may or may not be a specialist on the topic. In some instances prior knowledge of the subject will prove helpful, but every effort has been made to offer a clear and direct exposition of the material for the uninitiated reader and to avoid the use of undefined technical terms.

There is a total of 315 articles in the encyclopedia: 314 articles are included in the body of the work and an additional article introduces the Appendix. The articles range in length from 800 to 12,000 words, with an average length of 3,400 words.

Entries are arranged alphabetically. To achieve a systematic and multidisciplinary coherence among related topics, some *entries* are composed of several *articles*. For example:

REPRODUCTIVE TECHNOLOGIES
I. SEX SELECTION
II. ARTIFICIAL INSEMINATION
III. SPERM AND ZYGOTE BANKING
IV. IN VITRO FERTILIZATION
V. ASEXUAL HUMAN REPRODUCTION
VI. ETHICAL ISSUES
VII. LEGAL ASPECTS

In the above entry, the ethical principles that can be applied in the first five articles are discussed in depth only in the sixth article. We have followed this pattern on occasion throughout the encyclopedia: One or more articles on a given topic explain the scientific state of the art and present the ethical issues associated with the use of certain technologies or procedures, and a subsequent article in the same entry systematically discusses the relevant ethical principles.

Some entries name in their titles particular populations—e.g., CHILDREN AND BIOMEDICINE, ADOLESCENTS, WOMEN AND BIOMEDICINE, and AGING AND THE AGED. These articles contain discussions of ethical issues concerning both the therapeutic relationship and human research with these populations.

The encyclopedia contains no biographical articles, because the scholars who have made outstanding contributions to bioethics are identified with a great variety of disciplines, and their biographies are generally available in biographical dictionaries and other encyclopedias. Our contributors were asked simply to mention the names and contributions of those figures who have exerted a significant influence on the ethical principles pertinent to the life sciences and health care.

This encyclopedia appears at a time when many writers and publishers are attempting to avoid noninclusive ("sexist") language. The editors of this encyclopedia have urged the contributors to accept inclusive language wherever possible, but also made efforts to avoid the sometimes awkward and inaccurate alternatives to traditional usage.

An important resource of the encyclopedia is the bibliographies following each article. These select bibliographies were prepared by the contributors and were verified, edited, and occasionally supplemented by the encyclopedia's bibliographic staff. The bibliographic items refer the reader to sources used by the contributor, some of which have been cited in the text in parentheses, e.g., (Smith, 1972, p. 50); to further readings; and to works containing additional bibliographies.

Use of this encyclopedia is facilitated by a carefully worked out system of cross-references that lead the reader to other entries or to parts of the Appendix that offer further information relevant to the article at hand. The principal cross-referencing device is found in a paragraph following each article. Here the reader is referred to other articles, which are listed in categories of descending importance as regards their relevance to the present article. Occasionally the cross-references appear in an introductory paragraph preceding an entry, and some are located within the article itself.

In cross-references of every type we have used a uniform style to help the reader differentiate between the titles of entries and articles. Entry titles use large capitals for the first letter of each main word; article titles use all small capitals—e.g.:

> [*For further discussion of topics mentioned in this*
> *article, see the entry* HEALTH AND DISEASE, *article*
> *on* HISTORY OF THE CONCEPTS.]

The alphabetical arrangement of the entries and the various cross-referencing mechanisms make the entire body of the encyclopedia self-indexing. Nonetheless, an indispensable tool for the use of this encyclopedia is its thorough index: Many specific topics and names can be found only by making use of the index.

Further research aids, found in the last volume, include an "Alphabetical List of Articles" with contributors, a "Systematic Classification of Articles," and a list of "Additional Resources in Bioethics."

WARREN T. REICH
Editor in Chief

Contributors

Abdul-Rauf, Muhammad
Director, The Islamic Center (Washington, D.C.)
MEDICAL ETHICS, HISTORY OF, *section on* NEAR
AND MIDDLE EAST AND AFRICA, *article on* CON-
TEMPORARY MUSLIM PERSPECTIVE

Allen, David Franklyn
*Associate Professor of Psychiatry and Religion,
The Divinity School, Yale University*
MENTAL HEALTH SERVICES, *article on* EVALUATION
OF MENTAL HEALTH PROGRAMS

Amundsen, Darrel W.
*Associate Professor of Classics, Western Washing-
ton University*
MEDICAL ETHICS, HISTORY OF, *section on* NEAR
AND MIDDLE EAST AND AFRICA, *article on* AN-
CIENT NEAR EAST; *section on* EUROPE AND THE
AMERICAS, *articles on* ANCIENT GREECE AND
ROME *and* MEDIEVAL EUROPE: FOURTH TO SIX-
TEENTH CENTURY

Anderson, Odin W.
*Professor and Director, Center for Health Adminis-
tration Studies, University of Chicago*
HEALTH POLICY, *article on* HEALTH POLICY IN
INTERNATIONAL PERSPECTIVE

Annas, George J.
*Associate Professor of Law and Medicine, School
of Medicine, Boston University*
PATIENTS' RIGHTS MOVEMENT

Asper, Samuel P.
*Professor of Internal Medicine and Dean, School
of Medicine, American University of Beirut*
MEDICAL ETHICS, HISTORY OF, *section on* NEAR
AND MIDDLE EAST AND AFRICA, *article on* CON-
TEMPORARY ARAB WORLD

Aufhauser, Marcia Cavell
*Associate Professor of Philosophy, State University
of New York, College at Purchase*
SEXUAL DEVELOPMENT

Back, Kurt W.
*James B. Duke Professor and Chairman, Depart-
ment of Sociology, Duke University*
SELF-REALIZATION THERAPIES

Baier, Kurt
Professor of Philosophy, University of Pittsburgh
ETHICS, *articles on* DEONTOLOGICAL THEORIES *and*
TELEOLOGICAL THEORIES

Bailey, Lloyd
*Associate Professor of Old Testament, Duke Uni-
versity*
DEATH, *article on* WESTERN RELIGIOUS THOUGHT:
DEATH IN BIBLICAL THOUGHT

Bajema, Carl Jay
*Professor of Biology, Grand Valley State Colleges
(Allendale, Michigan)*
POPULATION POLICY PROPOSALS, *article on* GENE-
TIC IMPLICATIONS OF POPULATION CONTROL

Baker, Robert
*Assistant Professor of Philosophy, Union College
(Schenectady, New York)*
MENTAL ILLNESS, *article on* CONCEPTIONS OF MEN-
TAL ILLNESS; VIOLENCE AND THERAPY

Barbour, Ian G.
*Professor of Religion and Professor of Physics,
Carleton College (Northfield, Minnesota)*
ENVIRONMENT AND MAN, *article on* WESTERN
THOUGHT

Basham, A. L.
*Professor and Head, Department of Asian Civili-
zations, Australian National University*
HINDUISM

Bassett, William W.
Professor of Law, University of San Francisco
EUGENICS AND RELIGIOUS LAW, *article on* CHRIS-
TIAN RELIGIOUS LAWS

Bayles, Michael D.
 Professor of Philosophy, University of Kentucky
 POPULATION POLICY PROPOSALS, *article on* POPULATION DISTRIBUTION

Beauchamp, Tom L.
 Associate Professor, Department of Philosophy and Senior Research Scholar, Center for Bioethics, Kennedy Institute of Ethics, Georgetown University
 PATERNALISM

Bleich, J. David
 Professor of Talmud, Yeshiva University
 POPULATION ETHICS: RELIGIOUS TRADITIONS, *article on* JEWISH PERSPECTIVES

Block, Ned
 Associate Professor of Philosophy, Massachusetts Institute of Technology
 REDUCTIONISM, *article on* PHILOSOPHICAL ANALYSIS

Blomquist, Clarence
 Department of Psychiatry, Karolinska Hospital (Stockholm)
 MEDICAL ETHICS, HISTORY OF, *section on* EUROPE AND THE AMERICAS, *article on* WESTERN EUROPE IN THE TWENTIETH CENTURY

Bloom, Samuel W.
 Professor of Sociology and Community Medicine, City University of New York
 THERAPEUTIC RELATIONSHIP, *article on* SOCIOHISTORICAL PERSPECTIVES

Bok, Sissela
 Lecturer in Medical Ethics, School of Medicine, Harvard University
 DEATH AND DYING: EUTHANASIA AND SUSTAINING LIFE, *article on* ETHICAL VIEWS; TRUTH-TELLING, *article on* ETHICAL ASPECTS

Bole, Thomas J., III
 Assistant Professor of Philosophy, Auburn University
 OBLIGATION AND SUPEREROGATION

Bowker, John W.
 Professor of Religious Studies, University of Lancaster (England)
 PAIN AND SUFFERING, *article on* RELIGIOUS PERSPECTIVES

Branson, Roy
 Senior Research Scholar, Center for Bioethics, Kennedy Institute of Ethics, Georgetown University
 HEALTH CARE, *article on* THEORIES OF JUSTICE AND HEALTH CARE; PRISONERS, *article on* PRISONER EXPERIMENTATION

Brieger, Gert H.
 Professor and Chairman, Department of the History of the Health Sciences, University of California, San Francisco
 HUMAN EXPERIMENTATION, *article on* HISTORY

Brody, Baruch A.
 Professor and Chairman, Department of Philosophy, Rice University
 LAW AND MORALITY

Brody, Eugene B.
 Professor of Psychiatry and Human Behavior, University of Maryland
 MENTAL HEALTH SERVICES, *article on* SOCIAL INSTITUTIONS OF MENTAL HEALTH

Brown, Peter G.
 Director, Center for Philosophy and Public Policy, University of Maryland
 POPULATION ETHICS: ELEMENTS OF THE FIELD, *article on* ETHICAL PERSPECTIVES ON POPULATION

Bryant, John H.
 Professor and Director, School of Public Health, Columbia University
 POVERTY AND HEALTH, *article on* POVERTY AND HEALTH IN INTERNATIONAL PERSPECTIVE

Bürgel, J. C.
 Professor of Oriental Studies, University of Bern
 ISLAM

Burns, Chester R.
 Rockwell Associate Professor of Medical History and Associate Director, Institute for the Medical Humanities, University of Texas Medical Branch
 DENTISTRY, *article on* PROFESSIONAL CODES IN AMERICAN DENTISTRY; MEDICAL ETHICS, HISTORY OF, *section on* EUROPE AND THE AMERICAS, *article on* NORTH AMERICA: SEVENTEENTH TO NINETEETH CENTURY

Burrow, James G.
 Professor of History, Abilene Christian University
 MEDICAL PROFESSION, *article on* ORGANIZED MEDICINE

Burt, Robert A.
 Professor of Law, Yale University
 INFORMED CONSENT IN MENTAL HEALTH

Caplan, Arthur L.
 Instructor in the History and Philosophy of Medicine, School of Public Health, Columbia University; Associate for the Humanities, The Hastings Center, Institute of Society, Ethics and the Life Sciences (Hastings-on-Hudson, New York)
 GENETIC ASPECTS OF HUMAN BEHAVIOR, *article on* PHILOSOPHICAL AND ETHICAL ISSUES

Capron, Alexander Morgan
 Professor of Law and Professor of Human Genetics, University of Pennsylvania
 DEATH, DEFINITION AND DETERMINATION OF, *article on* LEGAL ASPECTS OF PRONOUNCING DEATH; HUMAN EXPERIMENTATION, *article on* BASIC ISSUES; RIGHT TO REFUSE MEDICAL CARE

Carney, Frederick S.
 Professor of Ethics, Southern Methodist University
 ETHICS, *article on* THEOLOGICAL ETHICS

Casebeer, Kenneth M.
Assistant Professor of Law, University of Miami
TECHNOLOGY, *article on* TECHNOLOGY AND THE
LAW

Cassell, Eric J.
Clinical Professor of Public Health, Medical College, Cornell University
INFORMED CONSENT IN THE THERAPEUTIC RELATIONSHIP, *article on* CLINICAL ASPECTS; THERAPEUTIC RELATIONSHIP, *article on* CONTEMPORARY MEDICAL PERSPECTIVE

Childress, James F.
Joseph P. Kennedy, Sr. Professor of Christian Ethics, Center for Bioethics, Kennedy Institute of Ethics, Georgetown University
RATIONING OF MEDICAL TREATMENT; RISK

Christiansen, Drew
Research Associate, Woodstock Theological Center, Georgetown University
AGING AND THE AGED, *article on* ETHICAL IMPLICATIONS IN AGING; ENVIRONMENTAL ETHICS, *article on* THE PROBLEM OF GROWTH

Clouser, K. Danner
Professor of Humanities, College of Medicine, The Pennsylvania State University
BIOETHICS

Cohen, Sidney
Clinical Professor of Psychiatry, Neuropsychiatric Institute, University of California, Los Angeles
DRUG USE, *article on* DRUG USE FOR PLEASURE AND TRANSCENDENT EXPERIENCE

Cole, Jonathan R.
Professor of Sociology, Columbia University
SCIENCE, SOCIOLOGY OF

Connery, John R.
Professor of Moral Theology, Loyola University (Chicago)
ABORTION, *article on* ROMAN CATHOLIC PERSPECTIVES

Cooke, Robert E.
President, Medical College of Pennsylvania
MENTALLY HANDICAPPED

Copenhaver, Brian P.
Director, Honors Program, Western Washington University
DEATH, *article on* WESTERN RELIGIOUS THOUGHT: ARS MORIENDI

Coulter, Harris L.
Washington, D.C.
DRUG INDUSTRY AND MEDICINE

Cowen, David L.
Professor Emeritus of History, Rutgers, The State University of New Jersey
PHARMACY

Creson, D. L.
Chief, Division of Community and Social Psychiatry, University of Texas Medical Branch
HOMOSEXUALITY, *article on* CLINICAL AND BEHAVIORAL ASPECTS

Curran, Charles E.
Professor of Moral Theology, The Catholic University of America
ABORTION, *article on* CONTEMPORARY DEBATE IN PHILOSOPHICAL AND RELIGIOUS ETHICS; ROMAN CATHOLICISM

D'Arcy, Eric
Reader in Philosophy, University of Melbourne (Victoria, Australia)
NATURAL LAW

DeBakey, Lois
Professor of Scientific Communication, Baylor College of Medicine and Tulane University School of Medicine
COMMUNICATION, BIOMEDICAL, *articles on* MEDIA AND MEDICINE *and* SCIENTIFIC PUBLISHING

DeBakey, Selma
Professor of Scientific Communication, Baylor College of Medicine
COMMUNICATION, BIOMEDICAL, *article on* MEDIA AND MEDICINE

De Graeve, Frank
Professor of Comparative Religion, University of Louvain
HEALTH AND DISEASE, *article on* RELIGIOUS CONCEPTS

Derr, Thomas Sieger
Professor of Religion, Smith College (Northampton, Massachusetts)
RELIGIOUS DIRECTIVES IN MEDICAL ETHICS, *article on* PROTESTANT STATEMENTS

Draguns, Juris G.
Professor of Psychology, The Pennsylvania State University
BEHAVIORISM, *article on* HISTORY OF BEHAVIORAL PSYCHOLOGY

Dubos, René
Professor Emeritus of Environmental Biomedicine, The Rockefeller University
GENETIC CONSTITUTION AND ENVIRONMENTAL CONDITIONING

Dukeminier, Jesse
Professor of Law, University of California, Los Angeles
ORGAN DONATION, *article on* LEGAL ASPECTS

Dummett, Clifton O.
Professor of Dentistry, University of Southern California
DENTISTRY, *article on* ETHICAL ISSUES IN DENTISTRY

Duncombe, David C.
Assistant Professor of Pastoral Theology, Lecturer in Medicine, and Chaplain, School of Medicine, Yale University
PASTORAL MINISTRY

Dyck, Arthur J.
Mary B. Saltonstall Professor of Population Ethics, Harvard University
POPULATION ETHICS: ELEMENTS OF THE FIELD, *article on* DEFINITION OF POPULATION ETHICS

Edel, Abraham
Research Professor of Philosophy, University of Pennsylvania
SCIENCE: ETHICAL IMPLICATIONS

Ehrman, Lee
Professor of Biology, State University of New York, College at Purchase
EUPHENICS

Emmott, Carol
Special Assistant to the Deputy Assistant Secretary of Legislation/Health, Department of Health, Education, and Welfare (Washington, D.C.)
HEALTH CARE, *article on* HEALTH-CARE SYSTEM

Engelhardt, H. Tristram, Jr.
Rosemary Kennedy Professor of the Philosophy of Medicine, Center for Bioethics, Kennedy Institute of Ethics, Georgetown University
HEALTH AND DISEASE, *article on* PHILOSOPHICAL PERSPECTIVES; MEDICINE, PHILOSOPHY OF

Epstein, Samuel S.
Professor of Environmental and Occupational Medicine, School of Public Health, University of Illinois (Chicago)
ENVIRONMENTAL ETHICS, *article on* ENVIRONMENTAL HEALTH AND HUMAN DISEASE

Erde, Edmund L.
Assistant Professor of the Philosophy of Medicine, University of Texas Medical Branch
FREE WILL AND DETERMINISM; MEDICINE, PHILOSOPHY OF

Eshraghi, Rahmatollah
Chairman, Department of Community Medicine, Ferdowsi University (Meshed, Iran)
MEDICAL ETHICS, HISTORY OF, *section on* NEAR AND MIDDLE EAST AND AFRICA, *article on* PERSIA

Faramelli, Norman J.
Chief of Environmental Management, Massachusetts Port Authority (Boston)
ENVIRONMENTAL ETHICS, *article on* QUESTIONS OF SOCIAL JUSTICE

Farley, Margaret A.
Associate Professor of Ethics, The Divinity School, Yale University
SEXUAL ETHICS

Feinberg, Joel
Professor of Philosophy, University of Arizona
BEHAVIOR CONTROL, *article on* FREEDOM AND BEHAVIOR CONTROL; JUSTICE; RIGHTS, *article on* SYSTEMATIC ANALYSIS

Feldman, David M.
Rabbi, Bay Ridge Jewish Center (Brooklyn, New York)
ABORTION, *article on* JEWISH PERSPECTIVES; EUGENICS AND RELIGIOUS LAW, *article on* JEWISH RELIGIOUS LAWS

Finnis, J. M.
Fellow and Praelector in Jurisprudence, University College, Oxford
ABORTION, *article on* LEGAL ASPECTS

Fletcher, John C.
Assistant for Bioethics, Office of the Director, Clinical Center, National Institutes of Health (Bethesda, Maryland)
PRENATAL DIAGNOSIS, *article on* ETHICAL ISSUES

Fletcher, Joseph
Professor of Medical Ethics, School of Medicine, University of Virginia
ETHICS, *article on* SITUATION ETHICS

Flew, Antony G. N.
Professor of Philosophy, University of Reading (England)
EVOLUTION

Foot, Philippa
Professor of Philosophy, University of California, Los Angeles; Senior Research Fellow, Somerville College, Oxford University
ETHICS, *article on* MORAL REASONING

Fost, Norman C.
Associate Professor of Pediatrics, University of Wisconsin, Madison
CHILDREN AND BIOMEDICINE

Fox, Renée C.
Professor and Chairman, Department of Sociology and Professor, Departments of Medicine and Psychiatry, University of Pennsylvania
KIDNEY DIALYSIS AND TRANSPLANTATION; ORGAN TRANSPLANTATION, *article on* SOCIOCULTURAL ASPECTS

Frankel, Mark S.
Assistant Professor of Political Science, Wayne State University
HUMAN EXPERIMENTATION, *article on* SOCIAL AND PROFESSIONAL CONTROL; REPRODUCTIVE TECHNOLOGIES, *articles on* ARTIFICIAL INSEMINATION *and* SPERM AND ZYGOTE BANKING

Freeman, John M.
Associate Professor of Neurology and Pediatrics, Johns Hopkins University; Director, Birth Defects Treatment Center, John F. Kennedy Institute (Baltimore)
INFANTS, *article on* MEDICAL ASPECTS AND ETHICAL DILEMMAS

French, Richard D.
Associate Professor, Faculty of Management, McGill University
ANIMAL EXPERIMENTATION, *article on* HISTORICAL ASPECTS

Fried, Charles
Professor of Law, Harvard University
HUMAN EXPERIMENTATION, *article on* PHILOSOPHICAL ASPECTS

Friedman, Jane M.
Professor of Law, Wayne State University
STERILIZATION, *article on* LEGAL ASPECTS

Fruchtbaum, Harold
Associate Professor of the History and Philosophy of Public Health, Columbia University
PUBLIC HEALTH

Garland, Michael J.
Bioethics Program Representative, School of Medicine, University of California, San Francisco
BLOOD TRANSFUSION

Gass, Ronald S.
Research Assistant, National Commission for the Protection of Human Subjects of Biomedical and Behavioral Research (Bethesda, Maryland)
APPENDIX: INTRODUCTION, *article on* CODES OF THE HEALTH-CARE PROFESSIONS

Gatch, Milton McC.
Professor of English, University of Missouri, Columbia
DEATH, *article on* WESTERN RELIGIOUS THOUGHT: POST-BIBLICAL CHRISTIAN THOUGHT

Gerson, Elihu M.
Lecturer in Psychiatry, University of California, San Francisco
CHRONIC CARE

Gert, Bernard
Professor of Philosophy, Dartmouth College (Hanover, New Hampshire)
ETHICS, *article on* OBJECTIVISM IN ETHICS

Gettner, Alan
Former Assistant Professor of Philosophy, State University of New York, College at Purchase
MENTAL HEALTH, *article on* MENTAL HEALTH IN COMPETITION WITH OTHER VALUES

Girardot, Norman J.
Assistant Professor of Theology, University of Notre Dame
TAOISM

Golding, Martin P.
Professor of Philosophy, Duke University
FUTURE GENERATIONS, OBLIGATIONS TO; POPULATION POLICY PROPOSALS, *article on* POPULATION DISTRIBUTION

Gordy, Michael
Assistant Professor of Humanities, University of Houston
SOCIALITY

Gorovitz, Samuel
Professor and Chairman, Department of Philosophy, University of Maryland
HEALTH AS AN OBLIGATION

Gottesman, Irving I.
Professor and Director, Behavioral Genetics Center, University of Minnesota
GENETIC ASPECTS OF HUMAN BEHAVIOR, *articles on* STATE OF THE ART *and* GENETICS AND MENTAL DISORDERS

Gray, Bradford H.
Professional Associate, Institute of Medicine, National Academy of Sciences (Washington, D.C.)
INFORMED CONSENT IN HUMAN RESEARCH, *article on* SOCIAL ASPECTS

Greenawalt, Kent
Professor of Law, Columbia University
PRIVACY

Gresson, Aaron D.
Assistant Professor of Humanistic and Behavioral Studies, Boston University
RACISM, *article on* RACISM AND MENTAL HEALTH

Grote, Jim
Graduate Student, University of Louisville
TECHNOLOGY, *article on* PHILOSOPHY OF TECHNOLOGY

Gruman, Gerald J.
Silver Spring, Maryland
DEATH AND DYING: EUTHANASIA AND SUSTAINING LIFE, *article on* HISTORICAL PERSPECTIVES

Gutmann, James
Professor Emeritus of Philosophy, Columbia University
DEATH, *article on* WESTERN PHILOSOPHICAL THOUGHT

Haddad, Fuad Sami
Clinical Professor of Surgery, American University of Beirut
MEDICAL ETHICS, HISTORY OF, *section on* NEAR AND MIDDLE EAST AND AFRICA, *article on* CONTEMPORARY ARAB WORLD

Hammer, A. G.
Professor of Psychology, MacQuarie University (North Ryde, Australia); Research Associate, The Institute of the Pennsylvania Hospital (Philadelphia)
HYPNOSIS

Harakas, Stanley S.
Dean and Professor of Christian Ethics, Holy Cross Greek Orthodox School of Theology (Brookline, Massachusetts)
EASTERN ORTHODOX CHRISTIANITY; POPULATION ETHICS: RELIGIOUS TRADITIONS, article on EASTERN ORTHODOX CHRISTIAN PERSPECTIVES

Hare, Peter H.
Professor of Philosophy, State University of New York at Buffalo
CIVIL DISOBEDIENCE IN HEALTH SERVICES

Hare, R. M.
White's Professor of Moral Philosophy, Oxford University and Fellow of Corpus Christi College, Oxford
ETHICS, articles on UTILITARIANISM and NON-DESCRIPTIVISM

Häring, Bernard
Professor of Moral Theology, Academia Alfonsiana, Lateran University (Rome)
RELIGIOUS DIRECTIVES IN MEDICAL ETHICS, article on ROMAN CATHOLIC DIRECTIVES

Hartt, Julian N.
William Kenan, Jr. Professor of Religious Studies, University of Virginia
MAN, IMAGES OF

Hauck, George H.
Lecturer in Law, University of California, Berkeley
MEDICAL MALPRACTICE

Hauerwas, Stanley
Associate Professor of Theology, University of Notre Dame
CARE

Havighurst, Clark C.
Professor of Law, Duke University
ADVERTISING BY MEDICAL PROFESSIONALS

Hayflick, Leonard
Senior Research Cell Biologist, Bruce Lyon Memorial Research Laboratory (Oakland, California)
AGING AND THE AGED, article on THEORIES OF AGING AND ANTI-AGING TECHNIQUES

Heelan, Patrick A.
Professor of Philosophy, Dean of Arts and Sciences, and Vice President for Liberal Studies, State University of New York at Stony Brook
PURPOSE IN THE UNIVERSE

Hehir, J. Bryan
Office of International Justice and Peace, United States Catholic Conference (Washington, D.C.)
POPULATION ETHICS: RELIGIOUS TRADITIONS, article on ROMAN CATHOLIC PERSPECTIVES

Hellegers, André E.
Director, Kennedy Institute of Ethics, Georgetown University
ABORTION, article on MEDICAL ASPECTS; FETAL RESEARCH

Hellman, Louis M.
Director of Health Information, Population Reference Bureau, Inc. (Washington, D.C.)
STERILIZATION, article on MEDICAL ASPECTS

Hemphill, John Michael
Department of Neurology, Johns Hopkins Hospital (Baltimore)
INFANTS, article on MEDICAL ASPECTS AND ETHICAL DILEMMAS

Henriot, Peter J.
Staff Associate, Center of Concern (Washington, D.C.)
FOOD POLICY

High, Dallas M.
Professor and Chairman, Department of Philosophy, University of Kentucky
DEATH, DEFINITION AND DETERMINATION OF, article on PHILOSOPHICAL AND THEOLOGICAL FOUNDATIONS

Himmelsbach, Kathryn K.
Chief, Cancer Social Work Section, Clinical Center, National Institutes of Health (Bethesda, Maryland)
MEDICAL SOCIAL WORK

Hook, Ernest B.
Chief, Epidemiology and Human Ecology, New York State Birth Defects Institute (Albany, New York); Associate Professor of Pediatrics, Albany Medical College, Union University
GENETIC ASPECTS OF HUMAN BEHAVIOR, article on MALES WITH SEX CHROMOSOME ABNORMALITIES (XYY AND XXY GENOTYPES)

Hovde, Christian A.
Chairman, Department of Religion and Health, Rush-Presbyterian-St. Luke's Medical Center (Chicago)
CADAVERS, article on GENERAL ETHICAL CONCERNS

Howard, Jan
Research Sociologist and Lecturer, School of Medicine, University of California, San Francisco
HEALTH CARE, article on HUMANIZATION AND DEHUMANIZATION OF HEALTH CARE

Howard, Richard J.
Assistant Professor of Surgery, University of Minnesota
ORGAN TRANSPLANTATION, article on MEDICAL PERSPECTIVE

Izen, Judith E.
Research Analyst, Psychiatry Service, Massachusetts General Hospital (Boston)
PSYCHOPHARMACOLOGY

Jaggi, O. P.
Head, Department of Clinical Research, University of Delhi
MEDICAL ETHICS, HISTORY OF, section on SOUTH AND EAST ASIA, article on INDIA

Jakobovits, Immanuel
Chief Rabbi of the United Hebrew Congregations of the British Commonwealth of Nations (London)
JUDAISM

Jameton, Andrew L.
Postdoctoral Fellow, Bioethics Program, School of Medicine, University of California, San Francisco
MEDICAL ETHICS, HISTORY OF, section on EUROPE AND THE AMERICAS, article on NORTH AMERICA IN THE TWENTIETH CENTURY;
ORGAN DONATION, article on ETHICAL ISSUES

Johnson, James T.
Associate Professor and Chairman, Department of Religon, Douglass College of Rutgers, The State University of New Jersey
PROTESTANTISM, article on HISTORY OF PROTESTANT MEDICAL ETHICS

Jones, James H.
National Endowment for the Humanities (Washington, D.C.)
RACISM, article on RACISM AND MEDICINE

Jonsen, Albert R.
Associate Professor of Bioethics, School of Medicine, University of California, San Francisco
HEALTH CARE, article on RIGHT TO HEALTH-CARE SERVICES; LIFE-SUPPORT SYSTEMS; MEDICAL ETHICS, HISTORY OF, section on EUROPE AND THE AMERICAS, articles on WESTERN EUROPE IN THE SEVENTEENTH CENTURY and NORTH AMERICA IN THE TWENTIETH CENTURY

Kalish, Richard A.
Professor of Behavioral Sciences, Graduate Theological Union (Berkeley, California)
DEATH, ATTITUDES TOWARD

Kanoti, George A.
Professor of Religious Studies, John Carroll University
HOMOSEXUALITY, article on ETHICAL ASPECTS

Kao, Frederick F.
Professor of Physiology, Downstate Medical Center, State University of New York
MEDICAL ETHICS, HISTORY OF, section on SOUTH AND EAST ASIA, article on CONTEMPORARY CHINA

Kao, John J.
Clinical Fellow, Department of Psychiatry, Harvard University
MEDICAL ETHICS, HISTORY OF, section on SOUTH AND EAST ASIA, article on CONTEMPORARY CHINA

Katz, Jay
Professor (Adjunct) of Law and Psychiatry, Law School, Yale University
INFORMED CONSENT IN THE THERAPEUTIC RELATIONSHIP, article on LEGAL AND ETHICAL ASPECTS

Kaufman, Martin
Professor of History, Westfield State College (Massachusetts)
ORTHODOXY IN MEDICINE

Keller, Mark
Professor Emeritus, Center of Alcohol Studies, Rutgers, The State University of New Jersey
ALCOHOL, USE OF

Kelman, Herbert C.
Richard Clarke Cabot Professor of Social Ethics, Harvard University
RESEARCH, BEHAVIORAL

Kitagawa, Joseph M.
Professor of History of Religions and Dean, The Divinity School, University of Chicago
MEDICAL ETHICS, HISTORY OF, section on SOUTH AND EAST ASIA, article on JAPAN THROUGH THE NINETEENTH CENTURY

Kittrie, Nicholas N.
Director, Institute for Advanced Studies in Justice, and Professor and Dean, School of Law, The American University
MENTAL ILLNESS, article on LABELING IN MENTAL ILLNESS: LEGAL ASPECTS

Klerman, Gerald L.
Professor of Psychiatry, Harvard University
PSYCHOPHARMACOLOGY

Konold, Donald
Professor of History, Arkansas State University
CODES OF MEDICAL ETHICS, article on HISTORY

Kosnik, Anthony R.
Professor of Moral Theology and Dean, SS. Cyril and Methodius Seminary (Orchard Lake, Michigan)
HOMOSEXUALITY, article on ETHICAL ASPECTS

Ladd, John
Professor of Philosophy, Brown University
ETHICS, article on THE TASK OF ETHICS

Laín Entralgo, Pedro
The Arnaldo de Villanova Institute (Madrid)
THERAPEUTIC RELATIONSHIP, article on HISTORY OF THE RELATIONSHIP

Landy, David
Professor of Anthropology, University of Massachusetts at Boston
DEATH, article on ANTHROPOLOGICAL PERSPECTIVE

Lappé, Marc
Chief, Office of Health Law and Values, California State Department of Health
EUGENICS, article on ETHICAL ISSUES

Largey, Gale
Associate Professor of Sociology and Anthropology, Mansfield State College (Pennsylvania)
REPRODUCTIVE TECHNOLOGIES, article on SEX SELECTION

Lebacqz, Karen
Associate Professor of Christian Ethics, Pacific School of Religion (Berkeley, California)
INFORMED CONSENT IN HUMAN RESEARCH, *article on* ETHICAL AND LEGAL ASPECTS; STERILIZATION, *article on* ETHICAL ASPECTS

Lee, Philip R.
Professor of Social Medicine and Director, Health Policy Program, University of California, San Francisco
HEALTH CARE, *article on* HEALTH-CARE SYSTEM

Leighton, Dorothea C.
Former Professor and Chairman, Department of Mental Health, University of North Carolina
MEDICINE, ANTHROPOLOGY OF

León C., Augusto
Professor of Medicine, Central University of Venezuela
MEDICAL ETHICS, HISTORY OF, *section on* EUROPE AND THE AMERICAS, *article on* LATIN AMERICA IN THE TWENTIETH CENTURY

Levine, Robert J.
Professor of Medicine and Lecturer in Pharmacology, Yale University
INFORMED CONSENT IN HUMAN RESEARCH, *article on* ETHICAL AND LEGAL ASPECTS; RESEARCH, BIOMEDICAL

Lieb, Irwin C.
Professor of Philosophy, Dean of Graduate Studies, and Vice-President, The University of Texas at Austin
PRAGMATISM

Lister, George
Assistant Professor in Residence, Departments of Pediatrics and Anesthesia, University of California, San Francisco
LIFE-SUPPORT SYSTEMS

Lloyd, Charles W.
Co-Director, Center for Study of Human Sexual Behavior, Professor of Clinical Psychiatry, and Professor of Obstetrics/Gynecology, University of Pittsburgh
SEX THERAPY AND SEX RESEARCH, *article on* SCIENTIFIC AND CLINICAL PERSPECTIVES

Lloyd, Kenneth E.
Professor and Chair, Department of Psychology, Drake University
BEHAVIORAL THERAPIES

Lloyd, Margaret E.
Associate Professor of Psychology, Drake University
BEHAVIORAL THERAPIES

Loehlin, John C.
Professor of Psychology, The University of Texas at Austin
GENETIC ASPECTS OF HUMAN BEHAVIOR, *article on* RACE DIFFERENCES IN INTELLIGENCE

London, Perry
Professor of Psychology and Psychiatry, University of Southern California
SEXUAL BEHAVIOR

Louisell, David W.
Elizabeth Josselyn Boalt Professor of Law, University of California, Berkeley
MEDICAL MALPRACTICE

Ludmerer, Kenneth M.
Instructor of Medicine, Washington University (St. Louis)
EUGENICS, *article on* HISTORY

Lynch, Abbyann
Associate Professor of Philosophy, St. Michael's College, University of Toronto
MEDICAL ETHICS, HISTORY OF, *section on* EUROPE AND THE AMERICAS, *article on* NORTH AMERICA IN THE TWENTIETH CENTURY

MacIntyre, Alasdair
University Professor of Philosophy and Political Science, Boston University
BEHAVIORISM, *article on* PHILOSOPHICAL ANALYSIS

McCarthy, Charles R.
Chief, Legislative Development Branch, Office of the Director, National Institutes of Health (Bethesda, Maryland)
RESEARCH POLICY, BIOMEDICAL

McCormick, Richard A.
Rose F. Kennedy Professor of Christian Ethics, Center for Bioethics, Kennedy Institute of Ethics, Georgetown University
ORGAN TRANSPLANTATION, *article on* ETHICAL PRINCIPLES; REPRODUCTIVE TECHNOLOGIES, *article on* ETHICAL ISSUES

McCullough, Laurence B.
Assistant Professor of the Philosophy of Medicine and Head, Department of Humanities in Medicine, College of Medicine, Texas A & M University
MEDICAL ETHICS, HISTORY OF, *section on* EUROPE AND THE AMERICAS, *articles on* INTRODUCTION TO THE MODERN PERIOD IN EUROPE AND THE AMERICAS, BRITAIN AND THE UNITED STATES IN THE EIGHTEENTH CENTURY, *and* INTRODUCTION TO THE CONTEMPORARY PERIOD IN EUROPE AND THE AMERICAS

Macklin, Ruth
Associate for Behavioral Studies, The Hastings Center, Institute of Society, Ethics and the Life Sciences (Hastings-on-Hudson, New York)
REDUCTIONISM, *article on* ETHICAL IMPLICATIONS OF PSYCHOPHYSICAL REDUCTIONISM; RIGHTS, *article on* RIGHTS IN BIOETHICS; SEX THERAPY AND SEX RESEARCH, *article on* ETHICAL PERSPECTIVES

Madden, Edward H.
Professor of Philosophy, State University of New York at Buffalo
CIVIL DISOBEDIENCE IN HEALTH SERVICES

Mahoney, Maurice J.
  Associate Professor of Human Genetics and Pediatrics, Yale University
  FETAL–MATERNAL RELATIONSHIP

Marshall, Carol Paul
  Former Coordinator for Program Planning and Special Services, Central Flushing–Upper Queens Medical Group (New York)
  POVERTY AND HEALTH, *article on* POVERTY AND HEALTH IN THE UNITED STATES

Marshall, Carter L.
  Professor of Preventive Medicine, College of Medicine and Dentistry of New Jersey (Newark)
  POVERTY AND HEALTH, *article on* POVERTY AND HEALTH IN THE UNITED STATES

Mastroianni, Luigi, Jr.
  Professor and Chairman, Department of Obstetrics and Gynecology, Hospital of the University of Pennsylvania
  REPRODUCTIVE TECHNOLOGIES, *article on* IN VITRO FERTILIZATION

May, William E.
  Associate Professor of Moral Theology, The Catholic University of America
  DOUBLE EFFECT

Mechanic, David
  John Bascom Professor of Sociology, University of Wisconsin, Madison
  MEDICINE, SOCIOLOGY OF; THERAPEUTIC RELATIONSHIP, *article on* CONTEMPORARY SOCIOLOGICAL ANALYSIS

Meister, Joel
  Assistant Professor of Sociology, Amherst College (Massachusetts)
  ELECTRICAL STIMULATION OF THE BRAIN

Michels, Robert
  Barklie McKee Henry Professor and Chairman, Department of Psychiatry, Cornell University
  MENTAL ILLNESS, *article on* DIAGNOSIS OF MENTAL ILLNESS

Milunsky, Aubrey
  Director, Genetics Division, Eunice Kennedy Shriver Center (Waltham, Massachusetts); Assistant Professor of Pediatrics, Harvard University
  PRENATAL DIAGNOSIS, *article on* CLINICAL ASPECTS

Mintz, Beatrice
  Senior Member, The Institute for Cancer Research (Philadelphia, Pennsylvania)
  GENE THERAPY, *article on* PRODUCTION OF FOUR-PARENT INDIVIDUALS

Missett, James R.
  Chief Resident in Psychiatry, Stanford University
  HEALTH, INTERNATIONAL; MASS HEALTH SCREENING

Mitcham, Carl
  Instructor of Philosophy and Psychology, St. Catharine College (Kentucky)
  TECHNOLOGY, *article on* PHILOSOPHY OF TECHNOLOGY

Molinari, Gaetano F.
  Professor and Chairman, Department of Neurology, The George Washington University
  DEATH, DEFINITION AND DETERMINATION OF, *article on* CRITERIA FOR DEATH

Moore, Harold F.
  Assistant Professor of Philosophy, University of Notre Dame
  ACTING AND REFRAINING

Morawetz, Thomas H.
  Associate Professor of Law and Adjunct Professor of Philosophy, University of Connecticut
  DYNAMIC THERAPIES

Murphy, Edmond A.
  Professor of Medicine, Johns Hopkins University
  DECISION MAKING, MEDICAL

Murray, Robert F., Jr.
  Professor of Genetics and Human Genetics and Professor of Pediatrics and Medicine, Howard University
  GENETIC DIAGNOSIS AND COUNSELING, *articles on* GENETIC DIAGNOSIS *and* GENETIC COUNSELING

Musallam, Basim F.
  Assistant Professor of History, University of Pennsylvania; Research Associate in Population Studies, Harvard University
  POPULATION ETHICS: RELIGIOUS TRADITIONS, *article on* ISLAMIC PERSPECTIVES

Nadelson, Carol C.
  Associate Professor of Psychiatry, Harvard University
  WOMEN AND BIOMEDICINE, *articles on* WOMEN AS PATIENTS AND EXPERIMENTAL SUBJECTS *and* WOMEN AS HEALTH PROFESSIONALS

Nagle, James J.
  Associate Professor of Zoology, Drew University
  EUPHENICS

Najarian, John S.
  Professor and Chairman, Department of Surgery, University of Minnesota
  ORGAN TRANSPLANTATION, *article on* MEDICAL PERSPECTIVE

Nakamura, Hajime
  Director, The Eastern Institute, Inc. (Tokyo); Professor Emeritus, University of Tokyo
  BUDDHISM; ENVIRONMENT AND MAN, *article on* EASTERN THOUGHT

Nelson, James B.
Professor of Christian Ethics, United Theological
Seminary of the Twin Cities (New Brighton,
Minnesota)
ABORTION, *article on* PROTESTANT PERSPECTIVES

Neufeld, Elizabeth F.
Chief, Section on Human Biochemical Genetics,
National Institute of Arthritis, Metabolism and
Digestive Diseases, National Institutes of Health
(Bethesda, Maryland)
GENE THERAPY, *article on* ENZYME REPLACEMENT

Neugarten, Bernice L.
Professor of Human Development, The University
of Chicago
AGING AND THE AGED, *article on* SOCIAL IMPLICA-
TIONS OF AGING

Neville, Robert
Professor of Religious Studies and Philosophy,
State University of New York at Stony Brook
BEHAVIOR CONTROL, *article on* ETHICAL ANALYSIS;
DRUG USE, *article on* DRUG USE, ABUSE, AND DE-
PENDENCE; PSYCHOSURGERY

Newman, Lucile F.
Assistant Professor of Community Health and
Anthropology, Brown University
MEDICAL ETHICS, HISTORY OF, *article on* PRIMI-
TIVE SOCIETIES

Ninomiya, Rikuo
Director, Ninomiya-Naika Clinic (Tokyo)
MEDICAL ETHICS, HISTORY OF, *section on* SOUTH
AND EAST ASIA, *article on* CONTEMPORARY JAPAN:
MEDICAL ETHICS AND LEGAL MEDICINE

Noonan, John T., Jr.
Professor of Law, University of California, Berke-
ley
CONTRACEPTION

Notman, Malkah T.
Associate Clinical Professor of Psychiatry, Har-
vard University
WOMEN AND BIOMEDICINE, *articles on* WOMEN AS
PATIENTS AND EXPERIMENTAL SUBJECTS *and*
WOMEN AS HEALTH PROFESSIONALS

Offer, Daniel
Professor of Psychiatry, The University of Chi-
cago; Chairman, Department of Psychiatry,
Michael Reese Hospital and Medical Center
(Chicago)
ADOLESCENTS

Offer, Judith B.
Research Associate in Psychiatry, Michael Reese
Hospital and Medical Center (Chicago)
ADOLESCENTS

Ost, David E.
Assistant Editor, Encyclopedia of Bioethics
INFANTS, *articles on* ETHICAL PERSPECTIVES ON
THE CARE OF INFANTS *and* PUBLIC POLICY AND
PROCEDURAL QUESTIONS

Page, Benjamin B.
Assistant Professor of Philosophy and Health Ser-
vices Administration, Quinnipiac College (Ham-
den, Connecticut)
MEDICAL ETHICS, HISTORY OF, *section on* EUROPE
AND THE AMERICAS, *article on* EASTERN EUROPE
IN THE TWENTIETH CENTURY

Panuska, J. A.
Former Professor of Biology, Georgetown Univer-
sity
CRYONICS

Parsons, Talcott
Professor Emeritus of Sociology, Harvard Univer-
sity
DEATH, *article on* DEATH IN THE WESTERN WORLD;
HEALTH AND DISEASE, *article on* A SOCIOLOGI-
CAL AND ACTION PERSPECTIVE

Pellegrino, Edmund D.
Professor of Medicine, Yale University; President,
Yale–New Haven Medical Center
MEDICAL EDUCATION

Perlin, Seymour
Professor of Psychiatry and Behavioral Sciences,
The George Washington University; Senior Re-
search Scholar, Center for Bioethics, Kennedy
Institute of Ethics, Georgetown University
SUICIDE

Pernick, Martin S.
Instructor of Social History, College of Medicine,
The Pennsylvania State University
MEDICAL PROFESSION, *article on* MEDICAL PROFES-
SIONALISM

Petersen, William
Robert Lazarus Professor of Social Demography,
Ohio State University
POPULATION ETHICS: ELEMENTS OF THE FIELD,
article on HISTORY OF POPULATION THEORIES;
POPULATION POLICY PROPOSALS, *article on* DIF-
FERENTIAL GROWTH RATE AND POPULATION POL-
ICIES: DEMOGRAPHIC PERSPECTIVES

Peterson, M. Jeanne
Assistant Professor of History, Indiana University
MEDICAL ETHICS, HISTORY OF, *section on* EUROPE
AND THE AMERICAS, *article on* BRITAIN IN THE
NINETEENTH CENTURY

Poste, George
Professor of Experimental Pathology, Roswell
Park Memorial Institute (Buffalo, New York)
GENE THERAPY, *article on* CELL FUSION AND HY-
BRIDIZATION

Potter, Ralph B.
Professor of Social Ethics, The Divinity School,
and Member, Center for Population Studies,
Harvard University
POPULATION ETHICS: ELEMENTS OF THE FIELD,
article on NORMATIVE ASPECTS OF POPULATION
POLICY

Powers, Charles W.
Cummins Engine Company, Inc. (Columbus, Indiana); Affiliate Professor of Social Ethics, Christian Theological Seminary (Indianapolis)
ENVIRONMENTAL ETHICS, *article on* QUESTIONS OF SOCIAL JUSTICE

Powledge, Tabitha M.
Research Associate, The Hastings Center, Institute of Society, Ethics and the Life Sciences (Hastings-on-Hudson, New York)
GENETIC SCREENING

Rao, K. L. Seshagiri
Professor of Religious Studies, University of Virginia
POPULATION ETHICS: RELIGIOUS TRADITIONS, *article on* A HINDU PERSPECTIVE

Redlich, F. C.
Professor of Psychiatry, University of California, Los Angeles
MEDICAL ETHICS UNDER NATIONAL SOCIALISM

Reich, Warren T.
Senior Research Scholar, Center for Bioethics, Kennedy Institute of Ethics, and Associate Professor of Bioethics, School of Medicine, Georgetown University
INFANTS, *articles on* ETHICAL PERSPECTIVES ON THE CARE OF INFANTS *and* PUBLIC POLICY AND PROCEDURAL QUESTIONS; LIFE, *article on* QUALITY OF LIFE

Restak, Richard M.
Instructor in Neurology, Georgetown University
ELECTROCONVULSIVE THERAPY

Reynolds, Frank E.
Associate Professor of History of Religions and Buddhist Studies, The Divinity School, The University of Chicago
DEATH, *article on* EASTERN THOUGHT

Richardson, William J.
Professor of Philosophy, Fordham University; Director of Research, Austen Riggs Center (Stockbridge, Massachusetts)
MENTAL HEALTH, *article on* RELIGION AND MENTAL HEALTH

Riesenfeld, Stefan A.
Professor of Law, University of California, Berkeley, and University of California, San Francisco
HEALTH INSURANCE

Risse, Guenter B.
Professor of the History of Medicine, University of Wisconsin, Madison
HEALTH AND DISEASE, *article on* HISTORY OF THE CONCEPTS; MEDICAL ETHICS, HISTORY OF, *section on* EUROPE AND THE AMERICAS, *article on* CENTRAL EUROPE IN THE NINETEENTH CENTURY

Robertson, John A.
Associate Professor of Law, University of Wisconsin, Madison
REPRODUCTIVE TECHNOLOGIES, *article on* LEGAL ASPECTS

Robinson, Daniel N.
Professor of Psychology, Georgetown University
PAIN AND SUFFERING, *article on* PSYCHOBIOLOGICAL PRINCIPLES

Roblin, Richard O.
Basic Research Program, Frederick Cancer Research Center (Frederick, Maryland)
GENE THERAPY, *articles on* GENE THERAPY VIA TRANSFORMATION *and* GENE THERAPY VIA TRANSDUCTION

Rosner, Fred
Associate Professor of Medicine, State University of New York at Stony Brook; Director, Division of Hematology, Queens Hospital Center (Jamaica, New York)
RELIGIOUS DIRECTIVES IN MEDICAL ETHICS, *article on* JEWISH CODES AND GUIDELINES

Russell, Paul S.
John Homans Professor of Surgery, Harvard University; Chief, Transplantation Unit, Massachusetts General Hospital (Boston)
SURGERY

Sagan, Leonard A.
Palo Alto Medical Clinic (Palo Alto, California)
PRISONERS, *articles on* MEDICAL CARE OF PRISONERS *and* TORTURE AND THE HEALTH PROFESSIONAL

Sai, Frederick T.
Assistant Secretary General, International Planned Parenthood Federation (London); Former Director of Medical Services (Ghana)
MEDICAL ETHICS, HISTORY OF, *section on* NEAR AND MIDDLE EAST AND AFRICA, *article on* SUBSAHARAN AFRICA

Sanders, Judith Rose
Co-Director, Health Education Resources (Brooklyn, New York)
SEXUAL IDENTITY

Savodnik, Irwin
Director of Medical Student Education, University of Pittsburgh
BIOLOGY, PHILOSOPHY OF

Schumacher, Sallie
Co-Director, Center for Study of Human Sexual Behavior and Associate Professor of Clinical Psychiatry, University of Pittsburgh
SEX THERAPY AND SEX RESEARCH, *article on* SCIENTIFIC AND CLINICAL PERSPECTIVES

Schumaker, Millard
Associate Professor of Religion and Ethics, Queen's Theological College (Kingston, Ontario)
OBLIGATION AND SUPEREROGATION

Shaffer, Jerome A.
Professor and Head, Department of Philosophy, University of Connecticut
PAIN AND SUFFERING, *article on* PHILOSOPHICAL PERSPECTIVES

Shaw, Margery W.
Director, Medical Genetics Center, The University of Texas Health Science Center
GENETICS AND THE LAW

Sherlock, Richard K.
Instructor of Philosophy and Religion, Northeastern University
POPULATION POLICY PROPOSALS, *article on* DIFFERENTIAL GROWTH RATE AND POPULATION POLICIES: ETHICAL ANALYSIS

Shinn, Roger L.
Reinhold Niebuhr Professor of Social Ethics, Union Theological Seminary (New York)
GENE THERAPY, *article on* ETHICAL ISSUES

Shoemaker, Sydney
Professor of Philosophy, Cornell University
MIND–BODY PROBLEM

Sidel, Victor W.
Professor of Community Health, Albert Einstein College of Medicine; Chairman, Department of Social Medicine, Montefiore Hospital and Medical Center (Bronx, New York)
WARFARE, *article on* BIOMEDICAL SCIENCE AND WAR

Sidel, Mark
Student, Princeton University
WARFARE, *article on* BIOMEDICAL SCIENCE AND WAR

Siegel, Seymour
Ralph Simon Professor of Theology, Jewish Theological Seminary of America (New York)
DEATH, *article on* WESTERN RELIGIOUS THOUGHT: POST-BIBLICAL JEWISH TRADITION; MEDICAL ETHICS, HISTORY OF, *section on* NEAR AND MIDDLE EAST AND AFRICA, *article on* CONTEMPORARY ISRAEL

Silver, George A.
Professor of Public Health, School of Medicine, Yale University
SOCIAL MEDICINE

Singer, Peter
Professor of Philosophy, Monash University (Melbourne, Australia)
ANIMAL EXPERIMENTATION, *article on* PHILOSOPHICAL PERSPECTIVES; LIFE, *article on* VALUE OF LIFE

Sinsheimer, Robert L.
Professor of Biology and Chancellor, University of California, Santa Cruz
REPRODUCTIVE TECHNOLOGIES, *article on* ASEXUAL HUMAN REPRODUCTION

Smith, David H.
Associate Professor and Chairman, Department of Religious Studies, and Director, Medicine and the Public Project, Indiana University
SUICIDE

Smith, Harmon L.
Professor of Moral Theology and Professor of Community Health Services, Duke University
HEART TRANSPLANTATION

Solomon, Wm. David
Milbank Research Fellow, Department of Philosophy, Boston University
ETHICS, *article on* RULES AND PRINCIPLES

Solomon, Robert C.
Professor of Philosophy, University of Texas at Austin
SEXUAL IDENTITY

Spengler, Joseph J.
James B. Duke Professor Emeritus of Economics, Duke University
POPULATION ETHICS: ELEMENTS OF THE FIELD, *article on* HISTORY OF POPULATION POLICIES

Stanley, Teresa
Kennedy Nursing Faculty Fellow in Bioethics; Director, Division of Nursing, Incarnate Word College (San Antonio, Texas)
NURSING

Strauss, Anselm
Professor of Sociology, University of California, San Francisco
CHRONIC CARE

Strickland, Stephen P.
Vice President, Aspen Institute for Humanistic Studies (New York)
HEALTH POLICY, *article on* EVOLUTION OF HEALTH POLICY

Sullivan, William M.
Assistant Professor of Philosophy, Allentown College of St. Francis de Sales (Center Valley, Pennsylvania)
MENTAL HEALTH THERAPIES

Swazey, Judith P.
Professor of Socio-Medical Sciences, School of Medicine, Boston University
KIDNEY DIALYSIS AND TRANSPLANTATION; SURGERY

Takemi, Taro
President, The Japan Medical Association (Tokyo)
MEDICAL ETHICS, HISTORY OF, *section on* SOUTH AND EAST ASIA, *article on* TRADITIONAL PROFESSIONAL ETHICS IN JAPANESE MEDICINE

Taylor, Carl E.
Professor and Chairman, Department of International Health, Johns Hopkins University
HEALTH, INTERNATIONAL; MASS HEALTH SCREENING

Teitelbaum, Michael S.
Fellow of Nuffield College, Oxford, and University Lecturer in Demography, Oxford University
POPULATION ETHICS: ELEMENTS OF THE FIELD, article on THE POPULATION PROBLEM IN DEMOGRAPHIC PERSPECTIVE

Thielicke, Helmut
Professor of Systematic Theology, University of Hamburg
MIRACLE AND FAITH HEALING, article on THEOLOGICAL PERSPECTIVE

Tooley, Michael
Research Fellow in Philosophy, Research School of Social Sciences, Australian National University
INFANTS, article on INFANTICIDE: A PHILOSOPHICAL PERSPECTIVE

Trainin, Isaac N.
Director, Federation of Jewish Philanthropies of New York
RELIGIOUS DIRECTIVES IN MEDICAL ETHICS, article on JEWISH CODES AND GUIDELINES

Trautmann, Joanne
Associate Professor of Humanities and English, College of Medicine, The Pennsylvania State University
MEDICAL ETHICS IN LITERATURE

Tribe, Laurence H.
Professor of Law, Harvard University
TECHNOLOGY, article on TECHNOLOGY AND THE LAW

Unschuld, Paul U.
Lecturer in Chinese, University of Marburg; Visiting Assistant Professor in Behavioral Sciences, Johns Hopkins University
CONFUCIANISM; MEDICAL ETHICS, HISTORY OF, section on SOUTH AND EAST ASIA, articles on GENERAL HISTORICAL SURVEY and PREREPUBLICAN CHINA

Vanderpool, Harold Y.
Assistant Professor of the History of Medicine, University of Texas Medical Branch
MIRACLE AND FAITH HEALING, article on CONCEPTUAL AND HISTORICAL PERSPECTIVES; PROTESTANTISM, article on DOMINANT HEALTH CONCERNS IN PROTESTANTISM

van Melsen, A. G. M.
Professor of Philosophy, University of Nijmegen
PERSON

Vastyan, E. A.
Professor and Chairman, Department of Humanities, College of Medicine, The Pennsylvania State University
WARFARE, article on MEDICINE AND WAR

Veatch, Robert M.
Senior Associate, The Hastings Center, Institute of Society, Ethics and the Life Sciences (Hastings-on-Hudson, New York)
CODES OF MEDICAL ETHICS, article on ETHICAL ANALYSIS; DEATH AND DYING: EUTHANASIA AND SUSTAINING LIFE, article on PROFESSIONAL AND PUBLIC POLICIES; MEDICAL ETHICS EDUCATION; POPULATION POLICY PROPOSALS, article on GOVERNMENTAL INCENTIVES; TRUTH-TELLING, article on ATTITUDES

Viederman, Stephen
Head, Social and Demographic Research Unit, United Nations Fund for Population Activities
POPULATION POLICY PROPOSALS, article on POPULATION EDUCATION

Walters, LeRoy
Director, Center for Bioethics, Kennedy Institute of Ethics, Georgetown University
TECHNOLOGY, article on TECHNOLOGY ASSESSMENT

Warwick, Donald P.
Institute Fellow, Harvard Institute for International Development
POPULATION POLICY PROPOSALS, articles on CONTEMPORARY INTERNATIONAL ISSUES and SOCIAL CHANGE PROPOSALS

Weber, Leonard J.
Associate Professor of Religious Studies, Mercy College of Detroit
SMOKING

Weiner, Dora B.
Associate Professor of History, Manhattanville College (Purchase, New York)
MEDICAL ETHICS, HISTORY OF, section on EUROPE AND THE AMERICAS, article on FRANCE IN THE NINETEENTH CENTURY

Wellman, Carl
Professor of Philosophy, Washington University (St. Louis)
ETHICS, articles on NATURALISM and RELATIVISM

Wexler, David B.
Professor of Law, University of Arizona
INSTITUTIONALIZATION

Williams, Kenneth J.
President, K. J. Williams and Associates, Inc., Hospital Consultants (Napa, California); Associate Professor of Hospital and Health Care Administration, St. Louis University
HOSPITALS

Winslade, William J.
> *Lecturer in Law, Lecturer in Psychiatry, and Co-Director, Program in Medicine, Law, and Human Values, University of California, Los Angeles*
> CONFIDENTIALITY

Wolf, C. P.
> *Associate Professor, Environmental Psychology Program, City University of New York*
> ENVIRONMENTAL ETHICS, *article on* THE PROBLEM OF GROWTH

Wolstenholme, Gordon
> *Director, The Ciba Foundation; President, The Royal Society of Medicine (London)*
> MEDICAL ETHICS, HISTORY OF, *section on* EUROPE AND THE AMERICAS, *article on* BRITAIN IN THE TWENTIETH CENTURY

Wurzburger, Walter S.
> *Rabbi, Congregation Shaaray Tefila (Far Rockaway, New York)*
> CADAVERS, *article on* JEWISH PERSPECTIVES

Yates, Wilson
> *Professor of Church and Society, United Theological Seminary of the Twin Cities (New Brighton, Minnesota)*
> POPULATION ETHICS: RELIGIOUS TRADITIONS, *article on* PROTESTANT PERSPECTIVES; POPULATION POLICY PROPOSALS, *article on* COMPULSORY POPULATION CONTROL PROGRAMS

Young, Ernlé W. D.
> *Lecturer in Medical Ethics and Chaplain, The Stanford University Medical Center*
> AGING AND THE AGED, *article on* HEALTH CARE AND RESEARCH IN THE AGED

Zaner, Richard M.
> *Easterwood Professor of Philosophy, Southern Methodist University*
> EMBODIMENT

Special Reviewers

To assure accuracy of content, articles in this encyclopedia were subject to review not only by the editors but by specialists in the numerous fields of learning discussed in the articles. More than 330 special reviewers were called upon to examine manuscripts for accuracy and comprehensiveness, and, on occasion, to recommend alternate authors and reviewers. These reviewers represent fields as diversified as surgery, Islamic studies, pediatrics, philosophy, environmental sciences, theology, psychiatry, philosophy, law, public health, anthropology of medicine, geriatrics, policy studies, genetics, history, psychology, demography, and health-care administration. We are indebted to the following scholars, from a number of different countries, who drew on their specialized knowledge to offer detailed assessments of this work:

Francisco Abel
Kenneth S. Abraham
Ruth D. Abrams
David C. Abramson
Leo Alexander
David Franklyn Allen
Gordon Allen
Darrel W. Amundsen
Odin W. Anderson
W. French Anderson
Paul H. Andreini
Judith Areen
Gordon Avery
Stephen Axelrad
Lloyd Bailey
Mitchell B. Balter
A. L. Basham
Donald Pates
Robert C. Baumiller
Tom L. Beauchamp
Alex Berman
Lyle W. Bivens
Peter Black
J. David Bleich
Ned Block
Samuel W. Bloom
Leon Bouvier

Joseph V. Brady
Gerard M. Brannon
Roy Branson
Lester Breslow
Harvey Brooks
Peter G. Brown
Walter Brueggemann
Mario Bunge
John Bunker
J. C. Bürgel
John C. Burnham
Chester R. Burns
Robert N. Butler
Jerome Bylebyl
Maureen Canick
Norman Cantor
P. V. Cardon
Frederick S. Carney
Charles Carroll
Kenneth M. Casebee:
Eric J. Cassell
Thomas Chalmers
Wing-tsit Chan
Satya N. Chatterjee
James F. Childress
Drew Christiansen
Ira Cisin

G. Mary Clinton
Mercedes Concepción
John R. Connery
Demetrios J.
    Constantelos
Robert E. Cooke
Harris L. Coulter
Austin B. Creel
D. L. Creson
Ralph C. Croizier
Barbara J. Culliton
Joseph Curl
Charles E. Curran
David Daube
Henry P. David
Kingsley Davis
Gerald Davison
Jean Robert Debray
Panagiotes Ch.
    Demetropoulos
Thomas Sieger Derr
Pat Diamond
Cornelia C. Dimmitt
Dennis J. Doherty
Raymond S. Duff
Clifton O. Dummett
David C. Duncombe

Arthur J. Dyck
Abraham Edel
Charles Edwards
R. G. Edwards
Barbara Ehrenreich
Anne H. Ehrlich
Paul R. Ehrlich
Bruce J. Ennis
L. Erlenmeyer-Kimling
Horacio Fabrega, Jr.
Richard M. Fagley
Margaret A. Farley
David M. Feldman
Mark G. Field
Max Fink
Norman J. Finkel
George Foster
Willard O. Foster, Jr.
Renée C. Fox
Donald S. Fredrickson
Daniel Freedman
John M. Freeman
Eliot Freidson
Paul A. Freund
Charles Fried
Jane M. Friedman
Arthur W. Galston
Edwin S. Gaustad
Willard Gaylin
Jack Geiger
Gerald L. Geison
Murray Gendell
Park S. Gerald
Norman J. Girardot
Barney G. Glaser
Bentley Glass
Holly Goldman
Byron J. Good
Irving I. Gottesman
Denis Goulet
Harold Green
Daniel Greenberg
Irving Greenberg
Otto E. Guttentag
John Whitney Hall
Bernard Häring
Bernice Catherine
    Harper
George T. Harrell
Harry Harris
Leston Havens
Robert Hayden
Leonard Hayflick
André E. Hellegers
Louis M. Hellman
Swailem S. Hennein
Richard J. Herrnstein
Ernest R. Hilgard
William J. Hill
Milton Himmelfarb
Kathryn K.
    Himmelsbach
P. Browning Hoffman
Frederick H. Holck

Edwin Holman
Ernest B. Hook
Rollin D. Hotchkiss
Lee Howard
Charles A. Hufnagel
Everett C. Hughes
David Lee Hull
Robert R. Huntley
E. P. Hutchinson
Warren F. Ilchman
Franz J. Ingelfinger
Charles Issawi
Immanuel Jakobovits
James T. Johnson
Renée Johnson
James H. Jones
Stephen Joseph
Michael Kaback
Richard A. Kalish
George A. Kanoti
John Karefa-Smart
Leon R. Kass
Jay Katz
Seymour S. Kety
Lester S. King
Dudley Kirk
Joseph M. Kitagawa
Nicholas N. Kittrie
Gerald L. Klerman
Martin Koen
Robert C. Kolodny
Donald Konold
Julius Korein
Samuel L. Kountz
Fridolf Kudlien
Stephan Kuttner
Marc Lappé
Donald V. Lassiter
Jérôme Lejeune
Charles Leslie
Charles W. Lloyd
George V. Lobo
Margaret Lock
John C. Loehlin
David W. Louisell
Paul Lowinger
Harold S. Luft
Edward Lurie
Abbyann Lynch
Arthur McCormack
Richard A. McCormick
James M. McCullough
Laurence B.
    McCullough
Thomas K. McElhinney
Peter J. M. McEwan
Jim McIntosh
Ronald W. McNeur
Francis MacNutt
Edward H. Madden
Jose Mainetti
David G. Mandelbaum
Herbert Joseph Manz
Vernon Mark

J. Donald Mashburn
Luigi Mastroianni, Jr.
William Maxted
Rollo May
William E. May
Jean Mayer
Ernst Mayr
David Mechanic
Zhores Medvedev
Thomas W. Merrick
John Meyendorff
David W. Meyers
Robert Michels
John Giles Milhaven
Aubrey Milunsky
Robert Mnookin
N. J. Modi
Gaetano F. Molinari
John W. Money
Richard T. Morris
Jerome A. Motto
Arno Motulsky
K. E. Moyer
Marjorie Smith Mueller
Charles W. Murdock
Edmond A. Murphy
Robert F. Murray, Jr.
Basim F. Musallam
Selma J. Mushkin
Henry L. Nadler
Ann Neale
Jacob Needleman
John R. Neil
D. R. Newth
Peter H. Niebyl
John T. Noonan, Jr.
Richard Norris
Frank W. Notestein
Thomas W. Ogletree
Marian Osterweis
Gene Outka
Larry I. Palmer
John Passmore
Edmund D. Pellegrino
Seymour Perlin
Martin S. Pernick
Josef Pieper
Harriet F. Pilpel
Robert Plotkin
Karl H. Pribram
David Rabin
Thomas A. Rakowski
Paul Ramsey
F. C. Redlich
James Reed
Nicholas Rescher
Frank E. Reynolds
Jeanne Clare Ridley
John A. Robertson
Daniel N. Robinson
Jonas Robitscher
Richard O. Roblin
George Rosen
Albert Rosenfeld

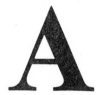

ABORTION

The article on MEDICAL ASPECTS *explains the physiological and medical data relevant to the ethical issues on abortion. The next three articles,* JEWISH PERSPECTIVES, ROMAN CATHOLIC PERSPECTIVES, *and* PROTESTANT PERSPECTIVES, *represent the consistent ethical methodologies in the dominant Western religious traditions through the mid-twentieth century. The fifth article,* CONTEMPORARY DEBATE IN PHILOSOPHICAL AND RELIGIOUS ETHICS, *continues the discussion of the religious traditions to the present and then compares them with the same points made in contemporary philosophical writings. The final article,* LEGAL ASPECTS, *offers a framework within which laws on abortion can be understood in an international perspective.*

I
MEDICAL ASPECTS

Medical context of abortion

The place occupied by the fetus in the thinking of the medical profession and the theological and philosophical professions has evolved along with the specialty of obstetrics or midwifery.

Thinking about the fetus as a human entity, separate from the mother, has a long tradition in both ethics and medicine. For ethics the subject of abortion has been discussed since pre-Christian days (Connery). For obstetrics, the concept of the fetus as an individual entity at first presented a philosophical problem of how it obtained its "vital spirit," later to be known as oxygen. The debate raged from the days of Greek philosophers until its final resolution when a separate fetal circulation was first described by William Harvey in 1651. Refinements in assessing fetal metabolism date largely to the twentieth century, when fetal physiology and neonatology emerged as distinct specialties.

The stimulus for a refined examination of the fetus in medicine and ethics followed a distinct drawn-out progression of events. At all times in medical practice, and mostly also in ethics, the mother has been considered more important than the fetus. In medicine the induction of death in the fetus to save maternal life has had a long tradition, ranging from the performance of embryotomy for cephalopelvic disproportion to the removal of pregnancies implanted in sites other than the uterus (ectopic pregnancies). For many decades also abortions were performed for a variety of maternal somatic diseases, especially of the lungs, heart, and kidneys, in which it was thought appropriate to perform abortions for the immediate relief of the perceived strains of pregnancy on the maternal renal, pulmonary, and cardiovascular systems. Only when medical institutions that refused to do such abortions on religious grounds adduced data to show that their maternal outcomes were no worse did a shift in thinking occur. It came to be understood that to perform surgical procedures, including abortions, on critically ill women was likely to induce death rather than to prevent it. A philosophy of first treating a critically ill woman medically, until she was fit enough to undergo surgery or abortion, evolved. Inevitably when she became fit enough to undergo surgery, the question arose why she was not sufficiently fit to complete the pregnancy, at least until the fetus was viable. What occurred, then, was a progressive questioning of the practice of deeming abortion necessary to save maternal life.

The questioning took place concurrently with considerable progress in the techniques of epidemiology and biostatistics. Those techniques permitted great refinements in assessing the long-term effects of acting or not acting obstetrically. Studies then became possible not just on the effects of abortion for the immediate saving of maternal life, but on the effects of aborting, or not aborting, on the subsequent life expectancy of women as well. As a result, the issue changed from one of aborting instantaneously to save maternal life to a matter of aborting to preserve an average life span. The new obstetrical question involved abortion for the maintenance of health in the long run, rather than for saving life in the short run.

Toward the middle of the twentieth century many epidemiological studies began to appear that related the quality of fetal outcome to the status of mothers in pregnancy. A key study performed in Australia related the incidence of congenital anomalies in infants to the occurrence of rubella, or German measles, in the first trimester of pregnancy (Gregg). A question arose as to whether abortions should be performed to prevent the birth of children who, by virtue of congenital anomalies, would be a handicap to their parents and at risk of suffering themselves. Thus, the question became whether abortions should be performed for "fetal indications." Proponents of the notion stressed the suffering, for both infant and parents. Antagonists stressed not only the value of any fetal life, but also the fact that, within the limits of the knowledge then available, several normal fetuses had to be aborted to ensure the abortion of the abnormal ones. With development of techniques for culturing amniotic fluid cells it became possible to diagnose fetal defects directly and to abort only defective fetuses, unless the diagnosis was inaccurate. Abortions performed acutely to save maternal life therefore decreased as abortions to prolong the life span or to avoid the birth of anomalous infants increased.

These trends in abortion practice were influenced not just by the availability of prognostic and diagnostic techniques, such as epidemiology and amniotic fluid analysis, but also by progress in obstetrical techniques of other kinds. Committees for analyzing each maternal death were established, and corrective measures and educational programs were instituted until, by 1974, total deaths associated with the pregnancy process had decreased to no more than a few hundred per year for the entire United States. As the obstetrical task of making pregnancy safe for women became almost fully successful, stress was increasingly laid on making it safe for fetuses as well. It became realized that many newborn infants who had not died had, nevertheless, been damaged. Prematurity and fetal distress in the labor process were discovered to be particularly productive of subsequent damage, especially to the brain. Progress in anesthesiology, in Caesarean section techniques, in blood transfusion, and in antibiotic therapy permitted increasing opportunities to perform Caesarean sections with relative impunity. Progressive decrease in perinatal and infant mortality also meant that women needed to undergo fewer pregnancies before desired family size was achieved. As a consequence, Caesarean section scars would be less frequently subjected to risk of rupture in subsequent pregnancies, another factor that fostered an earlier resorting to Caesarean section. The same relative certainty that almost all products of birth could be made to survive led to an increasing concern for the avoidance of infant morbidity as well as infant mortality. The focus of obstetrics and allied sciences, therefore, gradually changed from mothers to fetuses and to their quality.

As data became available to suggest that wanted babies fared better than unwanted ones, the stress on family planning increased. An ethos arose that proclaimed that parents should have the number of children they desired and at the time they desired. Thus the procedure of abortion, which originally was linked to the preservation of maternal life and health, gradually changed to become a backstop to, or an alternative to, other methods of family planning.

Definition of abortion

In medical parlance, abortion is defined as termination of pregnancy, spontaneously or by induction, prior to viability. Thereafter termination of pregnancy is called delivery. To the lay public the term spontaneous abortion is usually referred to as miscarriage. Induced abortions have been classified as therapeutic and non-therapeutic in the past, the terms often being used synonymously with legal and illegal abortion respectively. The synonymous use of the terms stemmed from the fact that licensed physicians, operating in hospitals, were not prosecuted for performing abortions where a threat to the life of the mother existed.

An induced termination of pregnancy prior to viability is not always regarded as an abortion in common parlance. For example, salpingectomy (removal of a fallopian tube) for ectopic pregnancy (pregnancy implanted in the tube) is a common, indeed a universal, practice, even in Catholic hospitals, where the operation is justified by the "principle of double effect" as an "indirect" abortion. Regardless of what the procedure is called in common parlance or in ethics, it conforms to the medical definition of induced abortion. Similarly, most diagnostic uterine curettages are performed in the late stages of the menstrual cycle, when a fertilized ovum may well be present in the tube, unless patients have been told not to have unprotected intercourse in that menstrual cycle. Such advice is rarely given, leading to the loss of thousands of fertilized eggs annually. Thus, the curettage will either not be regarded as an abortion at all or will be judged as "indirect" abortion, providing the curettage is justified on diagnostic, even though not directly therapeutic, grounds. Similarly again, it is often held, though far from settled, that intrauterine devices act by preventing implantation of fertilized eggs. Many disapprove of such "abortifacient" action, yet would not hesitate to do a curettage in the postovulatory (and hence potentially postfertilization) stages of the menstrual cycle. These are some of the vagaries in debates on what constitutes abortion.

Abortion procedures

Where there is an intention to procure an abortion, several procedures are available. The procedures are chosen largely on the basis of uterine size.

First trimester. In the first trimester of pregnancy, the uterine contents are of such size that they are easily evacuated through the cervix (mouth) of the uterus (womb). That is done by dilating the cervix and then emptying the uterus, either by strong suction ("suction curettage") into a bottle, or by scraping the uterine contents from its wall with a spoon-shaped instrument called a curette ("D & C" or dilation and curettage). In general, less uterine dilation is required for suction curettage than for a D & C, because the tubing through which the uterine contents are removed by suction is thinner than a curette. Also, since the pregnant uterus is very soft in consistency, the relatively soft tubing used in suction curettage presents fewer hazards of perforation of the uterus than the steel curette. Thus, suction curettage has become the commonest, safest, and fastest method of performing abortions in the first thirteen or so weeks of pregnancy.

Second trimester. Early in the second trimester uterine contents become of such size that rapid evacuation through the cervix becomes dangerous. Methods of uterine evacuation are therefore used, which increasingly resemble full-term delivery, surgically or medically.

Surgical. Surgical evacuation of the uterus prior to viability of the fetus is called hysterotomy (incision of the uterus) and is a miniature Caesarean section. Either the fetus is delivered first, the umbilical cord tied and cut, and then the placenta delivered, or the placenta is separated from the uterine wall first, thus delivering the placenta and fetus as one entity. The former procedure gives the fetus, if viable, a better chance of survival, for it can be better and earlier oxygenated if it is not retained *in utero* with its oxygen supply via the placenta cut off. Removal of the placenta and fetus simultaneously, however, gives the uterus a better chance of contracting down and stopping bleeding from the placental implantation site.

Medical. Medical evacuation of the uterus seeks to emulate the natural mechanism of labor and delivery at term by initiating uterine contractions, thereby dilating the uterine cervix and expelling the uterine contents. The initiation of contractions is induced by injecting into the amniotic fluid a concentrated solution of salt or twenty-five to forty mg. of a hormone called prostaglandin. The former is thought to act by destroying placental and fetal actions that tend to prevent the uterus from contracting, while the latter is thought to establish uterine contractions directly. Thus, the former tends to kill the fetus directly, while the latter does not. Upon occasion, both agents' action is augmented by the intravenous infusion into the maternal circulation of a pituitary gland extract called pitocin. Pitocin causes uterine contractions in its own right.

Sometimes, also, physicians will insert into the cervical canal laminar or tentlike structures that, by absorbing fluid, will enlarge and thus help dilate the cervix. Additional use of pitocin and laminaria is designed to speed up the time from the induction of abortion to its completion and also increases the percentage of abortions factually achieved by saline or prostaglandin. The disadvantage of added pitocin is that it may overstimulate uterine contractions, with the occasional occurrence of a uterine rupture.

Ethical considerations

It is a recognized fact that physicians often misjudge the existing duration of a pregnancy. In large part, this is because twenty percent of pregnant women bleed at some time during early pregnancy, often at the time of an expected menstrual period. Such bleeding episodes may be mistaken for a regular or slightly abnormal menstrual period. One such bleeding episode may cause the underestimation of gestational age by a month, and two episodes by even more. Occasionally, therefore, abortion procedures may produce live fetuses that approximate viability; in fact, some fetuses have survived abortion by these methods. At issue, then, ethically, is whether second-trimester abortions should be done only by those methods—hysterotomy with immediate fetal delivery, or prostaglandins—which constitute the least direct attacks upon the possibility of fetal survival, in contrast to saline injections. In part, the answer depends upon whether abortion is seen as a physical separation of mother and fetus, two parties who have a conflict of interest, or whether it is seen as a procedure that guarantees for a mother the destruction of her fetus. The American College of Obstetricians and Gynecologists, in a policy statement issued in 1976, takes the view that abortion is a process of separating conflicting parties and does not primarily aim at destruction of the fetus directly. It therefore implies that interruptions of pregnancy should, in the choice of methodology, maximize survival chances of the fetus, where this can be done without increasing the risk of the procedure to the mother. Courts of law have not expressed an opinion on whether abortion is a process of separating mother and fetus, or whether it may guarantee death of the fetus, whether necessary or not.

Complications

In general induced abortion, like any surgical or medical procedure, carries some risks. In general also, they are less frequent and of less severity than childbirth. A representation of those risks in terms of complication rates is contained in the following table. They refer to complications immediately incident to the various procedures. Still at issue are long-term sequellae of abortion, both physically and psychologically.

Complication Rates per 1000 Abortions by Type and Method of Termination, New York City

July 1, 1970–December 31, 1971

TYPE OF COMPLICATION	METHODS OF TERMINATION				
	TOTAL	DILATION AND CURETTAGE	SUCTION	SALINE	HYSTEROTOMY
Hemorrhage	1.1	1.0	0.5	4.0	3.7
Infection	1.5	0.9	0.8	5.4	11.0
Perforated uterus	1.3	1.9	1.3	0.2	5.1
Anesthesia	0.1	0.1	0.1	0.1	0.7
Shock	*	*	*	0.2	0.7
Retained tissue	2.3	0.5	0.5	14.7	1.5
Failure	0.3	*	*	2.4	–
Lacerated cervix	0.2	0.3	0.2	0.1	0.7
Other	0.4	0.3	0.3	1.0	4.4
Unspecified	0.1	0.1	*	0.2	–
Total	7.3	5.1	3.7	28.3	27.8

* Less than 0.05.
Source: J. Pakter and F. G. Nelson, "Effects of a Liberalized Abortion Law in New York City," *Mt. Sinai Journal of Medicine* 39 (1972): 535. Reprinted by permission of the publisher and the authors.

At the physical level, the main unresolved question is the effect of aborting one pregnancy on the outcome of subsequent pregnancies, particularly in teenagers (Russell). The problem seems to revolve around the degree of damage done to the uterine cervix in artificial dilation or by natural dilation occurring at an early age, through either abortion or childbirth. At the psychological level, the problem revolves around how the human mind views its own fetuses.

Finally, it should be realized that any medical procedure is limited by the total biological knowledge available at the time of its development. At all times medical science seeks to make its interventions effective with the least trauma. The psychological degree of trauma induced depends in large part upon the body image that the individual has of himself or herself. Because abortion is a procedure following upon one result of sexual activity, its effects depend, in part, upon the significance that may, from time to time, be attached to that sexual activity.

ANDRÉ E. HELLEGERS

[*While all the articles in this entry are relevant, see especially the articles* CONTEMPORARY DEBATE IN PHILOSOPHICAL AND RELIGIOUS ETHICS *and* LEGAL ASPECTS. *For further discussion of topics mentioned in this article, see the entries:* CONTRACEPTION; DOUBLE EFFECT; FETAL–MATERNAL RELATIONSHIP; GENETIC DIAGNOSIS AND COUNSELING; INFANTS; LIFE; PRENATAL DIAGNOSIS; *and* RISK. *See also:* EMBODIMENT; PERSON; POPULATION ETHICS: ELEMENTS OF THE FIELD; POPULATION ETHICS: RELIGIOUS TRADITIONS; *and* POPULATION POLICY PROPOSALS.]

BIBLIOGRAPHY

American College of Obstetricians and Gynecologists, Executive Board. "Some Ethical Considerations in Abortion." Chicago: 1975. Xeroxed.

CONNERY, JOHN. *Abortion: The Development of the Roman Catholic Perspective.* Chicago: Loyola University Press, 1977.

GREGG, N. MCALISTER. "Congenital Cataract Following German Measles in the Mother." *Transactions of the Ophthalmological Society of Australia* 3 (1941): 35–46.

HARVEY, WILLIAM. *Anatomical Exercitations Concerning the Generation of Living Creatures: To Which Are Added Particular Discourses of Births, and of Conceptions, etc.* London: Printed by James Young for Octavian Pulleyn, 1653.

PAKTER, JEAN, and NELSON, FRIEDA G. "Effects of a Liberalized Abortion Law in New York City." *Mt. Sinai Journal of Medicine* 39 (1972): 535–543.

RUSSELL, J. K. "Sexual Activity and Its Consequences in the Teenager." *Clinics in Obstetrics and Gynaecology* 1 (1974): 683–698.

II
JEWISH PERSPECTIVES

The abortion question in talmudic law begins for some with an examination of the fetus's legal status. For this the Talmud has a phrase, *ubar yerekh imo,* a counterpart of the Latin *pars viscerum matris.* The fetus, that is, is deemed a "part of its mother" rather than an independent entity. Of course, this designation says nothing about the right of abortion; the term is found only in more theoretical contexts. It defines ownership, for example, in the case of an embryo found in a purchased animal, that, as intrinsic to its mother's body, it belongs to the buyer. Moreover, in the religious conversion of a pregnant woman, her unborn child is automatically included and requires no added ceremony. Nor does the fetus have power of acquisition: Gifts or transactions made on its behalf, except by its father, are not binding; it inherits from its father only, in a natural rather than a transactional manner.

Germane as such information might seem to the question of abortion, it tells us little more than, in the words of a modern writer on Roman and Jewish law, Y. K. Miklishanski, that in both systems the fetus has no "juridical personality" of its own. The morality of abortion is a function, rather, of the legal attitude to feticide as distinguished from homicide or infanticide. The law of homicide in the Torah, in one of its several formulations (Exod. 21:12), reads: "*Makkeh ish* . . ." "He who smites a man . . ." Does this include *any* "man," say, a day-old child? Yes, says the Talmud, citing another text (Lev. 24:17): *ki yakkeh kol nefesh adam,* "if one smite *any nefesh adam*"—literally, any human person. The "any" is understood to *include* the day-old child, but the "*nefesh adam*" is taken to *exclude* the fetus in the womb, for the fetus in the womb is *lav nefesh hu* (not a person) until he is born. In the words of Rashi, the classic commentator on the Bible and Talmud, only when the fetus "comes into the world" is it a "person."

The basis, then, for denying capital-crime status to feticide in Jewish law is scriptural. Alongside the *nefesh adam* text is another basic one, in Exodus 21:22, which provides: "If men strive, and wound a pregnant woman so that her fruit be expelled, but no harm befall [her], then shall he be fined as her husband shall assess, and the matter placed before the judges. But if harm befall [her], then shalt thou give life for life."

The Talmud makes this latter verse's teaching explicit: Only monetary compensation is exacted of him who causes a woman to miscarry. And though the abortion spoken of in this biblical passage is accidental, the verse is still a source for the teaching that feticide is not a capital crime (since even accidental homicide could not be expiated by monetary fine).

This important passage in Exodus has an alternate version in the Septuagint, the Greek translation of the Bible produced in Alexandria in the third pre-Christian century. One word change there yields an entirely different statute on miscarriage. Prof. Viktor Aptowitzer's essays analyze the disputed passage; the school of thought it represents he calls the Alexandrian school, as opposed to the Palestinian—that is, the talmudic—view set forth above. The word in question is *ason*, rendered above as "harm," hence, "if [there be] no harm [i.e., death, to the mother], then shall he be fined. . . ." The Greek renders the word *ason* as "form," yielding something like: "if [there be] form, then shalt thou give life for life." The "life for life" clause is thus applied to the fetus instead of the mother, and a distinction is made—as Augustine will formulate it—between *embryo informatus* and *embryo formatus*, a fetus not yet "formed" and one already "formed"; for the latter, the text so rendered prescribes the death penalty.

Among the Christian Church Fathers, the consequent doctrine of feticide as murder was preached by Tertullian (160?–230?), who accepted the Septuagint, and by Jerome (340?–420), who did not. Jerome's classic Bible translation renders this Exodus passage according to the Hebrew text accepted in the Church. The Didache, a handbook of basic Christianity for the instruction of converts from paganism, follows the Alexandrian teaching and specifies abortion as a capital crime. Closer to the main body of the Jewish community, we find the doctrine accepted by the Samaritans and Karaites and, more important, by Philo, the popular first-century philosopher of Alexandria. On the other hand, Philo's younger contemporary, Josephus, bears witness to the Palestinian (halakhic) tradition. Aside from its textual warrant, the latter is the more authentic, according to Aptowitzer, while the other is a later tendency, "which, in addition, is not genuinely Jewish but must have originated in Alexandria under Egyptian-Greek influence" (Aptowitzer, p. 88).

In the rabbinic tradition, then, abortion remains a noncapital crime at worst. But a curious factor further complicates the question of the criminality of the act. This is the circumstance that one more biblical text, this one in Genesis and hence "before Sinai" and part of the Laws of the "Sons of Noah," served as the source for the teaching that feticide is indeed a capital crime—for non-Jews. Genesis 9:6 reads, "He who sheds the blood of man, through man [i.e., through the human court of law] shall *his* blood be shed." Since the Hebrew (*shofekh dam ha'adam, ba'adam . . .*) allows for a translation of "man, in man" as well as "man, through man," the Talmud records the exposition of Rabbi Ishmael: "What is this 'man in man'? It refers to the fetus in its mother's womb." The locus of this text in Genesis—standing as it does without the qualifying balance of the Exodus (Sinaitic) passage—made feticide a capital crime for non-Jews (i.e., those not heir to the Sinaitic covenant) in Jewish law. Some modern scholars hold this exposition to be more sociological than textually inherent, representing a reaction against abuses among the heathen. In view of rampant abortion and infanticide, they claim, Rabbi Ishmael "expounded" the above exegesis in the Genesis text in order to render judgment against the Romans.

Regardless of its rationale, the doctrine remains part of Jewish law, as Maimonides systematically codifies it: "A 'Son of Noah' who killed a person, even a fetus in its mother's womb, is capitally liable. . . . (The Jewish court is obliged to provide judges for the resident alien to adjudicate for them in accordance with these laws [of the Sons of Noah] so that society not corrupt itself. The judges may come either from their midst or from the Israelites.)" Lifesaving therapeutic abortion is not, of course, included in this Noahide restriction. Nor is an abortion during the first forty days of pregnancy included, according to some. The implications of this anomaly of a different law for "Sons of Noah" were dealt with in a Responsum of the eighteenth century: "It is not to be supposed that the Torah would consider the embryo as a person [*nefesh*] for them [Sons of Noah] but not a person for us. The fetus is not a person for them either; the Torah merely was more severe in its practical ruling in their [the Noahides'] regard. Hence, therapeutic abortion would be permissible to them, too."

In the rabbinic system, then, abortion is not murder. Nor is it *more* than murder, as would be the case if "ensoulment" were at issue. Talmudic discussions speak of the moment—conception, birth, postbirth, etc.—at which the soul joins the body. This is seen to be irrelevant to the abortion question, because the soul is immortal no matter when it enters or leaves the body. And, more important than being immortal, it is a pure soul, free of the taint of "original sin." In the sixth century, St. Fulgentius asserted that "original sin" is inherited by the soul of the fetus at conception. This made baptism *in utero* necessary in cases of miscarriage, and also made abortion worse than murder, in the sense that the fetus was being "killed in this world and the next." Judaism has no concept of "original sin" of this kind; in the words of the Talmud and Daily Prayer Book, "My God, the soul with which Thou hast endowed me is pure."

Murder (of the innocent) would be forbidden even to save life. But with abortion removed from the category of murder, therapeutic abortion becomes permissible and, in fact, mandated. The Mishnah sets forth the basic talmudic law in this regard: "If a woman has [life-threatening] difficulty in childbirth, the embryo within her should be dismembered limb by limb, because her life takes precedence over its life. Once its head (or its greater part) has emerged, it may not be touched, for we do not set aside one life for another" (Mishnah, Oholot 7:6).

In analyzing such provisions the Talmud suggested that the reason could well be that the fetus is in the category of an "aggressor"; that is, its life is forfeit under the law that permits killing a "pursuer" in order to save the intended victim. The Talmud, however, dismisses this reasoning, since the fetus is an innocent being, and since one cannot know "who is pursuing whom"; the pursuit must therefore be deemed an "act of God," and this factor does not apply. Yet, in his great Law Code, Maimonides reintroduced the term "aggressor"—his commentators explaining his qualified use of the concept. He formulates the Mishnaic provision as follows:

This, too, is a [Negative] Commandment: Not to take pity on the life of a pursuer. Therefore the Sages ruled that when a woman has difficulty in giving birth, one may dismember the child in her womb—either with drugs or by surgery—because it is like a pursuer seeking to kill her. Once its head has emerged, it may not be touched, for we do not set aside one life for another; this is the natural course of the world [Mishnah Torah, Laws of Murder and Preservation of Life, 1:9].

Some commentators to Maimonides's Code suggest that although abortion is not technically murder it is still so grave an act that Maimonides enlisted the aggressor argument to buttress the existing permission for abortion; its justification is that the fetus is at least *like* an aggressor.

The subsequent rabbinic tradition seems to align itself either to the right, in the direction of Maimonides; or to the left, in the direction of Rashi, above. The first approach can be identified especially with the late Chief Rabbi of Israel, Issar Unterman, who sees any abortion as "akin to homicide" and therefore allowable only in cases of corresponding gravity, such as saving the life of the mother. This approach then builds *down* from that strict position to embrace a broader interpretation of lifesaving situations, which include a threat to her health, for example, as well as a threat to her life. The second approach, associated with another former Chief Rabbi of Israel, Ben Zion Uziel, and others, assumes that no real prohibition against abortion exists—other than antiprocreational—and builds *up* from that lenient position to safeguard against indiscriminate abortion. This includes the example of Rabbi Yair Bachrach in the seventeenth century, whose classic Responsum saw no legal bar to abortion, in the case before him, but would not permit it on other grounds. The case was one of a pregnancy conceived in adultery; the woman, in "deep remorse," wanted to destroy the fruit of her sin. The author concludes by refusing to sanction the abortion, not on legal grounds but on sociological ones, as a safeguard against immorality. Other authorities disagreed on this point, reaffirming the legal sanction of abortion for the woman's welfare, whether life or health, or even avoidance of "great pain."

The criterion in both approaches remains maternal rather than fetal. A principle in Jewish law is *tza'ar gufah kadim*, i.e., that avoidance or prevention of "her pain should be the first consideration." The mother's welfare is primary, and hence maternal indications, rather than fetal—or even the husband's wishes—are determinative. Rabbinic rulings on abortion are thus amenable to the following generalization: If a possibility or probability exists that a child may be born defective, and the mother seeks abortion *on the grounds of* pity for a child whose life would be less than normal, the rabbi would decline permission. If, however, an abortion for that same potentially deformed child were sought on the grounds that the possibility is causing severe anguish to the mother, permission would be granted. The fetus is unknown, future, potential, part of the "secrets of God"; the mother is known, present, alive, and asking for compassion.

One rabbinic authority, writing in Rumania in 1940, responded to the case of an epileptic mother who wanted to interrupt her pregnancy for fear that her child too would be epileptic. He first discusses the question of epilepsy itself, then writes:

For fear of possible, remote danger to a future child that, maybe, God forbid, he will know sickness—how can it occur to anyone to actively kill him because of such a possible doubt? This seems to me very much like the laws of Lycurgus, King of Sparta, according to which every blemished child was to be killed. . . . Permission for abortion is to be granted only because of fear of mental anguish for the *mother*. But for fear of what might be the child's lot—"the secrets of God are none of your business" [Feldman, p. 292].

In the current Tay-Sachs genetic screening controversy, rabbinic authorities recommend screening before rather than during the pregnancy. This is because the alternative would be resort to amniocentesis after the first trimester of pregnancy, with possible abortion on the basis of its results. This abortion for fetal rather than maternal indications would not ordinarily be sanctioned by Jewish law. True, rabbinic opinion permitting abortion for fetal reasons alone is not altogether lacking, but the normative rabbinic view is to permit it for maternal indications only. Yet the one can blend into the other: Fetal risk can mean mental anguish on the part of the mother, so that the fetal indication becomes a maternal one. The woman's welfare is thus the key to warrant for abortion.

Implicit in the Mishnah above is the teaching that the rights of the fetus are secondary to the rights of the mother all the way up until the moment of birth. This principle is obscured by the current phrase "right to life." In the context of abortion questions, the issue is not the right to life, which is very clear in Jewish law, but the right to be born, which is not as clear. The right to be born is relative; the right to life, of existing persons, is absolute. "Life" may begin before birth, but it is not the life of a human person; animal life, plant life, or even prehuman life is not the same as human life. Rabbinic law has determined that human life begins with birth. This is neither a medical nor a court judgment, but a metaphysical one. In the Jewish system, human life in this sense begins with birth. Of course, potential life already partakes of the po-

tential sacredness of actual life, since the latter can have its inception only through the former.

Another slogan-like phrase is dealt with in the same Mishnah, wherein it is ruled that "once the fetus has emerged from the womb, it cannot be touched" even to save the life of the mother, "for we cannot set aside one life for another." The "quality of life" slogan or concept is thus inadmissible. The life of the mother has more "quality"; she is adult and has husband, children, and associations. Still, the *sanctity*-of-life principle means that life is sacred regardless of differences in quality: mother and newborn babe are equal from the moment of birth.

Talmudic statements do use the term "murder," in a figurative sense, of course, to describe even the neglect to conceive. Procreation is a positive mitzvah (commandment), and he who fails to fulfill this mitzvah is called "guilty of bloodshed." Much of the pronatalist attitude of Judaism helps account for its abhorrence of casual abortion. There may be legal sanction for abortion where necessary, but the attitude remains one of hesitation before the sanctity of life and a pronatalist reverence for potential life.

Accordingly, abortion for "population control" is repugnant to the Jewish mind. Abortion for economic reasons is also not admissible. Taking precaution by abortion or birth control against physical threat remains a mitzvah, but never to forestall financial hardship. Material considerations are improper in this connection. In the Jewish community today, with a conscious or unconscious drive to replenish ranks decimated by the Holocaust, contemporary rabbis invoke not the more lenient but the more stringent Responsa of the earlier authorities. The more permissive decisions, they point out, were in any case rendered against the background of far greater instinctive hesitation to resort to abortion. Against today's background of more casual abortion, rabbis are moving closer to the position associated with Maimonides and Unterman, allowing abortion only for the gravest of reasons.

DAVID M. FELDMAN

[*While all the articles in this entry are relevant, see especially the articles* ROMAN CATHOLIC PERSPECTIVES, CONTEMPORARY DEBATE IN PHILOSOPHICAL AND RELIGIOUS ETHICS, *and* LEGAL ASPECTS. *For further discussion of topics mentioned in this article, see the entries:* CONTRACEPTION; GENETIC DIAGNOSIS AND COUNSELING; INFANTS; LIFE; POPULATION ETHICS: RELIGIOUS TRADITIONS, *article on* JEWISH PERSPECTIVES; PRENATAL DIAG-

NOSIS; *and* RIGHTS. *Also directly related are the entries* JUDAISM; MEDICAL ETHICS, HISTORY OF, *section on* NEAR AND MIDDLE EAST AND AFRICA, *article on* CONTEMPORARY ISRAEL; *and* RELIGIOUS DIRECTIVES IN MEDICAL ETHICS, *article on* JEWISH CODES AND GUIDELINES. *See also:* PERSON; *and* POPULATION POLICY PROPOSALS, *article on* DIFFERENTIAL GROWTH RATE AND POPULATION POLICIES: ETHICAL ANALYSIS.]

BIBLIOGRAPHY

APTOWITZER, V. "Observations on the Criminal Law of the Jews." *Jewish Quarterly Review* 15 (1924): 55–118.

BLEICH, DAVID. "Abortion in Halakhic Literature." *Tradition* 10 (1968): 72–120.

FELDMAN, DAVID MICHAEL. *Birth Control in Jewish Law: Marital Relations, Contraception and Abortion as Set Forth in the Classic Texts of Jewish Law.* New York: New York University Press, 1968. Schocken Paperback, 1974.

JAKOBOVITS, IMMANUEL. *Jewish Medical Ethics: A Comparative and Historical Study of the Jewish Religious Attitude to Medicine and Its Practice.* New York: Bloch Publishing Co., 1962. Rev. ed. 1975.

KLEIN, ISAAC. "Abortion" (1959). *Responsa and Halakhic Studies.* New York: Ktav Publishing House, 1975, chap. 4, pp. 27–33.

ROSNER, FRED. *Modern Medicine and Jewish Law.* Studies in Torah Judaism, vol. 13. Edited by Leon D. Stitskin. New York: Yeshiva University, Department of Special Publications, 1972.

III
ROMAN CATHOLIC PERSPECTIVES

Scriptural influence

An understanding of the Roman Catholic perspective on abortion, if it is to be adequate, will call for an acquaintance with the Hebrew tradition that preceded the Christian era. One would expect to discover the source, or at least the expression, of this tradition in the Torah, the first five books of the Bible, which contains the fundamental law of the Jews. Unfortunately, an examination of this part of the Bible yields only one text that deals explicitly with abortion. It comes from Exodus (21:22–25), more specifically from that part of Exodus known as the Book of the Covenant, and imposes a penalty on a person guilty of what seems to be an accidental abortion. According to the law, if two men are fighting and one happens to strike a pregnant woman, causing an abortion, he will have to pay a fine. But if injury occurs (to the woman), he will have to pay in kind according to the *lex talionis,* that is, "an eye for an eye," etc. This has generally been interpreted to mean that the fetus was not considered a human being. If it

were, the *lex talionis* would apply and the penalty would be "a life for a life," which would be the penalty if the mother herself died.

Curiously enough, the Septuagint (Greek) version of the above text, made in the early third century B.C., is quite different. The case presented is the same, but the distinction made is not between an abortion and damage to the mother, but between the formed and unformed fetus. If the fetus is unformed, the one guilty will have to pay a fine; if the fetus is formed, the *lex talionis* will apply and he will have to pay a life for life. This statement of the law is quite different from that of the Hebrew text and coincides more with Greek, particularly Aristotelian, thought. According to Aristotle the human soul was infused into the fetus when it took on the human form and figure. This occurred forty days after conception in the male, and ninety days in the female. Before that time it did not have a human soul. The Septuagint makes no distinction between male and female but seems to consider the fetus a human being when it is formed and applies the *lex talionis* to the formed fetus just as the Hebrew text applied it to the mother. Since the lingua franca of the Roman world at the beginning of the Christian era was Greek, it was the Septuagint text that had the greater impact on the Christian tradition. The Vulgate of St. Jerome (Latin version of the Bible, A.D. 389?) followed the Hebrew text, but there is no evidence that the Roman Church ever accepted the view that the fetus is not a human being until it is born.

The Hebrew Bible says nothing about a woman causing an abortion on herself. It might be tempting to conclude from the rabbinic tradition, which considered the fetus a part of the mother, to a liberal attitude toward self-induced abortion. But this would be quite contrary to the entire Jewish tradition of respect for fertility. The only case mentioned in early (pre-Christian or early Christian) Jewish tradition in which it was permitted to sacrifice the fetus was to save the mother. Dismemberment of the fetus (at term) rather than abortion was involved in this case, but the principle was the same. Since the fetus was not considered a human being in the full sense, it was permissible to sacrifice it to save a human being.

There is another text (Gen. 9:6) that Jewish tradition applied to abortion, at least among the Romans. According to this text abortion would be considered a capital crime. No explicit use of this text was made in the Christian tradition but some of the early Fathers condemned abortion as murder without any distinction between the formed and the unformed fetus.

The New Testament says nothing explicit about abortion, but the incompatibility of abortion, as well as infanticide, with the Christian message, came through quite clearly. An explicit condemnation of both is found in the *Didache* and the *Epistle of Barnabas*, first- or early second-century writings. Although these were documents of the early Church, the part that contains these condemnations, known as the *Duae Viae*, seemed to belong originally to the Jewish community and was used to instruct converts to Judaism. If this is correct, these condemnations are as representative of the moral traditions of the Jews of the pre-Christian era as they are of the Christians themselves. Such explicit condemnations were necessary because of the tolerant attitude of the Roman world of the time toward both abortion and infanticide. The apologists of the early Church were able to point to their attitude toward these two practices to distinguish the Christians from the pagans of the times.

Foundations: status of the fetus

Later Christians were not always of the same caliber as the early Christians, but the Church in no way relaxed its attitude toward these practices. When at the beginning of the fourth century the first Church legislation appeared in connection with penitential discipline (reconciliation of sinners), a woman who committed abortion after adultery was not allowed back into the Church for the rest of her life. This legislation, which came from the Council of Elvira, was modified by a council held at Ancyra in A.D. 314 to allow reconciliation after ten years, but even this penance would be considered very severe by modern standards.

Early Church law regarding penance made no distinction between the formed and unformed fetus, but this distinction, already used by some of the Fathers, was introduced into the practice of private penance in the late seventh century. Although this practice differed considerably from the public or canonical penance mentioned above, it was basically the same practice of reconciling sinners to the Church. Formation of the fetus was significant because it was thought that the human soul was infused at that time. Abortion of the formed fetus was consequently considered homicide. But the distinction was not accepted universally on the level of Church law

until after the decree of Gratian in 1140. Official recognition of it came in the decree *Sicut ex* of Innocent III in 1211. The decree dealt with an irregularity, an impediment to the reception or exercise of clerical orders, which was incurred, among other reasons, for homicide. According to the decree the irregularity would not be incurred for abortion unless the fetus was animated. Since the time of animation was identified with formation, the decree implied that only abortion of the formed fetus was considered homicide, at least in reference to irregularities. Confusion arose, however, from a parallel tradition that extended the notion of homicide not only to the abortion of the unformed fetus but to sterilization as well. Nonetheless, the distinction was generally accepted during the late Middle Ages, and only abortion of the formed fetus was considered homicide even in reference to sacramental penances. Forty and ninety days were also accepted as the time of animation for the male and female fetus respectively. Aristotle claimed to base this time difference on evidence derived from aborted fetuses, but it may have been based more on false concepts of embryology.

Although the distinction between the animated and unanimated fetus was used as a canonical dividing line, it was never used during the early centuries of Christianity as a moral dividing line. Abortion was condemned as wrong, whether the fetus was animated or not. In the early fourteenth century, however, the Dominican theologian John of Naples introduced an exception into the condemnation. If the fetus was unanimated, he argued, it would be permissible to abort it to save the life of the mother when threatened by disease. This exception was accepted by another Dominican theologian, Antoninus, Archbishop of Florence (1389–1459), and subsequently by several other theologians. The original argument of John of Naples was that, since the unanimated fetus was not yet a human being, it would be permissible to sacrifice it, if necessary, to save a human being. Later theologians, particularly Thomas Sanchez (1550–1610), used the argument of self-defense against unjust aggression (considering the fetus an unjust aggressor in these circumstances) or the principle of totality (looking upon the fetus as a part of the mother). These arguments would give rise to difficulties at a later date.

In the early Church the penance for serious sins was exclusion from communion with the faithful for a determined period of time. By the end of the first millennium, however, sinners were reconciled to the Church immediately upon confessing their sins and before performing whatever penance was imposed on them. Excommunication from the Church then began to appear as a special penalty for certain sins. Excommunication for the sin of abortion was first imposed in the thirteenth century, but only on a local level. The penalty was extended to the whole Church in 1588 by Sixtus V. What is interesting about the decree (called *Effraenatam* from the introductory word) in which the penalty was legislated was that it imposed the penalty not only on the abortion of the formed fetus but on the abortion of the unformed fetus and sterilization as well. In doing this, it was going beyond the practice of the Church in dealing with irregularities. As already mentioned, from the time of Innocent III (1211), an irregularity was attached only to the abortion of the formed or animated fetus. Sixtus V (1588) was following more in the footsteps of the *Si aliquis,* a canon that originated with Regino of Prüm (d. 905) but was made official in the Decretals of Gregory IX (1234). This canon gave expression to the parallel tradition noted above, which classified all of these acts as homicide. The reason behind the rigid position taken by Sixtus V may have been the revival of pagan practices that accompanied the Renaissance in Europe. The legislation was soon modified, however, and in 1591 the excommunication was limited to the abortion of the animated fetus. The estimate of the time of animation was still the one generally accepted, that is, forty to ninety days. This legislation remained in effect until 1869, when Pius IX extended the excommunication to all abortion. By this time theories of delayed animation had given way to the proponents of early animation.

The question of intentionality

For centuries theologians distinguished between intentional and accidental abortion. They discussed at length the circumstances under which an abortion that was not intentional would be imputed to the person performing the act from which it followed. Initially, the person performing the act was not considered responsible for the abortion if what he was doing was necessary. Later the person was relieved of responsibility as long as what he was doing was licit. Generally speaking, in these cases the agent did not foresee the danger of abortion, but the question eventually arose about the responsibility of a person who would foresee such danger. At the end of the sixteenth century a Spanish Franciscan, Anthony of Cordova, set down the principle that, if the procedure was necessary to save the life of the mother and if its nature aimed principally at this goal, it would be permissible, even if it carried a danger of abortion. In this category he placed such remedies as bloodletting, baths, analgesics, and cathartics. But if the procedure in question was aimed principally at causing the abortion, e.g., striking the mother, giving her a poisonous drug, etc., it would not be permissible. This distinction met with immediate and universal acceptance by theologians of the time and has since that time been generally accepted. It has been formalized in the terms *direct* and *indirect* abortion.

Modern controversies: fetal and maternal factors

The exception made by John of Naples regarding the abortion of the unanimated fetus to save the life of the mother did not receive such universal acceptance as indirect abortion. Many important theologians of the seventeenth and eighteenth century argued against his exception: They refused to consider the fetus either an unjust aggressor or part of the mother. If the unanimated fetus could be considered an unjust aggressor, there might be more reason to regard the animated fetus as an aggressor and argue for abortion even of the animated fetus to save the life of the mother. Or if the fetus could be sacrificed as a part of the mother to save her from some intrinsic threat, it could also be sacrificed to save her from an extrinsic threat as well. But the authors who used these arguments rejected their extension to other cases. There were a few theologians during the seventeenth century who wanted to permit the abortion of the unanimated fetus to save the life or reputation of the mother from an extrinsic threat, e.g., from an angry father or husband, but the more important theologians of the period rejected this opinion. It was also condemned in 1679 by Innocent XI.

Another development that would influence the abortion debate began in the early seventeenth century. As mentioned earlier, theories of delayed animation, particularly that of Aristotle, were generally accepted throughout most of the Christian era. In the early seventeenth century a Belgian physician, Thomas Fienus (De Feynes), wrote a treatise on the formation of the fetus in which he defended the thesis that the human soul was infused into the fetus at least by the third day after conception. His basic argument is that since formation begins shortly after conception, some formative principle must be present. This can only be the human soul, unless one wants to admit, as Aristotle does, a succession of souls. Fienus argues at length that postulating a succession of souls leads to ridiculous conclusions. He concludes therefore that the human soul is infused within three days after conception. Another physician of the time, Paolo Zacchia, also came to the conclusion of immediate animation.

Oddly enough, about the same time a Prague physician, Ioannes Marcus, was arguing in favor of the position taken in Roman law, and perhaps in the Jewish Bible, that the fetus was part of the mother until birth and did not become a human being until that time. But this opinion gained no adherents among the theologians and was condemned by Innocent XI at the same time he condemned the opinion allowing abortion to save the mother's life from extrinsic threat, or even to save her reputation. The revival of this old opinion regarding the status of the fetus may well have been the product of Renaissance interest in the ideas of the Classic Age.

The opinion of Fienus and Zacchia on immediate animation, although not rejected by the Church, did run into considerable opposition from theologians. It was objected to on three specific grounds: It was contrary to the Scriptures, to the universal opinion of theologians, and to the practice of the Church. It might be surprising that an opinion that had so much authority against it could survive. But the fact is that it did take hold and gradually replaced theories of delayed animation. As might be expected, it was put into practice first in baptismal discipline. Since the benefit of any doubt was to be given to the fetus, the Church on the strength of this opinion allowed the conditional baptism of fetuses, no matter how early they were aborted, as long as they showed signs of life, or at least as long as certain death had not set in. Again, as might be expected in the area of penal law, where the benefit of any doubt is given to the culprit, the opinion was put in practice last in penal legislation regarding abortion. It was not until 1869 that excommunication was attached to all abortions without distinction. It is important, however, to distinguish here between Church practice or discipline and Church teaching. The Church has made no positive teaching statement regarding the time of infusion of the

human soul, and this is true of Vatican II as well as of earlier documents. Some have seen in the dogma of the Immaculate Conception an affirmation of immediate infusion of the human soul, but no such affirmation is implied in this teaching. The only opinion the Church has condemned is that of Ioannes Marcus, that the human soul is not infused until birth.

With the common acceptance of early animation the whole question regarding the abortion of the unanimated fetus to save the life of the mother lost its practical significance. Up to the middle of the nineteenth century theologians were almost unanimously opposed to the abortion of the fetus, once it was animated, even to save the mother's life. But in the middle of the nineteenth century a few theologians, particularly Ballerini, suggested that a medical abortion would be permitted to save the life of the mother. They argued that, since such an abortion did not involve an attack on the fetus, it would not be direct killing. It would involve moving the fetus from a place where it could not survive to another place where it would also die. The death of the fetus would result not from the operation itself but from the inability of the fetus to survive in a different medium.

There were also some theologians in the second half of the nineteenth century who argued in favor of craniotomy to save the life of the mother. They offered several arguments to justify their position, but their main defense seemed to be that the fetus in these circumstances was an unjust aggressor. When the Sacred Penitentiary, a Roman tribunal that among other functions handles cases of conscience, was first presented with a craniotomy case, its response was simply that the petitioners should consult the approved authors for their answer. It was probably the ambiguity of this response that gave rise to the controversy that ensued. The controversy was resolved finally by a response from the Holy Office, the Roman Congregation, which is entrusted with the protection of faith and morals. According to the response the opinion that craniotomy was permissible in this case could not be safely taught. In further responses the Holy Office condemned any kind of direct attack on the fetus, and even medical (therapeutic) abortion. In the response dealing with medical abortion it was refusing to accept the distinction Ballerini and others were trying to make between this procedure and those that would clearly involve a direct attack on the fetus, such as craniotomy.

In the first half of the twentieth century there was general acceptance by Catholic theologians of the condemnations of craniotomy and medical (therapeutic) abortion. A few still wanted to make exception for the case where without these procedures both the mother and the child would die—even after the 1930 encyclical *Casti Connubii*, which condemned direct abortion even in these instances—but they found little support among their confreres. As medical science learned how to handle complications of pregnancy and delivery, the issue of craniotomy and medical abortion was reduced largely to the realm of speculation.

The distinction between direct and indirect abortion would still give rise to difficulties in judging individual cases. A controversy arose in the 1930s over the removal of a cancerous but pregnant uterus. At an even earlier date a similar controversy began regarding ectopic pregnancies. Eventually a consensus developed in favor of considering abortion indirect in these instances—and therefore permissible to save the mother's life—because the direct intent would be the removal of a pathological, though pregnant, uterus or tube.

Conclusion

The abortion debate of the 1960s and 1970s, which is the subject of a separate article in this entry, makes clear that theologians have discussed and adopted a greatly expanded number of positions on the two historically significant focal points—namely, as regards both the value of fetal life and the resolution of conflict cases. Still, the Church's official teaching retains considerable continuity. The Second Vatican Council (1965) summarized in two brief sentences the commitment of the Church to the welfare of the fetus, condemning abortion as an unspeakable crime and asking that the fetus be given the greatest of care right from the moment of conception. This statement was in strict continuity not only with the remote past but also with more recent pronouncements by Pius XI, Pius XII, John XXIII, and Paul VI. These Pontiffs confirmed the traditional teaching in statements too numerous to mention.

JOHN R. CONNERY

[*While all the articles in this entry are relevant, see especially the articles* JEWISH PERSPECTIVES, *and* CONTEMPORARY DEBATE IN PHILOSOPHICAL AND RELIGIOUS ETHICS. *Other relevant material may be found under* DOUBLE EFFECT; FETAL–MA-TERNAL RELATIONSHIP; POPULATION ETHICS: RELIGIOUS TRADITIONS, *article on* ROMAN CATHOLIC PERSPECTIVES; RELIGIOUS DIRECTIVES IN MEDICAL ETHICS, *article on* ROMAN CATHOLIC DIRECTIVES; ROMAN CATHOLICISM. *For further discussion of topics mentioned in this article, see the entries:* INFANTS, *article on* INFANTICIDE: A PHILOSOPHICAL PERSPECTIVE; PERSON; POPULATION ETHICS: RELIGIOUS TRADITIONS, *article on* ROMAN CATHOLIC PERSPECTIVES; STERILIZATION, *article on* ETHICAL ASPECTS. *See also:* MEDICAL ETHICS, HISTORY OF, *section on* EUROPE AND THE AMERICAS, *article on* MEDIEVAL EUROPE: FOURTH TO SIXTEENTH CENTURY. *See* APPENDIX, SECTION I, ETHICAL AND RELIGIOUS DIRECTIVES FOR CATHOLIC HEALTH FACILITIES.]

BIBLIOGRAPHY

BEUGNET, A. "Avortement." *Dictionnaire de théologie catholique.* Paris: Librairie Letouzey & Ané, 1903, vol. 1, cols. 2644–2652.

BOUSCAREN, TIMOTHY LINCOLN. *Ethics of Ectopic Operations.* 2d ed., rev. Milwaukee: Bruce Publishing Co., 1944.

CANGIAMILA, FRANCISCO EMANUELLO. *Sacra embryologia* (1745). Venice: 1763, pp. 1–43.

ESCHBACH, ALPHONS. *Disputationes physiologico-theologicae tum medicis chirurgis tum theologis et canonistis utiles.* Rev. ed. Rome: Desclee, Lefebvre & Sacii, 1901.

FELDMAN, DAVID MICHAEL. *Birth Control in Jewish Law: Marital Relations, Contraception, and Abortion as Set Forth in the Classic Texts of Jewish Law.* New York: New York University Press, 1968, pp. 251–297.

FIENUS [FEYENS], THOMAS. *De formatrice foetus liber in quo ostenditur animam rationalem infundi tertia die.* Antwerp: Gulielmum á Tongris, 1620.

GRISEZ, GERMAIN G. *Abortion: The Myths, the Realities and the Arguments.* New York: Corpus Books, 1970, pp. 117–185.

HUSER, ROGER JOHN. *The Crime of Abortion in Canon Law: An Historical Synopsis and Commentary.* Catholic University of America, Canon Law Studies, no. 162. Washington: 1942.

NOONAN, JOHN T., JR. *The Morality of Abortion: Legal and Historical Perspectives.* Cambridge: Harvard University Press, 1970, pp. 1–59.

PALAZZINI, GIUSEPPE. *Ius fetus ad vitam eiusque tutela in fontibus ac doctrina canonica usque ad saeculum XVI.* Urbania: Bramantes, 1943.

VISCOSI, DANIELE. *L'Embryotomia nei suoi rapporti colla morale cattolica.* Naples: Tipografia & Libr. di Andrea & Salv. Festa, 1879.

ZACCHIA, PAOLO. *Questiones medico-legales* (1621). Lyons: 1701, pp. 51–53, 686–707.

IV

PROTESTANT PERSPECTIVES

Early Protestant perspectives

Early Protestant abortion attitudes show considerable continuity with those of the pre-sixteenth-century Church. The major reformers—Martin Luther (1483–1546), Philip Melanchthon (1497–1560), and John Calvin (1509–1564)—were at least as conservative as their Roman Catholic counterparts on the issues of ensoulment and the gravity of abortion. Indeed, some historians (e.g., Williams, pp. 13, 41) believe that they indirectly but significantly contributed to the present papal position on the subject.

The reformers insisted upon the full humanity of the fetus from the time of conception. Their insistence arose, however, less from attention to the abortion issue itself than from their concern about the doctrines of original sin and predestination. Full humanity of the conceptus was believed necessary if the mind and spirit as well as the body of nascent life were to be involved in the consequences of the human Fall.

Luther reclaimed the traducian position of the early Church Fathers in regard to ensoulment. This position held that the soul of the fetus along with its body was inherited from its parents. However, influenced by the embryology of Aristotle and Galen, Luther assumed that the semen alone contained life and that the woman provided only nourishment for that life. Hence, the father (through the power of God) was the source of the fetal soul. Melanchthon's theory of ensoulment was creationist, the belief that God directly creates the soul of each nascent life. Both of these reformers, however, insisted upon the full humanity of the conceptus regardless of its gestational stage.

With Melanchthon, Calvin was creationist concerning ensoulment. With Luther, Calvin was concerned about the depth of human need and the radical nature of God's grace in the face of original sin. His particularly strong doctrine of predestination gave additional force to the contention that the fetus from its earliest stage was already *homo,* fully a person, for this life was believed to be primordially destined to be saved or damned.

The major reformers, then, were rigorously opposed to abortion at any stage of pregnancy. Moreover, they had significantly enhanced the fetal status for reasons more basically doctrinal than for ethical reasons against abortion. Regarding fetal status, they were more conservative than the sixteenth-century Roman Catholic Church, which still maintained the Septuagint's distinction between the "unformed" and the "formed" fetus, and with it a consequent distinction in the gravity of abortion, depending upon

its timing. On the other hand, the Reformation's strong affirmations of justification by grace and forgiveness of sin were to provide many later Protestants with theological perspectives and religious resources for dealing with the potential abortion as a situation of ambiguity, compromise, and value conflict.

In seventeenth-century England, both Anglicans and Puritans continued the opposition to abortion, but with the distinction between the unformed and the formed fetus. At the same time, however, the English Puritans initiated changes in the traditional understanding of marriage. Companionship was now seen as marriage's primary end, to which the ends of procreation and the restraint of lust were believed subordinate. This companionate view gradually became the dominant Protestant interpretation, and with it came the groundwork for justifiable abortions in cases of mortal conflict between mother and fetus. Indeed, by the late eighteenth century, English physicians were commonly urging and performing abortions to save threatened mothers.

Eighteenth and nineteenth centuries

American Protestantism manifested at least three major developments relevant to the abortion issue during the eighteenth and nineteenth centuries. One was a loss of interest in the human status of the fetus. Puritan predestinationists pressed Calvin's position on salvation but with different results. Convinced that the individual's eternal destiny was fixed well before conception and gestation, the Puritans saw little to be gained from speculation about fetal ontology. Protestants generally lost touch with the earlier traditions on abortion and were inclined to appeal directly to Scripture, where the early Jewish view and most subsequent texts supported full humanity only at birth. The pietist and revivalist groups of this period were disinclined to reflect about fetal humanity, for they were principally concerned in adult conversion. While they continued the typical Protestant opposition to abortion, their emphasis was often more restricted and practical: Abortion was wrong because it was used, frequently at least, as a coverup for sexual sins.

A strong profertility norm emerged in large segments of nineteenth-century American Protestantism, further buttressing antiabortion sentiments. Women must bear children if they were to be fulfilled as women. Furthermore, as God's New Israel, America had a crucial destiny in the world's salvation, and population growth was desirable to that end. Abortion thus was not simply an individual sin but also a social evil which denied society its needed citizens, economic producers, and defenders.

A significant countervailing influence on the abortion issue also emerged in nineteenth-century American Protestantism, however: the rise of social idealism and the Social Gospel movement. Those trends were less concerned about abortion than about the more visibly disadvantaged. But their general support for the oppressed and their particular concern for women's dignity, expressed in the suffrage movement, laid important foundations for later theories of both justifiable abortion and abortion-on-request.

Twentieth-century influences

During the first half of the twentieth century, while official American Protestant opposition to abortion largely continued, the attitudes of numerous Protestant individuals were gradually being altered by several factors (Potter, pp. 88–89; Yates, pp. 63–78). Under the impact of secularization, certainties that once had undergirded theological opposition to abortion became less certain. If to an earlier Protestant the presence of each fetus in the womb was an expression of God's mysterious providence, to a later Protestant the fetal presence was explained by natural processes, including human mistakes as well as human planning.

Further, the mid-century abortion reform movement drew upon themes of great importance to the Protestant tradition itself, particularly human self-determination and the obligation to exercise rational control over nature. While the latter-day view of self-determination may have been a highly individualistic and secularized version of the Reformation's image of Christian liberty, it was nevertheless inexplicable apart from that historical connection.

A third factor was the waning of the vision of a Protestant America. The failure of the Protestant-inspired Prohibition law was a reminder that religious pluralism had replaced Protestant hegemony. America was no longer a society in which moral convictions that arose from particular Protestant theologies could be sanctioned by legislation. Thus, the distinction between a sin and a crime gained currency: What a particular religious group deemed sinful on its own doctrinal grounds ought not to be socially legislated as criminal without a much broader moral consensus on the issue. This distinction was further to erode Protestant support for anti-abortion legislation.

Patterns in contemporary Protestant thought

In their theological reasoning, Protestants tend to take the church's tradition less seriously than they take the Bible. However, those Protestants who look to Scripture for specific moral instruction rather than for more general ethical principles discover an absence of biblical texts specifically forbidding or permitting induced abortions. Indeed, the Old Testament does not typically view the fetus as fully human life. Exodus 21:22–25, for example, simply demands monetary compensation from the guilty party who causes a woman's miscarriage. Only if the woman herself dies does the charge become homicide and the offender sentenced to death. Nevertheless, there are significant themes in both Old and New Testaments upon which Protestants typically draw for guidance in the abortion question. Life is a gift from God, and human reproduction is a process of sharing in God's creative powers (Psalm 139:13). Human beings are created not simply for comfort and pleasure but more basically for fulfillment, which often involves sacrifice for others (John 15:13). Life and death belong to God's providence, and there is no human right to extinguish life apart from persuasive evidence that such action expresses God's will in a tragic situation (Phil. 1:21–24). However general these biblical principles are, many Protestants insist that even they must be understood within the framework provided by the central ethical norm of Scripture: the love commandment, which includes the dimensions of justice and mercy.

The major historical positions and influences earlier mentioned are present in the contemporary configurations of Protestant opinion on abortion. The perspectives range along a continuum from antiabortion to abortion-on-request, with perhaps the large number of ethicists and Protestant groups affirming the justifiable-but-tragic abortion in certain situations of value conflict.

The antiabortion position is voiced by Dietrich Bonhoeffer, Paul Ramsey, Helmut Thielicke, and, with qualification, Karl Barth. Regarding the ensoulment issue, these ethicists maintain that it is not necessary to describe the fetus as a person. Rather, it is crucial that the fetus be recognized as a human individual; it is en route to becoming personal, but at all times it possesses the full sanctity of human life. Thus, two arguments are interwoven. First, biological data, especially at the stage of segmentation, establish human individuality. Second, Christian faith insists that the dignity of human life is not founded upon the individual's utility but rather is an alien dignity conferred by God and not admitting relative degrees of worth. While additional antiabortion arguments are typically added to the two above, the central issue is held to be the inviolable right to life of the fetus as a human individual, and not the weighing of competing values. Antiabortion Protestants, however, usually incorporate some version of the traditional Roman Catholic "principle of double effect" to argue that in certain extreme situations (threat to the mother's life) abortion is permitted because it is not the direct and willful taking of innocent life but rather the indirect result of saving life.

Abortion-on-request is a more recent and less fully developed position in the literature of Protestant ethics, although it has its articulate defenders. Proponents of this position argue that only wanted babies should be born. They typically maintain that permissive legal systems better protect women's lives and health, minimize social discrimination, and protect the autonomy of the medical profession. However, like the antiabortion position, this stance finally elevates one human right to supremacy. In this instance it is the woman's right to control over her own body and its reproductive processes, against those double standards that would permit others (usually males) to make choices on her behalf. "[M]aybe an unexpressed and powerful objection is that responsible abortion, especially upon request, may give women the final control over reproduction" (Fletcher, p. 27). The earlier Protestant emphases upon self-determination, rational control of nature, equality, social justice, and the dignity of women enter strongly into this position. The real question, proponents argue, is not so much how we can justify abortion, but rather how we can justify compulsory pregnancy.

The third general approach, sometimes called the justifiable abortion, lies somewhere between the first two, affirming arguments of each but differing from both. Rights of both fetus and woman are to be highly valued, but in theory and in practice neither ought to be absolutized. The elevation of one single right, it is argued, removes the inherent moral ambiguity of abortion decisions and oversimplifies other relevant moral factors. Instead of absolute rights, it is better to speak of competing rights and values. Together with the woman's right to self-determination and the value of human fetal life, a complex range of relational, social, medical, economic, and psychological values must be weighed, inasmuch as God cares for all of these dimensions. Thus, each problem pregnancy has its own uniqueness, its own moral tragedy, and its possible alternatives. Christians must rely upon God's grace and forgiveness as they make these ambiguous decisions (Gustafson).

A number of issues related to public policy on abortion have concerned Protestant ethicists of all persuasions. Does a legally permissive policy tend to cheapen or enhance human dignity and the value of human life generally, and how can the evidence be assessed? Is abortion-on-request a disguised, genocidal attack on racial minorities, or does it enhance racial equality? What should be the relation of abortion policies to the population problem? What abortion policies best protect the freedoms of religion and conscience that belong both to those with problem pregnancies and to medical personnel?

In the decades of the 1950s and 1960s several American Protestant denominations and ecumenical groups publicly affirmed positions on the abortion issue. Since the 1973 U.S. Supreme Court rulings (*Roe* v. *Wade, Doe* v. *Bolton*) additional Protestant groups have issued policy statements. Most of these pronouncements affirm the recognition of competing values and the possibility of the justifiable abortion as the lesser of the evils in many situations. Some denominations, however, have remained officially silent, encouraging their members to exercise prayerful freedom of conscience in such decisions.

JAMES B. NELSON

[*While all the articles in this entry are relevant, see especially the articles* ROMAN CATHOLIC PERSPECTIVES, CONTEMPORARY DEBATE IN PHILOSOPHICAL AND RELIGIOUS ETHICS, *and* LEGAL ASPECTS. *For further discussion of topics mentioned in this article, see the entries:* DOUBLE EFFECT; PERSON; POPULATION ETHICS: ELEMENTS OF THE FIELD, *article on* HISTORY OF POPULATION THEORIES; POPULATION ETHICS: RELIGIOUS TRADITIONS, *article on* PROTESTANT PERSPECTIVES; PROTESTANTISM; *and* RELIGIOUS DIRECTIVES IN MEDICAL ETHICS, *article on* PROTESTANT STATEMENTS. *See also:* CIVIL DISOBEDIENCE IN HEALTH SERVICES; FETAL–MATERNAL RELATIONSHIP; LIFE; RIGHTS, *article on* RIGHTS IN BIOETHICS.]

BIBLIOGRAPHY

CALVIN, JOHN. *Institutes of the Christian Religion.* 2 vols. Translated by Henry Beveridge. Grand Rapids, Mich.: Wm. B. Eerdmans Publishing Co., 1957, vol. 1.

Doe v. Bolton. 410 U.S. 179. 35 L. Ed. 2d. 201. 93 S. Ct. 739 (1973).

FLETCHER, JOSEPH F. "A Protestant Minister's View." *Abortion in a Changing World.* 2 vols. Edited by Robert E. Hall. The Proceedings of an International Conference Convened in Hot Springs, Virginia, November 17–20, 1968, by the Association for the Study of Abortion. New York: Columbia University Press, 1970, vol. 1, pp. 25–29.

GUSTAFSON, JAMES M. "A Protestant Ethical Approach." *The Morality of Abortion: Legal and Historical Perspectives.* Edited by John Thomas Noonan. Cambridge: Harvard University Press, 1970, pp. 101–122.

LUTHER, MARTIN. *Luther's Works.* Edited by Jaroslav Pelikan. American ed. St. Louis: Concordia Publishing House, 1955–.

POTTER, RALPH B., JR. "The Abortion Debate." *Updating Life and Death: Essays in Ethics and Medicine.* Edited by Donald R. Cutler. Boston: Beacon Press, 1968, pp. 85–134.

Roe v. Wade. 410 U.S. 113. 35 L. Ed. 2d. 147. 93 S. Ct. 705 (1973).

SPITZER, WALTER O., and SAYLOR, CARLYLE L., eds. *Birth Control and the Christian: A Protestant Symposium on the Control of Human Reproduction.* Wheaton, Ill.: Tyndale House Publishers; London: Coverdale House Publishers, 1969.

WILLIAMS, GEORGE HUNTSTON. "Religious Residues and Presuppositions in the American Debate on Abortion." *Theological Studies* 31 (1970): 10–75.

YATES, WILSON. *Family Planning on a Crowded Planet.* Minneapolis: Augsburg Publishing House, 1971.

V
CONTEMPORARY DEBATE IN PHILOSOPHICAL AND RELIGIOUS ETHICS

Since approximately 1950, there has been an ongoing debate about abortion as the availability and public acceptance of abortion have increased considerably in most societies. Many religions consider abortion to be a significant moral issue, and religious ethicists have long been interested in the question. Philosophical ethicists generally have not given much consideration to abortion until the contemporary period. There is no agreement about the morality of abortion among either philosophical or religious ethicists, but religious ethicists as well as philosophical ethicists often appeal to rational arguments. This article will summarize and analyze the contemporary debate about abortion in philosophical and religious ethics.

Various reasons or indications have been proposed for justifying abortion: to protect the life of the mother, to safeguard the physical and mental health of the mother, to act as a remedy against injustices due to rape or incest, to prevent the birth of defective children, to vindicate the right of the woman to determine her own reproductive capacities and to have control over her body, to protect the reputation of the woman, and to alleviate economic, sociological, or demographic problems. These reasons all have some validity, but they must be seen in a larger context including the zygote-embryo-fetus and its value or rights.

Most philosophers and theologians recognize that the heart of the abortion problem is the difficult question of the beginning of human life, since human beings are treated differently from all other beings. A terminological problem exists in even framing the question, for some authors make a distinction between human life and personal life, between human being and human person, between biological existence and fully human existence. To avoid confusion the term "truly human being" or "truly human life" will be used and understood as that human life deserving the value, rights, and protection due the human person as such.

When does truly human life begin?

Opinions about the beginning of truly human life may be conveniently categorized in two ways: (1) in terms of the conclusions about the beginning of truly human life, which range from the moment of conception to various stages in fetal development, viability, birth, and for some time after birth; or (2) in terms of the criteria employed for determining the beginning of truly human life. The following types of criteria best categorize and summarize the abundant literature on the subject: (1) individual-biological, (2) relational, (3) multiple, and (4) the conferral of rights by society. There is no absolute correlation between the criterion employed and the conclusion about the beginning of truly human life; but the following tendencies exist: the individual-biological criterion tends to place the beginning of human life at conception or at early stages of development; the relational and conferral of rights criteria usually accept a rather late point in development for the beginning of truly human life; the multiple approach often results in an intermediary position.

One preliminary point is most important. Biological, genetic, or scientific data alone will not be able to solve the problem of when truly human life begins. The ultimate judgment remains truly a philosophical or human judgment, which gives meaning and interpretation to the biological and other data involved. Such a conclusion is based on the recognition that human existence involves more than just the biological and genetic and cannot be simply identified with just one aspect. However, it must also be pointed out that at times the human and the physical or biological are inseparable. Our personal existence as human beings is intimately connected with our physical-biological existence. Human beings do not exist without or apart from their bodies. Human personal death is described in accord with individual-biological categories—the cessation of brain activity accompanied by other signs, according to increasingly accepted criteria of human death.

Individual-biological criterion. The individual-biological approach generally sees the criterion of truly human existence in terms of some physical, biological, or genetic aspects of the individual. Exponents of the theory placing human life at an early stage based on the individual-biological criterion usually begin with the assumption that all humans accept the born child as a truly human being. The first serious question is raised about birth as the beginning of human life. But the fetus one day before birth and the child one day after birth are not that significantly or qualitatively different in any respect. Even outside the womb the newborn child is not independent but remains greatly dependent on the mother and others. Birth in fact does not really tell much about the individual as such but only where the individual is—either outside the womb or still inside the womb. Viability has often been proposed as the beginning of truly human life, but from the perspective of the individual-biological criterion viability again indicates more about where the fetus can live than what it is. The fetus immediately before viability is not that qualitatively different from the viable fetus. In addition viability is a very inexact criterion because it is intimately connected with rapidly changing medical and scientific advances. In the future it might very well be possible for the fetus to live in an artificial womb or even with an artificial placenta from a very early stage in fetal development.

There are two other stages in the development of the fetus that have been pointed out as marking the beginning of human life. Joseph Donceel has based a delayed hominization or delayed animation theory on the Thomistic concept of hylomorphism (viz., there is a complementarity between the material and formal aspects of being). The form, which in this case is the soul, is received only into matter capable of receiving it. Thomas Aquinas and many other medieval theologians and philosophers accepted a theory of delayed animation. According to Donceel, the insistence on immediate animation in Catholic circles in the last few centuries was based on the erroneous biological theory of preformation and was influenced by a Cartesian dualism. The unity of the human person demands that the bodily or material element be more highly organized in order to receive the truly human form or soul. The fertilized ovum, the morula, the blastula, and the early embryo cannot be animated by an intellectual soul. Donceel concludes that the least that must be present before admitting a human soul is the availability of these organs: senses, the nervous system, the brain, and especially the cortex. Since these organs are not ready during early pregnancy, there is no human person present until several weeks have elapsed. Others might want to insist on the incipient presence of the major organs as the determining point for the existence of truly human life.

Some (e.g., Grisez, p. 283) reply that Thomas Aquinas's own position was determined more by poor biological knowledge according to which the seed was the primary active element in human generation, the ovum was not known, and the seed had to die before new life could come into existence in the womb of the mother. Whether Aquinas's position is based on faulty biological knowledge which is corrected in the light of modern biology and genetics or is based on his philosophical theory will continue to be debated. However, it seems difficult to maintain that such early development of these organs constitutes the qualitative difference between truly human life and no truly human life. Self-awareness and reason are not actually present at this time, and much more growth and development are necessary. The appearance of these organs appears to mark just another stage in the ongoing development—a stage directed by an inner teleology already present in the embryo or fetus.

A somewhat similar theory (Ruff, and proposed but not accepted in practice by Häring, pp. 81–85) places the beginning of human life at the time of the formation of the cortex of the brain. Electrical brain activity is detectable at the eighth week. Personal life is characterized by consciousness and self-reflection which have their indispensable substratum in the cerebral cortex. Many accept brain death—a flat EEG—together with other signs of no responses as a criterion of death. Is it not logical to insist on the same criterion for determining when human life begins?

Within the individual-biological criterion the early formation of the cortex seems to be just another step in the ongoing development and does not constitute a qualitatively different threshold distinguishing truly human life from nonlife. There is validity in the plea for consistency in dealing with the beginning and end of life, but consistency does not necessarily call for the same material test at the beginning as at the end of life. The test really measures whether there is any immediate potentiality for spontaneous life functioning. At the beginning of life this can be present before electrical brain activity can be detected and measured.

Many proponents of the individual-biological criterion emphasize a continual, progressive development of the fetus without any obviously qualitatively different thresholds, concluding that the only logical place to mark the beginning of truly human life is conception. John T. Noonan (pp. 51–59) has accepted as the conclusion of his analysis of the Catholic tradition that whatever is conceived of human beings is human and buttresses his conclusion with three different reasons: the presence of characteristics in the embryo and adult which are similar, an argument based on probabilities which indicates the great difference between the sperm or ovum and the fertilized ovum or zygote, and a critique of alternative proposals. Modern genetics, according to Noonan, supports this position by showing that the zygote is a dynamic blueprint which if it receives proper nourishment and suitable environment grows and develops.

Germain Grisez (pp. 273–287) develops a two-stage argument for his opinion that truly human beings come into existence at conception. The first stage is factual. The fertilized ovum is a single thing derived from two sources. The facts of genetics indicate that a new being comes into existence with conception, for the fertilized ovum is continuous with that which develops from it, while the sperm and ovum which constitute the new being are themselves two different realities continuous with the duality of the two parents. This factual question leads to the moral question: Is this new individual to be regarded as a person? Anyone who recognizes the importance of the body and does not adopt a dualistic understanding of the person must acknowledge that development is a continual process from the time of fertilization so that the conceptus must be considered a truly human being.

Lately, some authors (for example, Chiavacci, Curran, and Ramsey) have proposed on the basis of the individual-biological criterion that an individual is not present until a certain development has occurred which is usually placed somewhere between the second and third week after conception and does not occur before nidation or implantation (*Aborto*, pp. 254–274; Curran, pp. 179–193; Noonan, pp. 60–100). Biological information heavily influences this judgment, but the ultimate reason rests on the recognition that individuality, which is a most fundamental characteristic of the truly human being, is not achieved before this time. Twinning and recombination can occur before this time. Before this time there is no organizer that directs the differentiation of the pluripotential cells so that without this organizer hominization cannot occur. Also this theory contends that the large number (perhaps as many as fifty percent) of fertilized ova that are spontaneously aborted without the mother's being aware of having conceived are not truly human beings. Rebuttal arguments downplay the fact of twinning and recombination, which are comparatively rare and can be explained in other ways, such as the direct infusion of a new soul in the case of twinning.

The reasons proposed thus far have been of a rational nature and not based on any particular religious or theological perspective. Paul Ramsey invokes the religious understanding that the value and sanctity of human life are not something intrinsic in the human being but result from the gift of God (1968, pp. 71–78). The sanctity of life is an alien dignity conferred by God so that even a small zygote can have that dignity and value. Interestingly, Roman Catholic ethics, which has often insisted on an early beginning of human life, usually appeals not to the alien dignity of human life but to its intrinsic dignity. God does bestow the gift of life, but the presence of human life can and should be proved by rational arguments.

The following arguments have been raised against the individual-biological criterion, especially the conclusion—often derived from this criterion—that truly human life has an early beginning. It goes against the common experience, which does not consider the embryo or early fetus to be a human being; it absolutizes the biological and genetic, not giving enough importance to broader understandings of the human; it fails to recognize that in addition to genetic factors environmental aspects are also necessary for human growth; it overemphasizes potentiality and does not give enough importance to development. Counterarguments can be proposed. Common human experience must always be subject to reflection, scrutiny, and critique. Granted that the human is more than just biological, at times the human and the biological are inseparable. The only human beings we know in this world are human beings in their physical and biological nature. Although environmental factors are important for human development, these factors also continue to be of great importance after birth. Potentiality based on something intrinsic in the being itself is a better criterion than a developmental approach that could open the door to differing value attributed to different human lives depending on their developed potential.

Relational criterion. A relational criterion for the beginning of human life generally sees truly human life coming into existence late in the development of the fetus—usually at the time of viability or even birth. The starting point of the relational school emphasizes the common experience, which rejects the notion that the embryo or early fetus is a truly human being and insists that the concept "truly human being" cannot be applicable by virtue simply of the genetic or biological features of a living thing. In fact it is futile to look for a biological moment when truly human life begins even if it were possible to determine such a moment. After brain waves or other acceptable criteria of human death are no longer present, lower biological life can continue to exist in the body even if truly human life is ended. These approaches frequently distinguish between human life and human person, between biological life and personal life, between human life and humanized life.

According to some French Catholic moral theologians, e.g., Pohier, Ribes, Roqueplo (*Avortement et respect de la vie humaine*), fully personal and humanized life must be seen in terms of relationships. An older objectivist epistemology sees the fruit of conception as a human being in itself, but contemporary epistemology insists on a more relational understanding, especially the relationship of the conceptus to the parents. There are economic, psychological, cultural, and even faith aspects of human life in addition to the biological. The mere fact of biological procreation does not constitute a truly human personal life, especially if the parents were not intending such a result and were trying to prevent it. The fetus must be accepted by the parents and also to some extent by the society into which it will be born.

One of the arguments frequently raised against the relational criterion is that the employment of such a criterion logically leads to infanticide and the killing of adult human beings who are no longer capable of entering into such human relationships. Some authors, such as Michael Tooley and Joseph Fletcher, are willing to admit infanticide and/or the killing of some biological adults who do not fulfill the criterion of the human, but most defenders of abortion based on a relational criterion of the beginning of human life do not want to admit such killing and make a distinct effort to show that acceptance of abortion does not logically entail acceptance of these other forms of killing.

It seems that truly human relationships cannot exist until after birth because full human relationships require a reciprocity of giving and taking in a human way that cannot be had until both partners have the requisite self-consciousness to enter into such a relationship. In a true sense fully personal life is not present at birth or even immediately thereafter. The infant does not possess the characteristics of rationality or self-consciousness that are generally proposed as definitive of the human person. Lederberg maintains that the infant becomes a human person only after the first year or so of life.

H. T. Engelhardt has addressed this particular question and proposed a second concept of person in addition to the strict concept used to identify actually self-conscious moral agents—a social category of person based on a social role or function which claims the intrinsic value of actual persons. The newborn infant, although not yet a full person, has such a potential personhood that it can play the role or function of a person within family and society. The mother–child relationship is a social relationship which depends upon the mother's agency and involves the child's being treated as if it were a person. The mother–child relationship is a social and willed structure of interaction and a cultural enterprise as contrasted with the mother–fetus relationship, which is a biological and imposed structure and a physiological enterprise. The biological reality of viability now becomes understood in broader social terms as indicating when the social role of a person can begin. This theory is thus based on two concepts of human life—biological and personal—and on a strict and social concept of person but insists that the social concept of person has exactly the same consequences as the strict concept of person.

Does the relational criterion avoid the danger of exposing infants and other adult human beings to being judged less than fully human persons and therefore killed or sacrificed for others? As a matter of fact it can be pointed out that many people, countries, and cultures which accept abortion do not endorse any form of infanticide or killing of the weak, the retarded and the defenseless. In theory most authors proposing a relational criterion oppose any extension to those who are already born, but there remains a grave doubt about the logic involved in such a criterion. Truly human relationships are not present immediately after birth, and often adult human beings seem to fall below the line of full human relationships. If one admits a distinction between a strict and a social concept of a person, it becomes very easy to say that a strict concept of a person results in more rights or more values than a social concept of a person, thus denying the basic realization that all persons have equal rights and equal values in terms of the fundamental question of life itself.

A multiple criterion. A third type of criterion tries to avoid some of the problems associated with both the individual-biological and the relational by calling for a criterion based on multiple indications. Daniel Callahan, in a well-documented monograph on abortion, argues for a consensus approach to the question which will do justice to all the values involved, and proposes a criterion for the beginning of human life based on biological, psychological, and cultural factors. Callahan (pp. 349–404, 493–501) maintains that even a zygote is individual human life, but full value should not be assigned at once to the life thus begun. Interestingly, he never explicitly develops or describes in great detail when truly human life which is to be valued as such does occur, but he seems to indicate the existence of brain activity as the distinguishing mark. Callahan's criterion enables him to do three things: to allow for the possibility of decisions in which the woman would want an abortion; to avoid the unilateral approach of the biological; and to avoid some of the dangers of the relational criterion, which if used alone could endanger the rights of the newborn and other marginal people in society.

There are many aspects of Callahan's mediating approach which are appealing, but in the last analysis doubts remain, perhaps increased somewhat by his apparent reluctance to discuss in greater detail precisely when human life is to be fully valued as such. The danger in an approach calling for the threefold criterion of biological, psychological, and cultural considerations is that the psychological and cultural aspects are really not all that present at the time of birth and might also cease to exist for some adults after birth. Callahan himself implies a comparatively early point at which full value is achieved (brain activity), and one could really question if enough cultural and psychological development have truly taken place to mark this as the beginning of fully valued human life. Any developmental theory also is going to open the door to the recognition that such a criterion can be employed even after birth to distinguish the values involved in different human lives depending upon their development in accord with psychological and cultural aspects.

Conferred rights criterion. Metaphysical considerations, the recognition that human beings must ultimately make the decision about when human life begins, and the difficulties involved with other criteria are some of the reasons proposed for a fourth type of criterion for the beginning of human life—the social conferral of rights. In the earlier years of the abortion debate after 1950, Glanville Williams and Garrett Hardin advocated such approaches. Williams contends that life is a continuum and the fundamental problem is to discover when human life begins. The basic criterion becomes what answer will have the best social consequences. Williams leans to viability as the dividing line. Hardin also acknowledges that whether or not the fetus is human is a matter of definition and not of fact.

More nuanced philosophical understandings of the same type of criterion have been advanced. R. B. Brandt proposes a contractual understanding of morality based on the criterion that what is right is fixed by what would be permitted in a moral code which rational, impartial persons, with no personal gain, living now or in the future, would prefer. The important condition emphasizes that these individuals would be totally impartial and would in no way know how they themselves as individuals might profit or suffer from their decision. It is prima facie wrong to kill a being that wants to live, Brandt contends, but the fetus is not sentient and cannot choose. Even if these people were altruistic, the fetus would not be an object of their sympathy. Nor can a human person ever truly put itself in the place of a fetus, for the precise reason that the human person is not a fetus. On this basis, Brandt concludes that abortion is not prima facie wrong.

R. M. Green proposed a similar approach of a rational theory of rights as a way of bypassing the thorny and seemingly insoluble problem of when human life begins. Understanding morality as a noncoercive means of settling disputes, Green identifies a class of agents who must have fundamentally equal rights—all those agents with whom we can possibly come into dispute, who display an elementary rational ability and who are capable of understanding and respecting moral rules. Such a broad understanding includes almost all human beings; but there are some who do not have these capacities so that rights in these cases are conferred at the behest of rational agents who are concerned about behavior with respect to third parties that have ultimate effects on their own lives. A threefold criterion is proposed for conferring rights on others: on the basis of the effect on our capacity for sympathy, on the effect on the possible interests of particular agents, and finally on the effect on the character or moral worth of rational agents generally. This threefold criterion would confer rights on the newborn but not on the eight-week-old fetus, although they would place some value on that life. Sissela Bok proposed somewhat similar standards as the reasons for protecting human life, most of which are absent in the case of prenatal life but some of which are clearly present with respect to newborn life, although not as fully as in the case of adult human beings.

Various reasons have been proposed against the criterion of conferred rights. Biological data are given little or no importance, even though such data can never be used by themselves to determine when truly human life begins. It seems one cannot avoid the question of when human life begins, for our sympathy and our concern depend primarily on what we believe the fetus to be. Proponents of this criterion are very conscious of the charge of arbitrariness which might allow many people to be excluded from human rights. One way to avoid the charge is to include as many as possible within the class of moral agents who confer the rights, thus including all races, colors, and creeds. Another approach appeals to the neutral observer who behind the "veil of ignorance" does not know what one's own position is. However, if agents put themselves in the place of the fetus, which all of them were at one time, it seems that they would be quite prone to protect the life of the fetus. One cannot exclude the rational agent from taking that position unless one first decides that the fetus is not a person. There always remains the philosophical problem that human rights must exist prior to any conferral of rights by the state or by individuals representing society.

Value and rights of the fetus

The question of the value and rights of the fetus is intimately connected with the question of when human life begins. For those who see the fetus as a truly human being, the fetus has all the rights and values of every other human being.

An opposite approach is taken by those who view the embryo or fetus as only tissue in the mother and give the mother the right to control her body as her personal property. If women are to be truly free and liberated, they must ultimately have full freedom to control their own reproductive capacities. The woman, according to Wahlberg, cannot truly experience the fetus as anything but a part of her own flesh. There can be no doubt that in practice emphasis on the right of the woman to control her own body has greatly contributed to a wider acceptance of abortion, but in the ethical literature the women's rights reasons have not been developed in great depth. This position seems to ignore the rights of the fetus. Although biological data alone cannot determine the existence of a truly human being, such data prove that the fetus is a biological individual and not merely maternal tissue.

The developmental school, as exemplified in Callahan (pp. 493–501) and others, views the fetus from conception as individual human life, but development counts in assigning value to the fetus. On the basis of this, there should be a strong bias against abortion; but the body life of the conceptus is not of the same value as the person life of the pregnant woman, so that many considerations would justify abortion. Relational approaches could give some value to the fetus as biological life, but fully human life becomes present only when the requisite relationship is present. Since the relational criterion does not generally give that much importance to biological life, the fetus before the time of becoming fully human would seem not to be of great overriding value. The conferred rights approach could also assign different meaning and value to the fetus; but generally speaking, since such an approach gives little significance to the biological aspects, the fetus does not have that much value in such a generic approach.

R. M. Hare in dealing with the issue of abortion wants to avoid both rights talk and the question of when human life begins. The proper question is whether there is anything about the fetus that says we should not kill it. The primary moral question results from the fact that the fetus has the potentiality of becoming a person in the full, ordinary sense of that word. The potentiality principle in the case of the fetus asserts a presumption against the permissibility of abortion, which is fairly easily rebutted if there are good indications, such as the interests of the mother. The above serve as illustrations of the various ways in which the value or rights of the fetus have been understood in the contemporary debate about abortion.

Solution of conflict situations. Various reasons have been proposed to justify abortion: medical, psychological, sociological, economic, humanitarian, fetal, feminist, and demographic. The moral decision involves a proper balancing of the reasons or indications proposed in relationship to the rights, value, or importance of the fetus. The position which regards the fetus as just tissue in the mother would then accept practically any reason the woman proposed based on her right to the control of her body and reproductive capacities. The vast majority of commentators would see abortion as somewhat different from artificial contraception, but reasons of family planning or population control would be a sufficient reason to justify abortion for some. The balancing and weighing of the various reasons ultimately depend upon the value which one attributes to the fetus. The greater the value given to the fetus, the greater the reason needed to justify abortion. Generally speaking, the solution to such conflicts is based on the proportion existing between the value given to the fetus and the indications or reasons proposed for the abortion.

The question most discussed in the literature is the solution to conflict situations if the fetus is looked upon as a truly human being with all the rights of human beings. This is the problem that has been traditionally discussed within Christian ethics and especially within Roman Catholic ethics down to the present. Recently some philosophers have given attention to the same question, often with the intention of showing that the abortion question is not morally closed once one accepts or asserts, without necessarily conceding, that the fetus has the rights of a human being.

Roman Catholic theology in its historical tradition has acknowledged that conflict situations arise in which human lives can be taken; e.g., war, killing in self-defense, capital punishment. In the question of abortion the hierarchical magisterium in the Roman Catholic Church taught that the fetus cannot be considered an unjust aggressor, since the fetus in the womb is just doing what is necessary to preserve its own life—hence the mother cannot kill the fetus in self-defense. Conflict situations involving abortion were dealt with in terms of the principle of the double effect which justified action producing evil effects as well as good effects if the following four conditions were fulfilled: (1) The action itself is good or indifferent; (2) the good effect and not the evil effect is the one sincerely intended by the agent; (3) the good effect is not produced by means of the evil effect (If the evil effect is not at least equally immediate causally with the good effect, then it becomes a means to the good effect and intended as such.); and (4) there is a proportionate reason for permitting the foreseen evil effect to occur.

The decisive criterion is the third—the causality of the act cannot be such that the good effect comes about by means of the evil effect. When applied to the question of abortion, this means that abortion cannot be the means by which the good effect is accomplished—for example, one cannot abort to save the life of the mother which might be endangered because her heart cannot take the pregnancy. The two most famous illustrations of indirect abortion are the removal of the cancerous uterus when the woman is pregnant and the removal of a fallopian tube or part of it that is threatened with rupture from an ectopic pregnancy in the tube.

The accepted Catholic teaching allows less conflict situations for the fetus in the womb than for human life outside the womb because outside the womb the possibility of killing in defense against an unjust aggressor is recognized. One can argue that the older teaching on unjust aggression was not referring to the subjective will of the aggressor nor even to an objectively unjust act, but to the reality of a conflict situation. In this perspective it is easier to see that the right of defense even to the killing of the fetus might be extended to the mother, for truly conflict situations can arise even though the fetus is just attempting to provide what is necessary for its own growth and continued existence.

The theory of double effect has come in for closer scrutiny in the last few years (McCormick; Schüller). Some Catholic scholars continue to uphold it, but often contemporary Catholic authors reject the theory, especially its third condition based on the causal structure of the act itself. Historical scholarship, with some dissenting voices, indicates that the third condition for the double effect was not found in Thomas Aquinas. There is also a strong tendency among Catholic theologians to reject the identification of the moral aspect of the act with the causal and physical structure of the act. In the abortion case where there is some conflict existing between the fetus and the mother, a good number of contemporary Catholic moralists would agree with the conclusion that the physical causality of the act has no moral significance. The human values involved must be carefully considered and weighed. In my judgment abortion can be justified for preserving the life of the mother and for other important values commensurate with life even though the action aims at abortion as a means to an end. The difficult problem concerns what values if any are commensurate with life. In the Catholic tradition, killing an aggressor was justified not only in defense of one's life but even in defense of earthly goods of great value. Obviously there is the danger here of opening the door for reasons that are truly not of grave seriousness, but within the Catholic tradition other values have been proposed as commensurate in some situations with the value of human life.

Protestant authors generally do not accept the principle of double effect and usually employ some type of proportionate reasoning to solve conflict situations involving abortion. Paul Ramsey, an American Protestant ethicist, originally praised the double effect theory, but later he abandoned the all-important third condition of the double effect (1968, p. 78; 1973, pp. 210–226). Some philosophers have lately discussed the principle of double effect in general and have often rejected the third condition, while calling for distinctions between positive and negative obligations, or between foreseen and unforeseen consequences. But even in philosophical circles there are some defenders of the principle of double effect (e.g., Finnis).

Judith Jarvis Thompson sparked an interesting exchange by proposing that, granted only for the sake of argument that the fetus is a truly human being, it does not follow that abortion is always wrong. She draws an analogy with a person who unknowingly and unwillingly is plugged into a famous violinist who has a fatal kidney ailment that can be overcome only by using the kidneys of the other person. Does the person in this case have the right to unplug the violinist even though it will bring about the death of the famous musician? A minimally decent Samaritan or the normal human being is not required to make such a huge sacrifice as being plugged into the violinist for nine months in order to sustain the life of another who has no right to demand this.

Thompson has raised the very important question of conflict situations, but her analogy with the person plugged into the violinist for nine months decidedly limps. It seems that only in the case of rape might one hope to find a comparison between the two cases. A woman has to assume responsibility for her previous actions, and likewise there is a significant difference between an obligation to save the life of another and an obligation not to take the life of another.

There is another possible approach in conflict situations involving abortion which to some extent is also acceptable within the traditional approach of Roman Catholic theology. James Gustafson (in Noonan, pp. 119–122), a Protestant ethicist, accepts the decision of a woman to have an abortion after she has been brutally raped by her former husband and acknowledges some financial and psychological problems in having the child. Bernard Häring (pp. 112–115) and even Gustafson himself recognize that from the viewpoint of Roman Catholic pastoral theology on the basis of an expanded notion of invincible ignorance, which prudently recognizes that one cannot ask another to do what is not possible, a counselor can accept the decision of the woman. Others are continuing to debate whether there are any real differences in the solutions proposed by Gustafson and Häring.

Survey of the contemporary debate

Protestant church teaching and Protestant ethicists until 1950 generally condemned abortion, but since that time many Protestant churches and groups have come out in favor of abortion in certain circumstances and rejected the concept that the fetus from the moment of conception is a truly human being. However, it would be wrong to say that all Protestants are in favor of abortion.

In Germany in 1973 a conference of German Bishops (Catholic) and of the Evangelical Church (Protestant) issued a common statement on abortion which insisted that all decisions that involved human life can be oriented only to the service of life. Generally speaking, more evangelical and conservative Protestant groups strenuously oppose abortion. Also a large number of respected Protestant ethicists in the United States oppose abortion although many others do not consider the conceptus from the time of fertilization to be a truly human being.

Developments have also occurred within Roman Catholicism. The hierarchical magisterium has continued to proclaim the accepted Catholic teaching. The Second Vatican Council's *Pastoral Constitution on the Church in the Modern World* (n. 51) taught that from the moment of its conception life must be regarded with the greatest care and that abortion and infanticide are unspeakable crimes. Pope Paul VI in his 1968 encyclical *Humanae Vitae* (n. 14) declared once again that both the direct interruption of the generative process already begun and every directly willed and procured abortion, even if for therapeutic reasons, are to be absolutely excluded as licit means of regulating birth. The Vatican's Sacred Congregation for the Doctrine of the Faith issued a Declaration on Procured Abortion, 18 November 1974, which reiterated the traditional teaching, and this has also been repeated by national conferences of Catholic bishops throughout the world.

The majority of Roman Catholic theologians still seem to uphold the traditional teaching that from the moment of conception the conceptus is to be treated as a truly human being. There is however some dissent on this issue, most publicized in France, where a small respected group of Catholic theologians has been proposing a relational criterion for determining when human life begins. While an increasing number of Catholic scholars claim that dissent on when truly human life begins is legitimate and justified (since, in this matter, it is impossible to arrive at a certitude that excludes the possibility of error), still the vast majority of Roman Catholic authors accept the traditional teaching or disagree only to the extent that the beginning of truly human life is placed in the second or third week after conception. A comparatively large number of Catholic theologians from all countries reject the traditional use of "double effect" to solve conflict situations involving the fetus.

Differences continue to exist within Judaism. The only authoritative text on therapeutic abortion in the Talmud recognizes that the fetus becomes truly human only if the greater part of it is already born. The controversy obviously centers on the value and importance of the fetus. All authors in the orthodox and conservative cultural tradition (e.g., Novak) accept the therapeutic abortion necessary for the life of the mother and, according to some, also for the mental health of the mother; but there is always a very strong emphasis in favor of the life of the fetus. Within the reformed branch of Judaism there is a greater willingness to attribute less value to the fetus. It is indistinguishable from the mother and may be destroyed for the mother's sake, just as a person may decide to sacrifice a bodily limb to cure a worse malady (Margolies in Hall, vol. 1, pp. 30–33).

One of the characteristics of the contemporary debate has been the interest shown by professional philosophers in the question of abortion. Until very recently, philosophers tended to neglect content questions such as abortion, but changes in philosophy and the strong interest within society on this question have changed this. The writings of the philosophers, while not numerous to date, have frequently added precision of thought to the contemporary debate. In general there is no doubt that in the contemporary debate since 1950 many voices have been raised in favor of the position that the fetus is not a truly human being from the moment of conception and therefore abortion is morally acceptable for various reasons. Such sentiments obviously have had an effect on public opinion and on changing abortion laws in a number of countries, even though there is not a strict correlation between questions of law and questions of morality. However, it is interesting to note in the last few years some former advocates of abortion have expressed either a change of mind or doubt about the morality of abortion, at least to the extent that they want to caution against a too ready acceptance of abortion. The general public, philosophers, and theologians continue to be divided on this issue.

CHARLES E. CURRAN

[*While all the articles in this entry are relevant, see especially the articles* JEWISH PERSPECTIVES, ROMAN CATHOLIC PERSPECTIVES, *and* PROTESTANT

PERSPECTIVES. *Also directly related are the entries* DOUBLE EFFECT; LIFE; PERSON; *and* PRENATAL DIAGNOSIS, *article on* ETHICAL ISSUES. *Other relevant material may be found under* FETAL–MATERNAL RELATIONSHIP; INFANTS, *article on* INFANTICIDE: A PHILOSOPHICAL PERSPECTIVE; RIGHTS; SEXUAL ETHICS; *and* WOMEN AND BIOMEDICINE, *article on* WOMEN AS PATIENTS AND EXPERIMENTAL SUBJECTS. *For discussion of related ideas, see the entries:* CONTRACEPTION; OBLIGATION AND SUPEREROGATION; STERILIZATION, *article on* ETHICAL ASPECTS.]

BIBLIOGRAPHY

Aborto questione aperta: Le Posizioni dei moralisti italiani. Introduction by Ambrogio Valsecchi. L'opinione religiosa in Italia, no. 1. Turin: Gribaudi, 1973.

Avortement et respect de la vie humaine. Colloque du Centre catholique des médecins français (commission conjugale). Paris: Éditions du Seuil, 1972.

BOK, SISSELA. "Ethical Problems of Abortion." *Hastings Center Studies* 2, no. 1 (1974), pp. 33–52.

BRANDT, RICHARD B. "The Morality of Abortion." *Monist* 56 (1972): 503–526.

CALLAHAN, DANIEL. *Abortion: Law, Choice and Morality.* New York: Macmillan, 1970.

CLOUSER, K. DANNER, and ZUCKER, ARTHUR, comps. *Abortion and Euthanasia: An Annotated Bibliography.* Philadelphia: Society for Health & Human Values, 1974.

CURRAN, CHARLES E. "Abortion: Its Legal and Moral Aspects in Catholic Theology." *New Perspectives in Moral Theology.* Notre Dame, Ind.: Fides, 1974, pp. 163–193.

DONCEEL, JOSEPH F. "Immediate Animation and Delayed Hominization." *Theological Studies* 31 (1970): 76–105.

ENGELHARDT, H. TRISTRAM, JR. "The Ontology of Abortion." *Ethics* 84 (1974): 217–234.

FEINBERG, JOEL, ed. *The Problem of Abortion.* Belmont, Calif.: Wadsworth Publishing Co., 1973.

FINNIS, JOHN. "The Rights and Wrongs of Abortion: A Reply to Judith Thompson." *Philosophy and Public Affairs* 2 (1973): 117–144.

FLETCHER, JOSEPH. "Medicine and the Nature of Man." *The Teaching of Medical Ethics.* Edited by Robert M. Veatch, Willard Gaylin, and Councilman Morgan. Hasting-on-Hudson, N.Y.: Institute of Society, Ethics, and the Life Sciences, 1973, pp. 47–58.

FLOYD, MARY K. *Abortion Bibliography for 1973.* Troy, N.Y.: Whitson Publishing Co., 1974. Similar volumes were published for 1970, 1971, and 1972.

GREEN, RONALD M. "Conferred Rights and the Fetus." *Journal of Religious Ethics* 2 (1974): 55–75.

GRISEZ, GERMAIN G. *Abortion: The Myths, the Realities, and the Arguments.* New York: Corpus Books, 1970.

GRÜNDEL, JOHANNES. *Abtreibung—Pro und Contra.* Würzburg: Echter, 1971.

HALL, ROBERT E., ed. *Abortion in a Changing World.* 2 vols. New York: Columbia University Press, 1970.

HARDIN, GARRETT. "Abortion—Or Compulsory Pregnancy?" *Journal of Marriage and the Family* 30 (1968): 246–251.

HARE, R. M. "Abortion and the Golden Rule." *Philosophy and Public Affairs* 4 (1975): 201–222.

HÄRING, BERNARD. *Medical Ethics.* Notre Dame, Ind.: Fides, 1973, pp. 75–119.

HAUERWAS, STANLEY. *Vision and Virtue: Essays in Christian Ethical Reflection.* Notre Dame, Ind.: Fides, 1974, pp. 127–165.

LADER, LAWRENCE. *Abortion.* Boston: Beacon Press, 1966.

LEDERBERG, JOSHUA. "A Geneticist Looks at Contraception and Abortion." *Annals of Internal Medicine* 67, supp. 7 (1967): 25–27.

McCORMICK, RICHARD A. *Ambiguity in Moral Choice.* The 1973 Père Marquette Theology Lecture. Milwaukee: Marquette University Press, 1973.

NOONAN, JOHN T., JR. *The Morality of Abortion: Legal and Historical Perspectives.* Cambridge: Harvard University Press, 1970.

NOVAK, DAVID. "A Jewish View of Abortion." *Law and Theology in Judaism.* New York: Ktav Publishing House, 1974, pp. 114–124.

RAMSEY, PAUL. "Abortion: A Review Article." *Thomist* 37 (1973): 174–226.

———. "The Morality of Abortion." *Life or Death: Ethics and Options.* By Edward Shils, Norman St. John-Stevas, Paul Ramsey, P. B. Medawar, Henry K. Beecher, and Abraham Kaplan. Introduction by Daniel H. Labby. Seattle: University of Washington Press, 1968, pp. 60–93.

RUFF, WILFRIED. "Individualität und Personalität im embryonalen Werden." *Theologie und Philosophie* 45 (1970): 24–59.

SCHÜLLER, BRUNO. *Die Begründung sittlicher Urteile: Typen ethischer Argumentation in der katholischen Moraltheologie.* Düsseldorf: Patmos, 1973.

THOMPSON, JUDITH JARVIS. "A Defense of Abortion." *Philosophy and Public Affairs* 1 (1971): 47–66.

TOOLEY, MICHAEL. "Abortion and Infanticide." *Philosophy and Public Affairs* 2 (1972): 37–65. Edited reprint. "A Defense of Abortion and Infanticide." Feinberg, *The Problem of Abortion,* pp. 51–91.

WAHLBERG, RACHEL CONRAD. "The Woman and the Fetus: 'One Flesh'?" *Christian Century* 88 (1971): 1045–1048.

WILLIAMS, GLANVILLE. "Euthanasia and Abortion." *University of Colorado Law Review* 38 (1965–1966): 178–201.

VI
LEGAL ASPECTS

In all developed legal systems, abortion has been and is more or less explicitly regulated by law. This can hardly fail to continue to be so, for reasons that emerge from an analysis of recent legal developments in the United States.

The specific legal norms in relation to abortion vary widely from country to country, and from one time to another. But three basic models can be discerned. Most actual schemes approximate to one or another of these three models, though of course some actual schemes are compromises between diverse models, and others are in transition from one model to another, so that their practical working differs from their formal legal framework. The characterization of these models will refer not only to the formal normative structure of prohibitions, permissions, and authorizations but also to the values or objectives to be realized or protected by way of that structure. The scope for variation is as wide as it actually is precisely because the functional objectives of a scheme, its formal normative structure, and the procedures for operating and policing that structure are three more or less independent variables, all of which must be taken into account in explaining and classifying any particular scheme.

In the first of the three basic models all abortions are legally prohibited, either absolutely or subject to an exception where continuation of the pregnancy would threaten the life of the pregnant woman. The characteristic objective of this type of scheme is to protect the interests of the unborn child, either for its own sake (as a matter of justice and respect for rights) or for the sake of the social interest in the maintenance or increase of the population, or sometimes (as in France in the first half of this century) for both reasons. In the past those two objectives were often supplemented by a concern to protect the pregnant woman from the medical risks involved in attempts to terminate pregnancy.

The second model is that in which abortion is permitted only with the prior authorization of independent officials, whose grant or refusal of permission is guided by standards relating to defined categories of medical, psychomedical, or quasi-medical conditions. Schemes with this type of formal normative structure are often in fact compromises or transitional phases between the first and the third models, that is to say, devices for relaxing the first scheme (in the interests, e.g., of women's freedom) or for tightening up the third scheme (in the interests, e.g., of women's health, or of stemming a decline in population or in birthrate). But the second model can have the distinctive goal of empowering the medical and psychiatric professions to apply representative standards of judgment—in a matter that deeply affects these professions—in order to maintain professional unity and standards.

In the third model all abortions are legally permitted if performed by medically qualified persons. The characteristic objectives are to give effect to the rights of the woman over her own body and to eliminate unskilled abortions with their attendant medical hazards.

First model: restriction for the sake of the child

Although the matter has been disputed, the better view appears to be that the law of England always adopted the first model. Abortion after quickening (about the sixteenth week of pregnancy) was, according to Chief Justice Coke (c. 1630), a "great misprision" (and he defines "misprision" as a high offense, under, but "nearly bordering" on, the "degree of capital" offense). This position was reaffirmed in judgments or scholarly expositions by all the great common-law writers—Hale, Hawkins, Blackstone. In the nineteenth century many American courts affirmed that in the common law of England, and of the American colonies and states, abortion after quickening was a serious (though not felonious) offense, and courts in two states ruled that the offense extended to abortion at all stages of pregnancy. However, it is also true that English criminal law as enforced in the common-law courts was, as in many other important matters, encumbered by procedural, evidential, and doctrinal rigidities. Prosecution directly for the offense itself was difficult if not impossible in those courts and was left to the ecclesiastical courts, whose law was accepted by common-law lawyers as an important part of the law of the land. But the common law's characterization of (postquickening) abortion as a serious offense appears quite clearly from the common-law rule that to cause accidentally the death of the mother in an effort to abort her was murder. The opinion expressed by the United States Supreme Court in 1973, that "it now appear[s] doubtful that abortion was ever firmly established as a common-law crime even with respect to the destruction of a quick fetus" gives a rather misleading impression of the state of scholarship on this matter, and the Court's conclusion that "at common law . . . a woman enjoyed a substantially broader right to terminate a pregnancy than she [did] in most States [in 1972]" would have been rejected as equivocal or mistaken by any common-law judge or scholar between the beginning of the seventeenth and the end of the nineteenth centuries, at least.

The decadence of the English ecclesiastical courts and the rigidities of the common law gave rise to statutory reform by the Parliament of Great Britain in 1803 (a time of extensive reform of the inadequate common law of crimes). The statute cut through the evidential encumbrances of the common law by penalizing (as felony) all attempts to procure abortion. All abortions were criminal, but postquickening ones were punishable more severely than prequickening ones; in 1837 this distinction disappeared from English law altogether. In 1861 the statutory abortion law of the United Kingdom reached the form it retained until 1967. Any act intended to cause abortion, whether induced by the woman herself (if she were pregnant) or by others (whether or not she was in fact pregnant) was a felony.

The first American legislation against abortion was passed in Connecticut in 1821. Many early American statutes did not penalize abortion before quickening. But in 1827 (Illinois) that restriction began to disappear; by 1860 twenty American states or territories, including Connecticut, had statutes against abortion at all stages of pregnancy. By 1868 thirty-six states or territories had antiabortion statutes. In 1965 all fifty states prohibited abortion and attempts to abort, at all stages of pregnancy. In forty-six states and the District of Columbia the relevant statute explicitly permitted abortion to save the mother's life, while in two of the other four states (as in England) judicial interpretation had recognized a similar exception to the statutory prohibition. A survey both of the legislative history and of accompanying judicial and professional statements leaves little room for the opinion, favored by the Supreme Court in 1973, that the primary intention of the law prevailing in the United Kingdom and the United States up to 1965 was to protect the pregnant woman against the medical risks that were inherent in abortion until the advent of modern medical techniques. On the contrary, the law's primary intention was plainly to prohibit what was considered a wrongful attack on human life in the womb.

Developments in the United States and the United Kingdom after 1965 are discussed below. In the early 1970s, schemes on the first model were legally in force in more than sixty countries, including more than twenty where the formal legal norms absolutely prohibited all abortions, even when performed to save the life of the mother. In some other jurisdictions—such as Belgium, most of the states of Australia, and to some extent New Zealand—judicial interpretation or prosecutorial policy had effected a substantial move toward the third model by permitting abortion when performed by a medical practitioner in order to avert any substantial risk (in the view of that practitioner) to the physical or mental health of the pregnant woman, or to prevent the birth of a handicapped child.

Second model: restriction for the sake of uniform medical practice

The earliest instance of a scheme of legal regulation on the second model—in which each abortion requires (save in emergency) the prior authorization of some official referee(s)—is afforded by the German law enacted shortly after the Nazi accession to power in 1933 and replaced after the Second World War by a law on the first model. Other early instances are the laws and administrative regulations in force in Denmark from 1937 to 1973 and in Sweden from 1939 to 1974. The criteria for authorization by the relevant committee or board in these Scandinavian countries included the principle that, in assessing how giving birth to and caring for the expected child would affect the mental or physical health of the woman, her actual and prospective living conditions are to be taken into account. The Swedish criteria were always a little more restrictive than the Danish, but in both countries the law and administrative practice were several times relaxed to allow wider medical, eugenic, sociomedical, or social "indications." Countries that adopted some form of the second model more recently include Turkey, Brazil, and Singapore.

Between 1967 and early 1973 a dozen jurisdictions in the United States adopted abortion laws more or less patterned on the model legislation suggested in 1962 by the American Law Institute, an unofficial voluntary association of lawyers. This permitted abortion when performed by a licensed physician who believed that there was a substantial risk that continuance of the pregnancy would gravely impair the physical or mental health of the mother, that the child would be born with grave physical or mental defect, or that the pregnancy resulted from rape, incest, or other felonious intercourse. However, although a few of the states amending their laws in this direction adopted somewhat looser categories of permitted circumstances, those few and almost all the others of the dozen reforming jurisdictions sought to strengthen the institutionalization of abortion practice by stipulating that an abortion would be lawful only if performed (in the permitted circumstances) in an accredited hospital after approval by a committee established in the hospital for that purpose. This institutionalization of an evolving consensus of professional medical judgment was stronger than in the Scandinavian countries, in that the hospital committees were to be composed entirely of medical practitioners, but also weaker, in that the hospital committees were subject to no central appointment, direction, or control. A scheme of this kind was adopted by legislation in Canada in 1969.

In retrospect it is difficult to see the Scandinavian and American experiments with prior authorization as anything other than unstable compromises adopted along a society's path from the first to the third model. But it would be wrong to deny that many people genuinely believed that abortion was a matter that society should leave to medical judgment—not individual, but *representative* medical judgment. This belief was rooted in the assumption that the medical profession had an ethic, autonomous and distinct from society's general laws and mores, which, when combined with medical knowledge and technical expertise, would generate a code of practice that society would do well to follow. Traces of this assumption can still be found in the decisive role accorded to "the physician" in the judgments of the United States Supreme Court in 1973—a role that on any other assumption is difficult to reconcile with the Court's basic reliance on the *woman's* constitutional right of personal privacy.

In Eastern European countries such as Hungary, Rumania, and Bulgaria, abortion is lawful only if approved by a state board. Here the objective is to free women for employment while at the same time giving effect to the state's population policy. The general policy has usually been to permit abortion in almost every case, at least up to the sixteenth week of pregnancy. But from time to time a government's concern about falling population growth, or about the medical side effects of repeated abortions, has inspired a severe restriction on the number of authorizations of abortion (e.g., in Rumania in 1966).

Third model: general availability for the sake of women's freedom

The earliest instance, in the modern world, of a scheme on the third model is afforded by the decree of the Soviet Union, in November 1920, that made lawful any abortion performed by a physician in a state hospital. The expressed objective of the decree was to protect women from unskilled abortionists, to whom they resorted because of "moral survivals of the past" (presumably shame at illegitimate pregnancy) and "the difficult economic conditions of the present." But the decree was also part of a general program of women's liberation and sexual equality in work, education, and marriage. In June 1936 the decree was replaced by a law that

prohibited abortion except where pregnancy threatened the life or seriously threatened the health of the woman, or when a serious disease of the parents could be inherited. The shift back to a form of the first model seems to have been motivated by concern primarily about declining birthrates, and secondarily about medical side effects and increasingly irresponsible attitudes toward marriage and childbearing. But in November 1955 the decree of 1936 was repealed, for the express reasons of reducing the harm done by unskilled abortionists and giving women "the possibility of deciding by themselves the question of motherhood."

Japan adopted, in 1948, a scheme on the second model but in 1952 amended it to a scheme on the third model, not by extending the grounds for abortion specified in the Eugenic Protection Law but simply by removing the control of district Eugenic Committees over individual physicians' decisions. The primary objective appears to have been population control; a secondary objective was reduction in unskilled abortions.

The Abortion Act 1967, which came into effect in Great Britain in April 1968 and has been copied in Hong Kong, Zambia, and South Australia, amounts in practice to a scheme of the third type: In practice abortion is freely and openly available, at least to anyone who can pay the fees charged by licensed private institutions. Indeed, even in theory the law is on the third model (though this seems not to have been the intention of many of the legislators who supported it), for it permits an abortion where any two medical practitioners are of the opinion, formed in good faith, that continuance of pregnancy "would involve risk to the life of the pregnant woman, or of injury to the physical or mental health of the pregnant woman or any existing children of her family, *greater than if the pregnancy were terminated.*" The last words are here emphasized because they mean that the legal justification of abortion depends on nothing more than the medical evaluation that controls any surgical procedure: The risk of performing it must be less than the risk of omitting it, but neither risk need be in any way serious. Official analysis of the medical data, supplied by medical practitioners to the relevant government department, suggests that in 1973, in the nongovernment institutions in which two-thirds of all notified abortions were performed, ninety-nine percent of the abortions were performed primarily or exclusively for reasons of "risk to mental health" of the mother; in National Health Service hospitals the corresponding proportion was over eighty percent. Abortion is also lawful where two physicians believe that "there is substantial risk that if the child were born it would suffer from such physical or mental abnormalities as to be seriously handicapped." Responsible medical opinion in Great Britain considers that a risk of one in ten is certainly "substantial."

Since 22 January 1973, when the Supreme Court decided *Roe* v. *Wade* and *Doe* v. *Bolton,* the law throughout the United States has been on the third model. In those cases, the Court by majority of seven to two decided that the constitutional right to privacy, protected by the due process clause of the Fourteenth Amendment to the Constitution, entails that (1) no law can restrict the right of a woman to be aborted by a physician during the first three months (trimester) of her pregnancy; (2) during the second trimester the abortion procedure may be regulated by law only to the extent that the regulation reasonably relates to the preservation and protection of maternal health; (3) at the point at which the fetus becomes viable (not before the beginning of the third trimester) a law may prohibit abortion but only subject to an exception permitting abortion wherever necessary to protect the woman's life or health (including any aspects of her physical or mental health); (4) no law may require that all abortions be performed in accredited hospitals (where accreditation has no particularized concern with abortion as a medical or surgical procedure), or that abortions be approved by a hospital committee, or by a second medical opinion, or that abortions be performed only on women resident in the state concerned. The effect of these decisions was to invalidate the laws regulating abortion in every state, except perhaps the already very permissive laws adopted in 1969 and 1970 in New York, Alaska, Hawaii, and Washington.

The theory underlying the Supreme Court's division of pregnancy into three trimesters of differing constitutional status is that during the first trimester the mortality rates for women undergoing abortion "appear to be as low as or lower than the rates for normal childbirth"; as one moves into the second trimester the health risks of abortion begin (on the average) to exceed those of childbirth; and as the third trimester begins the fetus is becoming viable and a state's interest in protecting it, *should the state legislature choose to do so,* overrides the woman's right to privacy in deciding for or against maternity.

Within two years of the Supreme Court's decisions, cases in lower federal courts appeared to have established the following implications or consequences: (1) During the first trimester abortions are exempt from any legal or licensing requirements that do not apply to medical facilities generally, and from any regulations other than those applicable to all other relatively minor operations. (2) Advertisements of medical facilities for first-trimester abortions may not be prohibited. (3) No law may require the consent of the husband or of the parent or guardian of a pregnant, unmarried minor (even where the motive for requiring consent of the parent or guardian is to protect the health of the minor—at least during the first trimester). (4) During the second trimester the decision about abortion must remain absolutely with the woman and her physician; only procedures for carrying out the operation may be regulated, and these only where necessary to protect the woman's health. (5) A state law may not truncate the woman's constitutional rights by declaring that a fetus is to be deemed viable at twenty weeks, or by requiring medical personnel to seek to preserve the life of an aborted fetus between the twentieth and the twenty-fourth week. (6) It is unconstitutional to restrict third trimester abortions to cases where the woman's *physical* health is threatened. (7) Any denial of public assistance funds for abortion is unconstitutional. (8) Public hospital facilities must be made available for abortions, and it is unconstitutional for a state to enact a conscience clause specifying that "no person or hospital or institution shall be coerced, held liable or discriminated against in any manner because of a refusal to perform, accommodate, assist or submit to an abortion for any reason"; for such a clause tends to limit the availability of hospital facilities for abortion. (9) Where a state fails to enact a constitutionally valid abortion statute, there is no restriction on the availability of abortion, performed by a physician, at any time during pregnancy. (10) Subject to the foregoing nine points, there is no legal right to abortion on demand.

Not all the foregoing points, perhaps, are established with equal certainty. In any event, a large number of legal questions remain to be resolved. The following are examples of these questions, most of which would need to be the subject of explicit legal decision (i.e., regulation by law) however widely abortion is permitted. (1) What are the implications of *Roe* v. *Wade* in relation to rights of the unborn child, other than its now legally unrecognized right not to be aborted? There is a considerable body of law granting rights to sue to persons who were tortiously injured before birth, and this law is in many jurisdictions expressly founded on the theory that a human life begins at conception. In *Roe* v. *Wade* the Supreme Court recognized without approving or disapproving that body of law but did declare that "the judiciary, at this point in the development of man's knowledge, is not in a position to speculate as to the answer" to "the difficult question of when life begins." (2) Does the woman's right to privacy really entail that a state is powerless to require medical personnel to make reasonable efforts to save fetuses that are aborted before the end of the second trimester (cf. point [5] above)? In general, is the Supreme Court's theory of viability open or impervious to future advances in medical techniques (artificial wombs, etc.)? In connection with these questions, note that several states require abortion procedures be used which will preserve the life of a viable fetus, and several also provide that a fetus surviving an abortion may be made a ward of the state. (3) Is it lawful for a woman to self-induce an abortion during the first trimester? On the one hand, the Supreme Court said that a state may proscribe any abortion by a person who is not a physician. On the other hand, the Court's basic theory is of the woman's right to privacy, and moreover the Court takes for granted "new medical techniques such as menstrual extraction [and] the 'morning-after' pill," which might well be used without medical supervision (the Court's reference to these new techniques was, oddly, as posing a "substantial problem for precise definition of [the] view" that human life begins at conception). (4) Can a state prohibit all, or some, or any forms of experimentation on fetuses before, during, or after abortion? Is a fetus to be treated as a part of the pregnant woman which she can dispose of at will, at least during the first two trimesters? (5) What is the legal liability of a physician who fails to advise, or to perform, an abortion? (6) What forms of conscientious objection are available to physicians, nurses, hospitals, or other institutions unwilling to perform any or some abortions (cf. point [8] above)? (7) Does the father of an unborn child, even during the third trimester, altogether lack any rights that might prevail against the mother's constitutionally recognized rights? (8) What forms of assistance is a state or federal agency bound to afford to a woman who wants an abortion? (9) Could a state validly *require* a woman

to undergo an abortion, whether to prevent the birth of a handicapped child, to protect the health of the woman, or to advance a state policy of population control? The question can arise because in 1973 the Supreme Court refused to consider that another human life (that of the unborn) is involved, and appeared to accept the 1927 decision of the Supreme Court upholding compulsory sterilization of imbeciles afflicted with hereditary forms of insanity or imbecility.

During the early 1970s a number of countries adopted laws approximating the third model. The theory that during the first trimester abortion ought to be available without any restrictions gained popularity; it was adopted in East Germany in 1972, Denmark in 1973, Sweden in 1974, and France in 1975. "Viability," the point at which, in most of these schemes, the interests of the woman cease to be accorded overriding weight, is variously fixed at twenty weeks (Sweden, India), twenty-four weeks (Singapore), and twenty-eight weeks (in the United Kingdom, in practical effect). The French law of 17 January 1975 is representative of much international opinion in the wake of the judicial transformation of United States law in 1973. The French enactment begins with a declaration that the law guarantees respect for every human being from the beginning of life, and that this principle is to be departed from only in case of necessity and according to the conditions defined by the present enactment. But the law authorizes any pregnant woman whose condition puts her in a situation of hardship to request a physician for abortion. Provided that the abortion is performed before the end of the tenth week of pregnancy, there are no preconditions other than: (1) The physician must inform the woman of the medical risks to herself and her future pregnancies, and give her an official guide to the forms of assistance available to all families, mothers, and children, and to relevant social service organizations; (2) the woman must consult one of the listed social services; (3) if the woman still wishes to proceed to an abortion she must confirm this in writing, not earlier than one week after her first request; (4) the abortion must be performed by a physician in a public or recognized private hospital and must be reported to the regional health authorities; (5) the hospital must provide the aborted woman with birth control information. But the law also removes, for a period of five years, all penalties against a doctor who performs an abortion, in a public or recognized private hospital, on any woman before the end of the tenth week. After that stage of pregnancy, right up to the moment of birth, abortion is lawful if two physicians, one of them from an official list, certify that continuation of pregnancy would put the woman's health gravely in peril, or that there is a strong possibility that the child would suffer from an incurable condition. The law concludes with the declaratory statement that in no case should termination of pregnancy be used as a means of birth control.

J. M. FINNIS

[*While all the articles in this entry are relevant, see especially the articles* MEDICAL ASPECTS, *and* CONTEMPORARY DEBATE IN PHILOSOPHICAL AND RELIGIOUS ETHICS. *For further discussion of topics mentioned in this article, see the entries:* CONTRACEPTION; FETAL–MATERNAL RELATIONSHIP; FETAL RESEARCH; GENETIC DIAGNOSIS AND COUNSELING; INFANTS; LIFE; POPULATION POLICY PROPOSALS; PRENATAL DIAGNOSIS; PRIVACY; *and* RIGHTS. *Other relevant material may be found under* LAW AND MORALITY.]

BIBLIOGRAPHY

BYRN, ROBERT M. "An American Tragedy: The Supreme Court on Abortion." *Fordham Law Review* 41 (1973): 807–862.

CALLAHAN, DANIEL J. *Abortion: Law, Choice, and Morality.* New York: Macmillan Co., 1970. Chapters 5, 6, and 7 survey "restrictive," "moderate," and "permissive" codes in various countries.

DELGADO, RICHARD, and KEYES, JUDITH DROZ. "Parental Preferences and Selective Abortion: A Commentary on Roe v. Wade, Doe v. Bolton, and the Shape of Things to Come." *Washington University Law Quarterly* 1974 (1974): 203–226.

Doe v. Bolton. 410 U.S. 179. 35 L. Ed. 2d. 201. 93 S. Ct. 739 (1973).

ELY, JOHN HART. "The Wages of Crying Wolf: A Comment on Roe v. Wade." *Yale Law Journal* 82 (1973): 920–949. Perhaps the most damaging critique of the Supreme Court's decision, by a constitutional lawyer not opposed to abortion.

EPSTEIN, RICHARD A. "Substantive Due Process by Any Other Name: The Abortion Cases." *1973: The Supreme Court Review.* Edited by Philip B. Kurland. Chicago: University of Chicago Press, 1974, pp. 159–185.

FINNIS, JOHN M. "Three Schemes of Regulation." *The Morality of Abortion: Legal and Historical Perspectives.* Edited by John T. Noonan, Jr. Cambridge: Harvard University Press, 1970, pp. 172–219.

GRISEZ, GERMAIN G. *Abortion: The Myths, the Realities and the Arguments.* New York: Corpus Books, 1970. Chapters 5 and 8 contain the best available discussion of the legal questions discussed in this article.

MALEDON, WILLIAM J. "The Law and the Unborn Child: The Legal and Logical Inconsistencies." *Notre Dame Lawyer* 46 (1971): 349–372.

MEANS, CYRIL C., JR. "The Law of New York Concerning Abortion and the Status of the Foetus, 1664–1968: A Case of Cessation of Constitutionality." *New York Law Forum* 14 (1968): 411–515.

———. "The Phoenix of Abortional Freedom: Is a Penumbral or Ninth-Amendment Right About to Arise from the Nineteenth-Century Legislative Ashes of a Fourteenth-Century Common-Law Liberty?" *New York Law Forum* 17 (1971): 335–410. Means's views on the history of the common law, which differ in his two articles, appear to have considerably influenced the Supreme Court in 1973. For a preliminary reply, see Byrn, "An American Tragedy."

QUAY, EUGENE. "Justifiable Abortion—Medical and Legal Foundations." *Georgetown Law Journal* 49 (1960): 173–256, 395–538. Appendix I reproduces all the enactments on abortion in the United States and its territories, as of 1960.

REBACK, GARY L. "Fetal Experimentation: Moral, Legal, and Medical Implications." *Stanford Law Review* 26 (1974): 1191–1207. Analysis in the light of *Roe v. Wade* and its legislative aftermath.

Roe v. Wade. 410 U.S. 113. 35 L. Ed. 2d, 147. 93 S. Ct. 705 (1973).

VEITCH, EDWARD, and TRACEY, R. R. S. "Abortion in the Common Law World." *American Journal of Comparative Law* 22 (1974): 652–696.

World Health Organization. *Abortion Laws; A Survey of Current World Legislation.* Geneva: World Health Organization; London: Her Majesty's Stationary Office, 1971. Surveys legislation up to 1970. Original appearance. *International Digest of Health Legislation* 21 (1970): 437–512.

ACTING AND REFRAINING

It is often claimed that there is a radical difference, from the moral point of view, between making something happen and merely letting something happen. It has been argued that there are instances where taking overt direct action to bring some state of affairs about would be wrong, while merely refraining from preventing the same result is at least sometimes permissible. Important moral consequences are based on the general distinction that directly killing someone is prohibited, while letting someone die, at least in some circumstances, is permissible. Claims like this have direct bearing on medical practice in general and on issues like abortion and euthanasia in particular. The aim of this essay is to trace the outlines of the development of the distinction between acting and refraining, with special attention to two particular issues: the conceptual basis of the distinction and the moral significance of the distinction.

One might begin by considering the difference among (1) shooting someone with the intention of killing him, (2) letting someone die and intending that he die, (3) letting someone die but not intending that he die, and (4) killing someone, but not intending to kill him (e.g., using a high dose of narcotics to ease the pain of a terminal cancer patient which may also depress the respiration of the patient and actively hasten death). Granted that each case involves a death, the issue is whether there is any significant *moral* difference exemplified by these four cases. Prima facie, (1) seems to be morally unacceptable, (2) perhaps less clear. For present purposes (3) and (4) are more significant, for many philosophers and theologians argue that there are decisive moral differences between (1) on the one hand and (3) and (4) on the other. But what could this difference be?

In (1), the model of a prima facie unacceptable act, there is a direct, willing, causal assault on someone's life. In (3) and (4), some or all these features are missing. In (3), there is no overt causal intervention on another's life, rather a mere letting something occur or a refraining from preventing; nor in (3) is the effect an intended one. In (4), although there is causal intervention, the claim is made that the causal intervention bearing on death does not fall within the range of what is intended by the agent, and therefore cannot be analyzed as (1) is analyzed. The morally relevant difference then between (1) and (3) and (4) could be defended by appealing to two different claims: (a) there is a moral difference between "acting" and "refraining," or (b) there is a decisive difference between the consequences of our "actings" and "refrainings" that we directly intend to happen and those consequences that we merely foresee, but don't intend. If both (a) and (b) are indefensible, then it is not clear how moral differences between (1) and (3) and (4) could be established.

Let us begin the discussion with an analysis of (b), for it provides the conceptual link between (3) and (4), both of which presuppose that there is a distinction between what we foresee and what we intend, or between what we "obliquely intend" and "directly intend." The best defense of such a distinction is to be found in the tradition of Catholic moral theology and its development of the so-called principle of double effect.

The principle of double effect in Catholic moral theology

Directly intending and causing the death of an innocent individual is prima facie forbidden in the tradition of Catholic moral theology. Yet the very same tradition permits a physician to "pyramid" painkilling drugs that will have the net effect of shortening the life of the patient. Furthermore, the performance of a hysterectomy on a pregnant woman in the case of uterine cancer is also permitted.

Critics of the tradition, like Glanville Williams, argue that exceptions like these are simply inconsistent and cast serious doubt on the viability of the tradition of moral theology (Williams). Defenders of such exceptions, on the other hand, argue that it is of the utmost moral significance that one individual must always refrain from taking direct action against the life of another. Clearly some principle that will maintain the general prohibition against the taking of life and that can make such exceptions intelligible is needed. Why is it morally justifiable that the doctor refrain from taking direct action against a life, while it is permissible in some circumstances to hasten the moment of death? The principle of double effect (PDE) has been employed to answer questions like these.

Thomas Aquinas is probably the first theologian who articulated both the principle and the general conditions for its use. Aquinas formulated the principle to deal specifically with the issue of whether it is ever morally justifiable to take the life of another in self-defense. Aquinas answered affirmatively, on the general grounds that sometimes one action had more than one consequence, and that some of these further consequences might themselves be evil. Some scholars believe that the four conditions later associated with the principle of double effect were at least implied in Aquinas's argument. Those conditions, according to which an action that results in undesirable consequences was judged permissible, were the following: (1) the act itself must be morally good or indifferent; (2) only the good consequences of the action must be intended; (3) the good effect must not be produced by means of the evil effect; and (4) there must be some grave reason for permitting the evil (Aquinas). (1) and (4) are certainly acceptable principles. The difficulty in interpreting the principle seems to hang on the intelligibility of (2) and (3). Aquinas is relying on two things in accepting both constraints: with regard to (2) he is appealing to the difference between foresight and intention; with respect to (3) he is relying on a principle that had substantial theological and moral weight, "Never do evil so that good might result." Both constraints have in common a plausible moral principle: a moral agent should never intentionally do something that is evil. PDE, in its original formulation, is neither bizarre nor mysterious; whether it can carry the heavy conceptual and moral weight it is made to bear by the Catholic tradition is an issue on which we can reserve judgment temporarily.

The development of the principle from Aquinas bears witness to the ambiguity of (2) and (3) and to the difficulty of applying the principle in a plausible way. Cajetan (1468–1534), for example, in his commentary on Aquinas's *Summa,* was the first to apply the principle explicitly to the killing of the innocent (Mangan). The casuists Sanchez (1550–1610) and Lessius (1554–1623), among others, applied the principle in great detail to the problem of abortion (Grisez, chap. 4). And yet Aquinas does not do so, even though he was not unaware of its relevance (Noonan). Whether or not there is an entirely consistent application of the principle to be found in Aquinas is not clear.

What is clear is that the casuists of the sixteenth and seventeenth centuries did extend the principle to the taking of innocent life. These discussions centered on issues like the just war theory and the conditions under which abortion might be legitimate. A second key transition in the application of the principle emerges here: the introduction of the distinction between direct and indirect means. In general, casuists like Sanchez and Lessius condemned any means of abortion that tended to kill the fetus directly, while under certain conditions means that did not "tend directly" toward the taking of life were permissible. Much the same position was endorsed by St. Alphonsus Ligouri (1696–1787) (Mangan; Noonan). The moral significance of the direct–indirect distinction was debated even at that point in history: Gabriel Vasquez, a Jesuit casuist of the seventeenth century, argued that any abortion that resulted from any overt positive act, even one that employed indirect means, was immoral (Grisez). Most moral theologians, however, have accepted the significance of the direct–indirect distinction. In summation, there seem to have been three roughly distinct periods involved in the development of the principle: its formulation by Aquinas, the extension of the principle to moral problems other than self-defense, and the interpretation of the principle in terms of the direct–indirect distinction.

The modern period has seen almost no serious conceptual development of the principle, but is marked by debate over the correct scope and application of the principle. The principle itself has been accepted by many moral theologians and implicitly endorsed by two popes, Pius XI and Pius XII, but precisely which actions fall under the principle is not yet clear. There seems to be some consensus on its application to the issue of painkilling drugs that hasten death, so-called indirect euthanasia, and there also seems to be consensus on the issue of abortion in ectopic pregnancy and in the case of cancer of the uterus. The application of the principle to the moral issues of modern warfare is a matter of some contention. Contrary to Williams, then, the consistency of PDE over a period of roughly seven centuries is remarkable; the historical difficulties with PDE seem to lie not so much with the principle as with how it is to be applied.

In the contemporary period, the principle of double effect is subject to three sorts of attack: (1) it generates ridiculous consequences; (2) it rests on an untenable distinction between intention and foresight, and (3) the principle is itself morally insignificant. The first two criticisms can be coped with, while the third is more troublesome.

Duff has generated an attack on PDE along the lines suggested by (1). He appeals to the Dudley and Stephens case. Lost at sea on a raft, Dudley and Stephens ate their cabin boy in order to survive. Couldn't they argue, if PDE is an acceptable principle, that they in no way intended the foreseen death of the boy, and hence that their action was justifiable? A second supposed counterexample is a medical one: a doctor removes the heart, lungs, and liver of one patient in order to save the lives of three others. Is it not possible to argue that the death of the first patient was foreseen but unintended and that such a procedure is morally justifiable? Surely the number of such cases can be multiplied indefinitely, and, as Duff argues, if PDE can be used to justify such actions then it is an untenable moral principle.

These alleged counterexamples put little pressure on PDE, however, for they involve misapplication of the principle. In neither case is there one action with good and bad results: the killing and eating in the first case and the killing and the transplantation in the second are distinct and separable actions in both cases. Therefore, the only rational way to regard the killing in both instances is as a means to an end and consequently as falling within the range of the agent's intention. Hence the principle could not be employed to generate this sort of counterexample. It can be said with some confidence that PDE, in general, will not have the outrageous results it is alleged to have by this sort of counterexample. For PDE is not an act-utilitarian principle whereby any particular means might in principle be used to bring about some independent result. To interpret it as such would be to ignore all the constraints Aquinas placed on PDE.

A second distinct attack is the claim that PDE is unacceptable because the distinction between intention and foresight it rests on cannot be defended. While any number of philosophers have attacked the distinction, the claims made by Bentham and Aune are typical. The basic line of argument may be reconstructed as follows: If a person (P) is (a) doing an action A; (b) knows that he is doing A; (c) intends to do A; (d) knows that doing A will bring about event B; and (e) knows that B will not occur unless he does A, then it cannot be claimed that he refrained from B; rather the agent acted and intended in such a way that B obtained. Bentham calls this an instance of "oblique intention." Aune argues similarly that it is only by taking a too narrow view of practical reason that we come to make such a distinction in the first place. Clearly, if this line of counterargument succeeds, PDE must be rejected.

Such an attack could be forestalled, however, if there were at least a general way to indicate why it is conceptually important not to collapse the difference between intention and foresight, and this can be done. We need to consider whether there is a difference between (f) P does A, intending that B will result; and (g) P does A, knowing that B will result.

The difference can in general be marked by discovering the reasons that P has for doing A. In the first instance, one might say that P does A because it will bring about B. In the latter case, the occurrence of B is in *no way a reason for* performing A. The agent might do A and be entirely indifferent to the occurrence of B; he might do A in spite of the fact that it will bring about B because on balance he might think that A is the best action to perform, whatever the consequences of his doing so. Insofar as it is possible to understand way an agent is doing something, intention and foresight should be distinguished. It may, of course, not always be possible to specify what the reasons are for P's performing any given action; perhaps the reasons are unconscious, perhaps they are indeterminate. Insofar, however, as it is important to

understand the behavior of an individual by understanding his reasons for performing or refraining from any given act, intention should be distinguished from foresight.

Even if one is able in a particular instance to distinguish intention from foresight, however, the moral dimension of the problem remains open. For the principle of double effect to be of any moral significance the following principle seems to be presupposed, and is explicitly held by at least one defender of PDE (Geddes): *One is not morally responsible for the foreseen but unintended consequences of an action.* Prima facie, however, it seems that this principle is false, for we are in general responsible for the foreseen consequences of our action. That a given action was unintended might be a good excuse for what we did or permitted, but that hardly renders us free from our responsibility to account for what we did or permitted. Consider the example of the shopkeeper who sells poisons knowing full well the consequences of such an act (Foot). Even if this case could be made out that the merchant in no way intended anyone's death, this would hardly constitute an adequate moral justification for such an action. And it is just here that PDE seems to flounder. For what seems to be of paramount moral interest is the character of the action being performed or refrained from and not the narrower issue of whether or not the consequence was merely foreseen and not intended. At best the moral theologian could argue that it is only *sometimes* morally justifiable to appeal to PDE, but this has yet to be done, and it is not clear that it could be done in a way that would render clear and concrete guides to action.

"Killing" and "letting die": contemporary debate

Even though PDE is an intrinsically interesting and historically influential principle, its development and debate have precipitated an even more important moral issue, especially for medical practice. Any defense of PDE presupposes that there is an important moral difference between directly acting to bring something about and merely letting (allowing, permitting) something come about; it is just the prohibition against direct, intentional killing, for example, that makes PDE such an important principle for the justifiable taking of life.

Yet it is just the assumption that there is a morally significant difference between "acting" and "refraining" that has been the center of much recent debate. In particular, the debate has centered on the difference between "killing" and "letting die." A number of philosophers and theologians have defended the distinction in various ways (Anscombe; Casey; Dinello; Ramsey); others have argued that no special moral significance is to be attributed to such a distinction (Bennett; Tooley). In examining the issue, I shall argue that the distinction is not, in general, of decisive moral significance; there is, however, one way of interpreting the distinction that makes it more credible.

Consider the following four examples: (1) directly killing someone; (2) refusing to operate on a (retarded) child; (3) suspending treatment for a terminal disease; (4) not using all the life-support measures available for a terminally ill patient. In terms of currently accepted law and medical practice in most countries, the only item in the series that is categorically forbidden is (1). There may be any number of ways of explaining the different stances taken with respect to these particular actions, including historical and psychological reasons. If the difference is to be of any substantial *moral* weight, though, there should be some significant *moral* difference between (1) and the other items on the list.

Now the central difference between (1), on the one hand, and (2), (3), and (4), on the other, is that (1) involves the notion of making something happen while (2), (3), and (4) do not. This in turn suggests that, if there is a significant moral difference between the first instance and the others, there ought to be a difference between causing something to happen and merely letting something happen. Now surely the decision to let something happen is going to have consequences, but these consequences are nonetheless not, in general, going to be *causal* consequences of actions initiated by the agent. Hence, it is reasonable to assume that, if there is a significant moral difference between (1) and (2), (3), and (4), it has something to do with the idea that (1) involves "killing" while (2), (3), and (4) all seem to involve the notion of "letting die." And this seems to presuppose, in turn, that there is a moral difference between initiating a chain of events and forbearing from preventing a chain of events that has already been initiated.

This move has some plausibility, but how is it to be interpreted? One way to mark this difference might be to contrast "action" and "inaction" and argue that moral responsibility, properly analyzed, attaches only to instances of positive action. If "refraining" is interpreted as "not acting," however, then this distinction is of little moral interest because it surely cannot be sustained. Refraining from something might often, though not always, involve *not moving*, but it surely cannot be analyzed as a species of inaction. This is perhaps best seen by comparing refraining with inadvertence. My behavior is inadvertent if I fail to pay attention to something or if I do something unintentionally. But it would not make sense to say that I refrained from something unintentionally or "by accident." The conceptual feature of "conscious attention" precludes analyzing "refraining" as a kind of inaction. Just the opposite is true, for refraining is not only an action but a special kind of action, one that involves reference to a conscious intention. Since we are prima facie responsible for the consequences of our actions one might argue, then, we are prima facie responsible for the consequences of our forbearing.

One might conclude on the basis of considerations like these that there is no significant moral difference between acting and refraining. This is essentially the position taken by Jonathan Bennett and Michael Tooley. Although they defend the position differently they both seem to agree that if the *only* difference between two courses of action is the difference between acting and refraining, then there is no significant *moral* difference between the two courses of action. This suggests that there is no significant moral difference between "killing" and "letting die," which in turn suggests that there is no defensible *moral* basis for analyzing (2), (3), and (4) as issues that are morally different from (1).

The conclusion is tempting for several reasons. The discussion of "refraining" seems to support strongly the claim that there is no intrinsic conceptual feature possessed by instances of forbearance that could underwrite the derived distinction. And surely it is the sheerest form of self-deception to assume that not feeding a child is somehow more "morally responsible" than "directly killing" it.

If we bracket (2), however, which it would be very difficult to defend, and restrict the further discussion to the killing involved in (1) and the letting die involved in (3) and (4), there is something to be said in defense of current medical practice. In particular, the difference between (1), on the one hand, and (3) and (4), on the other, bears directly on the justifiability of euthanasia.

It is typically argued by those in favor of euthanasia that there is a "right to die." The extreme thesis that all rights can be analyzed into obligations does not seem to be either a logical or a moral truth. However, there are a significant number of rights, typically those which depend on the performance or nonperformance of a particular action, which do underwrite obligations. In these performance situations, usually underwritten by either contract or positive law, for A to have a right means A's ability to *claim* something from B, to have something to press against him that, in justice, he owes to A. To assert this sort of right then is to assert something about the prima facie obligations of others.

The notion of "right to die" interpreted as "right to euthanasia" clearly falls under the classification of claims *to* a certain kind of performance. But if this is so then the coherence of "right to die" depends on the following assumption: if an individual has a right to euthanasia, then someone is obliged to kill him. This assumption, however, is extremely implausible. For it is not clear what it would mean to say that one individual is morally obliged to kill another. There are all sorts of reasons one might bring to bear on why it is merciful or perhaps kind to end someone's life. One might even argue that a doctor ought to, when requested by a patient, end the patient's suffering. Yet in each instance the doctor could deny that he is *obliged* to kill the patient, that is, he is not depriving the patient in justice of anything that is due to him. But if this is so then the concept of "right to die" loses it hold.

Some people might find this argument counterintuitive, that is, they might argue that from "A ought to do X for B" it follows, as a logical or moral truth, that B has a right against A. There is an important reason for not accepting any such claim. Basically we should keep distinct the issue of having good or even compelling reasons for doing something (i.e., "X ought to be done") from the issue of whether or not any individual has a right to X. The coherence of the latter notion, unlike the former, is contingent on the ability to assign a reasonable obligation, and it is just this that seems to be lacking with respect to the euthanasia issue.

The notion of "right to X" then is used to underwrite a rational demand that something be done to a specific individual. Insofar as it is

possible to defeat the latter demand, the claim to possess a right is cast in doubt. The instances that involve "letting die," on the other hand, place no such extraordinary demand on a doctor or any other person and hence are not contingent on the existence of such rights. There is, then, at least one interesting conceptual difference between acting and refraining and hence at least one prima facie reason for analyzing the issues in different ways. Hence, a doctor can reject a patient's claim to have a "right to die" if this means that the doctor is *obliged* to kill him. It is precisely because he is under no such obligation that there is no such right.

The assignment of obligations, of course, does not yet *settle* anything significant about the moral issues, but rather throws into sharp relief what is often really at issue in such discussions. We tend to assign obligations in terms of what we normally expect from one another, and such expectations often take the form of fairly determinate rules. A doctor who refrains from giving insulin to a diabetic is doing something wrong because of the reasonable expectations and assumptions of the doctor–patient relationship. A doctor who forbears from using all the available measures on a hopeless terminal case is not breaking any obligation because usually no one expects him to make use of them. What such observations show (as the discussion of PDE also shows) is that the issue that should play a central role in this moral discussion is not so much the narrow one of acting or refraining, but rather the rules that will define an appropriate and justifiable set of expectations. Since we are not, in the normal course of events, usually called on or required to account for the things that we let happen, then the claim that we merely "let something happen" is often a perfectly good and relevant moral reason for justifying our behavior. However, it is just as clear (for example, as articulated in child neglect laws) that the appeal to "letting something happen" is contingent for its moral justification on our understanding of what is and is not required or expected of one individual toward another.

Substantial moral progress on these questions, then, demands a careful and detailed account of what individuals *ought* to *expect* from one another, of what ought to be required from both sides of the doctor–patient relationship. What is the nature of "care," what limits does it have, what limits should it have? In short, complete and adequate understanding of the issues raised by the "acting–refraining" problem, as with virtually every other problem in medical ethics, presupposes an account of a humane, reasonable, and morally acceptable set of assumptions about medical care and treatment. If the debate on these issues is to continue, it should focus on the articulation of a reasonable set of presuppositions and not on the narrow issue of "acting" and "refraining."

HAROLD F. MOORE

[*Directly related is the entry* DOUBLE EFFECT. *This article will find application in the entries* ABORTION; *and* DEATH AND DYING: EUTHANASIA AND SUSTAINING LIFE, *article on* ETHICAL VIEWS. *For further discussion of topics mentioned in this article, see the entries:* CARE; RIGHTS; *and* THERAPEUTIC RELATIONSHIP. *Other relevant material may be found under* ETHICS, *article on* UTILITARIANISM; INFANTS, *articles on* ETHICAL PERSPECTIVES ON THE CARE OF INFANTS, *and* INFANTICIDE: A PHILOSOPHICAL PERSPECTIVE; *and* LIFE, *article on* VALUE OF LIFE.]

BIBLIOGRAPHY

ANSCOMBE, G. E. M. "Modern Moral Philosophy." *Philosophy* 33 (1958): 1–20.
AUNE, BRUCE. "Intention and Foresight." *Journal of Philosophy* 60 (1963): 652–654.
BENNETT, JONATHAN. "Whatever the Consequences." *Analysis* 26 (1966): 83–102.
BENTHAM, JEREMY. *Introduction to the Principles of Morals and Legislation* (1780). New York: Humanities Press, 1970.
CASEY, JOHN. "Actions and Consequences." *Morality and Moral Reasoning.* Edited by John Casey. London: Methuen, 1971, pp. 155–205.
DINELLO, DANIEL. "On Killing and Letting Die." *Analysis* 31 (1971): 84–86.
DUFF, R. A. "Intentionally Killing the Innocent." *Analysis* 34 (1973): 16–19.
FOOT, PHILIPPA. "Abortion and the Doctrine of Double Effect." *Moral Problems: A Collection of Political Essays.* Edited by James Rachels. New York: Harper & Row, 1971, pp. 28–41.
GEDDES, LEONARD. "On the Intrinsic Wrongness of Killing Innocent People." *Analysis* 33 (1973): 93–97.
GRISEZ, GERMAIN G. *Abortion: The Myths, the Realities, and the Arguments.* New York: Corpus Books, 1970.
HUGHES, GERARD J. "Killing and Letting Die." *Month* 2d n.s., 8 (1975): 42–45.
KNAUER, PETER. "The Hermeneutic Function of the Principle of the Double Effect." *Natural Law Forum* 12 (1967): 132–162.
MAGUIRE, DANIEL C. *Death by Choice.* Garden City, N.Y.: Doubleday & Co., 1974.
MANGAN, JOSEPH T. "An Historical Analysis of the Principle of Double Effect." *Theological Studies* 10 (1949): 41–61.
NOONAN, JOHN T., JR. "An Almost Absolute Value in History." *The Morality of Abortion: Legal and Historical Perspectives.* Edited by John T. Noonan, Jr. Cambridge: Harvard University Press, 1970, pp. 1–59.
RACHELS, JAMES. "Active and Passive Euthanasia." *New England Journal of Medicine* 292 (1975): 78–80.
RAMSEY, PAUL. *The Patient as Person.* New Haven: Yale University Press, 1970.
THOMAS AQUINAS. *Summa Theologiae*, II–II 64,6 and 64,7.
TOOLEY, MICHAEL. "Abortion and Infanticide." *Philosophy and Public Affairs* 2 (1972): 37–65.
WILLIAMS, GLANVILLE. *The Sanctity of Life and the Criminal Law.* New York: Knopf, 1957.

ADOLESCENTS

Adolescents (ages thirteen to eighteen) have been regarded as minors who need the consent of parents for most forms of medical treatment. This categorization of adolescents together with other minors is, however, controversial because the issues regarding the necessity of parental consent for the medical treatment of adolescents are different from those for children. Attention is rarely paid to the rights of adolescents vis-à-vis their parents, their physicians, and society (e.g., Katz).

This article is concerned with areas where ethical conflicts arise concerning the accepted cultural norm, the parents' wishes, the physicians' recommendations, and the adolescents' wishes and needs. Further, guidelines for adolescents within treatment and research programs are given. These are similar to those utilized when an adult is the patient or subject. The guidelines are presented in order to underscore their importance in the ethical treatment of each adolescent as an individual with rights for self-determination and needs for guidance.

Conflicts between adolescents' rights and the need for parental consent occur in connection with providing contraceptive devices, abortion, medical treatment for chronic drug or alcohol usage, and psychiatric treatment. These are the areas where adult ethical judgments are most widely divided. Treatments relating to sexuality are particularly frequent both because of cultural taboos (along with implicit encouragements for sexual experimentation) and because sexual maturity represents an area in which adolescents' capacities unquestionably differentiate them from younger minors. At times the need for parental consent is an issue because of parental disapproval of the treatment which the adolescent is requesting; but often it is the adolescent who wants to keep the medical treatment confidential because of fear or shame related to confiding in the parent.

The American Academy of Pediatrics Model Act of 1973, providing for consent of minors for health services, recommends that minors should be allowed to give consent for health services when they are "pregnant or afflicted with any reportable communicable diseases including venereal diseases, or drug and substance abuse including alcohol and nicotine. This self consent only applies to the prevention, diagnosis, and treatment of those conditions." Taken in its broadest context, the Model Act may be read as an advocacy of adolescent self-determination on the use of contraceptives and on the procedure of abortion, as one relates to "prevention" and the other, at least tangentially, to either "prevention" or "treatment" of pregnancy.

There are legal guidelines for certain medical treatments that are generally accepted. The age of the patient is not considered for some treatments. If the patient is below eighteen, parental consent is automatically required for other treatments. As an example of the former, in most states adolescents can obtain treatment for venereal disease without the knowledge and consent of their parents. The therapeutic contract is made between the physician and the adolescent with society's sanction and legal protection. Similarly, any treatments deemed to be emergency procedures do not require parental consent for any minors, be they adolescents or children. On the opposite end of the spectrum are other areas of medical treatment for which the consent of the parent is not considered an issue of controversy but accepted as necessary. As a seldom disputed example, if an adolescent wants to have plastic surgery for cosmetic reasons, almost all physicians would require consent from the parents or legal guardians. In relation to the need for parental consent, age or psychological variables such as levels of maturity become issues of ethical concern when the treatment requested is not seen to have a fairly clearly definable physical necessity.

Relationship between age and psychological maturity

Legislators and citizens are continuously grappling with the extent to which the state serves as a protector by legislating "rights" through arbitrary points such as age. Except in unusual cases where parents are deemed incompetent, parents assume the responsibility for their children under the age of thirteen. The law ought to differentiate the youth who attains biological and possibly cognitive maturity during adolescence (Inhelder and Piaget), both from the child whose capacities are less developed and from the adult who has had more years of experience. Adolescents' rights, however, have been minimized, or simply not considered apart from those of minors in general. The legal profession and society at large have, because of a lack of better criteria, used the arbitrary age of eighteen as representing maturity. One reason suggested for the failure to regard adolescents as different from younger children has been a fear that the result would be the deterioration of the family unit (Emson).

Within the period of adolescence, the mere age of an individual may not reflect adequately the level of psychological and physiological maturity. Recent research in a small subsample of adolescents has demonstrated that certain adolescents develop cognitively and emotionally at age fifteen far beyond their peers at age eighteen (Hatcher). Hatcher's study of a homogeneous population of thirteen unwed pregnant adolescents suggested a strong developmental determinant in how the young women reacted to the pregnancies and abortions. From an analysis of interviews and projective test material, three clinical and statistical patterns of adjusting to the experience emerged. The ability to cope with both the pregnancy and subsequent abortion related to the maturity level of the adolescent girls, whereas coping capacities did not correlate with age of the adolescent.

Maturity as a measure of self-determination?

Even if the intent were to correct for the psychological differences among peers of the same age, methodological complications interfere. How confident are we of the reliability and validity of psychological measurements? Within the behavioral and social sciences, when reliable and valid measurements of maturity are attainable, further questions have to be asked: For whom is the treatment, under what circumstances, and what are the personal values of the people involved? These determinations involve definitions or conceptualizations of normality, health, and maturity that can relate the type of treatment sought to the context in which the adolescent is functioning. Is a consensual understanding of what is normal or healthy for a particular adolescent obtainable?

Normality has been described as having four perspectives: (1) *Normality as health* is the traditional medical approach to health and illness; behavior is within normal limits when no gross psychopathology is present. (2) *Normality as utopia* conceives of normality as a harmonious and optimal blending of diverse elements of the mental apparatus that culminates in optimal functioning. (3) *Normality as average* is based on a mathematical principle of the bell-shaped curve; the middle range is normal and both extremes are deviant. (4) *Normality as transactional systems* defines normality as an integration of bio-psychosocial variables over a period of time (Offer and Sabshin). Definitions of normality or health will differ according to the perspective utilized for the definition, the particular cultural contexts, and the psychology of the individual adolescent within the sociological and cultural context (ibid.).

The range in conceptualizations of normality makes elimination of age-related restrictions problematic. However, our inability clearly to define measurable criteria of maturity, to determine a stage where a person is cognitively and emotionally able to make relatively sound decisions concerning his or her physical and emotional welfare, does not mean that we have to maintain the legal status quo. The difficulties in replacing age-related laws requiring parental consent do not mean that these laws should be retained without qualification.

What is the effect of a request for parental consent? Is the adolescent being protected by the request for parental consent or is this request a denial of one's rights as a person separate from one's parents? Does abdicating the need for parental consent give too much power to the physician vis-à-vis the relatively inexperienced adolescent, and, alternatively, is it justifiable to assume that the parent provides reasonable protection?

Judgment by the physician on the "mature minor"

Particularly in the areas which we have mentioned above, the physician needs to evaluate the adolescent's capacity to make reasonable decisions concerning his or her future. If the physician believes that the adolescent is capable of making sound decisions, the patient, at the very least, ought to be classified under the category of "mature minor" (American Academy of Pediatrics, 1974). Similarly, the American Academy of Pediatrics Model Act of 1973 recommends that the minor assume responsibility for medical treatment when he or she seems to the physician to "be capable of making rational decisions."

Recognizing the maturity of the adolescent patient renders treatment of the adolescent subject to the same potential judgmental biases as are present in the treatment of the adult patient. If the physician feels that the adult patient or research subject cannot grasp the significance of the situation, the physician consults relatives (or in extreme situations, the courts) to act on behalf of the best interests of the patient. This same procedure can be followed for the adolescent patient. If the physician has serious doubts about the appropriateness of treatment of an adolescent, the physician ought to consult colleagues, parents, and in some cases the courts. An adolescent should be encouraged to proceed with parental knowledge and consent but not required to do so unless, in the physician's opinion, the individual case necessitates parental consent. Thus, the physician's judgment is substituted for state or federal laws, in which individual personality assessments are not taken into consideration.

There are no scientifically based criteria to aid the physician in deciding the level and extent of maturity. It is frequently assumed that the physician will automatically know when a minor is mature enough to make the "rational decision." The further question to be asked is, How often are individuals of any age who are coming for treatment in a position to be able to use their capacities for making rational and abstract judgments when their own bodies or minds are the "patients"?

Ideally, of course, "rational decision" should be reached by all parties: the patient, the family, the physician, and the society. Where differences arise concerning the nature of rationality, the weight ought to go to the adolescent patient's decision, with the agreement of a qualified physician. The physician, in turn, should examine the decision in the light of recommendations from his or her medical specialty.

What criteria do physicians use to arrive at these decisions? At times, factors other than the welfare of the patient are likely to be involved in the physician's decision to proceed without the consent of the adolescent's parents. Physicians, for example, might be influenced by their own inability to communicate effectively with parents or by an identification with some young patients and their overt rebellion against parental authority. On the other hand, there may be a psychological need on the part of the physician, in order to feel justified in his decision, to share all his knowledge concerning the adolescent patient with the parents. In the latter case, if this might be to the detriment of the patient's well-being, an ethical problem arises.

The physician has an obligation to adolescents not to abuse their confidence; yet the physician should respond when the adolescent's statement seems to contain an indirect plea to the physician to intervene and provide the patient with familial or legal supports which the adolescent has been emotionally unable to request directly. These are the cases where the physician judges that the patient wants guidance. Then, the doctor ought to require some sort of adult consent. This would come from the parents or, in special circumstances, from a "patient advocate." The patient should be refused treatment when the doctor believes that the greater harm would come from performing the treatment without parental or other guidance than from the neglect of the treatment requested.

In some cases, physicians' ethical beliefs prevent them from complying with adolescents' medical requests; this is most prevalent in cases involving requests for abortions or contraceptive pills. Here the physician is responding neither to the maturity level of the patient nor to the legal status of the treatment. Under these circumstances, physicians should discuss their beliefs with the adolescent patients. When the physician's ethical beliefs conflict with those of the adolescent, the patient should be referred to a medical colleague who does not share the physician's ethical beliefs and who can act in accordance with both good medical judgment and the rights of the patient involved.

The adolescent in psychotherapy

Under what conditions should an adolescent be allowed to obtain psychiatric treatment without the knowledge and consent of parents or legal guardians? Is it only when a medical emergency is involved that endangers the young person's life, such as a suicidal patient?

The high school student can consult his or her high school counselor, who is paid by the Board of Education. The student sees the counselor once or twice a week for therapy or counseling. These sessions are not labeled as psychiatric treatment and, therefore, there is no need to obtain permission from the parents. Most of these counselors do practice psychodynamically or behaviorally oriented psychotherapy. But because they are not psychiatrists, they

are not, by definition, delivering medical care, and hence no consent is needed. Is there really a significant difference between the adolescent choosing therapy in the high school and the teenager going to a mental health clinic—a difference significant enough to make parental consent necessary for the one treatment and not for the other?

The adolescent may go to a medical clinic seeking psychiatric treatment for relief of depression. The depression may not be severe enough to endanger the teenager's life with suicide, yet there is much discomfort and agitation. The parents of this adolescent may be unwilling to let their child undergo psychiatric treatment because of a disbelief in the validity of psychiatric treatment, an unwillingness to accept the fact that they, the parents, cannot help their own child, or a resentment against the child, feeling that he or she is not "trying" hard enough to function adequately. Here the adolescent's rights conflict with parental judgments. Is it for the society to legislate or for the physician to decide based on his or her knowledge of the case? If the latter, there would be a bias in favor of treatment, as this is the tool the physician has been trained to value and provide. Yet the laws in most states are explicit in stating that the parents have the right to decide whether their child will enter psychotherapy or not (Shlensky). This legal bias seems to collide with the rights of adolescents and generally to disregard their ability to seek help in situations where parents or parental decisions may be irrational. Thus, the parents' irrationality may be legally sanctioned while the rights of the adolescent are ignored.

The right of adolescents to refuse therapy is less clear cut. They can refuse therapy and can make the therapist's role meaningless if they choose not to cooperate. Most psychiatrists know that they cannot effectively treat an adolescent without his or her consent. However, parents, physicians, and courts together can require psychotherapy in the face of the adolescent's refusal when the adolescent is adjudged to be incapable of recognizing his or her needs. Thus, the adolescent's right to refuse psychotherapy is a right which, under certain circumstances, can be countermanded.

Confidentiality

Once treatment has begun, the physician should have absolute protection under the law regarding confidentiality. After proper consent has been given, the patient and the physician enter into a mutual contract of confidentiality. Medical records should not be released to a third party without the written consent of the adolescent patient (Hofmann). This means that the physician's obligation is to the adolescent patients, and only when patients agree should physicians communicate with families, insurance investigators, or educational institutions.

Informed consent within treatment and research programs

In any treatment, objective information must be provided in a manner understandable to both adolescent and parents, where parents are involved. Where a patient is a control for a research project, knowledge of an involvement as a control and of the research as a whole must be provided. Patients should have the knowledge that enables them to accept or reject the treatment program in which they are involved. In areas of insufficient knowledge, patients should be informed of the parameters of what is known and what is hypothesized.

In situations where current theory and practice provide any indication that one treatment is preferable to another, the more generally accepted treatment should be given to the patient unless there is truly informed consent for being a part of an experimental program, where the results have not been demonstrated.

The word "demonstrated" is undoubtedly open to a sliding scale of truths. We must continue our research while treating patients according to our most educated guesses. How best to protect the interest and well-being of the individual yet not stagnate or eliminate research has been a burning issue for some years (Duffy). The American Medical Association has set relatively strict ethical guidelines for clinical investigation (American Medical Association, pp. 10–12). One of the crucial requirements is for the adolescent patient to be informed of the limitations and potential dangers of research undertaken. Consent for participation is meaningless unless it is informed consent.

As psychiatric researchers we suggest the use of empathy, of putting oneself in the other's place, when deciding how much should be told. A study of doctors at Michael Reese Hospital in Chicago reported that ninety percent of doctors did not believe in telling their patients that they had cancer. However, sixty percent of doctors said that they themselves would, in a similar situation, prefer to be told the truth (Oken). A

conclusion might be that doctors are not identifying with their patient population but rather consider themselves to be in a class by themselves.

In research on normal adolescent subjects, who have not approached the physician with a request for treatment, knowledge of the use of the data must form a part of a "research alliance" between adolescent and physician. The physician should assess the psychological significance of the relationship with the subject and take precautions against creating situations in which the subject's coping may be threatened without adequate supports applied. When a normal subject in a research project requests aid, the role of the physician–researcher must shift to provide the necessary humane aid or referrals. In cases where requests have not been made but the physician sees a dangerous situation developing, he or she owes it to the subject to intervene. Above all, however, the researchers working with a normal adolescent population must be careful not to intervene too much, intervention being the role to which the physician is more accustomed. Medical researchers must be aware of personal value judgments and must try to empathize with the subject, in this case the adolescent, without influencing the subject where no psychological issue of danger is involved. The physician should not be engaged in sociological engineering unless that has been the stated purpose of the research, and informed consent has been obtained.

In our study of normal male adolescents (Offer and Offer) we followed the guidelines stated above. The investigation began when the subjects were fourteen and continued until the young men were twenty-two. During the selection process, schools, parents, and the high school freshmen were informed of the purposes and extent of the study, and their consents were obtained. We developed the concept of a research alliance, contrasted to a therapeutic alliance. We wanted to gain the subjects' trust and cooperation but were not providing the usual contracts for psychiatric treatment. We needed to be careful not to seduce the subjects into cooperation by allowing them to assume that, since the interviewers were psychiatrists, there was an implicit agreement to treat them. In addition, the psychiatrists had to change their usual role orientation. This was done through the timing of interviews. Throughout the high school years we saw the young men once every four months in order to encourage continued long-term involvement of the teenagers; we believed that this interval was infrequent enough to avoid interfering with their own modes of functioning. The interviews were semi-structured, and care was taken not to delve too deeply when resistance became manifest. In psychiatric research, the resistance would be noted; in psychiatric therapy, it might have been challenged.

Where are the physicians' values and the values of the parents most likely to collide? In our research on normal adolescents, we found the adult population to take most offense when questions about sexual behavior were asked. Here, it was our value judgment that the adolescents would not become sexually active just because they were questioned about their sexuality. Further, we believed that our inquiries would, and did, provide relief to the subject in an area where discussion had often been taboo. This is an example of the predominance of the researcher's value judgments, which are operative within any study. They can, and should, be checked through peer and institutional review in order to ensure that the researchers do not act in a way that is considered to be professionally deviant. Where general societal dictates are contradictory, the researchers' point of view should be ethically acceptable within their field of specialization. What is most necessary is for researchers to be aware of influences upon their subjects and to understand their own biases while logically defending the tactics being utilized to the satisfaction of a professionally accredited medical society.

The researcher and the clinician

Need there be a conflict between researcher and clinician? Within medicine, and certainly within patient care, the researcher and the clinician are often the same individual. The major difference between the labels "researcher" and "clinician" is the systematized way in which data are used, observed, and communicated; possibly, there is also a difference in selectivity of populations treated. These differences should not affect quality of treatment; they are pertinent to use of data rather than to quality of care. Dangerous situations may arise when the researchers disregard the informed consent strictures mentioned above. Advantages for the patient within the research setting must also be noted. These may be provided through the sophistication of knowledge within a highly specialized area that researchers may have or

through possible benefits arising from experimental situations. Here we speak of the individual adolescent patient. Clearly, for the society research must be continued in order to advance clinical care. Without it, we can only repeat the same mistakes. In this section attention has not been directed to the need for research, which ought to be self-evident. Our consideration is for the rights of the adolescent patient within the research program, the research itself being a necessity for the advancement of knowledge in any scientific field (Offer, Freedman, and Offer).

Conclusion

Adolescence should be understood as a separate stage of human development with its own tasks and solutions, its specific problems, and moral and legal considerations that differentiate it from both childhood and adulthood.

Decisions on the appropriate response to an adolescent requesting medical care ought to be flexible enough to take into consideration variances pertaining to the individual's level of maturity and the nature of the treatment requested. The need for parental consent for adolescent medical treatment may serve as a detriment to the adolescent, rather than as a protection for the youth's health. Although many adolescents do not attain cognitive and emotional maturity, this does not differentiate them from much of the adult community. Maturity cannot be defined by age alone. The concepts of "mature minor" and "rational decision" are particularly applicable to the adolescent years. In all research and treatment cases the right of the adolescent to give informed consent must be respected. A plan has been entered for the treatment of the psyche as well as the soma of the adolescent patient. The ability to put oneself in the place of the adolescent and of the adolescent's parents might well be the most important determinant in the physician's ethical–medical judgments.

Daniel Offer and Judith B. Offer

[*For further discussion of topics mentioned in this article, see the entries:* Abortion; Confidentiality; Contraception; Informed Consent in Human Research; *and* Informed Consent in the Therapeutic Relationship. *Also directly related are the entries* Children and Biomedicine; Paternalism; Person; Right to Refuse Medical Care; Rights; Sexual Development; Therapeutic Relationship; *and* Truth-Telling. *See* Appendix, Section III, pediatric bill of rights.]

BIBLIOGRAPHY

American Academy of Pediatrics, Committee on Youth. "The Implications of Minor's Consent Legislation for Adolescent Health Care: A Commentary." *Pediatrics* 54 (1974): 481–485.

————. "A Model Act Providing for Consent of Minors for Health Services." *Pediatrics* 51 (1973): 293–296.

American Medical Association, Judicial Council. *Opinions and Reports of the Judicial Council.* Chicago: 1971.

DUFFY, JOHN C. "Research with Children: The Rights of Children." *Child Psychiatry and Human Development* 4 (1973): 67–70.

EMSON, H. E. "The Age of Consent." *Canadian Medical Association Journal* 109 (1973): 687–688.

HATCHER, SHERRY L. M. "The Adolescent Experience of Pregnancy and Abortion: A Developmental Analysis." *Journal of Youth and Adolescence* 2 (1973): 53–102.

HOFMANN, ADELE D. "Confidentiality and the Health Care Records of Children and Youth." *Psychiatric Opinion* 12, no. 1 (1975), pp. 20–28.

INHELDER, BÄRBEL, and PIAGET, JEAN. *The Growth of Logical Thinking from Childhood to Adolescence.* New York: Basic Books, 1958.

KATZ, JAY, with the assistance of CAPRON, ALEXANDER, and GLASS, ELEANOR S. *Experimentation with Human Beings.* New York: Russell Sage Foundation, 1972.

OFFER, DANIEL; FREEDMAN, DANIEL X.; and OFFER, JUDITH L. "The Psychiatrist as Researcher." *Modern Psychiatry and Clinical Research.* Edited by Daniel Offer and Daniel X. Freedman. New York: Basic Books, 1972, pp. 208–233.

————, and OFFER, JUDITH L. *From Teenager to Young Manhood: A Psychological Study.* New York: Basic Books, 1975.

————, and SABSHIN, MELVIN. *Normality: Theoretical and Clinical Concepts of Mental Health.* Rev. ed. New York: Basic Books, 1974.

OKEN, D. "What to Tell Cancer Patients—A Study of Medical Attitudes." *Journal of the American Medical Association* 175 (1961): 1120–1128.

SHLENSKY, RONALD. "Minors' Rights to Psychiatric Outpatient Treatment without Parental Consent in Illinois." *Illinois Bar Journal* 61 (1973): 650–652.

ADVERTISING BY MEDICAL PROFESSIONALS

Advertising by medical professionals is adjudged to be generally unethical in all countries where physicians have established their professional identity. The International Code of Medical Ethics, adopted by the World Medical Association in October 1949, declares unethical "any self-advertisement, except such as is expressly authorized by the national code of medical ethics" (World Medical Association).

Professional codes of ethics typically adopt broad definitions of prohibited advertising. Thus, for example, the British General Medical Council defines "the professional offence of advertising . . . [as arising] from the publication (in any form) of matter commending or drawing attention to the professional skill, knowledge, services, or qualifications of one or more doctors, when the doctor or doctors concerned have instigated or sanctioned such publication primarily or to a substantial extent for the purpose of obtaining patients or otherwise promoting their own professional advantage or financial benefit" (British Medical Association, p. 52). Professional organizations typically attempt to justify such strictures on public interest grounds. Thus, the British Medical Association expresses the conviction that "in taking up the attitude of determined opposition to undesirable methods of publicity it is acting in the best interests of the public as well as of the medical profession" (ibid., p. 42).

Restrictions in the United States

Advertising of physicians' services in the United States has long been restricted by the Principles of Medical Ethics of the American Medical Association (AMA). Formulation of the ethical principle has varied over time, but since 1957 it has read simply, "He [the physician] should not solicit patients." State and local medical societies have maintained similar restrictions and are recognized by the AMA as having the responsibility for giving specific content to the general principles to reflect "local custom" and "local ideals." Though long accepted and actively enforced, the professional restriction against advertising has recently come under attack in the United States and may be subject to significant curtailment under emerging legal principles.

On numerous occasions, the AMA Judicial Council has expressed its views on the meaning and purpose of the AMA rule against solicitation of patients: "The practice of medicine should not be commercialized or treated as a commodity in trade. Respecting the dignity of their calling, physicians should resort only to the most limited use of advertising and then only to the extent necessary to serve the common good and improve the health of mankind" (American Medical Association, p. 27). "Self-laudations defy the traditions and lower the moral standard of the medical profession; they are an infraction of good taste and are disapproved" (ibid., p. 23). The Judicial Council defines *advertising* as "making information or intention known to the public" and contrasts it with *solicitation*, which involves "the attempt to obtain patients by persuasion or influence" through the use of "testimonials," creating "unjustified expectations," implying superior skills, or deceiving the consumer ("AMA Clarifies Policy"). This fuller delineation of "solicitation" was provided in a 1976 statement issued following the filing of an antitrust action against the AMA's restrictions by the Federal Trade Commission. Though offered as a clarification, this statement may have liberalized the AMA's earlier position.

With respect to the scope of the ethical constraint, the Judicial Council concludes that "the public is entitled to know the name of physicians, the type of their practices, the location of their offices, their office hours," and the like (American Medical Association, p. 24). Increased specificity is supplied in the 1976 statement, which allows the giving of some fee information and "biographical and other relevant data." This seeming liberalization is qualified, however, by the use of such unspecific terms as "relevant data" and the requirement that information not be "misleading or deceptive," formulations that would allow professional societies considerable leeway to challenge individual doctors' attempts to convey information to the public.

Physicians "may furnish this information through the accepted local media of advertising and communication . . . [such as] dignified announcements, telephone directory listings and reputable directories" ("AMA Clarifies Policy"). Newspapers are not mentioned, though "the particular use to be made of any medium of communication and the extent of that use are . . . matters to be determined according to local ideals" (American Medical Association, p. 24).

Enforcement of the restriction on advertising may be by the local medical society itself, through means ranging from informal warnings to termination of society membership. In some thirty-four states, however, a statutory prohibition of advertising by physicians allows the state board of medical examiners also to police excesses. Where the law prohibits merely "unprofessional conduct" or the like, the state board will frequently define such conduct in accordance with ethical codes of state or local medical societies. Normally the threat of being charged with unethical conduct is an effective enough deterrent to physicians, although stronger punishments are occasionally imposed.

One area of frequent difficulty has been how to regard publicity given to a physician for either medical or nonmedical accomplishments. The AMA states that a physician's name may appear in "the reporting of proper news" and in connection with civic projects, but that he may not initiate or encourage its use in a news story (ibid., p. 29). Televised interviews with physicians in various capacities are now common and present recurrent problems, especially where the interview appears to boost the physician's book on a medical topic or his style of medical practice.

Justifications for restrictions on medical advertising

The historical justification for the ban on advertising was the perceived need to distinguish quackery from ethical professionalism. The 1920 Code of Ethics of the Massachusetts Medical Society stated, "The distinction between legitimate medicine and quackery should be clearly maintained. Physicians should not advertise their methods of practice" (Massachusetts Medical Society). In the years prior to 1920, when medical science had relatively little to offer to patients in comparison with today, the profession sought to enhance its reputation by substituting cooperation for competition, repressing extramural criticism of individual physicians, and cultivating primary consumer reliance on the profession's image and the individual practitioner's general reputation rather than on his advertised specific qualifications. The Massachusetts code of 1920 provided that "a spirit of competition considered honorable in purely business transactions cannot exist among physicians without diminishing their usefulness and lowering the dignity and standing of the profession" (ibid.). In contrast, the AMA Judicial Council says, "Freedom of choice of physician and free competition among physicians are prerequisites of optimal medical care" ("AMA Clarifies Policy").

Although the policy against advertising originated as part of the early strategy of raising the practice of medicine to "professional" status, the asserted justifications for a restrictive policy have not changed much today. Even though licensure laws have long since removed most unqualified practitioners and the profession has gained the power to remove any remaining ones, the AMA Judicial Council still contends that the advertising ban "protects the public from the advertiser and salesman of medical care by establishing an easily discernible . . . distinction between him and the ethical physician" (American Medical Association, p. 23). Though now conceding that competition has a role, the Judicial Council's position is still that "[s]ome competitive practices accepted in ordinary commercial and industrial enterprises . . . are inappropriate among physicians" ("AMA Clarifies Policy"). The extent of the difference between professional and commercial standards is likely to be established ultimately by the courts, which have frequently conceded that such a difference exists.

While the profession's concerns are largely unchanged, modern conditions may put advertising in a somewhat different light. For example, the technical advances in medicine, in addition to increasing the patient's stake in the physician's skill, may have strengthened the argument that the consumer cannot make the necessary judgments concerning quality of care and should therefore not be trusted with possibly misleading information. Price information in particular may be regarded as difficult to evaluate and misleading in view of the widely variable content and quality of the services rendered. To compensate for the consumer's presumed inadequacy, the medical profession has purported to accept primary responsibility for maintaining the quality of care through peer oversight of practitioners. Moreover, in lieu of expecting consumers to find attentive care through the trial-and-error process of shopping, ethical standards are supposed to assure the consumer of the physician's commitment and concern. The profession is regularly criticized, however, for failing to police the quality of care effectively and for not sharing information with patients in the course of treatment in accordance with the legal and ethical requirements of informed consent. The ethical limitation on advertising, in denying consumers quality-related information and the opportunity to exercise judgment, may thus be seen as part of the larger ethical issue of professional dominance.

The repression of advertising can also be seen as an important aspect of the broad policy issue in medical care of the role and reliability of consumer choice and market forces on the one hand versus efficacy of regulatory and professional cost and quality controls on the other. Inflation in the mid-1970s caused heightened concern that regulatory restraints of all kinds, including restrictions on professional advertising, tend to increase prices, a fear confirmed in a widely cited study of state restrictions on opticians' advertising of eyeglass prices (Benham, p. 344). If primary reliance is to be placed on regulation and controls to guide the health industry's per-

formance, then advertising's utility will be limited, but questions currently being raised about advertising restrictions may reflect distrust of these mechanisms.

Impact on institutional providers

In recent years some important changes have taken place in the organization of medical care delivery and in the nature of financing mechanisms. Advertising has been important in informing consumers of some of these developments. The AMA's 1953 principles held that "solicitation of patients, directly or indirectly, by a physician, by groups of physicians or by institutions or organizations, is unethical." After the formulation of the basic principle was shortened in 1957, the AMA restated the foregoing language as part of its textual explication, omitting the reference to "institutions and organizations." This omission suggested that the new principles were addressed to medical practitioners alone and were not to govern institutional behavior, but group practices were advised that "no physician-member of a clinic may permit the clinic to do that which he may not do" (American Medical Association, p. 3). Advertising by prepaid group practices and—to use the newer, broader term—health maintenance organizations (HMOs), has been actively restricted by some medical societies under this principle. In some areas flexibility has prevailed, but HMOs have generally confined themselves to advertising only the availability of their services and perhaps the monthly rate, eschewing mention of their physicians' qualifications.

Some states have enacted legislation clarifying HMOs' right to advertise. California's Knox–Keene Health Care Service Act of 1975, following earlier legislation, imposes some controls while generally permitting the practice. Most important, the federal Health Maintenance Organization Act of 1973 explicitly declared inoperative with respect to certain HMOs those state laws which would prevent such HMOs from "soliciting members through advertising its services, charges, or other nonprofessional aspects of its operation." Significantly, however, it specifies that it "does not authorize any advertising which identifies, refers to or makes any qualitative judgment concerning, any health professional."

Legal issues

Until 1975 restrictions on advertising appeared to be immune from legal attack. "Free speech" arguments against statutory or regulatory restrictions appeared to be foreclosed by a 1942 Supreme Court ruling that suggested that advertising, as "commercial speech," was outside the scope of First Amendment protection (*Valentine* v. *Chrestensen*). Restrictions imposed through professional societies' ethical codes also appeared valid because the antitrust laws, prohibiting anticompetitive agreements, had never been held to apply to the so-called learned professions.

Both of these immunizing doctrines were subsequently discredited by the Supreme Court. In 1975 the antitrust laws were held to apply to the legal profession (*Goldfarb* v. *Virginia State Bar*), and shortly thereafter the Federal Trade Commission, following this lead, instituted an action against the AMA and professional associations in Connecticut, charging that their efforts to prevent their members from "soliciting business, by advertising or otherwise," violated federal law (Federal Trade Commission, 1975, p. 2). In a 1976 case the Supreme Court held unconstitutional a Virginia law prohibiting the advertising of prescription drug prices, stressing the consumer's First Amendment right to receive useful information through advertising; the Court discounted the state's argument that advertising was antithetical to high professional standards in pharmacy (*Virginia State Board of Pharmacy* v. *Virginia Citizens' Consumer Council*). In 1977, the Court extended this analysis to the legal profession, holding in a five-to-four decision that lawyers cannot be prohibited from using newspaper advertisements to disclose the price of routine services (*Bates* v. *State Bar of Arizona*).

The meaning of these developments for the advertising of medical services is not clear. One lower court has recognized consumers' right not to be denied the basic facts to be included in a physician directory prepared by a health planning agency (*Health Systems Agency of Northern Virginia* v. *Virginia State Board of Medicine*). More commercial types of advertising may still be subject to curtailment, however, under arguments different from those advanced against lawyers' advertisements in the *Bates* case. For example, a nontraditional but possibly convincing argument might focus on the danger of inducing overutilization of medical services by beneficiaries of insurance plans or governmental programs. Finally, advertising that in any way touts the quality of professional services is likely to be regarded with particular suspicion.

Issues about professional advertising that were long dormant seem now to be open for public debate and ultimate judicial resolution. The renewal of interest in this subject caused an apparent liberalization of the AMA's position in 1976 and changed the focus from whether doctors should be permitted to advertise to how they should be permitted to do so. New guidelines, developed not by the profession unilaterally but under public pressure and with some public input, appear to be in the offing.

CLARK C. HAVIGHURST

[*For the proscriptions against advertising medical and other health-care professions, see:* CODES OF MEDICAL ETHICS, *article on* ETHICAL ANALYSIS; DENTISTRY, *article on* ETHICAL ISSUES IN DENTISTRY; PHARMACY; APPENDIX, INTRODUCTION, *article on* CODES OF THE HEALTH-CARE PROFESSIONS. *For the text of such codes, see* APPENDIX, SECTION I: GENERAL CODES FOR THE PRACTICE OF MEDICINE; *and* SECTION IV: CODES OF SPECIALTY HEALTH-CARE ASSOCIATIONS. *See also:* COMMUNICATION, BIOMEDICAL; MEDICAL PROFESSION; *and* ORTHODOXY IN MEDICINE. *For a discussion of advertising of drugs by pharmaceutical companies, see:* DRUG INDUSTRY AND MEDICINE.]

BIBLIOGRAPHY

"AMA Clarifies Policy on Advertising by MDs." *American Medical News*, 19 April 1976, p. 9.

American Medical Association, Judicial Council. *Opinions and Reports of the Judicial Council, Including the Principles of Medical Ethics and Rules of the Judicial Council.* Chicago: American Medical Association, 1971, pp. 22–29.

"The American Medical Association: Power, Purpose, and Politics in Organized Medicine." *Yale Law Journal* 63 (1954): 937–1022.

Bates v. State Bar of Arizona. 45 U.S.L.W. 4895 (1977). U.S. Sup. Ct. Dkt. No. 76-316, argued 18 January 1977.

BENHAM, LEE. "The Effect of Advertising on the Price of Eyeglasses." *Journal of Law and Economics* 15 (1972): 337–352.

British Medical Association. *Medical Ethics.* London: 1974.

Federal Trade Commission, Complaint. *In Re American Medical Association, Connecticut State Medical Society, and New Haven Medical Association.* Docket no. 9064, filed 19 December 1975. Available on request from the Federal Trade Commission.

Goldfarb v. Virginia State Bar. 421 U.S. 773. 44 L.Ed.2d 572. 92 S. Ct. 2004 (1975).

Health Systems Agency of Northern Virginia v. Virginia State Board of Medicine. 424 F. Supp. 2d 267 (1976).

KESSEL, REUBEN A. "Price Discrimination in Medicine." *Journal of Law and Economics* 1 (1958): 20–53.

"Knox–Keene Health Care Service Plan Act of 1975." *California Health and Safety Code.* § 1340–1395 (Supp. 1975).

Konold, Donald. *A History of American Medical Ethics 1847–1912*. Madison: State Historical Society of Wisconsin, 1962.

Massachusetts Medical Society. "Code of Ethics of the Massachusetts Medical Society." *Massachusetts Medical Society: Its Services and Functions*. Boston: 1961, p. 48. Adopted 9 June 1920.

"Restrictive State Laws and Practices." "Health Maintenance Organization Act of 1973." Pub. L. 93–222 Sec. 1311 § 2(b); 87 Stat. 931; 42 U.S.C. § 300e–10(b) (1974).

Semler v. Oregon State Board of Dental Examiners. 294 U.S. 608. 79 L.Ed. 1086 (1935).

Valentine v. Chrestensen. 316 U.S. 52. 86 L.Ed. 1262 (1942).

Virginia State Board of Pharmacy v. Virginia Citizens Consumer Council. 425 U.S. 748. 48 L. Ed. 2d 346. 96 S. Ct. 1817 (1976).

World Medical Association. *International Code of Medical Ethics*. London: Third General Assembly of The World Medical Association, 1949. Printed single sheet. Text in Appendix. Also in *World Medical Association Bulletin* 1 (1949): 109, and in *World Medical Journal* 3 (1956), Supplement, p. 12.

ADVERTISING OF DRUGS

See Pharmacy; Communication, Biomedical, *article on* Media and Medicine; Drug Industry and Medicine.

AFRICA

See Medical Ethics, History of, *section on* Near and Middle East and Africa, *article on* Sub-Saharan Africa.

AGING AND THE AGED

I
THEORIES OF AGING AND ANTI-AGING TECHNIQUES

Theories of aging

Probably no other area of biological inquiry is susceptible to so many theories as is the science of gerontology. This occurs not only because of a lack of sufficient fundamental data but also because manifestations of biological changes with time affect almost all biological systems from the molecular level up to that of the whole organism. It is therefore easy to construct a theory of aging based on a biological decrement (or decline) that may be observed to occur in time in any system at the level of the molecule, cell, tissue, organ, or whole animal. The significant question will always be: Is the change observed a direct cause of aging or is it the result of changes that may be occurring at a more fundamental level?

If the modern notions of biological development are rooted in signals originating from information-containing molecules, then it would seem reasonable to attribute postdevelopmental changes to a similar system of signals occurring at the molecular level. The following example might be illustrative: One current theory of aging rests on decrements occurring with time in the immune system such that individuals are less able to deal with infections or antibodies "mistakenly" produced against their own cells. Either or both of these events would lead to a reduced ability to deal with environmental insults, and thus an increasing force of mortality would result. That such events might occur cannot be wholly denied, but this logic would suggest that, conversely, "maturation" of the immune system in early life controls development of the animal. Conventional wisdom does not accept this as a likely possibility.

If age changes are caused by fundamental changes in information-containing molecules that result, in chain-reaction fashion, in physiological decrements at higher organizational levels—that is, cell, tissue, organ, whole animal—then the most tenable theories of aging are those based on molecular events occurring in the genetic apparatus.

Error theories. Orgel developed a model for biological aging that is dependent upon a decrease in the fidelity of protein synthesis. In this way an accumulation of errors is thought to occur in enzyme synthesizing systems such that faulty proteins would be specified leading to decrements in cell function. Evidence both for and against this hypothesis has been obtained, although there is currently (1976) a greater preponderance of negative data.

Redundant message theory. Although partly based on error accumulation, Medvedev suggests an interesting alternative hypothesis (Medvedev). His conceptions are based on the fact that within each cell the genetic message is written in a highly redundant fashion. That is, each bit of information can be specified by a number of genes, only one of which functions at any given time. As errors accumulate in the expressed gene, it is repressed, and a second gene providing the same information becomes expressed, once again maintaining the fidelity of protein synthesis. This cycle can occur repeatedly as reserve genes become expressed after functioning genes accumulate errors and become repressed. The well-recognized differences in the life spans of animal species are conjectured to be a manifestation of the degree of gene repetition. Engineers are very familiar with the principle whereby the greater the number of "back-up" systems available for an essential function, the greater the likelihood that the total machine will not fail. A repeated information system simply has a greater chance of preserving intact the integrity of any complex system, although with time ultimate failure is inescapable.

The theory that aging is caused by gene mutations has several advocates (Burnet; Curtis; Szilard), yet the failure of this theory to explain the quantitative aspects of normal and radiation-accelerated aging has been repeatedly observed (Alexander; Clark; Strehler, 1959).

Molecular cross-linking. This thesis, championed by von Hahn, is based on several a priori assumptions, the most important of which is that there exists a universal physiological aging process due to intrinsic causes that is deleterious to the cell and acts progressively with chronological age (von Hahn). These are the essential criteria characterizing biological aging that have been proposed by Strehler (1962) and appear to be generally valid.

The central event of aging, at whatever level of biological complexity, seems to be a progressive diminution of adaptation to stress and of the capacity of the system to maintain the homeostatic equilibrium characteristic of the adult animal at the peak of growth and full development (Comfort).

Von Hahn suggests that information-containing molecules, specifically DNA, can accumulate linkages between adjacent portions of the folded molecule. Such binding will prevent the maintenance of fidelity of daughter molecules produced by this self-duplicating molecule, or it will interfere with the transcription of essential genetic information. Evidence has been reported that points to the occurrence of an age-related increase in the cross-linking of the DNA double helix, dependent on the presence and degree of binding of certain associated proteins. Since DNA strand separation is an essential step in transcription of genetic information, any process that blocks this step will lead to a loss of genetic information within the cell. An accumulation of these events, it is thought, could lead to functional decrements resulting in age changes.

The increased cross-linking with time of the protein collagen is also thought to provide a mechanism for age changes. Collagen constitutes twenty-five to thirty percent of the total body protein and is found in extracellular spaces. Cross-linking of this molecule increases with time and is thought to interfere increasingly with the flow of nutrients and waste products between cells, resulting in age-associated physiological decrements. The increasing flaccidity of the skin by which wrinkling occurs, and the decrease in elasticity of the lung and similar alterations in the vascular system over time are attributed to greater cross-linking in collagen molecules (Kohn).

The physiological changes that can be attributed to cross-linked molecules are analogous to similar changes that occur in a crowd of people who slowly join hands in random fashion until all are so linked. Individual members thus lose their mobility, and the flow of objects between them is slowly reduced. Although cross-linking of molecules undoubtedly occurs, its role as a direct cause of aging is still uncertain.

Programmed genetic events. A final proposition offered to explain age changes at the genetic level is based upon a continuation of those genetic events that result in the development and maturation of any animal. This notion assumes that the switching on and switching off of genes during developmental processes also determines age changes. That is, age changes, like developmental changes, are "programmed" into the original pool of genetic information and are "played out" in an orderly sequence just as developmental changes are. The graying of the hair is not generally thought of as a disease associated with the passage of time. It is regarded as a highly predictable event that occurs later in life after the genetic expression of myriad other programmed developmental events that occur in orderly sequences.

This example may be analogous to attributing the cause of aging to a similar series of orderly programmed genetic events that shut down or slow down essential physiological phenomena after postreproductive age is reached. The programming may be the result of specific gene determinants that, like the end of a tape recording, simply trigger a sequence of events to shut the machine down. Alternatively, the universality of aging might be attributed to functional failures arising from the random accumulation of "noise" in some vulnerable parts of the system, which ultimately interfere with optimum function and produce all of the well-known physiological decrements.

"Mean time to failure." If the "noise" is randomly accumulated, then why do members of each species appear to age at specific, highly predictable times? We may call the span of time during which "noise" accumulates and becomes manifest in some functional decrement the "mean time to failure." This concept is applicable to the deterioration of mechanical as well as biological systems and can be illustrated by considering the "mean time to failure" of, for example, automobiles. The "mean time to failure" of the average machine may be five to six years, which may vary as a function of the competence of repair processes. Barring total replacement of all vital elements, deterioration is inevitable. Similarly, failure of cell function may occur at predictable times that are dependent upon the fidelity of the synthesizing machinery and the degree of perfection of cellular repair systems. Since biological systems do not appear to function perfectly and indefinitely, we are led to the conclusion that the ultimate death of a cell or loss of function is genetically programmed and has a "mean time to failure." The "mean time to failure" may be applicable to a single cell, tissue, organ, or the intact animal itself. It is proposed that the genetic apparatus simply runs out of accurate programmed information that might result in different "mean times to failure" for all of the dependent biological systems. The existence of different life spans for all species may be the reflection of more perfect repair systems in those animals of greater longevity.

Finally, one must consider the two-cell lineages that seem to have escaped from the inevitability of aging or death. These are the continuity of the germ cells (precursors of egg and sperm cells) and continuously reproducing cancer cell populations. It may be possible to explain the immortality of cancer cell populations by suggesting that genetic information is exchanged between these cells in the same way that the genetic cards are reshuffled when egg and sperm fuse. Thus exchange of genetic information may serve to reprogram or reset a more perfect biological clock.

Anti-aging techniques

It is generally believed that the approximately maximum human life span of about 100 years has not changed since recorded history, but what has changed is the larger number of people who approach this apparent limit. Medical achievements have simply resulted in the fact that more people are reaching the limit of what appears to be a fixed life span. Deaths in the early years are becoming progressively less frequent, so that in many privileged countries one can now reasonably expect to become quite old, which is a very new phenomenon.

In a world where the leading current causes of death are resolved, the elimination of cardiovascular diseases, stroke, and cancer in, for example, the United States, would yield a net increase of about eighteen years in life expectation at birth and only slightly less at age sixty-five. This figure is almost identical to the net increase in life expectation at birth achieved in the United States from 1900 to 1950. The increase in life expectation at birth during the first half of this century resulted mainly from the resolution of deaths from infectious diseases occurring before the age of sixty-five. The gain in life expectation in the United States at ages sixty-five and seventy-five from 1900 to 1950 was, respectively, only 1.9 and 1.3 years.

If there is reason to believe that deaths from cardiovascular diseases, stroke, and cancer will be eliminated in the next fifty years, then life expectation will show an increase by A.D. 2025 as profound as that which has occurred since 1900. After that spectacular accomplishment, the leading cause of death will be accidents, which because of their random nature are not likely to yield to total elimination. Thus the social, psychological, political, and economic impacts of resolving the leading causes of death on life expectation in the next fifty years can be reasonably assessed by studying like changes that have occurred in the first seventy-five years of this century, when a similar increase in life expectation occurred.

Let us also consider a world in which all causes of death resulting from disease and accidents are totally eliminated. The theoretical effect on human longevity would be to find all citizens living out their lives, free of the fear of premature death, but with the likely fate that on the eve of their one-hundredth birthday they would suddenly die.

This situation will continue to evolve because

biomedical research has confined its efforts almost exclusively to causes of death associated with what have traditionally been thought of as diseases. Scant attention has been paid to the underlying causes of biological aging that are not disease-associated, which, in clock-like fashion, dictate for each species a specific maximum life span. To be sure, the physiological decrements that occur in advancing years increase vulnerability to disease, but unless more attention is paid to the fundamental non-disease-related biological causes of aging, then our inexorable destiny will be death on or about our one-hundredth birthday.

Prospects for increasing human longevity. As a consequence of these considerations there are two general ways in which biomedical research can be expected to extend human longevity in the next fifty years. The first is to reduce or eliminate the major particular causes of death, such as cardiovascular diseases, stroke, and cancer. The results of ameliorating minor diseases will be minimal. For example, if tuberculosis were completely eliminated in the United States, there would be a mere 0.1 year gain in life expectation at birth. Thus it could be argued that if an increase in life expectation becomes the main goal of biomedical research, most research should be directed toward the elimination of the major causes of death. This position, although less than humane (because it would reduce current research investments proportionally to diseases other than heart disease and stroke), and not likely to attract many adherents, is nonetheless the most logical conclusion to be reached.

The second way in which biomedical research can deal with human longevity is to address itself specifically to the underlying non-disease-related fundamental biological changes that occur with time. These are not diseases but are the basic biological changes that result in those physiological decrements characteristic of aging and upon which are often superimposed an increasing vulnerability to disease. Such an approach, then, does not directly concern itself with efforts to increase human life expectation but rather to extend what appears to be a fixed human life span.

Some immediate possibilities. Of all the areas of human health care, there is probably no other arena of greater quackery than the legion of alleged life-extending nostrums, diets, exercises, injections, and other procedures foisted on a gullible public. Most gerontologists agree that none of these claims has been authenticated by following sound principles of scientific proof. There is, in the judgment of some gerontologists, at least one comparatively innocuous way in which the human life span probably might be extended significantly. The method is based on classic studies made in the 1930s and since confirmed in many laboratories for a number of animal species including rats, in which it was first described (McCay, Pope, and Lunsford). The method is simply to reduce the caloric intake to such a level that undernutrition but not malnutrition occurs. This is done by providing an animal with a diet sufficient in all necessary nutrients but very low in calories. Longevity can then be increased by as much as fifty percent. The effects are most pronounced if caloric restriction diets are initiated when animals are very young. This results in a stretching out of the developmental stages; infancy, puberty, maturity, adulthood and aging simply occur at later than usual points in time, so that the total life span is increased.

On the assumption that undernutrition in man would yield similar results, it is of interest to observe that, in the forty years since this has been known, no human has consciously chosen to do it, even the biologists who know the data best. Considering the number of nostrums and treatments that have been foisted on a gullible public as anti-aging regimens, the lack of interest in underfeeding is, upon superficial consideration, remarkable. On the supposition that the method is widely known, that it works, and that it is not dangerous, the main conclusion that can be drawn from the notable lack of interest in it is that for most people the quality of life is more important than its quantity.

If this is so, then an important lesson can be learned. Any method that might increase human longevity could be unacceptable if it affects the enjoyment of life.

To sleep, perchance to dream. There remains yet another method for increasing life expectancy that bears consideration. Although it will not result in an extension of life on an absolute time scale, it is interesting to consider a form of increased longevity based on the self-evident supposition that life can be lived only when individuals are both physically and mentally active. Since, for most individuals, sleep consumes nearly one-third of our lives, a reduction in the time spent sleeping should result in an increase in productive occupation and the enjoyment of life, that is, if sleep itself is not considered to be either productive or enjoyable. Sleep researchers tell us that no detectable negative effect on health has been observed in those individuals who have learned how to make a modest reduction in the length of time usually spent asleep. The impact of this change would be profound, for if we were to reduce by one half hour the average of eight hours spent sleeping, the net effect on "life-extension" would be an increase of more than two years. This increase in "life expectancy" is equivalent to living in a society where cancer deaths have been totally eliminated.

Instead of any biological advances resulting in the prolongation of human life, this scenario could result from a social movement of an organization of "Awakists," whose members will have learned to do with less sleep in order to gain additional time and, it is to be hoped, spend it productively.

Reduced metabolic rates. Another similar approach to prolongevity would be to mimic in man the reduced metabolism of those animals that pass the winter in hibernation or the summer in estivation. The value of this method presupposes that a slowing of metabolic rates for prolonged periods of time could, in the long run, extend the life span.

Although no compelling evidence exists that a reduced metabolic rate might extend the human life span, this approach has the merit of likely feasibility since the state could probably be induced by drugs or by cold treatment, producing a controlled inhibition of the sympathetic nervous system and a twilight sleep resembling narcosis. Assuming that this were feasible, significant questions of the ethics and societal consequences of such an action must be considered. If it were possible to reduce the metabolic rate in man over a span of, say, ten years, with the result that five more years would be added to the life span, would this be useful? What ten-year period of hibernation would a subject choose in order to effect a gain in years at some future time? One might choose to arrest oneself in a sleep-like trance for, say, ten years, beginning at the age of forty, with instructions to be awakened in a decade so as to enjoy ten more years with one's grandchildren as young adults rather than as infants. The potential societal dislocations resulting from such a scenario are awesome. Family councils might have to be held in order to determine who should be al-

lowed to hibernate, when, and for how long, so as to avoid Father's being awakened at a biological age of forty only to celebrate Mother's eightieth birthday. Other variations on these kinds of asynchronous scenarios can lead to terrible consequences, although others might lead to amusing solutions of current problems. Consider those societies with negative attitudes toward May–December marriages. The older partner might hibernate for a few decades in order to allow the younger partner to either grow up or catch up.

Tampering with our biological clocks

If the control of aging is dependent upon an understanding of basic biological processes, one profoundly important question arises: How desirable is it to gain this understanding and to be able to manipulate our biological clocks? The answer is not simple. The fact that it must be asked is further evidence of the distinction that must be made between disease-oriented biomedical research and gerontological research. Who asks: What are the goals of cancer research, or what are the goals of cardiovascular or stroke research? The answers are so obvious as to preclude asking the question. But the goals of gerontological research are quite a different matter, because we are not certain whether the "resolution" of the physiological decrements of old age will indeed benefit the individual or society as a whole. Take, for example, the possibility that research into the biology of aging might result in the total elimination of all age-related physiological decrements. If this were achieved and no control were established over the biological clock itself, the result might be a society whose members would live full, physically vigorous, youthful lives until their one-hundredth birthday—at which time they would die.

If, on the other hand, we were to learn how to tamper with our biological clocks, with what goal in mind would one choose to reset his clock? Surely one wouldn't choose to spend ten additional years suffering from the infirmities of old age; yet that might, initially, be the only way to intervene. Is society prepared to cope with individuals whose only choice might be between naturally occurring death and ten or more years spent with the vicissitudes of old age? We can hardly deal with a mean maximum life span of, say, 100 years, not to mention the further social, economic, and political dislocations that might occur if we add a decade to this figure.

Aside from this possibility, it is also worth considering the prospect of clock-tampering in which the choice would be to spend more years at a particular stage of our lives than we now do. The clock might be stalled for ten years at, for example, a chronological age of twenty. Is this desirable? Each of us, after pondering this provocative question, would be likely to agree that the time at which we would like our biological clocks arrested should correspond to those years in which maximum life-satisfaction and productivity occurred. Yet if we were forced to make such a decision, it would probably have to be made prospectively. Even more complex is the question of when in the human life span individuals are most productive. An interesting and exhaustive study of this question was made in 1953 by Lehman, whose data showed that, depending upon the particular area of human endeavor, the time of maximum productivity can occur throughout the human life span. Thus clock-tampering becomes a game that very few of us are capable of playing.

In spite of the apparent dilemma in stating goals for gerontological research, there is one goal that appears to be wholly desirable and even attainable as a short-range objective. That would simply be to reduce the physiological decrements associated with biological aging so that vigorous, productive, nondependent lives would be led up until the mean maximum life span of, say, 100 years. Implicit in this notion is that the quality of life is more important than its quantity.

If tampering with our biological clocks ever becomes a reality, it would be tragic if such clock-tampering, instead of extending our most vigorous and productive years, served only to extend the years of our infirmities.

LEONARD HAYFLICK

[*Directly related are the other articles in this entry:* SOCIAL IMPLICATIONS OF AGING, ETHICAL IMPLICATIONS IN AGING, *and* HEALTH CARE AND RESEARCH IN THE AGED. *For discussion of related ideas, see:* LIFE, *article on* QUALITY OF LIFE; *and* POPULATION ETHICS: ELEMENTS OF THE FIELD, *article on* THE POPULATION PROBLEM IN DEMOGRAPHIC PERSPECTIVE.]

BIBLIOGRAPHY

Advances in Gerontological Research. Edited by Bernard L. Strehler. New York: Academic Press, 1964–. Irregular.

ALEXANDER, PETER. "Is There a Relationship between Aging, the Shortening of Life-Span by Radiation and the Induction of Somatic Mutations?" *Perspectives in Experimental Gerontology: A Festschrift for Doctor F. Verzár.* Edited by Nathan Wetheril Shock with F. Bourliere, H. von Hahn, and D. Schlettwein-Gsell. Springfield, Ill.: Charles C. Thomas, 1966, pp. 266–279.

BURNET, F. M. "A Genetic Interpretation of Ageing." *Lancet* 2 (1973): 480–483.

CLARK, A. M. "Genetic Factors Associated with Aging." *Advances in Gerontological Research* 1 (1964): 207–255.

COMFORT, ALEX. *Ageing: The Biology of Senescence.* Rev. ed. New York: Holt, Rinehart & Winston, 1964.

CURTIS, H. J. "The Possibility of Increased Longevity by the Control of Mutations." *Perspectives in Experimental Gerontology: A Festschrift for Doctor F. Verzár.* Edited by Nathan Wetheril Shock with F. Bourliere, H. von Hahn, and D. Schlettwein-Gsell. Springfield, Ill.: Charles C. Thomas, 1966, pp. 257–265.

FINCH, CALEB, and HAYFLICK, LEONARD, eds. *The Handbook of the Biology of Aging.* The Handbooks of Aging, vol. 3. Edited by James Birren. New York: Van Nostrand Reinhold, 1977.

GRUMAN, GERALD J. *A History of Ideas about the Prolongation of Life. Transactions of the American Philosophical Society,* n.s. vol. 56, pt. 9. Philadelphia: 1966.

HAYFLICK, LEONARD. "The Biology of Human Aging." *American Journal of the Medical Sciences* 265 (1973): 432–445.

———. "The Strategy of Senescence." *Gerontologist* 14 (1974): 37–45.

KOHN, ROBERT R. *Principles of Mammalian Aging.* Foundations of Developmental Biology Series. Edited by Clement L. Markert. Englewood Cliffs, N.J.: Prentice-Hall, 1971.

LEHMAN, HARVEY CHRISTIAN. *Age and Achievement.* Memoirs of the American Philosophical Society, vol. 33. Princeton: Princeton University Press, 1953.

McCAY, CLIVE M.; POPE, FRANK; and LUNSFORD, WANDA. "Experimental Prolongation of the Life Span." *Bulletin of the New York Academy of Medicine* 32 (1956): 91–101.

MEDVEDEV, ZHORES A. "Repetition of Molecular-Genetic Information as a Possible Factor in Evolutionary Changes of Life Span." *Experimental Gerontology* 7 (1972): 227–238.

ORGEL, L. E. "Aging of Clones of Mammalian Cells." *Nature* 243 (1973): 441–445.

STREHLER, BERNARD L. "Origin and Comparison of the Effects of Time and High-Energy Radiations on Living Systems." *Quarterly Review of Biology* 34 (1959): 117–142.

———. *Time, Cells and Aging.* New York: Academic Press, 1962.

SZILARD, LEO. "On the Nature of the Aging Process." *Proceedings of the National Academy of Sciences of the United States of America* 45 (1959): 30–45.

United States Bureau of the Census. *Some Demographic Aspects of Aging in the United States.* Current Population Reports, ser. P-23, no. 43. Washington: Government Printing Office, 1973.

VON HAHN, H. P. "The Regulation of Protein Synthesis in the Aging Cell." *Experimental Gerontology* 5 (1970): 323–334.

II
SOCIAL IMPLICATIONS OF AGING

Sociologists do not deal directly with ethical principles or with the determination of the values that ought to be respected in society. They can, however, supply data and interpretation of social trends that are important in understanding the complexity of ethical issues. This article is intended to highlight some of the implications of rapid social change as they have given rise to new ethical issues regarding aging and the aged.

Long life expectancy is a decidedly modern achievement. At the turn of this century, four of every hundred persons in the United States were sixty-five or older. Now it is ten of every hundred. Although the proportion of older people is not expected to rise a great deal more in the next few decades, their absolute numbers will grow rapidly. By the year 2000 the number is expected to surpass thirty million, and by the year 2020, when persons born in the "baby boom" of the 1950s and 1960s reach old age, the number is expected to surpass forty-two million.

These projections are relatively safe, because everybody who will be old by the year 2020 is already alive, and the numbers therefore depend only upon mortality rates. The projections are made by the U.S. Bureau of the Census, based on only slight declines in death rates to the year 2000, and they assume no new basic biological or medical discoveries.

The same general picture is true of other countries of the world. There are a dozen or more industrialized countries in which the proportions of the old are at present higher than in the United States, and although each nation will have a somewhat different age distribution over time, the world trend is toward "aging societies" in which the proportion of the old is increasing in comparison to the proportion of children and adolescents. That is true because populations, like individuals, age as the benefits of industrialization, rising standards of living, and modern medical research lead to longer life expectancy. In the more economically developed regions of the world, it is anticipated that between the years 1970 and 2000 there will be a 50 percent increase in the numbers of persons sixty and over, and, more strikingly, in the less developed regions of the world, a 158 percent increase (United Nations Report).

Changing relations between age groups

The increasing number of older persons is not itself a social problem. On the contrary, nations prize longevity and regard it as an outstanding accomplishment when, as in the United States, the majority of citizens live to old age. Average life expectancy, or average age at death, is often regarded as the single most important index of the overall quality of life of a society. The social problems arise in adapting social and economic institutions to the needs of older people at the same time that the needs of younger people are being met.

The relative numbers of young, middle-aged, and old affect every aspect of life, including the relations among age groups. In most societies in most periods of history, an equilibrium becomes established whereby all age groups receive a stable share of goods and services that is regarded as equitable. However, in countries where the appearance of large numbers of older persons has been relatively sudden, as in the United States within the past seventy-five years, social dislocations occur, because such societies have been unprepared by prevailing value systems to meet the newly emerging needs.

In many countries the aging society has brought with it varying proportions of older persons who suffer from poverty, preventable illness, and social isolation. Those persons, who can be called the needy aged, create acute problems in the field of social and health care. But broader issues stem from the needs of all individuals, young and old, to adjust to the new rhythms of life that come with increased longevity: multigenerational families, retirement, increased leisure, changing health status, and new opportunities and new problems of adaptation that accompany a long life. For the society at large innumerable policy questions arise as the whole social fabric accommodates itself to the changing age distribution.

In oversimplified terms the contemporary American society faces two different sets of issues. On the one hand, there are increasing numbers of the "young-old": persons in their late fifties, sixties, and early seventies who are relatively healthy and vigorous, a large number of whom are retired, who seek meaningful ways to use their time, either in self-fulfillment or in community participation, and who represent a great resource of talent for society. On the other hand, there are even more dramatic increases in numbers who might be called the "old-old": persons in their mid-seventies, eighties, and nineties, an increasing minority of whom remain vigorous and active, but a majority of whom need a wide range of supportive and restorative health services and social services (Neugarten).

For various historical reasons, the old-old of the 1970s in the United States represent a disproportionately disadvantaged group. Many were immigrants who had little formal education; many worked most of their lives at low-skill occupations; many lost their occupational moorings during the Great Depression and did not recoup in the period of prosperity ushered in by the Second World War, nor did they build up sizable equities under the social security program as it developed in the 1940s and 1950s.

In succeeding decades more and more older people will have been native-born, will have grown up in urban areas, will have had the advantages of regular medical care during their lifetimes, will have had high school and college educations, and will take for granted pension programs, social security, and government service programs of all types. Thus persons growing old in the future will have very different characteristics, different values and expectations, from those who are currently old.

The relations among age groups are also influenced by changing perceptions of the life cycle and the periods of life. Age groups have become increasingly differentiated over time. It was not until the seventeenth century that childhood became a discernible period of life with its special needs and characteristics (Ariès). Adolescence, socially defined, can be viewed as an invention of the late nineteenth century, and "youth" an invention of the twentieth century (Coleman et al.). In the past few decades middle age has become a newly delineated stage in the life cycle. Persons no longer move abruptly from adulthood—the period of full commitment to work and family responsibilities—into old age, but they move instead through a relatively long interval of middle age when family responsibilities are diminished but work continues, even though specific work roles may change—for example, women reentering the labor market in their forties and fifties—and when physical vigor remains high. Still another meaningful division is now appearing between the young-old and the old-old.

The young-old

Although age is not, in itself, the distinguishing characteristic, the young-old are drawn mostly from those who are fifty-five to seventy-five. Retirement is the primary event that distinguishes the young-old from the middle-aged. Granted that it is arbitrary to use a single life event as the criterion, retirement is nevertheless a meaningful marker, just as the departure of children from the home is a useful marker with regard to middle age.

This fifty-five to seventy-five grouping is not one to which we are accustomed. Age fifty-five is becoming a meaningful lower age limit because of the lowering age of retirement. Many workers are now voluntarily retiring just as soon as they can live comfortably on their retirement incomes. The 1970 U.S. census indicates that only eighty-one percent of fifty-five- to sixty-four-year-olds were in the labor force, as compared to ninety-two percent of the next younger group.

Whether this trend toward earlier retirement will continue depends upon rates of economic and technological growth, the number of young workers, the number of women workers, increases in part-time work opportunities, the development of share-the-work programs, and so on. Most observers predict, however, that the downward trend will continue over the next two or three decades (Jaffe). By and large, then, the young-old will increasingly become a retired group. It is already a relatively healthy group. It is estimated that, while a large number have one or more chronic illnesses, only twenty to twenty-five percent of persons aged fifty-five to seventy-five need to limit their major activities for reasons of health.

Because of the enormous diversity of lifestyles among the young-old, meaningful differences are obscured in aggregated data. Nevertheless, the gross characteristics of this age group are worth noting. At present the young-old constitute more than fifteen percent of the U.S. population, as compared with the old-old, who constitute less than four percent.

Because mortality rates for women are lower, women considerably outnumber men, and this imbalance is expected to grow even larger. Nevertheless, because most men marry women somewhat younger than themselves, the young-old as a total group are more like their younger than their older counterparts with regard to family relationships. About eighty percent of the men and well over half the women were married in 1970 and living with their spouses. (The rates of widowhood are very different for the two sexes; about seven percent of the men, but more than thirty percent of the women, were widowed.) By far the most common pattern is husband-wife families who live in their own households—some seventy percent own their own homes—and only a small minority who move from one house to another within a five-year interval.

The young-old see their children frequently,

and some seventy-five to eighty-five percent of those who have children live within thirty minutes of the nearest child (Shanas et al.). They expect that when they grow to advanced old age and can no longer manage for themselves their children will come to their aid—not financially, for the government is looked to as the expected source of financial and medical assistance, but emotionally. As a number of studies have shown, these expectations are usually met. Various forms of assistance and services are being exchanged across generational lines, ties of affection and obligation are strong, and the family continues to be an important part of daily life.

It is noteworthy that a large proportion of young-old have a living parent. The estimate in 1972 was one of every three sixty-year-old Americans; and this proportion will increase, because the numbers of old-old are growing faster than the numbers of young-old.

The economic status of the young-old is not easily summarized. Income from work is a major factor in economic status, and for many persons income drops precipitously upon retirement, despite public and private pensions. If present trends continue, the adjustment to lower incomes may be timed closer to age fifty-five than to age sixty-five. Nor is the economic status of the young-old easily described compared to other age groups, for satisfactory data are available only with regard to current money income, and money income is only part of total economic resources. For instance there is Medicare, the value of rent to homeowners, tax adjustments for those sixty-five and over, intrafamily transfers, and other assets that create differences between age groups. Overall, the majority of the young-old in the United States are currently neither poor nor "near-poor," and most likely the trend toward improved economic status for older people will continue, given the increases in social security and the growing number of public programs directed at protecting the financial security and general well-being of older people. Other programs, such as national health insurance, already provided in other Western countries, and improvements in private pension and profit-sharing plans, can be anticipated. The likely outcome is that not only will the future young-old be more financially secure than their predecessors, but their economic position will continue to improve when compared to younger adults. The ethical question nevertheless arises: What proportion of the gross national product should go into private and public pension systems?

The young-old are already much better educated than the old-old, but the more important fact is that successive cohorts will be in a less disadvantaged position in comparison to the young. So marked are the gains in educational level that by 1980 the average fifty-five-year-old in the United States will be a high school graduate; by 1990 this will be true of all the fifty-five-to-seventy-five group. Furthermore, with the growth in adult education programs, it can be anticipated that the educational differences that now exist between young, middle-aged, and young-old will be much reduced (Carnegie Commission).

With regard to political participation there is no evidence that age blocks are forming or that a politics of age is developing in the United States (Hudson and Binstock). A quite different picture emerges, however, when general political participation and voting patterns are examined. When national data are corrected for income and education, overall political participation is highest for the age group fifty-one to sixty-five. It falls off only a little for persons over sixty-five (Verba and Nie). Thus, the young-old are disproportionately influential in the electorate.

What do the young-old want?

A vigorous and educated young-old group can be expected to develop a variety of new needs with regard to the meaningful use of time. They are likely to want a wide range of options and opportunities for self-enhancement and for community participation—in general, for what might be called an age-irrelevant society in which arbitrary constraints based on chronological age are removed.

The young-old want a wide range of choices with regard to work. Some opt for early retirement; some want to continue working beyond age sixty-five; some want to undertake new work careers at one or more times after age forty. Even more in the future than in the present, they are likely to encourage economic policies that hasten the separation between income and work and that move toward the goal of providing retirees with sufficient economic resources to maintain their preretirement living standards.

We are already seeing a wider range of life patterns with regard to the related areas of work, education, and leisure. More middle-aged and older people are returning to education, some because of obsolescence of work skills and others for recreation or self-fulfillment. Plans are now going forward in various parts of the United States to create intergenerational educational campuses.

While age-segregated communities are on the increase, they now accommodate only a small percentage of the older population. Their growth will depend upon the extent to which the young-old will be provided opportunities for meaningful community participation in their present locations.

The vast majority of the young-old will continue to live as married couples, but the large number of widows and the increased number of single and divorced persons among them will probably lead to the formation of more group households composed of nonfamily members. At the same time, many will want housing arrangements that make it possible to maintain an aged parent at home. Family interactions of other types may also increase rather than decrease. Contrary to the concerns often expressed over the "vanishing" family, some observers now predict that, as the more instrumental aspects of life—education, income maintenance, health services—are shifted to other social institutions, the family may become more rather than less important with regard to the expressive aspects of life—that is, in providing lasting emotional ties, a sense of identity and self-worth, and respect for the worth of others.

Overall, as the young-old articulate their needs and desires, the emphasis is likely to be upon improving the quality of life and upon increasing the choices of life-styles.

The old-old

The number of those over seventy-five is growing at a more rapid rate than the young-old. Their claims upon the society are at least as morally compelling as those of other age groups.

The prevailing assumptions are that life expectancy will continue to increase, although slowly, and that in general older persons will have improved health in the future. But this says little regarding the period of disability that can be expected to occur for most people in the very last phase of life. There is little basis at present for predicting that this period will become shorter by the year 2000. Most persons would probably regard it as their goal to maintain physical and psychological intactness through their eighth or ninth decade, then die relatively quickly without a long period of terminal illness. (An example is Picasso, who reputedly main-

tained his full physical, mental, and creative abilities to the day before his death.) But the prospect may be the opposite: With increasing age, people may have a drawn-out period of physical and psychological debility, with medical services that can keep them alive but neither healthy nor happy. The latter is the specter that haunts most persons when they think of their own old age, and it is the specter that haunts medical and social planners when they ponder the implications of the aging society. For the latter, the question arises, for example, whether ours is an equitable distribution, with thirty percent of all health services now going to the ten percent who are over sixty-five. Is this too much or too little?

Whatever the uncertainties regarding the period of disability, the needs of the old-old for meaningful ways of spending time, for special housing, and for transportation will depend in large measure upon health status. The majority will probably live independently in the future, as now, but they will need both supportive social services and special features in the physical environment to enable them to function as fully as possible. The old-old require not only health services aimed at slowing physical and mental deterioration, but social services designed to prevent unnecessary decline in the individual's feelings of self-worth and dignity. Can opportunities for social interaction and social contributions be provided?

Some of the old-old will require nursing home care; others will require new forms of home health services. Will a larger share of the public budget go to meeting these needs of the old-old?

For persons who are terminally ill or incapacitated, the problems are likely to multiply with regard to providing maximum social supports, the highest possible levels of care and comfort, the assurance of dignified death, and, at the same time, an increasing element of choice for the individual himself or for members of his family in deciding how and when his life shall end. New ethical issues will arise over ways of achieving a "best death" for each individual.

Other social and ethical questions will become more pressing: What will be the principal deleterious and the principal beneficial effects of increased numbers of older persons on the society at large? Will vigorous older persons wish to employ their newly won leisure to become important agents of social change? Will they create an attractive image of aging, thus allaying the fears of the young about growing old? Will they be provided with the necessary resources? Or will their increased numbers so aggravate the problems of income maintenance, housing, health care, and social services that their situation will become generally worse rather than better?

In considering what proportion of the society's resources should go to the young, to adults, and to the aged, the question arises whether age itself constitutes a meaningful basis for categorizing people. Should public programs be addressed to the needs of persons who are ill or poor, but not to persons who happen to be old? Just as we have tried to erase distinctions based on sex or on race, should we try to erase distinctions based on age?

Finally, an additional set of value issues arises with regard to the aged: to what extent society should follow a cost-benefit analysis, with benefits to older people weighed in terms of their past or potential productivity; whether the analysis can be based on the very fact that the old are equal members of the society; and whether societies will (or should) develop higher forms of culture where the aged are cherished because their very presence symbolizes man's most humane values.

BERNICE L. NEUGARTEN

[*Most directly related to this article are its companion articles in this entry:* THEORIES OF AGING AND ANTI-AGING TECHNIQUES, ETHICAL IMPLICATIONS IN AGING, *and* HEALTH CARE AND RESEARCH IN THE AGED. *For discussion of related ideas, see the entries:* ADOLESCENTS; *and* CHILDREN AND BIOMEDICINE. *See also:* DEATH; *and* RATIONING OF MEDICAL TREATMENT.]

BIBLIOGRAPHY

ARIÈS, PHILLIPE. *Centuries of Childhood: A Social History of Family Life.* Translated by Robert Baldick. New York: Alfred A. Knopf, 1962.

Carnegie Commission on Higher Education. *Toward a Learning Society: Alternative Channels to Life, Work, and Service: A Report and Recommendations by the Carnegie Commission on Higher Education.* New York: McGraw-Hill, 1973.

COLEMAN, JAMES S.; BREMMER, ROBERT H.; CLARK, BURTON R.; DAVIS, JOHN B.; EICHON, DOROTHY H.; GRILICHES, ZVI; KETT, JOSEPH F.; RYDER, NORMAN B.; DOERING, ZAHAVA BLUM; and MAYS, JOHN M. *Youth: Transition to Adulthood—Report on Youth of the President's Science Advisory Committee.* Chicago: University of Chicago Press, 1974.

HUDSON, ROBERT B., and BINSTOCK, ROBERT H. "Political Systems and Aging." *Handbook of Aging and the Social Sciences.* Edited by Robert H. Binstock and Ethel Shanas. Handbooks of Aging Series, vol. 1. Edited by James E. Birren. New York: Van Nostrand Reinhold Co., 1976, chap. 15, pp. 369–400.

JAFFE, A. J. "Has the Retreat from the Labor Force Halted? A Note on Retirement of Men, 1930–1970." *Industrial Gerontology,* no. 9 (1971), pp. 1–12.

NEUGARTEN, BERNICE L. "Age Groups in American Society and the Rise of the Young-Old." *Annals of the American Academy of Political and Social Sciences* 415 (1974): 187–198.

SHANAS, ETHEL; TOWNSEND, PETER; WEDDERBURN, DOROTHY; FRIIS, HENNING; MILHØJ, POUL; and STEHOUWER, JAN. *Old People in Three Industrial Societies.* New York: Atherton Press, 1968.

United Nations, General Assembly. *Question of the Elderly and the Aged: Conditions, Needs and Services, and Suggested Guidelines for National Policies and International Action: Report of the Secretary General.* A/9126. New York: 1973.

VERBA, SIDNEY, and NIE, NORMAN H. *Participation in America: Political Democracy and Social Equality.* New York: Harper & Row, 1972.

III
ETHICAL IMPLICATIONS IN AGING

Ethical issues related to aging and old age—problems pertaining to the qualities of life of the elderly, the use of anti-aging technologies, etc.—are ultimately influenced by values (or disvalues) associated with longevity and aging.

Values and longevity: a history

Throughout the course of Western civilization complaints over the pains and disabilities of old age mix with exhortations to virtuous resignation and praise for old people who lead lives of strength and dignity. Generally, elderly men and women are given the most esteem when they continue to carry on the roles of adult life. Conversely, the loss of capacity through old age is often the occasion of ridicule and complaint.

In premodern Europe, four principal cultural traditions on aging are to be found: (1) The early Greeks regarded a happy old age as a fortuitous blessing. (2) With the spread of philosophical theories of virtue, the circumstances of old age became less important than one's attitude and bearing toward them. (3) The Hebrew tradition took note of the religious fidelity of old people and showed greater appreciation of the aged couple than Greco-Roman culture. Early Christianity, moreover, established a special status for older women as "widows." Medieval monasticism developed the ideal of old age as a preparation for death but also carried on the late classical ideal of leisured retirement. (4) In the later Middle Ages and the Renaissance old women lost the protection of the Church through the rise of bourgeois mores, and with the Reformation the work ethic eclipsed leisured retirement as a life task of old people.

Classical Greece.   Solon summarized an early Greek view of life in a terse sentence, "Man is accident." A happy old age was not something to be expected (Herodotus), and especially not something to be planned for. Life was an aesthetic whole, which misfortune could mar irreparably. The tragedians reminded their audiences of the sober dictum, "Call no one happy until he dies." Not length of life but its quality counted. Stories related by Herodotus in *The Histories* show that in Solon's time a happy old age consisted in favorable circumstances, success in multiple roles, and an honorable death. Fortune, however, not human wit, was regarded as the decisive factor for a happy old age.

Sophocles' *Oedipus at Colonus* is the first major literary work with an old person as hero. Sophocles wrote the play when he was past ninety, and legend says that he presented it for the first time in court as a defense against the charge of senility. In terms of the development of moral stances toward aging, the most important theme of the play is the coincidence of heroic choice and resignation in the old Oedipus. Willing consent to the sufferings of age marks a departure from the activist naturalism of the lyric age toward the ideal of spiritual appropriation of old age, which would dominate the classical period.

With Socrates' account of virtue in Plato's early dialogues the new attitude has fully emerged. In Aristotle's discussion of happiness in the *Nichomachean Ethics*, a generation later, virtue rather than fortune appears as the key to a successful life. The philosopher acknowledges that men can show nobility even in misfortune, not out of insensitivity to pain but through greatness of soul.

Rome.   Virtue is a key idea in Roman views of old age too. Cicero's *De Senectute (Old Age)*, the fullest treatment of the topic from antiquity, notes that responses to old age generally reflected life-long dispositions. People who never showed self-control found their last years troublesome. Those who practiced virtue found no evil in aging, because they viewed it as a natural process.

Cicero also informs us about the sociology of aging among the upper classes of his day. Continuance in public service was highly admired, and control over one's family nearly an imperative. Cicero himself retired for political reasons, and he describes with pleasure the enjoyments of literature and gardening. His description of those avocations served as a model of leisured retirement (*otium*) for centuries and was an important influence on the monasteries and convents of the early Middle Ages.

He also records Stoic attitudes toward health and death. To resist old age and compensate for its defects is a duty. Aging is to be combated as one would a disease, with moderate exercise and a spare diet. His readers were admonished to take no thought of death; when it was time to die, they should not vainly cling to life. The Stoic value of unimpassioned judgment gave old age a prized status.

Hebrew and Christian values.   The Jewish and Christian traditions show even greater tolerance for the difficulties of the last stages of life. Old people who have been faithful to God, the Law, and the coming Messiah are presented as models of devotion. Stories about the afflictions of age stress constancy in adversity as a basic disposition. Care of parents was valued (Exod. 21:15, 21:17; Lev. 20:91; Deut. 27:16; cf. Matt. 15:3–7); yet the usual form of the commandment to "honor thy father and thy mother" indicated a broader, more inclusive ideal than simple support (Exod. 19:3). It enjoins an attitude of reverence and affection akin to worship, and the promise of long life for those who observe it made it a solemn covenantal obligation.

From an early date, the Christian Church assigned a position of special esteem to widows. Women sixty years and older without family to support them could give themselves to a life of prayer and good works in return for maintenance by the early Christian Church (1 Tim. 5:3–16). Widowhood was a significant and flexible social invention: By the second century, it included both genuine widows who carried out works of mercy and unmarried women living a secluded life of prayer; and by the twelfth century, women who had been released from their marriage vows, e.g., to found convents, could be admitted to formal widowhood (*Monumenta de viduis . . .*). But the bourgeois customs associated with the rise of a new middle class (Harksen) and the revival of Roman law and of Greco-Roman family styles during the Renaissance (Sachs) contributed to the decline of widowhood as a distinctive status by reasserting the domestic duties of women and their subordination to their husbands.

In late antiquity and the Middle Ages, Christianity developed still another role for old age: preparation for death. Death after the model of Jesus was a religious ideal. With the passing of persecution, the enthusiasm that had been attached to martyrdom was transferred to monasticism and the ascetic life generally. Lives of saints from Anthony of Egypt in the fourth century to Aelred (or Ethelred) of Rievaulx in Yorkshire in the twelfth century record highly active old people who retire to a life of prayer and asceticism in their very last years in anticipation of death. The later manuals on the art of dying were popularizations of a way of life that first arose in the monasteries.

Transition to modernity. Through the late Middle Ages religious and humanistic ideals of retirement mix easily with one another. The iconography of the period pictures the old man as a scholar, indicating the social role that at least some elderly persons were expected to play. With the advent of Protestantism, and Puritanism in particular, this ideal fades in favor of continued participation in the roles of adult life. The activism never wholly absent from Western ideals of aging reasserts itself over more contemplative models of old age (Demos).

Moral confusion in modern societies. Values are intimately related to social structure. The most relevant fact about modernity, first in the West but increasingly in all industrialized nations, is the dominance of economic over other social factors. The debate between segregationists and integrationists among social gerontologists reflects a basic disagreement about the effects of economic structures and values on old age (Shanas et al.). The segregationists stress the disengagement of the elderly from their primary roles, especially employment, while the integrationists emphasize continued participation in a wide range of social involvements, generally outside the market place. Because of the dominance of job-related roles, the first group downplays nonpublic, personal pursuits and has little positive to say about old age and retirement. Looking to the family, the neighborhood, and voluntary associations, the second group sees the possibility of a shift of roles and goals in old age with an increase in the intensity of interpersonal relations and the expansion of personal pursuits. Both groups represent one face of aging in modern societies, but their differences expose the moral ambivalance of old age in modern times. The work ethic makes adjustment to nonwork roles problematic. Workers are unused to managing large periods of leisure time. Strong career identification builds barriers against fostering personal goals, and the nuclear family and antinatalist trends make it less easy to enjoy being a grandparent.

Ethical dilemmas with respect to aging concern maintaining a balance between work and leisure, freedom and dependence, economic enterprise and interpersonal life, health care and the acceptance of impairment.

Work and leisure. In advanced industrial societies, the balance between work and leisure is again shifting. Social security, retirement plans, associations of old people, and other factors open possibilities of rich retirement experiences even in nations where the work ethic is strongest. Both the place of work in contemporary notions of worth and identity and the difficulties of many in facing retirement suggest that adjustment to new roles may be eased by extended or part-time employment, or by gradual shortening of the workweek. A less problematic old age, however, will demand changes in social attitudes: appreciation of leisure, the acceptance of personal goals and private time, belief in the potentialities of old persons, and encouragement to participate in cultural and religious activities. Psychologists have noted life review and integration as tasks of old age, and sociologists have suggested the resumption of interrupted interests (Markson; Erikson, 1968, 1976; Havighurst and Albrecht). But these are yet to become accepted and supported patterns of aging.

Freedom and dependence. A peculiar difficulty of aging in many societies, and Western societies particularly, is the assumption that freedom means independence and mastery. This conviction makes it exceedingly difficult to accept the losses and dependence that accompany aging. The same attitude causes strain for people who are faced with the subtle changes of more intimate personal relations—for example, extended daily contact with spouse and relatives—after years of involvement in the impersonal activity of economic life. Conflicts arise because cooperation at an interpersonal level and acceptance of diminution are alien attitudes in modern culture where unimpeded freedom is the paramount value. Affirmation of interdependence with others and of resignation to necessity, therefore, is a constituent of an adequate philosophy of human freedom forced on our attention by the losses of old age.

Interpersonal life. The return to active social relations in old age is also an unsettled area. Despite myths of abandonment and segregation, the vast majority of old people in the United States are in contact with their families and receive support from them in time of need (Shanas et al.). Still, the transition to a more intense social life is not easy. In old age, women adjust more readily than men, because they are usually responsible for maintaining familial and kin ties. Accordingly, male retirement sometimes suffers from reverse sexual discrimination and the stereotyping of social activity as a feminine role. Another severe strain on the elderly in many places is the denigration of family values. Although in Eastern Europe and elsewhere grandparents seem to have a respected role, grandparenting has lost some of its important functions in the United States, where peer relations have emerged as a substitute involvement.

Attitudes toward sickness. Attitudes toward sickness and impairment are related to independence as a dominant value. Fears of dependency due to chronic disability are common, particularly in the United States. Materialism and the cult of youth reinforce preoccupation with bodily health and aggravate feelings of chagrin and indignation when they accompany age (ibid.). An important area of concern, therefore, is the set of values one brings to aging. It is relevant to consider whether any set of values is appropriate to only one or two stages of life and not to others, whether it engenders the moral strength needed in adversity, and whether it overcomes preoccupation with the body.

Against the background of the foregoing values and value conflicts associated with aging, an ethical analysis will be offered of two sets of problems that can be properly understood only in conjunction with each other: first, problems related to the general condition and care of the aged, and second, issues raised by the use of anti-aging and other life-prolonging techniques.

Ethical analysis of problems of the aged

When old people are a marginal group, as they have been until recently in industrial countries, they tend to be penalized like any marginal group. Social losses are heaped onto the natural losses of age. The most general rule of geriatric ethics is that losses should not be compounded (Christiansen). Principles that apply to others in the wider society should apply equally to old people. They include principles of justice, rules against discrimination, and codes of medical ethics. There are at least three areas, however, in which general ethical principles can be given specification with respect to common problems of aging: dependency, financial and moral support, and medical care.

Autonomy. General aversion to dependency and to the real but often unexpected burdens it creates frequently leads to undue loss of dignity by the aged, as measured in terms of their actual need. In such cases the general moral rule attempts to ensure that dependency does not turn into humiliation. Respect for the autonomy of the elderly remains an important factor in their ability to age with full dignity. In the family situation, the ability of old people to direct their own affairs is a matter of some importance (ibid.). Family members are helpers; preempting responsibilities older members can still fulfill is a serious infringement of the rights of the elderly. Conversely, retaining powers of decision, especially over health care, enhances their dignity. In many cases at least, aging is a gradual process with an incremental scale of loss. It helps, therefore, to adjust the withdrawal of responsibility to the degrees of impairment. At every stage of senescence the moral optimum is attained when the aged themselves and their families foster that range of personal autonomy which remains to them after their other losses.

Familial justice. With respect to support of the elderly, equitable sharing of the burden among relatives is a grave but seldom treated issue. Psychologically and sociologically it is understandable that care for aged parents usually falls on one family member, generally a daughter. But that burden can seem excessive, especially where self-fulfillment is a value and women have access to professional careers. Graduated retirement might assist in alleviating financial problems for at least some period of time. When the support does fall to adult children, however, the monetary burden needs to be shared more equitably and compensation given for service rendered. One solution might be the encouragement of a temporary career, discontinuous with other life careers, which would have as its purpose the care of the elderly infirm, similar to a career in the care of children. Yet if such a career is to have social approval and ease the burden of care, it should be accorded suitable tax preferences. Similarly, temporary care institutions would allow necessary time for rest, illness, and recreation for the children, so that uninterrupted care does not become oppressive. It should be noted, too, that the needed support is not simply monetary. Since older people have more personal time, there is a need for social exchange that cannot be satisfied by one or two close relatives.

Medical care. Finally, the principle that losses ought not to be compounded in reference to the aged may be applied to the medical context.

First, health policy should not overlook basic services. Old people need simple things: eyeglasses, false teeth, comfortable shoes, and foot care. The structure of technological medicine, however, often prevents the serving of these needs. Similarly, rehabilitation and quality home care would seem to merit priority over research and development of technology for treating catastrophic illness. Second, since communication of health information is critical to the disposition of the lives of old people themselves, reports on their condition and prognosis ordinarily ought to be made to them fully and without mediation. Family members are helpers and as such are not entitled prima facie to privileged access or control of health information. Third, instead of the elderly infirm finding themselves in the sick role for an indefinite period, health professionals should encourage them to resume as much responsibility as their condition allows. Fourth, in view of the personal crises brought on by impairment in old age, professionals should regard the psychological and religious growth of the aged as an important aspect of care.

Anti-aging techniques: ethical assessment

The quest for immortality is as old as Western culture, but so also is the acceptance of mortality as the highest wisdom. With the dawn of scientific knowledge, Francis Bacon proposed that prolongation of life could be the highest gift of scientific medicine (Bacon). During the last hundred years, the curbing of infectious diseases has extended life expectancy by many years. More recently, organ transplants, renal dialysis, heart-lung machines, and other advanced techniques have given extended life to many, and developments in molecular biology offer the promise of controlling at least some aspects of the aging process itself. Forecasts as of 1975 suggest that adequately funded research on such methods could increase life expectancy once more from fifteen to thirty years (Segerberg).

Moral assessment of anti-aging techniques—which are but one issue of an emerging geriatric ethics—includes the following considerations: (1) the use of various kinds of anti-aging techniques and their place in overall health priorities; (2) their social impact, and (3) their moral and anthropological effects.

Use of anti-aging techniques. Anti-aging techniques include everything from intelligent nutrition and physical fitness programs to advanced prosthetic devices, new treatments for catastrophic diseases such as heart disease and stroke, and yet undeveloped but plausible techniques to inhibit cytolysis, the breakdown in cellular life, which comes with age.

Little or no objection can be raised to the simple techniques of improved nutrition and exercise programs. Indeed many moral traditions view such prudent health measures as a moral imperative. Because these practices would improve the lives of those already living at relatively low cost, there is reason to give them greater weight than more exotic techniques that may reach only select populations at some future time. In addition, such limited techniques tend to involve people in their own care, reduce dependence on experts, and circumvent large expenditures on technologies that are only marginally useful (Illich, 1975).

The development of prosthetic devices is a more ambiguous matter. Medicine's capability of preserving life even though conscious, meaningful existence has ceased has created situations in which neither patient nor family is permitted to accept the reality of death and the burden of moral responsibility. Techniques like renal dialysis raise very difficult questions of just allocation of scarce resources and moral-psychological problems about man–machine synergies. Again, there are important issues of complex dependence on societal resources with related issues of cost–benefit analysis (Arrow; Rice and Cooper). Simple devices, such as pacemakers, offer the least difficulty in that they involve only limited institutional commitments and allow patients to function on their own with only intermittent hospitalization.

Evaluation of advances in cellular biology is difficult. Knowledge of the aging process is rapidly increasing, but specific techniques to counteract the ill effects of aging are still to be developed. In general, proposals for research and development of anti-aging techniques should weigh: (1) the degree of availability that will be feasible with a given technique; (2) the impact of the techniques on the just allocation of all biomedical resources and on the quality of overall health care; (3) the degree of dependence on experts, institutions, and technologies; and (4) the utility of the invention in relation to the general health and full life of the patient.

A variety of life-prolonging technologies is already in use and under development. In some areas, such as cancer and cardiovascular ailments, public commitment is substantial. Should applied research aimed specifically at inhibiting the aging process itself be added to existing programs to fight the major age-related diseases? To answer this question, choices must be made about the lines of research to be adopted, about the structure of a desirable pattern of health care, and about the allocation of resources. Basic research on aging will be important. But should higher priority be given to study and relief of infirmities like arthritis that now afflict old people? What is the proper balance between resources employed for rehabilitation now and those applied to research that will benefit future generations? Is there a just allocation of resources when the poor lack basic nutrition and health services and at the same time sophisticated medical technologies are developed at public expense? Will a majority of the population benefit from these new technologies, or will extended life be a boon only to an elite? Will life-extending technologies lead to a fuller, healthier life for the elderly, or only to prolonged illness and suffering? Answers to such questions will disclose important differences in value judgments concerning the weight given the present generation over the future, the drive for scientific breakthroughs vis-à-vis the demand for the relief of suffering, the relative power of technological versus human imperatives, and the balance between health maintenance and crisis medicine as ideals of health care.

Social impact. Prolongation of life carries with it the potential for massive economic, social, political, and psychological dislocations. Life-extension at the far end of the life cycle could place an immense financial burden on the middle generation. Opportunity for retirement might be reduced simply to offset the cost of subsidizing the elderly. The demographic shifts resulting from anti-aging policies could also lead to political upheavals. The elderly, with larger numbers and resources, might press for greater services, and younger people might rebel at having to support a large, unproductive class of people. One solution would be to focus on the middle years as the phase of life that would be prolonged. But this too would have its difficulties, such as providing employment for the increased pool of workers.

The psychological impact of life extension must also be assessed. Some techniques, such as low-temperature hibernation, would result in gaps in an individual's life experience and in disconnections in relations with others. These side effects seem to provide occasion for identity conflicts and social tensions. Furthermore, when compared with old people in traditional societies,

the aged in modern industrial countries already live in a relatively anomic social situation. Meaningful, socially sanctioned ideals and roles are not available for them (Callahan and Christiansen). Without consensus on the values of old age, life extension offers potential for great personal disorientation among the elderly.

Life extension has serious effects on demographic policy too. If stabilized population size is a matter of policy, life extension would have to be compensated for by further curtailment of births. Accordingly life tasks related to child care and the family would be reduced. Other forms of mutual support and bonding would arise and would be of special significance in providing companionship and care for the elderly infirm. But with fewer children proportionally in the population, society's ability to renew itself generally in ideals and ideas might be jeopardized. This is a cost that must be weighed in terms of an overall demographic policy. Where the threat of "overpopulation" has not yielded a coherent government population policy, the imbalances threatened by wide use of anti-aging techniques may well force the development of such plans.

Moral and anthropological effects. Scientific immortality is not in prospect, but significant delays in aging and dying are near. Such human power over death poses substantive questions about morality and human nature. New questions arise about the termination of human life. Will people be permitted to choose a natural death? Will their choices be classified as suicides? At what point will cessation of life-prolonging treatment be allowed? Will society set upper limits to the extension of life, and by what criteria? In short, anti-aging technology will force redefinition of suicide and euthanasia.

Extended life may also bring substantive changes in the structure of moral life. A decline in fertility may mean a decrease in intergenerational responsibility, the paradigm case of altruistic behavior and moral obligation. Will prolonged life lead to an increase in the excesses of individualism, indifference to the weak and powerless, increased competitiveness, and a consequent increase in legal control of interpersonal relations? What areas will remain for moral responsibility in the traditional sense?

Summary approaches

Two approaches to humanism conflict in weighing the prospects for life-prolonging technologies. One attitude might be called neonaturalism, because it regards old age and death as natural events that are to be freely appropriated by the aging and the dying (Kübler-Ross). Others argue for natural limits to technological innovation on the grounds that those satisfactions which can be legitimately expected from technology must be distinguished from those that are unrealistic in light of the human condition (Callahan), such as immortality. The second approach, technological humanism, insists to the contrary that the control of death is a desirable goal, and that there is no warrant for depriving people of realizing the ancient longing for immortality (Harrington).

The debate over natural death and the prolongation of life concerns the desirability of certain sets of virtues and alternative views of human nature, especially of freedom. For the humanism that sees death as natural, old age places activism and individualism proper to the other phases of the life cycle in perspective. Trust, sociality, and contemplation reassert themselves over the drives for mastery and aggressive self-fulfillment. The passive virtues are necessary for coping with the limits of the human condition.

For technological humanism, however, restraint and resignation are values only when there are no alternatives. The role of technology is to push back the limits of human life and increase the opportunities for growth and enrichment. In the new world of technological immortality, passive virtues, such as contemplation and moderation, are merely optional matters of life-style. Technological developments give people a choice. They can continue their pursuit of self-fulfillment or not, as they choose. On this view, anti-aging techniques would increase the freedom of individuals to realize their own desires. For this group, then, human nature is defined by freedom as a power of self-fulfillment, a power greatly and rightly enhanced by technology. For neonaturalism, however, humanity is differently defined. It consists in the coincidence of freedom with natural and social limitations (Ricoeur). As a result, individual fulfillment is realized in a moral universe that sets important limits to one's desires and power (Callahan).

DREW CHRISTIANSEN

[*Most directly related to this article are its companion articles in this entry:* THEORIES OF AGING AND ANTI-AGING TECHNIQUES, SOCIAL IMPLICATIONS OF AGING, *and* HEALTH CARE AND RESEARCH IN THE AGED. *For further discussion of topics mentioned in this article, see the entries:* KIDNEY DIALYSIS AND TRANSPLANTATION; LIFE-SUPPORT SYSTEMS; *and* ORGAN TRANSPLANTATION. *Other relevant material may be found under* DEATH; HEALTH AND DISEASE; JUSTICE; *and* RATIONING OF MEDICAL TREATMENT. *See also:* DEATH AND DYING: EUTHANASIA AND SUSTAINING LIFE; POPULATION ETHICS: ELEMENTS OF THE FIELD, *article on* THE POPULATION PROBLEM IN DEMOGRAPHIC PERSPECTIVE; POVERTY AND HEALTH, *article on* POVERTY AND HEALTH IN THE UNITED STATES; RISK; *and* SUICIDE.]

BIBLIOGRAPHY

ARROW, KENNETH J. "Government Decision Making and the Preciousness of Life." With commentaries by Guido Calabresi and Edmund D. Pellegrino. Tancredi, *Ethics of Health Care*, pp. 33–64.

BACON, FRANCIS. *Historia Naturalis: Historia Vitae et Mortis* (1623). "Historia Vitae et Mortis." *The Works of Francis Bacon.* 15 vols. Edited by James Speddings, Robert Leslie Ellis, and Douglas Denon Heath. Vol. 2: *Philosophical Works, Vol. II.* London: Longman & Co., 1887–1901, pp. 89–226. Translation. "The History of Life and Death, or the Second Title in Natural and Experimental History for the Foundation of Philosophy: Being the Third Part of the Instauratio Magna." *The Works of Francis Bacon*, Vol. 5: *Translations of the Philosophical Works, Vol. II*, pp. 215–335.

BLAU, ZENA SMITH. *Old Age in a Changing Society.* New York: New Viewpoints, 1973.

CALLAHAN, DANIEL. *The Tyranny of Survival.* New York: Macmillan Co., 1973.

CALLAHAN, SIDNEY, and CHRISTIANSEN, DREW. "Ideal Old Age." *Soundings* 57 (1974): 1–16. Special Issue: Leisure, Retirement and Aging.

CHRISTIANSEN, DREW. "Dignity in Aging." *Hastings Center Report* 4, no. 1 (1974), pp. 6–8.

CICERO, MARCUS TULLIUS. *De Senectute, De Amicitia, De Divinatione.* Translated by William Armistead Falconer. Loeb Classical Library. Cambridge: Harvard University Press, 1938, pp. 1–99.

COWGILL, DONALD O., and HOLMES, LOWELL D., eds. *Aging and Modernization.* New York: Appleton-Century-Crofts, 1972.

CUMMING, ELAINE, and HENRY, WILLIAM E. *Growing Old: The Process of Disengagement.* New York: Basic Books, 1961.

DEMOS, JOHN. *A Little Commonwealth: Family Life in Plymouth Colony.* New York: Oxford University Press, 1970.

ERIKSON, ERIK H. "The Life Cycle: Epigenesis of Identity." *Identity: Youth and Crisis.* New York: W. W. Norton & Co., 1968, chap. 3, pp. 91–141.

———. "Reflections on Dr. Borg's Life Cycle." *Daedalus* 105, no. 2 (1976), pp. 1–28.

HARKSEN, SIBYLLE. *Women in the Middle Ages.* Translated by Marianne Herzfeld. The Image of Woman. New York: Abner Schram, Universe Books, 1975.

HARRINGTON, ALAN. *The Immortalist: An Approach to the Engineering of Man's Divinity.* New York: Random House, 1969. Paperback ed. New York: Avon, Discus Books, 1970.

HAVIGHURST, ROBERT J., and ALBRECHT, RUTH. *Older People.* New York: Longmans, Green, 1953.

HERODOTUS. *Herodotus.* Translation by A. D. Godley. Loeb Classical Library. New York: Putnam, 1931, vol. 1, bk. 1, nos. 30–32, pp. 32–41.

ILLICH, IVAN D. *Medical Nemesis: The Expropriation of Health.* London: Calder & Boyars, 1975.

———. "The Political Uses of Natural Death." *Hastings Center Studies* 2, no. 1 (1974), pp. 3–20.

KÜBLER-ROSS, ELIZABETH, ed. *Death: The Final Stage of Growth.* Human Development Books: A Series in Applied Behavioral Science. Englewood Cliffs, N.J.: Prentice-Hall, 1975.

KAPLAN, JEROME. "In Search of Policies for Care of the Aged." With commentary by Sissela Bok. Tancredi, *The Ethics of Health Care,* pp. 281–313.

MARKSON, ELIZABETH WARREN. "Readjustment to Time in Old Age: A Life Cycle Approach." *Psychiatry* 36 (1973): 37–48.

Monumenta de viduis, diaconissis virginibusque tractantia. Edited by Josephine Mayer. Florilegium Patristicum tam veteris quam medii aevi auctores complectens, vol. 42. Bonn: Peter Hanstein, 1937.

RICE, DOROTHY P., and COOPER, BARBARA S. "The Economic Value of Human Life." *American Journal of Public Health and the Nation's Health* 57 (1967): 1954–1966.

RICOEUR, PAUL. *Freedom and Nature: The Voluntary and the Involuntary.* Translated, with an introduction, by Erazim V. Kohák. Evanston, Ill.: Northwestern University Press, 1966.

ROSENFELD, ALBERT. *Prolongevity: A Report on the Revolutionary Scientific Discoveries Now Being Made about Aging and Dying, and Their Promise of an Extended Lifespan, without Old Age.* A Borzoi Book. New York: Alfred A. Knopf, 1976.

SACHS, HANNELORE. *The Renaissance Woman.* Edited by Bernhardus Geyer and Johannes Zellinger. Translated by Marianne Herzfeld. Revised by D. T. Rice. The Image of Woman. New York: McGraw-Hill, 1971.

SEGERBERG, OSBORN, JR. *The Immortality Factor.* New York: Dutton, 1974.

SHANAS, ETHEL, and STREIB, GORDON F., eds. *Social Structure and the Family: Generational Relations.* Englewood Cliffs, N.J.: Prentice-Hall, 1965.

———; TOWNSEND, PETER; WEDDERBURN, DOROTHY; FRIIS, HENNING; MILHØJ, POUL; and STEHOUWER, JAN. *Old People in Three Industrial Societies.* New York: Atherton Press, 1968.

TANCREDI, LAURENCE R., ed. *Ethics of Health Care.* Conference on Health Care and Changing Values, Institute of Medicine, 1973. Washington: Academy of Sciences, 1974.

IV

**HEALTH CARE AND RESEARCH
IN THE AGED**

This article will deal with (1) the provision of health care for the aged, with special consideration.of medical and hospital services, nursing home care, and mental health care in the United States, and (2) experimentation involving the aged.

Health care for the aged

Medical and hospital services. The majority of older Americans below the age of seventy-five are independent. Among those not in this majority, and among those seventy-five years of age and older, intractable problems of ill health are prevalent, straining to the limit the resources of the health-care delivery system, and exposing its deficiencies. In the United States the sick aged (bedfast and housebound) number more than three million, or between twelve and fourteen percent of those over sixty-five (Anderson, pp. 89 f.). Elderly patients remain in hospital twice as long and require hospitalization twice as often as those under sixty-five. They account for one-fourth of the nation's health expenditures, are the prime users of long-term care facilities, and consume twenty-five percent of all drugs (Butler, p. 174). Unfortunately, the emphasis in American society has been on "high medical technology" designed to meet acute, episodic needs, rather than on adequate care for the chronically ill. Yet, as one commentator observes, "while the aged have need for acute medical care, their major requirement is in the continuum of services for the chronically disabled that will enable them to function optimally" (Brody, p. 414).

Our ability to respond to this principal requirement by managing the chronic ailments associated with aging is disastrously poor. This is evident in a widespread apathy toward the old within the medical profession. House-call services are rare. Emergency room treatment is typically depersonalizing. Doctors' fees are beyond the means of many (Butler, pp. 183 f.). Medicare, with its array of deductibles, coinsurances, and rising premiums, meets less than forty percent of the costs of health care (Corman, pp. 83 ff.). As the 1976 report by the Congressional Subcommittee on Health and Long-term Care of the Select Committee on Aging points out, this situation is exacerbated by two underlying factors. One is that "both government and carriers of health insurance accept as given a tightly defined medical model as the premise for defining benefits and payments" (*New Perspectives,* p. 2). This medical model "has severe limitations which hamper its application in designing benefits for chronic illness, geriatrics and long-term care services" (ibid.). The other factor is that the scope of and eligibility for health-care services are normatively designated in terms of levels. "The levels of care needed by the users and the level of services provided by classes of providers not only have complicated and limited the provision of patient care, but have also created an administratively cumbersome mechanism for monitoring the quality and quantity of services" (ibid.).

Together, those two factors contribute to the following problems: delayed entry into the health-care system because of constraints on early detection and treatment; lack of incentives for optimum use of health resources and cost-efficient use of home health services; increased dependency upon institutionalization for persons whose needs are for maintenance and rehabilitation; perpetuation of minimum standards for providers, which discourage the provision of individualized care; overemphasis on quantitative factors (such as size of physical facilities) rather than a qualitative concern; and the neglect of the needs of a sizable patient population whose requirement for care does not conform to the artificial structure of the reimbursement systems. In practice this means, inter alia, that the elderly encounter obstacles when they require hospitalization. Acute brain syndromes are frequently overlooked in emergency rooms; chronic brain syndromes are commonly dismissed as "senility." Older patients are treated symptomatically and released, or transferred from voluntary to overburdened and underfinanced community hospitals. Nor have Medicare and Medicaid succeeded in eradicating a double standard in medicine, whereby younger and less impecunious patients receive better hospital care than those both aged and poor.

This generally dismal situation calls for a review of methods of medical and hospital practice, fee schedules, reimbursement formulae, and incentive grants, and of the universal applicability of the medical model. The moral imperative is to develop a more adequate system of medical and hospital services to the aged. The ethical principles of respect for persons and distributive justice might serve as criteria for doing this (Jonsen, pp. 97 ff., 100 ff.). These norms underlie many of the recommendations made by the 1976 congressional subcommittee in the report, among the more significant and far-reaching of which are the following: a system of community long-term care centers to coordinate the provision of health services for older Americans, allowing to the elderly high-quality care in the setting of their choice; a revision of the congressional committee structure to provide better coordination of legislation affecting the aged; and legislation to provide for the gathering and disseminating of information concerning the various public and private agencies delivering home health care and correlative services to the elderly (*New Perspectives*).

Nursing homes. Nonprofit and government homes, providing residential and personal care rather than nursing services, accommodate twenty percent of those older persons who are in institutions. The remaining eighty percent are in commercial or proprietary nursing homes, which now constitute a $9 billion industry (ibid., p. x). Despite exceptions, it is in this latter category that gross abuses occur in the wake of a conflict between profit and service. This has led one commentator necessarily to conclude that "a nursing home is a facility that has few or no nurses and can hardly qualify as a home" (Butler, p. 263). Another investigator and her collaborators document Butler's view in devastating terms (Townsend). Of the persons residing in nursing homes, seventy percent are female; fifty percent either have no living relatives or contact with even distant relatives; the average age is seventy-eight; ninety-six percent are white—because of the shorter life expectancy of minorities and widespread discrimination against them; sixty to eighty percent are poor; eighty-five percent die in nursing homes; almost all have more than one physical ailment; about thirty-two percent have either serious hearing defects or visual disabilities (Butler, p. 267). Considering that in 1969 there were approximately 815,000 residents sixty-five years of age and over in 18,000 nursing and personal care homes (Anderson, p. 91), and that those figures have now increased appreciably, one can see that victimization of the elderly is occurring on a massive scale. Federal programs have not only contributed to making nursing homes profitable to the owners; they have also failed to enforce with any rigor the comprehensive national standards. There is a dearth of audits of nursing homes across the nation (*New Perspectives*, p. 29). Many government surveys, such as the Office of Nursing Home Affairs' 1975 Facility Improvement Survey (United States), and many of the state fiscal audits of nursing homes are confidential, ensuring the anonymity of the institutions being surveyed. In many cases this policy does not serve the best interests of the public: Disclosure of information "may encourage action that will result in correction of deficiencies and improvement of life safety conditions for residents" (*New Perspectives*, p. 31).

The use of nursing homes as extended-care facilities providing skilled nursing has been hampered by the arbitrary, inflexible, and inconsistent nature of social security guidelines in the United States, and by the fact that the most obdurate conditions do not fall into the "acceptable" category or, if they do, do so for a limited time only. This has led one author to assert that

"Medicare essentially ends when long-term help-lessness and need for surveillance starts" (Anderson, p. 90). Aggravating this bleak state of affairs is the propensity of associations of homes for the aged to seek to perpetuate the status quo (Butler, pp. 285 ff.).

The profound deficiencies in nursing homes and Medicare-approved homes thwart the ideal of adequate medical care for the elderly. Reforms are long overdue. Several eminently reasonable proposals have been made in this regard (ibid., pp. 295–299). A massive enlistment of public support for radical change is both warranted and wanting. One of the more acute moral questions concerns the propriety of placing home health services, a logical alternative to nursing homes, under the jurisdiction of the Office of Nursing Home Affairs. Since "the nursing home industry and the home health industry are, at least theoretically, competing for the same market" (New Perspectives, p. 8), present policy seems clearly to involve a substantial conflict of interest.

Mental health care.   Given the conditions described briefly above, and similar formidable difficulties encountered in respect to housing, transportation, the cost of living, family and societal segregation and consequent isolation, and employment, and consequent upon the deterioration of physical functions, it is not surprising that those sixty-five and over are the most susceptible to mental illness, with males the most prone to committing suicide (ibid., p. 37).

There is a disproportionately high number of elderly in mental hospitals: the total population over 65 in mental hospitals ranges from 28 to 40 percent although the elderly comprise only about 10 percent of the total population. And while there are only about 5 percent of the total population in all forms of institutions at any one point in time, almost 1 in 4 elderly persons will be institutionalized at some point in their later years [ibid., p. 34].

In spite of this situation, substantial increases of funds, personnel, and facilities for matching the mental needs of the aged have not been forthcoming.

Psychiatry as a whole "shares a sense of futility and therapeutic nihilism about old age" (Butler, p. 231). The label "senility" is often indiscriminately applied as a means of evading thorough diagnosis and treatment. Drugs are often used to pacify, control, and treat symptomatically aged persons with remediable disorders (ibid., pp. 235 f.). Federally funded community health centers provide deficient care because of budgetary constraints and a lack of trained staff. Private mental hospitals, affording the best care, are beyond the means of most of the elderly. State and county hospitals thus become their chief resource, but most are dubiously effective in respect to basic services, trained psychiatrists, and their environment. Transfer out of these institutions to boarding homes is often precipitous and more in the interest of cutting costs than of benefiting mental patients (ibid., pp. 225–259). On the other hand, "it is clear that many elderly persons are in mental hospitals, not because of severe mental impairment, but because there is no other place for them to go" (New Perspectives, p. 34). The President's Task Force on Aging in 1970 expressed concern about the use of state mental hospitals as custodial facilities for the elderly who are not in need of psychiatric care simply because of the absence of alternative living arrangements and psychological support.

Ethical considerations.   This unexaggerated delineation of shortcomings in the provision of medical and hospital services, nursing homes, and mental health care for the aged gives weight to the moral arguments advanced by Jonsen and others. Not only is the form of care in the United States, being predominantly acute rather than chronic, unsuited to the elderly; it also compromises their individuality and diversity. Instead of respecting and enhancing their autonomy, it contributes to their deterioration and dependency and, in so doing, compromises their constitutional right to liberty. In addition, it raises sharply the question of allocating limited resources. The principle of distributive justice, of which John Rawls is an outstanding contemporary exponent, gives grounds for contesting productivity as a preferred societal value, for challenging our cultural equation of age with obsolescence and ordering our priorities accordingly, for claiming that the aged represent the acme of our human vulnerability to physical and psychological insult, and for urging that we should not invoke "lifeboat ethics" until we have exhausted other, less desperate alternatives. But distributive justice is a philosophical concept beyond the immediate horizons of those engaged in politics. "It is largely impotent unless it attracts the force of constituencies' interests and social urgency" (Jonsen, p. 103). Therefore, it is not merely hortatory but strategically necessary for Jonsen to pose the moral question: "Who will raise the cry of injustice that the sick aged cannot utter? How can their injustices outweigh the competing injustices of other more vocal groups, not to say the competing claims of the already powerful?" (Ibid., p. 103.)

Experimentation involving the aged

Not only is research into the processes and experiences of aging requisite as a means to providing better care, but it promises benefits to society as a whole, all of whose members are ineluctably growing older. In order to extend and improve the life of the general population, as well as of those now aged, we need to know more about the multifarious ramifications of aging. At present, disproportionately small amounts of time and money are spent on such work. Much research can and is being done in vitro and with animal models. Moreover, many gerontological studies do not place subjects at risk. However, because it is not possible simply to extrapolate from animal or in vitro findings to human beings, and because geriatric research involves risks of harm as well as potential benefits, experimentation with elderly persons is fraught with moral dilemmas. Of these, three of the more important deserve mention.

Therapeutic and nontherapeutic research involving the aged. The Declaration of Helsinki, adopted in June 1964 by the World Medical Association and endorsed by the major American investigative and medical associations, makes a clear and crucial distinction between therapeutic research, in which investigation occurs coincidentally with the provision of care, and nontherapeutic research, in which the element of care for the individual is absent. The full text of the Declaration will be found in the Appendix to this encyclopedia. Sections II and III are relevant to this discussion.

I have already alluded to the need for investigation with this segment of the total population, but what of its ethical propriety? Therapeutic research raises fewer objections in this regard than experimentation of a nontherapeutic nature. Provided that the potential benefits of the therapy are greater than or equal to those of alternative modalities of treatment, and provided that the informed consent of the patient-subject is obtained, there is little to impugn the moral acceptability of therapeutic research. However, nontherapeutic research with the elderly as subjects is a more controversial matter. Such research involves an inescapable conflict of values: the potential benefits for aged persons, present and future, as a group versus respect for the dignity, security, and well-being of the individual.

The aged as a captive population. Should the aged be regarded as a controlled or "captive" population and, as such, be exempt from research, or at least receive special consideration? A case might be made for outright exemption. Most aged persons are deprived, not only economically, but because of social, cultural, administrative, and political exigencies as well; they are thus more controlled than the general population. The elderly are institutionalized more than any other group and, as "captives," are vulnerable to studies of questionable ethicality. Moreover, those suffering from diagnosed organic brain syndromes might be regarded as among the mentally incompetent, commonly excluded from research. These factors, however, seem to warrant special consideration for the aged as research subjects, rather than exemption. To exclude all because some have an impaired capacity to comprehend or by virtue of their external circumstances cannot make autonomous decisions would be to stereotype and degrade many. Recognizing that the aged constitute a heterogeneous group should cause us instead to urge extreme caution in their involvement in research. Jonas's principle of a descending order of permissibility ought to be applied with particular care: "The poorer in knowledge, motivation, and freedom of decision . . . the more sparingly and indeed reluctantly should the reservoir be used" (Jonas, p. 20).

Informed consent and the aged. If it is discriminatory to exempt all elderly persons from research because some are incapable of comprehending information about the risks and benefits of, and alternatives to, contemplated studies, or incapable of consenting freely to participate, the onus should be on investigators to distinguish between those who are competent and uncoerced and those who are not, and to apply Jonas's principle with discretion and restraint. This presupposes that researchers will establish genuine interpersonal relationships with those to be involved in experimentation, in which their abilities or disabilities to comprehend and consent can be assessed and in which, if they are judged competent, their collaboration can be enlisted without constraint. Consideration should also be given to the establishment of proxy or surrogate consent mechanisms as a means for providing additional protection to elderly research subjects.

Conclusion

While it is true that the aged have special needs, it is not clear that special ethical principles are needed to respond to the moral dilemmas raised by health care and biomedical research in the aged. Biomedical policies and practices affecting the aged should be scrutinized in light of an ethic of caring, of distributive justice, and of respect for the autonomy of the individual in a context of reasonable advances in scientific knowledge.

ERNLÉ W. D. YOUNG

[In addition to the foregoing three articles on aging in this entry, the following are directly related: HEALTH CARE; CHRONIC CARE; and POVERTY AND HEALTH. See also HOSPITALS; HUMAN EXPERIMENTATION, articles on BASIC ISSUES, PHILOSOPHICAL ASPECTS, and SOCIAL AND PROFESSIONAL CONTROL; INFORMED CONSENT IN HUMAN RESEARCH; INSTITUTIONALIZATION; JUSTICE; and PATIENTS' RIGHTS MOVEMENT.]

BIBLIOGRAPHY

ANDERSON, ODIN W. "Reflections on the Sick Aged and the Helping Systems." Neugarten, Social Policy, pp. 89–96.

BERNSTEIN, JOEL E. "Medical Experimentation in the Elderly." Journal of the American Geriatrics Society 23 (1975): 327–329.

BEAUVOIR, SIMONE DE. The Coming of Age. Translated by Patrick O'Brian. New York: Warner Paperback Library, 1973.

BRODY, STANLEY J. "Comprehensive Health Care for the Elderly: An Analysis." Gerontologist 13 (1973): 412–418.

BUTLER, ROBERT N. Why Survive? Being Old in America. New York: Harper & Row, 1975.

Commission on Chronic Illness. Chronic Illness in the United States. 4 vols. Vol. 2: Care of the Long-Term Patient. Cambridge: Commonwealth Fund, Harvard University Press, 1956.

CORMAN, JAMES C. "Health Services for the Elderly." Neugarten, Social Policy, pp. 81–88.

COWDRY, EDMUND VINCENT, and STEINBERG, FRANZ U. The Care of the Geriatric Patient. 4th ed. St. Louis: Mosby Co., 1971.

Group for the Advancement of Psychiatry, Committee on Aging. "The Aged and Community Mental Health: A Guide to Program Development." Group for the Advancement of Psychiatry. Report 8 (1971): 1–96. Report no. 81.

——. "Toward a Public Policy on Mental Health Care of the Elderly." Group for the Advancement of Psychiatry. Report 7 (1970): 651–700. Report no. 79.

JONAS, HANS. "Philosophical Reflections on Experimenting with Human Subjects." Experimentation with Human Subjects. Edited by Paul A. Freund. New York: George Braziller, 1969, pp. 1–31.

JONSEN, ALBERT R. "Principles for an Ethics of Health Services." Neugarten, Social Policy, pp. 97–104.

KATZ, JAY, ed. Experimentation with Human Beings: The Authority of the Investigator, Subject, Professions, and State in the Human Experimentation Process. New York: Russell Sage Foundation, 1972.

LASAGNA, LOUIS. The Conflict of Interest between Physician as Therapist and as Experimenter. Philadel-phia: Society for Health and Human Values, 1975. Originally prepared for the Committee on Human Experimentation of the Society for Health and Human Values, 1971.

MENDELSON, MARY ADELAIDE. Tender Loving Greed: How the Incredibly Lucrative Nursing Home "Industry" Is Exploiting America's Old People and Defrauding Us All. New York: Alfred A. Knopf, 1974.

National Academy of Sciences. Experiments and Research with Humans: Values in Conflict. Academy Forum, 3d, 1975. Washington: 1975.

NEUGARTEN, BERNICE L., and HAVIGHURST, ROBERT J., eds. Social Policy, Social Ethics, and the Aging Society. NSF/RA 76–000247. Washington: Government Printing Office, 1976. Report prepared by Committee on Human Development, University of Chicago, for the National Science Foundation, RANN-Research Applications Directorate.

New Perspectives in Health Care for Older Americans: Recommendations and Policy Directions of the Subcommittee on Health and Long-term Care: Report, Together with Additional and Supplemental Views. Subcommittee on Health and Long-term Care, Select Committee on Aging, House of Representatives. 94th Cong., 2d sess. Washington: Government Printing Office, 1976.

Older Americans Act of 1965. Pub. L. No. 89–73. 79 Stat. 218 (1965).

President's Task Force on the Aging. Toward a Brighter Future for the Elderly: A Report. Washington: Government Printing Office, 1970.

RAWLS, JOHN. A Theory of Justice. Cambridge: Belknap Press, Harvard University Press, 1971.

SLOATE, NATHAN. "Old Age." A Concise Handbook of Community Psychiatry and Community Mental Health. Edited by Leopold Bellak. New York: Grune & Stratton, 1974, pp. 91–104.

TOWNSEND, CLAIRE, project director. Old Age: The Last Segregation. New York: Grossman Publishers, 1971.

United States, Office of Nursing Home Affairs. Long-Term Care Facility Improvement Study: Introductory Report. DHEW Publication no. (OS) 76–50021. Washington: Government Printing Office, 1975.

WOODRUFF, DIANA S., and BIRREN, JAMES E., eds. Aging: Scientific Perspectives and Social Issues. New York: D. Van Nostrand Co., 1975. Project of the Ethel Percy Andrus Gerontology Center, University of Southern California.

ALCOHOL, USE OF

Three behaviors with alcoholic beverages pose ethical issues: drinking, drunkenness (getting drunk), and alcoholism. Numerous secondary ethical issues derive from attitudes toward and responses to these behaviors by individuals and by agencies of society.

Drinking

Many people see drinking itself as an ethical issue. The classical antialcohol (temperance) movement perceived that biological as well as social harms result from intake of alcohol and drew its moral conclusions from that fact. It held, first, that harm to the self was inherently wrong, and second, that even those who drank most moderately, so that self-harm could not be presumed, were nevertheless practicing an inessential indulgence that could harm others and were thus under an ethical imperative to desist. The harm to others was seen as in the nature of setting an example that the "weak brother" might follow to a harmful degree ("Wesley").

The morality of drinking and the belief that any drinking of alcoholic beverages may be immoral or unethical are subjects still discussed by many. Some old religions and some comparatively new religious developments forbid alcohol: Buddhism, Brahmanism, Islam, and, among Christian groups, the Baptists, Christian Scientists, Mormons, Quakers, Seventh-Day Adventists, and Witnesses. The Methodists only relatively recently modified the doctrine that made drinking a sin. Thus, for multitudes of religious people drinking itself is the ethical issue, and the alcohol industry is tainted with immorality. The ethical problems connected with alcoholism, then, are derivative. In addition, some churches that do not require abstinence advocate it as morally desirable (Cherrington).

Religions and churches were not alone in perceiving a moral issue in drinking. Social reformers, often religiously inspired (for example, Frances Willard, founder of the Women's Christian Temperance Union), often proclaimed the harm and recognized no compensatory virtue in alcohol. In addition, some nonreligious and even antireligious reformers also opposed drinking and the drink trade as social evils, ethically reprehensible. These latter included a portion of the nineteenth- and early twentieth-century socialist and labor leadership. And while in the United States labor generally opposed the imposition of national prohibition, seeing it as representing exploitative interests, in several European countries labor and socialist support helped to impose prohibition or stringent legal controls on the availability of alcohol, which was seen as compounding the workers' economic disadvantagement.

On the other side, against the outlook of the alcohol-rejecting groups, were the views of those who held drink to be either neutral or good—"The Good Creature of God"—to be used, in moderation, for man's benefit. They had reason to think that in moderate drinking there was not only no harm but positive benefit. The possibility of harmful misuse was recognized, but that was true of many things on earth and did not demand abstinence by the majority who did not misuse.

The question whether a primary ethical issue exists apparently hinges on whether any drinking, even in unchallengeable moderation, can be injurious to health. At present the consensus among health and biological authorities is that moderate drinking—here defined arbitrarily as small amounts of alcohol taken occasionally, for example, within the famed Anstie's (1864) limit of 1 1/2 ounces of absolute alcohol per day— causes no demonstrable injury to health. Whether the moderate drinker sets a seductive example, and whether this constitutes an ethical obligation to refrain entirely, are questions not answerable by present scientific knowledge. The problem is not the same as with moderate smoking, where it is argued that the smoker (at least in public places) pollutes the air that others must breathe. But it is a problem that may confront many potentially example-setting behaviors.

Whatever applies to the ethical problems connected with drinking is relevant also to engaging in the drink trade. At a time when alcohol—the substance itself, personified as the Demon Rum —was seen as the enemy of the good life, the Methodist Church in America, for example, doctrinally held traffic in alcohol to be sinful. Yet the Mormon Church, which forbids drinking, holds it no sin to sell alcohol to gentiles who want to drink.

Universal conflict thus exists about the rightness of drinking and of engaging in the drink trade. In the United States some 95 million adults and an additional nineteen million persons aged over thirteen but under twenty-one years are drinkers. Nearly one-third of the adults abstain, however (Keller and Gurioli). In other English-speaking countries, and in the Germanic, Romance, and Slavic lands; even larger majorities are drinkers. Thus it seems that the vast multitudes in these countries recognize no inherent wrong in drinking itself and consequently, it seems reasonable to presume, in the trade.

Drunkenness

Almost universally regarded as wrong is overdrinking—variously expressed as excessive, immoderate, heavy, irresponsible drinking—and, especially, getting drunk. A distinction is here made between drunkenness and alcoholism. People who do not have the disease of alcoholism (as defined below) may on occasion drink enough to achieve an alcoholic "high"—marked by some functional impairment—or even enough to get drunk, for a variety of reasons or purposes.

Although most people apparently regard drinking for the explicit purpose of getting drunk to be wrong on the grounds that it impairs a person's self-control and poses a risk to the well-being of others, there are some who believe that even this type of behavior can be justified on occasions. Thus, for example, some condone fiestal drinking, often to drunkenness sometimes lasting several days, practiced by whole communities (Washburne). Such may be the overdrinking required, by consensus, of the young man being initiated into a college fraternity, or expected by the friends of the bridegroom at his "bachelor party." Thus even drunkenness evokes equivocal responses, for in the eyes of some it too has its season.

Despite this benign view condoning occasional drunkenness, it is important to recognize that the intake of alcohol in beverages (as beer, wine, distilled spirits) beyond some safe quantity (or combination of quantity and frequency) can certainly injure the human biological organism. It can cause or contribute to the development of many physical and behavioral or mental disorders. On this ground, excessive drinking (here defined as that which is sufficient to cause drunkenness or other psychic or physical disorder) is condemned by ethicists who believe that self-indulgence which leads to self-injury is wrong. This position is the same as the moral teaching of the religions that do not forbid moderate drinking.

Alcoholism

Drinking and alcoholism. If drinking has been a source of conflict in the realm of ethics—churches and citizens seeing it as both right and wrong—alcoholism has been even more divisive of attitudes.

From ancient times, drinking has been connected with excess and derived troubles (Keller, 1974, pp. 442–443). Drunkenness seems to have occurred early, and for the most part most people did not distinguish between drunkenness and alcoholism as it is understood today—that is, a psychobiological disease (a drug addiction or drug dependency) marked by an inconsistent helplessness of the victim to refrain from re-sorting to alcohol, and inconsistent helplessness to refrain from drunkenness (Keller and McCormick, p. 12). It was therefore natural to condemn all drunkenness as wrongdoing. Yet an insightful first-century philosopher already made the distinction between drunkenness and addiction (Seneca, Epistle lxxxiii), and a long line of thinkers, including physicians, agree with him to this day.

Alcoholism as a disease. Alcoholism, conceptualized as alcohol addiction (Keller and McCormick, p. 14), or alcohol dependence, or the alcohol-dependence syndrome (Edwards et al., p. 1364), is regarded as a disease by most authorities; it is so classified in the nomenclatures of the authoritative American and international medical organizations (United States; National Conference; American Psychiatric Association; World Health Organization). The disease of alcoholism, so conceptualized, is thus to be distinguished from drinking as such and even from drunkenness. Of course, if drinking as such caused alcoholism, then it would come under the ethical ban of self-injurious behavior. But most authorities regard as simplistic the idea that drinking or alcohol alone is the cause of alcoholism. They hold that, while there is no alcoholism without drinking, the fact that the vast majority of drinkers—perhaps ninety-five percent in the United States (Keller and Gurioli) —do not develop alcoholism indicates that another cause must operate to induce addiction, and that the uncontrollable alcohol ingestion by alcoholics is not the same thing as the normal personal and social behavior of drinking (Bacon).

From the viewpoint of those who demand abstinence (and abolition of the alcohol trade) on account of the weak brother, the fact that most drinkers do not develop alcoholism is irrelevant. No one would develop alcoholism if alcohol were banished utterly. The problem, however, is not so simple. What would happen to the people who develop alcoholism if there were no alcohol? Would they escape trouble and harm? What does happen to such people in societies that do not have alcohol? There is evidence that some people, especially women, by way of "choice of symptoms," develop affective disorders rather than alcoholism (Winokur et al., p. 110), and this is suggested as one explanation of the higher frequency of alcoholism among men in contrast to the higher frequency of affective disorders among women. There are also indications in the medical literature that for some people alcoholism is a disorder that enables them to avert other psychic traumas that are more serious (Bird; Smilde). If, then, the abolition of alcohol would only prevent alcoholism but not alternative illness in susceptible people, the argument for an ethical imperative to abolish alcohol in order to prevent alcoholism loses its force.

The moral issue. If alcoholism is illness, can it still be immoral? Courts have sometimes struggled with the problem of self-inflicted disease—after all, alcoholics voluntarily "put an enemy in their mouths to steal away their brain" (Shakespeare, *Othello,* II, 3, 293) and their good health. A Catholic theologian, John Ford, has put the ethical issue well: The alcoholic may have been at fault, guilty of the sin of gluttony (by drunkenness), when he was still able to choose whether or not to drink, and how much. But once he has become addicted, once he has passed a line that marks him off as diseased and by reason of his disease no longer always has freedom with respect to alcohol—if under the compulsion of his disease he now gets drunk—he is guiltless. In recent years this understanding has been written into many state laws explicitly defining alcoholism as a disease and has been confirmed in decisions of high courts (Ford).

But this view is not accepted universally, not even by physicians. A surviving body of opinion holds that alcoholism is not a disease, an opinion apparently based on the belief that alcoholics are able to control their behavior but fail to make an adequate effort to do so (Todd; Schmidhofer). Some of this opinion appears to be based on misunderstanding of the conception of "loss of control over drinking." If "loss of control" is understood, according to one definition, to mean inability to stop drinking once it is started, then, the argument goes, the alcoholic is blameworthy for taking the first drink. But the more sophisticated conception of "loss of control" emphasizes the fundamental incapacity or disablement of the addict, at times, to choose whether to drink—to resist an overwhelming inner drive (Keller, 1972; Glatt; Ludwig and Wikler), possibly the effect of biodynamic changes in central neurons (Kesner, Priano, and DeWitt; Gross).

At one stage of alcoholism, at least, the behavior of alcoholics in resorting to alcohol, in drinking to and beyond drunkenness, seems surely a consequence as well as a manifestation of disease. At this point the alcoholic seems not to be free in his choices. This occurs in the course of a bout—whether or not its initiation is seen as blameworthy—when the alcoholic, pausing in alcohol intake, experiences the beginning of the alcohol withdrawal syndrome. The symptoms, unrelieved, may become intolerably painful, even threatening to sanity and life. The desperate resort to alcohol then, which may be the only reliable and effective medicine available to the alcoholic, appears to be beyond censure.

Of course, those who recently have challenged all belief in mental or behavioral illness reject utterly a conception of alcoholism as disease (Szasz). They are followed by a new trend in social science and behavioral psychology to reject what is perceived as "the medical model" of behavioral disorders. It is not yet clear where this trend leads with respect to the ethical issues of alcoholism. Those who refuse to grant that alcoholism is a disease would leave alcoholics alone: Certainly they would be against any compulsory treatment. Others, in particular the psychologists who believe that the behavior is environmentally induced, advocate behavioral therapies.

Some ethicists would question the ethics of leaving alcoholics alone. As against the idea that it is wrong to interfere with nonconformist behavior, they question the morality of not helping sick people but leaving them to inevitable disaster. The fate of alcoholics who recover is extremely different from that of those who suffer the severe and fatal consequences of unrelieved alcoholism. Is "leave them alone" a humane attitude?

Problems of response to the alcoholic

Renewal of the historical disagreement over whether alcoholism is a disease has raised questions about the ethical response to alcoholics and other drunken persons by various professions, by numerous social institutions, by related and unrelated individuals. Foremost among the concerned professions is medicine. The accusation has often been leveled that physicians try to avoid treating alcoholics, because alcoholics are difficult persons, unresponsive to sound medical advice (especially "you must stop drinking"), usually incurable, and unreliable in paying their bills. Physicians have been accused of being motivated to assume a moralistic view of alcoholism as an excuse for avoiding alcoholics. Nurses and other health professionals, as well as social workers, have been depicted similarly. To the extent that these accusations may be true of a part of the personnel of the health professions, a serious breach of professional ethics would prevail.

Among the social institutions, hospitals and clinics have been accused of refusing admission to alcoholics, sometimes even when they are acutely ill, if "drunkenness" is obvious. In 1956 the American Medical Association through its officers found it necessary to urge hospitals to admit alcoholics like other sick people ("Reports of Officers"), and subsequently the American Hospital Association echoed this sentiment.

Both public and private social service agencies have at times by policy refused to help alcoholics and families in which the perceived cause of distress was the drunkenness of the man of the house. Most social caseworkers in the field considered this policy to be wrong and frequently countered it by benignly (if unethically) neglecting to record the alcoholism in their reports to the agencies. Even jails, one social institution to which at least lower-class alcoholics are referred with special frequency, have been accused of discrimination against alcoholics by confining them in the infamous "drunk tanks" and failing to provide urgently needed medical care to the severely ill, sometimes with resulting fatalities. Jails and mental hospitals have been accused of seeking alcoholics as inmates so as to exploit them for housekeeping tasks. Clearly failures of normal humane treatment by health and social personnel and institutions are related to beliefs about drunkenness as a form of wrongdoing, deserving only punishment, and ignorance about or disbelief in the reality of alcoholism as a disease compelling the drunkenness of the alcoholic.

The belief that his repetitive ingestion of harmful amounts of alcoholic beverage is willful drunkenness, which the alcoholic could stop by sheer will power, is at the root of the discriminatory treatment of alcoholics. In the eyes of those who believe that alcoholism is a disease that most alcoholics are unable to overcome without therapeutic help, the result is unjust, inhumane, and unethical treatment of the alcoholic. The conflict of beliefs, whether it is the behavior of the alcoholics which is immoral, or the behavior of those who deny them help, remains an open challenge in ethics.

Experimentation and therapeutics

Biological and psychological interest in effects of alcohol on the organism and on behavior, and in the causes and treatments of alcoholic diseases and of alcoholism itself, evokes the same ethical issues with respect to experimentation and therapeutic approaches as interest in other biological–psychological functions and disorders. In addition, alcoholism presents some unique ethical problems.

A serious question seems to arise with informed and free consent, but there is really no difficulty in answering that question. Alcoholics may have a mental illness, one of the special alcoholic disorders, or coincidentally a psychosis such as schizophrenia. In such cases their capacity to decide and consent is presumably impaired. But otherwise, alcoholism is not in the class of psychic illnesses that render a person mentally incompetent, and alcoholics are capable of giving informed consent. In this connection it needs to be borne in mind that they are often found in mental hospitals only because that is where some authorities have found it convenient to situate treatment and rehabilitative programs for alcoholics.

A more serious issue arises when the experiment involves giving people large amounts of alcohol repeatedly and over prolonged periods, with the possibility of inducing addiction. With nonaddicted subjects this would presumably be ethically impermissible, regardless of informed consent, since here it is not a question of risking a curable disorder but of acquiring a catastrophic chronic disease that at present is rarely curable. Such experiments were conducted in the past, the subjects being either alcohol addicts or addicted to other drugs, with resulting induction of withdrawal symptoms (interpreted by the experimenters as indicative of physical addiction). It is unlikely that such an experiment would be undertaken nowadays in human subjects who are not already specifically alcohol addicts. But in the case of alcohol addicts who are going to ingest all the alcohol they can get and hold in any event, experimenters argue that to provide them with the alcohol under ideal, controlled, metabolic-ward conditions, with twenty-four-hour-a-day nursing supervision, medical care, and nutritional protection, is to their advantage rather than harmful.

It had been generally accepted throughout the world that the aim in treating alcoholism was not cure, which would allow normal drinking, but remission through total abstinence. A number of behavioral psychologists have reported experiments, with some claims of success, in treating alcoholic patients so that they could resume moderate drinking. But some have questioned such attempts and claims. They note that success in the relief of alcoholism has been almost exclusively based on the work of Alcoholics Anonymous, a self-help fellowship whose program is firmly rooted in the abstinence ideology, and on treatments by professionals who likewise have helped alcoholics to avoid any drinking. Further, they hold that remission into moderated drinking is classically temporary; only very rarely have reliable cases been reported of alcoholics who returned to normal drinking for several years. The treatment of alcoholics with a controlled-moderate drinking goal has therefore been challenged as both impractical and unethical.

The psychologists who have experimented with behavioral techniques to moderate the uncontrolled alcohol intake of alcoholics believe that the idea of hopeless, permanent incurability of alcoholism is illogical, and that past failure to cure it was due to failure to apply appropriate techniques. They consider it a necessary enterprise, from the viewpoint of public health, and of a majority of alcoholics who cannot achieve permanent total abstinence, or will not try it, to seek ways of achieving controlled drinking by alcoholics, or even moderated drinking that would at least reduce the harm.

MARK KELLER

[*Directly related are the entries* BEHAVIOR CONTROL; DRUG USE; HEALTH AND DISEASE; *and* HEALTH AS AN OBLIGATION. *See also:* BEHAVIORAL THERAPIES; HUMAN EXPERIMENTATION; INFORMED CONSENT IN THE THERAPEUTIC RELATIONSHIP; *and* PUBLIC HEALTH.]

BIBLIOGRAPHY

American Psychiatric Association, Committee on Nomenclature and Statistics. *Diagnostic and Statistical Manual: Mental Disorders with Special Supplement on Plans for Revision.* Washington: 1965. 2d ed. 1968.

ANSTIE, FRANCIS EDMUND. *Stimulants and Narcotics, Their Mutual Relations: With Special Researches on the Action of Alcohol, Aether, and Chloroform on the Vital Organism.* London: Macmillan & Co., 1864. Sets a limit of 1.5 ounces of absolute alcohol per day, which was newly confirmed in United States, Department of Health, Education, and Welfare, Public Health Service, National Institute on Alcohol Abuse and Alcoholism. *Second Special Report to the U.S. Congress on Alcohol and Health from the Secretary of Health, Education, and Welfare: New Knowledge.* Morris E. Chafetz, chairman of the Task Force. Edited by Mark Keller. DHEW Publication no. (ADM) 75-212. Washington: Government Printing Office, 1974.

BACON, SELDEN D. "Alcoholics Do Not Drink." *Annals of the American Academy of Political and Social Science* 315 (1958): 55–64.

BIRD, BRIAN. "One Aspect of Causation in Alcoholism." *Quarterly Journal of Studies on Alcohol* 9 (1949): 532–543. This wise psychiatrist wrote, "If all the help you have to offer an alcoholic is to stop him from drinking, you might as well leave him alone."

BOWMAN, KARL M., and JELLINEK, E. MORTON. "Alcoholic Mental Disorders." *Quarterly Journal of Studies on Alcohol* 2 (1941): 312–390. On "ethical degeneration" in alcoholism these reviewers quote from Eugen Bleuler's *Lehrbuch der Psychiatrie.* 6th ed. Berlin: J. Springer, 1937.

CHERRINGTON, ERNEST HURST, ed. *Standard Encyclopedia of the Alcohol Problem.* 6 vols. Westerville, Ohio: American Issue Publishing Co., 1924–1930. Details the history of the world temperance movement, the tenets of the churches, and the work of individual adherents and reformers.

EDWARDS, GRIFFITH; GROSS, MILTON M.; KELLER, MARK; and MOSER, JOY, eds. "Alcohol-Related Problems in the Disability Perspective: A Summary of the Consensus of the WHO Group of Investigators on Criteria for Identifying and Classifying Disabilities Related to Alcohol Consumption." *Journal of Studies on Alcohol* 37 (1976): 1360–1382.

FORD, JOHN C. *Depth Psychology, Morality, and Alcoholism.* Weston, Mass.: Weston College, 1951.

GLATT, MAX M. "Loss of Control: Extensive Interdisciplinary Borderland, Not a Sharp Pharmacological Borderline." *Alcoholism: A Medical Profile.* Edited by Neil Kessel, Ann Hawker, and Herbert Chalke. London: B. Edsall & Co., 1974, pp. 122–132.

GROSS, MILTON M. "The Psychobiological Contributions to the Alcohol Dependence Syndrome: A Selective Review of Recent Research." *Alcohol-Related Disabilities.* Edited by Griffith Edwards, Milton M. Gross, Mark Keller, Joy Moser, and Robin Room. WHO Offset Publication, no. 32. Geneva: 1977, pp. 107–131.

KELLER, MARK. "Alcohol Consumption." *The New Encyclopaedia Britannica.* 15th ed. 30 vols. Chicago: Encyclopaedia Britannica, 1974, vol. 1, pp. 437–450.

———. "On the Loss-of-Control Phenomenon in Alcoholism." *British Journal of Addictions* 67 (1972): 153–166.

———, and GURIOLI, CAROL. *Statistics on Consumption of Alcohol and on Alcoholism.* New Brunswick, N.J.: Rutgers Center of Alcohol Studies, 1976. Basic numerical data on drinking and alcoholism.

———, and McCORMICK, MAIRI. *A Dictionary of Words about Alcohol.* New Brunswick, N.J.: Rutgers Center of Alcohol Studies, 1968.

KESNER, RAYMOND P.; PRIANO, D. J.; and DeWITT, J. R. "Time-Dependent Disruption of Morphine Tolerance by Electroconvulsive Shock and Frontal Cortical Stimulation." *Science* 194 (1976): 1079–1081.

LUDWIG, ARNOLD M., and WIKLER, ABRAHAM. " 'Craving' and Relapse to Drink." *Quarterly Journal of Studies on Alcohol* 35 (1974): 108–130.

National Conference on Medical Nomenclature. *Standard Nomenclature of Disease and Operations.* 5th ed. Edited by Edward T. Thompson. New York: McGraw-Hill, 1961.

"Reports of Officers: Hospitalization of Patients with Alcoholism." *Journal of the American Medical Association* 162 (1956): 750.

SCHMIDHOFER, ERNST. "Alcoholism is NOT a Disease." *Maryland State Medical Journal* 18, no. 3 (1969), pp. 59–64. Example of the contemporary opposition to the concept of alcoholism as disease. See also Todd.

SMILDE, J. "Risks and Unexpected Reactions in Disulfiram Therapy of Alcoholism." *Quarterly Journal of Studies on Alcohol* 24 (1963): 489–494. Reports on alcoholics who, deprived of alcohol by pharmacological intervention and lacking other support, committed suicide.

SZASZ, THOMAS STEPHEN. *The Myth of Mental Illness: Foundations of a Theory of Personal Conduct.* New York: Hoeber-Harper, 1961.

TODD, JOHN EDWARD. *Drunkenness a Vice, Not a Disease.* Hartford, Conn.: Case, Lockwood & Brainard, 1882. Example of the historic, extremely moralistic view. See also Schmidhofer.

United States, Public Health Service. *Manual for Coding Causes of Illness According to a Diagnosis Code for Tabulating Morbidity Statistics.* Miscellaneous Publication, no. 32. Washington: Government Printing Office, 1944.

WASHBURNE, CHANDLER. *Primitive Drinking: A Study of the Uses and Functions of Alcohol in Preliterate Societies.* New York: College & University Press, 1961. Describes the survival and contemporary forms of drinking practices of early social groups.

"Wesley, John." Cherrington, *Standard Encyclopedia of the Alcohol Problem,* vol. 6, p. 2816.

WINOKUR, GEORGE; REICH, THEODORE; RIMMER, JOHN; and PITTS, FERRIS N., JR. "Alcoholism. III. Diagnosis and Familial Psychiatric Illness in 259 Alcoholic Probands." *Archives of General Psychiatry* 23 (1970): 104–111.

World Health Organization. *Manual of the International Statistical Classification of Diseases, Injuries, and Causes of Death: Based on the Recommendations of the Eighth Revision Conference, 1965, and Adopted by the Nineteenth World Health Assembly.* 2 vols. Geneva: 1967–1969.

ALLOCATION OF MEDICAL TREATMENT

See RATIONING OF MEDICAL TREATMENT; HEALTH CARE, *articles on* RIGHT TO HEALTH-CARE SERVICES *and* JUSTICE AND HEALTH CARE; JUSTICE.

ALLOCATION OF SCARCE RESOURCES

See RATIONING OF MEDICAL TREATMENT; JUSTICE; KIDNEY DIALYSIS AND TRANSPLANTATION; HEART TRANSPLANTATION.

ALLOWING TO DIE

See DEATH AND DYING: EUTHANASIA AND SUSTAINING LIFE; RIGHT TO REFUSE MEDICAL CARE; ACTING AND REFRAINING.

AMNIOCENTESIS
See PRENATAL DIAGNOSIS.

ANIMAL EXPERIMENTATION

I. HISTORICAL ASPECTS   *Richard D. French*
II. PHILOSOPHICAL PERSPECTIVES   *Peter Singer*

I
HISTORICAL ASPECTS

Man's use of animals for experimental purposes—to understand form, function, and their relationship in the animal and the human body—dates from pre-Christian times. Its nature and frequency have varied with the intellectual predispositions and technical capacities of biomedical scholars and have been strongly affected by the religious, philosophical, and political atmosphere in which those scholars have practiced. This article describes: (1) the rise of animal experimentation as a method in biological and medical research, (2) its institutionalization in the latter part of the nineteenth century, (3) the emergence of opposition to animal experimentation, the modern antivivisection movement, and (4) the current situation in animal experimentation and recent developments in antivivisectionism.

Origins of animal experimentation

The dissection of the dead animal body, incidental to the activities of hunters and cooks since the dawn of human existence, was carried out from motives of curiosity by the Greeks as early as five hundred years before Christ (Singer). The objective was essentially improved understanding of the internal structure of the body. When living animals were first used—probably by the Alexandrian physicians Herophilus and Erisistratus in the third century B.C.—the approach was similarly anatomical and morphological rather than physiological in nature. Death was understood to cause physical changes in internal organs such that observation in vivo rather than by dissection provided a more accurate sense of the shape, texture, color, interconnections, and other characteristics of the organs. From such observations, analogical reasoning based on the similarity between the viscera and everyday objects guided speculation as to the functions of the former.

Our knowledge of the medical researches at Alexandria derives from the works of later writers, especially the Roman physician Galen of Pergamum (A.D. 129–199), who codified the medical writings of the ancients. At least as important, his own researches dominated the biomedical theory that emerged in the rediscovery of the classical authors after the Dark Ages. Galen was a superb operator who dissected a variety of animals. His *De anatomicis administrationibus* [On anatomical procedures] described for the first time the methods and instruments used in specific experiments on living animals. This work recorded his observations on the effect of section at various points of the spinal cord in the living animal—a state of knowledge only modestly increased in the seventeen hundred years that followed.

The Dark Ages saw little development in what we recognize as the Western medical research tradition. Dissection of the human body —for purposes of postmortem and illustration of the classical and Arabic authorities rather than for research per se—seems to have emerged in the Northern Italian universities toward the end of the thirteenth century. By the fifteenth century it had become accepted in the leading medical schools, though hardly common and not without having attracted the attention of the ecclesiastical authorities from time to time.

Andreas Vesalius (1514–1564) created the first modern anatomy by systematic dissection, direct observation, and precise illustration. He experimented on living animals, as did a number of his contemporaries (Schiller, 1967). Francis Bacon (1561–1626), prophet of the scientific revolution, argued the value of animal experiment for scientific knowledge of the human subject in his *De augmentis scientarum* [The advancement of learning] in 1623.

Wherefore that utility may be considered as well as humanity, the anatomy of the living subject is not to be relinquished altogether . . . since it may be well discharged by the dissection of beasts alive, which, notwithstanding the dissimilitude of their parts to human, may, with the help of a little judgment, sufficiently satisfy this inquiry [Bacon].

The seventeenth century saw an enormous outburst of scientific activity—not least in the biomedical sciences, where new instruments and techniques were developed for experimentation on living animals. William Harvey's epochal demonstration of the circulation of the blood in 1628 was only the most important of a series of discoveries made by a combination of dissection and animal experimentation during the seventeenth and eighteenth centuries (Schiller, 1967). Harvey's example inspired a host of medical men and natural philosophers to imitate his logical exposition and brilliantly conceived and executed experiments. For the first time the practice of experimentation upon living animals impinged on the consciousness of the educated elite in general.

In the 1820s and 1830s extensive animal experiments by François Magendie (1783–1855) finally destroyed the anatomically based notions of structure–function relationships in favor of the concept of a function as the product of several organs. No longer were elaborate physiological systems to be developed from speculation and analogy applied to the structures of the body. Rather, physiological ideas would have to be developed empirically, by systematic operations on living animals and observation of the results (Schiller, 1967, 1973). The introduction of anesthesia in 1847 was at least as important for experimental medicine as it was for surgery, for it made feasible and humane a great many experiments previously impossible because of the pain and trauma they inflicted on the experimental subject (Cranefield).

Claude Bernard's classic, *Introduction à l'étude de la médecine expérimentale*, published in the 1860s, embodied the full technical sophistication and philosophical rationale for the new physiology. During the same mid-century period, the spread of the critical research tradition from biblical and classical studies through other disciplines in the highly competitive German university system affected the medical sciences just as it affected all of the natural sciences. The establishment of new university positions required aspirants to establish competence by virtue of successful experimental research. Laboratories in physiology spun off research traditions in the sciences of pathology, pharmacology, bacteriology, and the like, all of them invigorated by the practice of animal experimentation.

Institutionalization of animal experimentation

The new methodology involved the control of variables affecting a physiological system, isolating one variable, that one to be affected by experimental intervention—be it by ablation or extirpation, pharmaceutic agent, or introduction of an infectious agent—in order to observe the precise impact of the intervention. Propagandists since at least the seventeenth century had been promising great benefits to the clinical practice of medicine from the experimental approach, but it was not until the last decades of the nineteenth century that support among the great bulk of the medical profession and the university and bureaucratic authorities was such that resources were available for experimental medicine, and professional standards began to demand systematic knowledge of it. The newly recognized and reorganized medical professions of Northern Europe and America successively took up the standard of experimental medicine not only because they were convinced of its value but because they could use it as a kind of acid test for professionalism with which to exclude the unorthodox and isolate the older and more traditional members of the profession.

Spectacular medical advances attracted enormous public attention and acclaim. The emergence of the science of immunology in the 1880s was probably the most important single accomplishment to demonstrate in convincing fashion not only the intellectual validity but the practical benefit to the public of the experimental approach. There could be no denying that the discoveries involved were based on experiments on living animals. The consequences for medical practice eventually affected the lives of millions of people and received unequivocal endorsement from the medical establishment and governments. Similar advances in chemotherapy, surgery, and preventive medicine, among many others, stimulated a commitment to experimental medicine in virtually every developed nation by the third decade of the twentieth century.

In one hundred years, experimental research had emerged from the dingy back rooms of clinic and lecture theater and the scarcely read pages of arcane journals to recast the fundamentals of medical practice on the basis of laboratory research with living animals and of new techniques with vastly improved instrumentation. The power and prestige gained for the medical profession by the demonstrable public benefits of these research advances in turn made of it, for good or ill, the prototype of the modern profession in terms of independence and self-governance, state recognition, control over admission, and sole guardianship of its intellectual and political legacy.

Opposition to animal experimentation

Emergence of antivivisection movement. Early discussion of the ethics of vivisection was largely confined to its use on humans, a practice that was occasionally ascribed to the anatomists of antiquity, and more frequently to those of the sixteenth century. At least as far as the Renaissance anatomists were concerned, it is doubtful whether there was much validity to the charge, but they were anxious to avoid even the appearance of experimentation on humans, and this concern may have had some inhibiting effect on the resort to animal experimentation.

Opposition to the use of living animals in experimental procedures paralleled the spread of the practice following William Harvey's demonstration of the circulation of the blood in the early seventeenth century. One hundred years later, the experiments of the Reverend Stephen Hales and others inspired disapproving comments from literati like Alexander Pope, Joseph Addison, and Samuel Johnson. François Magendie and his French successors were likewise attacked on grounds of cruelty, but it was only when the research tradition of experimental medicine was imported from France and Germany to Great Britain—the birthplace of anticruelty movements of all kinds—that an organized movement against experiments on living animals emerged.

Led by Frances Power Cobbe (1822–1904), a skillful propagandist, the British movement created in the mid-1870s substantial public concern over vivisection—a term used to denote all animal experimentation, including the administration of drugs or bacteria where the literal implication of surgical incision is not present. A Royal Commission called by Disraeli's government in 1876 found no specific evidence of abuse by British experimenters but recommended regulation of the practice. After considerable political maneuvering, the Cruelty to Animals Act of 1876 was passed (French). The act, in force in Great Britain to the present day, required the registration of places where experiments on living animals were to take place, the licensure of experimenters, certification for particular kinds of experiments, and meticulous record-keeping and reporting on the part of licensees. British antivivisectionists have never been happy with the act or its administration, and, in part because of their pressure, subsequent government inquiries reported on the issue in 1913 and 1965.

As with the humane movement in general, other countries took up the style and philosophy of the activists who created the British antivivisection agitation. The campaign spread through Northern Europe (Bretschneider), to America (Dennis) and to the other English-speaking countries. Experiments on animals are illegal in Liechtenstein and are regulated in Austria, Denmark, Norway, Sweden, Poland, the Bahamas, Jamaica, Argentina, and parts of Switzerland and Australia (Lapage). Anticruelty statutes exist in most countries, and certain of these also have statutes covering the provenance and care of experimental animals. Historically, the Western anticruelty and antivivisection movements have had greater success in Protestant than in Catholic countries (Passmore; Stevenson, 1956).

The campaign against the use of animals for experiments stimulated the political development of the scientific and medical communities (French) and resulted in the establishment of organizations such as the Association for the Advancement of Medicine by Research and its successor, the Research Defence Society, in Great Britain and the National Society for Medical Research in the United States.

Antivivisection arguments. Antivivisectionists have attacked experimental medicine from two basic lines of argument. First, they have argued from the immorality of the method: In their view, whatever the medical or scientific benefits of scientific experiments, such benefits are too dearly bought at the price of complicity in a brutal and degrading practice. This line of argument has tended to coincide with the view that abolition of all experiments on animals—including painless ones—is the only legitimate objective. This approach has sought intellectual support in religion and philosophy (Passmore; Stevenson, 1956).

A second line of argument has been from the inutility of the results of the method. Antivivisectionists, both medical and lay, have ransacked the technical literature to deny the scientific validity of conclusions drawn, to deny the medical value of knowledge gained, or to contend that methods other than those using living animals, such as dissection or clinical research, would have resulted in the same conclusions. Regular themes in such critiques were that the trauma resulting from experimental incursion into the subject organism invalidated any conclusions that could be drawn, or that species error—arising from the difference between the experimental animal and the human patient—provided an ipso facto negation of any practical clinical benefit. As medical research became increasingly inaccessible to the uninitiated, this style of polemic became relatively rare; still, it has not fallen into complete disuse, especially with respect to the use of animals in experimental psychology. The argument from the inutility of the method has appealed both to total abolitionists and to those who seek more stringent regulation of experiments on animals.

On the whole, medical scientists have preferred to ignore antivivisectionist attacks, except when they manifest themselves in legislative initiatives. A small literature of experimental apologetics does, however, exist (e.g., Lapage; Visscher; White).

Antivivisection is a complex phenomenon: varied in form and impact by time and national context; rent by internal divisions and subject to that classical affliction of voluntary movements, the iron law of oligarchy; motivated at various times by myriad social, political, and psychological forces, from antiscientism to evangelicalism to feminism to simple love of animals. In the end its failure to achieve anything resembling its ultimate objectives would seem to depend upon broad public confidence in the medical profession and in the profession's claim that animal experimentation conduces to human health (National Opinion Research Center).

The current situation

The use of living animals for purposes of research in the biosciences, experimental medicine, and experimental psychology, as well as in medical technology—the production of biological extracts and the testing and standardizing of extracts, of drugs, of consumer products, of clinical samples, of water, and of food—is well entrenched in virtually all developed countries. The subjects used number in the millions per year, though precise statistics are available only for Great Britain. The main constraining factor in the growth of animal experimentation has historically been, and remains, the amount of resources available to the research community. The objective of total abolition of such experiments appears more distant today than when first fully articulated in the nineteenth century.

Two major responses to this situation may be detected among those concerned with the promotion of the anticruelty and antivivisection issues. The first is the attempt by intellectuals to construct a defensible philosophical underpinning for the movement, in the recognition that the attack on the medical and scientific utility of experimental medicine has failed, and that ethics rather than epistemology provides the only route of potential advance for the issue.

The second is the attempt by moderate antivivisectionists to promote the use of tissue culture and other nonvivisectional means of biomedical investigation by funding and publication of research developing or using such methods (Fund for the Replacement of Animals in Medical Experiments).

RICHARD D. FRENCH

[*Directly related is the other article in this entry:* PHILOSOPHICAL PERSPECTIVES. *Other relevant material may be found under* LIFE, *article on* VALUE OF LIFE; *and* RESEARCH, BIOMEDICAL. *For discussion of related ideas, see:* HUMAN EXPERIMENTATION. *See also:* RESEARCH, BEHAVIORAL; *and* RESEARCH POLICY, BIOMEDICAL.]

BIBLIOGRAPHY

BACON, FRANCIS. *De augmentis scientarum* (1623). Translated as "Of the Dignity and Advancement of Learning." *The Works of Francis Bacon.* Edited by James Spedding, Robert Leslie Ellis, and Douglas Denon Heath. Vol. 4: *Translations of the Philosophical Works, Vol. I.* London: Longman & Co., 1860, bk. 4, chap. 2, p. 386. Bacon says much the same thing in an earlier English work *The Twoo Bookes of Francis Bacon of the Proficience and Advancement of Learning: Divine and Humane* (1605). *The Works of Francis Bacon,* vol. 3, bk. 2, p. 374.

BRETSCHNEIDER, HUBERT. *Der Streit um die Vivisektion im 19. Jahrhundert: Verlauf, Argumente, Ergebnisse.* Medizin in Geschichte und Kultur, vol. 2. Stuttgart: G. Fischer, 1962.

CRANEFIELD, PAUL F. *The Way In and the Way Out: François Magendie, Charles Bell and the Roots of the Spinal Nerves: With a Facsimile of Charles Bell's Annotated Copy of His Idea of a New Anatomy of the Brain.* Mount Kisco, N.Y.: Futura, 1974.

DENNIS, CLARENCE. "America's Littlewood Crisis: The Sentimental Threat to Animal Research." *Surgery* 60 (1966): 827–839.

FRENCH, RICHARD D. *Antivivisection and Medical Science in Victorian Society.* Princeton: Princeton University Press, 1975.

Fund for the Replacement of Animals in Medical Experiments (FRAME). *Is the Laboratory Animal Obsolete?* London: 1970.

Great Britain, Home Department, Departmental Committee on Experiments on Animals. *Report of the Departmental Committee on Experiments on Animals Presented to Parliament by the Secretary of State for the Home Department by Command of Her Majesty, April, 1965.* Cmnd. 2641. London: Her Majesty's Stationery Office, 1965.

LAPAGE, GEOFFREY. *Achievement: Some Contributions of Animal Experiment to the Conquest of Disease.* Cambridge: W. Heffer, 1960.

National Opinion Research Center. *Animal Experimentation: A Survey of Information, Interest, and Opinion on the Question among the General Public, High School Teachers and Practicing Physicians.* Report no. 39. Chicago: 1949.

PASSMORE, JOHN. "The Treatment of Animals." *Journal of the History of Ideas* 36 (1975): 195–218.

SCHILLER, JOSEPH. "Claude Bernard and Vivisection." *Journal of the History of Medicine* 22 (1967): 246–260.

——. "The Genesis and Structure of Claude Bernard's Experimental Method." *Foundations of Scientific Method: The Nineteenth Century.* Edited by Ronald N. Gieve and Richard S. Westfall. Bloomington: Indiana University Press, 1973, pp. 133–160.

SINGER, CHARLES JOSEPH. *A Short History of Anatomy from the Greeks to Harvey.* 2d ed. New York: Dover Publications, 1957.

STEVENSON, LLOYD G. "Anatomical Reasoning in Physiological Thought." *The Historical Development of Physiological Thought: A Symposium Held at the State University of New York Downstate Medical Center.* Edited by Chandler McC. Brooks and Paul F. Cranefield. New York: Hafner Publishing Co., 1959, pp. 27–38.

——. "Religious Elements in the Background of the British Anti-Vivisection Movement." *Yale Journal of Biology and Medicine* 29 (1956): 125–157.

——. "Science down the Drain." *Bulletin of the History of Medicine* 29 (1955): 1–26.

VISSCHER, MAURICE B. "Medical Research and Ethics." *Journal of the American Medical Association* 199 (1967): 631–636.

WHITE, ROBERT J. "Antivivisection: The Reluctant Hydra." *American Scholar* 40 (1971): 503–507.

II

PHILOSOPHICAL PERSPECTIVES

Although the practice of conducting scientific experiments on living animals, vivisection, goes back at least to Galen (A.D. 130?–200?), the modern period of experimentation stems from the seventeenth century, when scientific inquiries were beginning to be made in many fields. This was the period of the philosopher and scientist René Descartes (1596–1650). For Descartes and the physiologists who declared themselves his followers, cutting open a fully conscious animal posed no ethical problem, since, Descartes said, animals are mere machines, more complex than clocks but no more capable of feeling pain.

If this convenient view of the nature of nonhuman animals is rejected, however, a serious ethical problem about experimenting on animals does arise, because the infliction of suffering and death on an animal seems, in itself, to be an evil. On the other hand, supporters of vivisection argue that such experiments provide great benefits for humans. Animal experimentation, therefore, raises the issue of whether the end justifies the means (an issue also raised by experiments on humans) and in addition forces us to consider what place nonhuman animals have in our ethical deliberations.

The nature and extent of experiments on animals

The number of experiments performed on animals has increased remarkably in the last hundred years. The present extent of experimentation, worldwide, is impossible to ascertain with accuracy, since few countries compile the necessary statistics. In the United Kingdom, according to an annual statement published by the Home Office, more than five million experiments "calculated to cause pain" are performed on live vertebrate animals every year. This figure is low compared to that of the United States, where the number of animals used yearly has been reliably estimated as being in excess of sixty million (Singer). Other countries using large numbers of animals include Russia, Japan, West Germany, and France. The worldwide tendency of smaller nations to follow Western scientific techniques has meant that there are now very few nations in which animal experiments are not being performed.

The animals most often used are mice and rats, but dogs, cats, and monkeys are also used in large numbers. It is commonly assumed that animals are experimented upon only for important medical research, but closer scrutiny reveals that only a minority of experiments can be classified as "medical" at all (Ryder). Many of the most painful experiments are carried out by psychologists and are intended to test theories about learning, punishment, maternal deprivation, and so on. Millions of animals are used to test foodstuffs, pesticides, industrial products, weapons, and even nonessential items like cosmetics, shampoos, and food-coloring agents.

Many of these experiments involve severe and lasting pain for the animals. To test the safety of a foodstuff or cosmetic, the substance is fed in concentrated doses to a group of animals, until a level is found at which half of the sample dies. This means that most of the animals become very sick before some die and others pull through. The dose at which half of the sample dies is supposed to give an indication of the toxicity of the substance, but, since different species have different tolerances, it is at best a very rough guide to the safety of the product for humans (thalidomide, for instance, was tested on several species of animals before being released to humans, and no deformities were found) (Ryder).

Psychologists' experiments about punishment or learning may involve hundreds of severe and inescapable electric shocks. Some psychologists have made monkeys permanently neurotic by rearing them in total isolation (these experiments have been repeated, with minor variations, over and over again). In experiments on stress, monkeys have been locked into iron chairs for more than a year and made to perform tasks in order to avoid electric shock. To study the effects of heatstroke, medical researchers have slowly heated fully conscious dogs to death. Further examples, drawn from recent scientific journals, may be found in Ryder and in Singer.

On the other hand, it is true that many experiments involve little or no suffering for the animals involved. This may be because the experiment is of a harmless nature (such as running a rat through a maze) or because the animal is totally anesthetized during the operation and killed painlessly afterward.

Moreover, some animal experimentation has been of considerable benefit to humans. In such areas as the identification of necessary vitamins and minerals and the development of new surgical techniques and new drugs, discoveries have been made through animal experimentation that could not have been made, or would have been much more difficult to make, had animals not been used. Diabetes is often cited as an example of a disease that has lost its terror through a cure first developed on animals ("Vivisection-Vivistudy").

Legislation

Laws governing experiments on animals vary from country to country, but in no country does the law prohibit outright painful experiments or require that the experiment be of sufficient importance to outweigh the pain inflicted.

The first law specifically regulating experiments was the British Cruelty to Animals Act of 1876. This law, which has never been amended, requires the use of an anesthetic, except where "insensibility cannot be produced without necessarily frustrating the object of such experiments"; but neither the statute itself nor the officials who administer it make any attempt to assess whether the object of the experiment is itself worth the pain caused. Clearly, a psychologist wishing to test the effects of electric shock on the behavior of dogs cannot anesthetize the animals without frustrating the object of his experiment. Even in toxicity tests of cosmetics anesthetics are not used, because it is thought that they might distort the result of the test. Therefore such experiments are permitted in Britain.

In the United States, the Animal Welfare Act of 1970 sets standards for the housing, transportation, and handling of animals; but the Act does not control the nature of the experiments performed, except to the extent of requiring research facilities to lodge a report stating that, when painful experiments were performed without the use of pain-relieving drugs, this was necessary to achieve the objectives of the research project. Again, no attempt is made to assess the importance of these objectives, and in fact one section of the law specifically disavows any intention of interfering with the design or performance of research or experimentation. Moreover, since the law is a federal one, facilities not receiving federal funds and not involved in interstate commerce do not have to comply.

A 1972 West German law requires the use of alternatives to experiments on animals whenever possible. Amendments to the same effect have been proposed in Britain, Denmark, and Holland, but it remains to be seen how effective the West German provision will be. Much depends on what is deemed to be a "possible alternative." Many countries, including France, Spain, Brazil, and Japan still have no legislation regulating experiments on animals.

The case for experimenting on animals

The simplest argument for the permissibility of experiments on animals is the Cartesian one: animals do not suffer, and so there is nothing wrong with experimenting upon them. But both common sense and the great majority of experts agree that mammals and probably other vertebrate animals, at least, are capable of suffering both physical pain and some kinds of emotional distress, such as fear.

If animals do suffer, how is their suffering to be justified? The usual justification offered is that the suffering of animals is outweighed by the benefits, for humans, of the discoveries made by the use of animals. Sometimes, however, it is said that the goal of increasing our understanding of the universe is sufficient justification.

Behind these justifications may lie one of a variety of philosophical positions. For instance, it may be said that, as related in Genesis, God has given man "dominion" over the other animals to use as man pleases. Combined with other theological notions, such as the idea that man, alone of all animals, has an immortal soul, this idea has been influential throughout the Christian world. But it can also be turned the other way: as long ago as 1713, Alexander Pope argued against cruel experiments on the grounds that man's dominion requires him to play the role of the good shepherd, caring for his flock (Turner, p. 48).

It has also been said, by writers as diverse as St. Thomas Aquinas, Immanuel Kant, and D. G. Ritchie, that animals are not "ends in themselves" or that they have no rights (Passmore; Regan and Singer). In support of this it is alleged that the status of a being that is an "end in itself," or has rights, belongs only to a being that is rational, capable of autonomous action, or a moral agent. Whereas humans satisfy this requirement, animals, it is alleged, do not. A difficulty with this argument is that *some* humans come no closer to satisfying the requirement than the animals experimented upon. Mentally retarded human beings, for instance, may be no more rational than a dog; yet we do not consider that they are entirely devoid of rights. Other writers have denied that rationality, autonomy, or moral agency is required before we can grant that a being has rights (Feinberg). Still others have taken the approach that we have obligations not to inflict suffering, irrespective of whether we can meaningfully attribute rights to the being in question (Singer).

A utilitarian case for animal experimentation is based on the idea that more suffering is alleviated by it than is caused by it. The classical utilitarian writers, however, all accepted that a utilitarian must take *all* suffering—human and animal—into consideration, and this makes the factual claim that animal experimentation relieves more suffering than it causes more difficult to defend. Nevertheless, there are probably some experiments—those that do not involve much suffering for the animals and promise major benefits for humans or animals—that can be defended on this ground.

Finally, defenders of experimentation often accuse their opponents of inconsistency in objecting to the deaths of animals in laboratories while continuing to participate in the practice of rearing and killing animals for food. This argument holds no validity for antivivisectionists who are also vegetarians. Even when directed against someone who does eat meat, it hardly amounts to a positive defense of experimentation.

The case against experimenting on animals

Opponents of experiments on animals tend to divide into two groups: absolute abolitionists and reformers. Absolute abolitionists usually rely on the principle that the end does not justify the means. To inflict pain and death on an innocent being is, they maintain, always wrong. They point out that we do not think the possibility of advancing scientific knowledge justifies us in taking healthy human beings and inflicting painful deaths upon them; similarly, they say, the infliction of suffering on animals cannot be justified by reference to future benefits for human or other animals.

The weakness of the absolutist position is that, when the end is sufficiently important, we do sometimes think otherwise unacceptable means are justifiable if there is no other way of achieving the end. We do not like invasions of privacy, but we countenance telephone taps on suspected criminals. Similarly, if the prospects of finding a cure for cancer depended upon a single experiment, should we have any doubt about its justification?

Reformers usually take a more utilitarian line. They concede that some experiments may be justifiable but contend that most are not, because the experiments bring certain suffering and death to animals with no likelihood of significant benefits. In reply to the general argument that experiments on animals benefit humans, the reformers demand that any such benefits be sufficient to offset the costs to the animal subjects; they urge that every experiment come under close prior scrutiny to determine if the benefits are likely to outweigh the costs. Were this done, they maintain, only a small fraction of the experiments now performed would be seen to be justifiable.

Reformers claim (like Ryder and Singer) that alternative methods, not involving animals, could replace many of the experiments now being carried out on animals. Techniques using tissue cultures, for instance, have already replaced animals in the production of certain vaccines, and opponents of animal experimentation suggest that other alternative methods would be developed more rapidly if they were to receive government support (Ryder, chap. 12).

Although the absolutists and reformers disagree in important respects, they are united in seeking to narrow the ethical gulf that now separates humans from other animals in our conventional morality. This may be the most philosophically interesting question raised by the vivisection controversy, and it has implications that go beyond experimentation to our treatment of animals in general.

The moral status of animals

Is there any ethical justification for the sharp distinction we now make between our treatment of members of our own species and members of other species? Although it is commonly said that humans are superior to other animals in various respects, or that humans are "persons," while animals are not, both Ryder and Singer have pointed out that certain categories of human beings—infants and mentally retarded humans—actually fall below some adult dogs, cats, pigs, or chimpanzees on any test of intelligence, awareness, self-consciousness, moral personality, capacity to communicate, or any other capacity that might be thought to mark humans as superior to other animals. Yet we do not think it legitimate to experiment on these less fortunate humans in the ways in which we experiment on animals. Ryder and Singer claim that our respect for the interests of these humans, and our neglect of the interests of members of other species with equal or superior capacities, is mere "speciesism"—a prejudice in favor of "our own kind" that is analogous to, and no more justifiable than, racism.

Certainly it does seem that those supporters of experimentation who have cited the benefits the experiments may bring to humans would need to explain whether this argument also justifies experiments on mentally retarded humans, and, if not, why not. The fact that a being is not a member of our own species does not, in itself, seem to be a sufficient reason for experimenting upon it, if we would refuse to perform a similar experiment upon a member of our own species with similar potentialities.

Defenders of vivisection have had surprisingly little to say about their reasons for disregarding or discounting the interests of nonhuman animals. R. J. White, who has himself carried out experiments in which the heads of monkeys are kept alive and conscious after being severed from their bodies, is perhaps representative of many experimenters when he writes that "the inclusion of lower animals in our ethical system is philosophically meaningless" (White, p. 507). But White does not explain why the clear proposal of utilitarian writers from Jeremy Bentham onward that pain, as such, is an evil, whatever the species of the being that suffers it, is devoid of meaning. It may sometimes be difficult to compare the suffering of a human and, say, a dog; but if rough comparisons can be made, surely the mere fact that the dog is a "lower animal" is no reason to give less weight to its suffering.

Seen in this light, the argument that restricting experiments on animals interferes with scientific freedom and medical progress also appears less conclusive. We do not grant scientists the freedom to experiment at will on humans, although such experiments might advance medical knowledge. It would seem, therefore, to be incumbent upon the defenders of experiments on animals to show that there is a relevant difference between humans and other animals that justifies experiments on the latter, but not the former; but this is a question to which the experimenters have not addressed themselves.

Conclusion

While there has been considerable controversy over the ethics of experiments on humans, there has been little serious discussion of the morality of the far more numerous experiments on animals in recent years. Antivivisectionists have, by and large, been regarded as oversentimental animal lovers or as eccentrics. In the first half of the 1970s, however, three books have appeared containing criticisms of animal experimentation based on carefully reasoned ethical considerations. It would not be surprising if these books provoke a more serious consideration of the entire issue.

PETER SINGER

[*For further discussion of topics mentioned in this article, see the entries:* PAIN AND SUFFERING; PERSON; *and* RIGHTS. *Also directly related are* LIFE, *article on* VALUE OF LIFE; *and* RESEARCH, BIOMEDICAL. *For discussion of related ideas see* HUMAN EXPERIMENTATION. *See also* APPENDIX, SECTION IV, AMERICAN PSYCHOLOGICAL ASSOCIATION.]

BIBLIOGRAPHY

FEINBERG, JOEL. "The Rights of Animals and Unborn Generations." *Philosophy and Environmental Crisis.* Edited by William T. Blackstone. Athens: University of Georgia Press, 1974. Argues that animals can possess rights.

GALTON, LAWRENCE. "Pain is Cruel, But Disease is Cruel Too." *New York Times Magazine*, 26 February 1967, pp. 30–31. A sympathetic view of animal experimentation.

GODLOVITCH, STANLEY; GODLOVITCH, ROSLIND; and HARRIS, JOHN, eds. *Animals, Men and Morals.* New York: Taplinger, 1972. A collection of essays by philosophers and others on our treatment of animals. Two essays by Richard Ryder and Brigid Brophy are concerned specifically with experimentation.

PASSMORE, JOHN. "The Treatment of Animals." *Journal of the History of Ideas* 36 (1975): 195–218. Treats the historical ethical issues in cruelty to animals.

REGAN, THOMAS, and SINGER, PETER, eds. *Animal Rights and Human Obligations.* Englewood Cliffs, N.J.: Prentice-Hall, 1976. An anthology of writings, ancient and modern, on ethical aspects of our relations with animals.

Report of the Departmental Committee on Experiments on Animals. Sir Sydney Littlewood, Chairman. London: Home Office, Her Majesty's Stationery Office, 1965. The result of an official inquiry into animal experiments in Britain; popularly known as the "Littlewood Report," after the committee chairman.

RYDER, RICHARD DUDLEY. *Victims of Science: The Use of Animals in Research.* London: Davis-Poynter, 1975. The most comprehensive account yet published of experiments on animals, the legislation governing experiments, and the case for reform, with principal focus on Britain.

SINGER, PETER. *Animal Liberation.* New York: Random House, New York Review of Books, 1975. Argues for a radical revision of our attitudes to animals; contains a long chapter discussing experiments, including descriptions of experiments in America and Britain.

TURNER, ERNEST S. *All Heaven in a Rage.* London: Michael Joseph, 1964. A historical account of the growth of compassion for animals, with sections on the beginning of vivisection and the antivivisection movement.

"Vivisection–Vivistudy: The Facts and the Benefits to Animal and Human Health." *American Journal of Public Health* 57 (1967): 1597–1626. In four separate papers presented at a symposium, medical and veterinary specialists discuss some of the benefits of animal experimentation for human and animal health.

VYVYAN, JOHN. *In Pity and in Anger.* London: Michael Joseph, 1969. A historical account of experiments on animals and the opposition to such experimentation.

———. *The Dark Face of Science.* London: Michael Joseph, 1971. A continuation of the above.

WESTACOTT, E. *A Century of Vivisection and Anti-Vivisection.* Ashingdon, England: C. W. Daniel & Co., 1949. Account of vivisection controversy from the beginnings to the time of publication, including a full account of the evidence presented by both sides to the British Royal Commission on Vivisection of 1875 and 1906.

WHITE, ROBERT J. "Anti-Vivisection: The Reluctant Hydra." *American Scholar* 40 (1971): 503–512. One of the few articles in which an experimenter defends his right to use animals.

ANTHROPOLOGY OF MEDICINE
See MEDICINE, ANTHROPOLOGY OF.

ANTIVIVISECTION
See ANIMAL EXPERIMENTATION.

ARAB NATIONS
See MEDICAL ETHICS, HISTORY OF, *section on* NEAR AND MIDDLE EAST AND AFRICA, *articles on*

CONTEMPORARY ARAB WORLD *and* CONTEMPORARY MUSLIM PERSPECTIVE. *See also* ISLAM; POPULATION ETHICS: RELIGIOUS TRADITIONS, *article on* ISLAMIC PERSPECTIVES.

ARTIFICIAL INSEMINATION
See REPRODUCTIVE TECHNOLOGIES, *articles on* ARTIFICIAL INSEMINATION, ETHICAL ISSUES, *and* LEGAL ASPECTS.

ARTIFICIAL ORGANS
See LIFE-SUPPORT SYSTEMS; ORGAN TRANSPLANTATION; KIDNEY DIALYSIS AND TRANSPLANTATION.

ASEXUAL HUMAN REPRODUCTION
See REPRODUCTIVE TECHNOLOGIES, *articles on* ASEXUAL HUMAN REPRODUCTION, ETHICAL ISSUES, *and* LEGAL ASPECTS.

ASIA
See MEDICAL ETHICS, HISTORY OF, *sections on* NEAR AND MIDDLE EAST AND AFRICA *and* SOUTH AND EAST ASIA.

AUSTRIA
See MEDICAL ETHICS, HISTORY OF, *section on* EUROPE AND THE AMERICAS, *article on* WESTERN EUROPE IN THE TWENTIETH CENTURY.

AUTOPSY
See CADAVERS.

B

BEHAVIOR CONTROL

This encyclopedia includes three entries on behavior. The first, BEHAVIOR CONTROL, *is divided into two articles:* ETHICAL ANALYSIS, *which gives a general definition of behavior control, and* FREEDOM AND BEHAVIOR CONTROL, *which describes the ways in which behavior control both enhances and threatens different kinds of freedom. This entry is related to, but distinct from, the entry on* BEHAVIORAL THERAPIES, *which raises the ethical issues created by the practices of behavioristic therapies, such as the freedom of the therapist–client relationship and questions concerning the mechanistic approach to training and curing. The final entry,* BEHAVIORISM, *offers a set of theories that are relevant for understanding the conceptual background of the other two entries. It accomplishes this in two articles— one that traces the history of the various schools of behavioral psychology and the issues of ethical interest under the title* HISTORY OF BEHAVIORAL PSYCHOLOGY, *and the other,* PHILOSOPHICAL ANALYSIS, *which discusses the philosophical and ethical implications of behavioristic schools of thought.*

I. ETHICAL ANALYSIS   *Robert Neville*
II. FREEDOM AND BEHAVIOR CONTROL

                             Joel Feinberg

I
ETHICAL ANALYSIS

Behavior control in its most general sense is "the ability to get someone to do one's bidding" (London, p. 3). Ethical issues emerge concerning behavior control when questions are asked about just who has the ability to control, whose bidding is served, and whose behavior is controlled. What values should shape the controlled behavior? Who determines and approves these values? What is the relation between valuable behavior and freedom?

Innovations in behavior control

Two general classes of innovations give behavior control its currency as a special problem in bioethics. First and most obvious is the invention of technologies for control. For example, behavior can be intentionally modified by direct manipulation of the brain, as in psychosurgery, electrical stimulation of the brain (ESB), or the infusion of chemicals through cannulas or hollow tubes leading to specific organs of the brain. Other behavioral effects can be obtained by indirectly manipulating the brain through drugs. Although the brain mediates all behavior, some new technologies such as those associated with behaviorism focus instead on the manipulation of environmental stimuli and reinforcements. Yet other new technologies, for instance those employed by various forms of dynamic psychotherapies, manipulate the affective and cognitive symbols structuring behavior. Even the technologies that have no new hardware, such as hypnosis and psychoanalysis, have new techniques, e.g., the diagnostic use of word association and the interpretation of dreams and slips, that systematically do what was usually only coincidentally done before the nineteenth century.

The second class of innovations augmenting behavior control consists of theoretical advances in the understanding of human behavior. As quite ordinary processes of behavior are understood theoretically, it becomes possible to control them more. For instance, as Perry London has shown, understanding how people deal with information makes it possible partially to control their responses by manipulating the information (London, chaps. 3 and 4).

There may be nothing new in the methods of controlling information, but there is much that is new in the use of those methods of control. Furthermore, new media of information, such as television, which were developed for reasons having little to do with behavior control, can now be used for that purpose with some effect (or so the advertising agencies tell their clients). Another example of control made possible by new knowledge is that in "total institutions." Erving Goffman has described some of the ways by which total environments such as prisons or mental hospitals determine behavior simply by their institutional structures, over and above specific therapies within the institution. Now that these are somewhat understood, the institutions can be deliberately arranged so as to produce effects intentionally. Early childhood education affords yet another example of an area where increased knowledge leads to greater possibilities of control. Observation of such unconscious communication between parent and child as eye contact or method of touch has led to increased understanding of the conditions for enhanced alertness and capacity for affection. Obstetric wards and play schools can now be ordered to certain behavioral goals.

For the most part the new technologies and the new uses of scientific knowledge for behavior control have been developed for benevolent purposes. As is usual with technologies, however, they can also be used malevolently, and they can cause great harm even with the best of intentions.

But there is an even greater dimension to the problem. Every society civilizes to some degree the powers functioning within it; that is, socially effective powers are put in contexts that define their acceptability, that set limits to their use, and that provide countervailing forces where the powers transcend proper limits. The older forms of behavior control, such as they are, have been more or less civilized; most societies have moral customs as well as legal traditions that civilize the power of parents over children, the use of weapons, and the application of the criminal sanction, to name only a few traditional behavior controls. But many of the newer forms of behavior control have not been civilized. At best, people reason from uncertain analogies, for instance when control of television news is considered as a First Amendment problem of free speech. The civilizing structures that ordered practitioners when their powers were not very effective may not do the same when their powers are great. Physicians treating the mind, for example, were civilized by the Hippocratic Oath when they could in fact do little and merely avoided doing harm; but more is needed now, when tranquilizers and electroshock are at their disposal. The general problem of behavior control is to understand its forms, assess its cumulative effects, and civilize its powers.

Dimensions of behavior control

Spelling out some elementary value dimensions of situations in which behavior control is possible is a first step toward understanding the importance of behavior control. Ethical judgments must balance the values involved in these many situations.

Of the many aspects of behavior that can be controlled overt public behavior comes first to mind. But there are also more internal senses of behavior. Thinking is a kind of behavior and it can be controlled sometimes through the manipulation of information. Emotion and affect are also inner sorts of behavior and are subject to control by drugs, psychoanalysis, or good or bad news. Perhaps even more inward are moods such as depression or feeling "high"; these are similar to but not identical with moods such as alertness, dullness, and feelings of vitality that are closely allied with physiological states and that also can be technologically modified.

Clearly one of the most morally weighty problems of behavior control is the theoretical one of conceiving the relations among these senses of behavior. For different technologies affect behavior at different points. Any harmonious full human action rises from the base of a person's mood and affect, involves deliberate thought reflecting emotional valuations, and makes its mark in a public environment in proximate and remote ways. It can be analyzed from inside to outside by terms meaningful within certain physical systems, and it can also be analyzed by terms taking their meaning from the realm of human interests and symbols. In common experience these all ordinarily interact.

Overt behavior reflects inner states and intentions, which in turn are responsive to overt stimuli and rewards. Bad news turns the bowels to water, and an undigested bit of beef is a plausible explanation of Marley's ghost. The ancient philosophical problem of the relation between mind and body is of utmost practical urgency if the connections between the various senses of behavior that might be subject to control are to be conceived coherently.

Behavior control, at least of the sort important to bioethics, is a technological ability. A technology is an organized, socially learnable way by which people can attain an effect. Behavior can be determined in part by factors other than behavioral technology—for instance, by conscious free choice, according to some thinkers, or by a chance concatenation of events. The determination of behavior by a technology requires a *method*, an organized way of attaining the behavioral effect. Hardware is a common connotation of technology in the twentieth century, particularly instruments using electricity. Psychosurgery, electroshock, and television are instances of hardware behavioral technologies. But many new technologies of behavior control are ways of organizing the preexisting social and physical environment, such as the talk in psychoanalysis or the manipulation of a total institution. The novelty in a method without hard tools is not the appearance of a new device but rather a new organization of the determinants of a person's behavior, for instance, conversation with the person so as to bring about the effect with some predictable regularity.

It is sometimes thought that behavior control implies someone who wants to control, that there is someone responsible who is potentially morally responsible. But sometimes no one intends to control, as when the behavioral effects of a drug are unknown or when the determinants of a total institution's structure are too diverse. The ethical dimensions of behavior control, however, arise because someone's behavior is controlled, not because someone actually controls it. If the control is technological, then perhaps someone wields the technology and in this sense, of course, is a controller. But even if the controller does not intend what he does, the control is a moral problem because of its effect upon the controlled party. Perhaps because of that effect the control should itself be brought under control or undertaken with greater deliberate effort. Even when deliberate,

the use of a behavior control technology in a given case is not necessarily moral; the deliberation may involve bad judgment, as when it mistakes the cost or serves bad purposes, or the use may be in willful contradiction to the results of deliberation, as when the controller knows he is doing wrong.

The use of a technology, while intentional, may be *unconscious*. One does not have to be a Freudian to accept the notion that people systematically pursue intentions of which they are not aware, or of which their awareness is the peculiar sort they themselves cannot admit. Hardly anyone consciously intends to drive another person crazy, for instance, yet many act so as to do so, and in methodical ways such as establishing pathological dependencies or creating double binds. Unconscious employment of behavior control technology is not always a bad thing; parents, for example, should shape their children's behavior unconsciously as well as consciously, for otherwise all parties would go mad.

Whether the use of a technology is intentional does not of itself, then, determine either morality or responsibility. The morality is determined by a cumulative assessment of the worth of all the effects and of the legitimacy of the agent employing controls relative to the party controlled. Responsibility is determined by an even more complex assessment of causal determinations, of authority, and of rights. Nevertheless, the intentionality of a use of a behavior control technology is frequently an important factor in composing a picture of the relevant factors to be assessed.

Controlled and free behavior

The first impression most people have of the ethical dimension of behavior control is that it conflicts with freedom. On second thought, this is seen to be an oversimplification. Some forms of control provide greater freedom, particularly those aiding self-control; others, such as some of the forms of social control, aid in establishing contexts where greater freedom is possible. Behavior control may, however, run into direct conflict with freedom when it takes a technological form that may enslave the controlled person to the will of others; this is discussed below in connection with the role-systems of behavior control. It may also contradict freedom in a subtler sense, namely, when it leads to behaviors or experiences that themselves are not free, that exclude freer ways of behaving and experiencing. The controlled person who lives in a vegetative state or acts like an automaton, or even who is led into an extreme dependency on the controller, is made unfree by the control technology, however many other benefits may be achieved. This distinction between controlled and free behavior is our concern here.

Controlled behavior differs from free behavior, according to many thinkers, in that the latter is motivated at some relevant stage by the appeal of the behavior itself. The general line of argument is that unfree behavior is performed without the person's motives being relevant to the worth of the behavior; either he is deceived about its worth, is motivated by someone's threat, or is acting mechanically without a motive. Of course, some thinkers object to the concept of free behavior. They believe that all behavior is learned in a sense that allows in principle for the learning process to be controlled. Whether or not responding to the appeal of something is a form of learning in the requisite sense is a complicated question not to be dealt with here. But it is possible to describe various senses in which the appeal of behaviors can be responded to, senses that constitute aspects of what some, though not all, thinkers call free behavior.

At one extreme is a rather unreflective, immediate appeal, such as a baby's grab at something bright, new, and moving. Immediate appeal frequently determines such behavior as eye movements, body posture, scratching, laughing, and, in general, one's comportment to the aesthetic aspects of the physical and social environment; the train of associations in one's inner psychological environment may also at times approach the immediate extreme.

Moving away from this extreme, there is a class of behaviors whose appeal includes the fact that they would satisfy intentions. That is, the behaviors are viewed symbolically in reference to the agent's purposes and intentions. It makes sense to say of these behaviors that people engage in them because they "mean" such and so to the people. Of course, there is a wide range of symbolic functions in the appeal of projected behavior, from the most rudimentary to the very complicated, from the confused and inarticulate to the highly refined. Perhaps even the unreflective and immediate behaviors discussed previously have a symbolic element, although that is not the important part of their appeal.

Yet another complicating dimension to the appeal of behaviors, over and above their symbolic promise of fulfilling intentions, may be their worth as self-chosen. That is, some aspect of their appeal may consist in the fact the chooser constitutes himself to be the chooser of the behaviors in the acts of choosing. For this dimension of appeal to be real and not merely illusion, as some people believe, it must be possible for the chooser to have chosen something else; his choice could not have been completely necessitated by antecedent factors, however influential they may have been. Whatever other aspects of appeal it has, a freely chosen behavior has a special appeal bestowed upon it by the chooser in adopting it as his choice. Whether this is real, of course, is the old problem of free choice, and some people believe this kind of appeal is necessarily illusory.

A further dimension of behavioral appeal can roughly be called "good reasons." This is the appeal that deliberation uncovers in a prospective behavior. Again, the forms of this appeal vary from the rudimentary to the sophisticated. Some behaviors have appeal stemming from a crude felt comparative evaluation with alternatives. Others derive from careful moral analysis, reflective of ethical theory and of scientific study of the contours of causation. Sophisticated deliberation includes evaluation of the behavior in reference to the identity of the performer as well as in reference to its particular world context.

More complex yet are the dimensions of appeal that stem from the performer's developing character. An action that may or may not be appealing in its own right has an added appeal when it expresses the ongoing character of the actor as a person. This dimension is connected with the fact that the element of the environment most frequently and seriously affected by a person's behavior is his own character. Related to this is the appeal a behavior has resulting from its being a continuation of the work of the agent in the past, whatever its own particular merits. Insofar as an action connects with a person's personality and past work, it has a special appeal because of its place in his career.

The far end of the spectrum of appeal is reached in those behaviors that are part of the tissue of creative life, where aesthetic responsiveness, intention, choice, deliberation, and connection with self and world have been internalized to the behavioral process. A creative person seems to come full circle to immediacy again with actions that seem to others and himself to be as spontaneous as the baby's reach yet to incorporate all the disciplines of maturity.

Behavior is itself free and perhaps responsible, many people believe, when it arises out of one or several of the senses of appeal mentioned above (and perhaps other senses). A person behaves freely upon presentation of the relevant appeal if his body and character have sufficient conditions to make that response possible. The appeal alone does not cause the behavior, but only in conjunction with the state of the person. The state of a person's actual conditions, however, may not allow him to behave according to the relevant appeal. This discordance of appeal and response provides much of the ambiguous ethical quality of behavior control technology.

On one hand, behavior control is inimical to free behavior when it affects the body or character so that there are insufficient conditions for response. For instance, drugs or surgery can stupify, psychotherapy can create enslaving dependencies, information control can mislead people about the true worth of things. On the other hand, behavior control is among the means people employ to make themselves free to respond to what appeals to them. A person drinks coffee (for its caffeine) to become alert enough to do his work when the appeal of the work is insufficient to overcome his groggy mind. A person goes to a psychologist or psychiatrist for behavioral help in overcoming his actual conditions which prevent him from doing what appeals to him.

Most of the biological technologies of behavioral control have been developed to give people more freedom, particularly psychological freedom. Some of these have effects that themselves make people's behavior less free. The ethical question is whether the benefits deriving from the use of those technologies outweigh the deficits, case by case. Freedom is not the only advantage to be gained by behavior control, nor the only loss that might be suffered.

The role-systems of behavior control

The technologies of behavior control do not merely happen to people. They are employed in the context of various social systems, and serious ethical questions arise from the fact that those systems distribute the power people have over each other and themselves.

Who desires a behavior to be controlled? Who exercises the control? Over whom? In whose interests? By what right? There are three broad classes of role systems in regard to motive: (1) self-control or control of oneself for one's own interest; (2) social control or control of individuals by a group of which they are members for the good of the group; and (3) other-control or the control of one party (a person or group) by another party in the interest of the latter. In all these role-systems, technical experts such as physicians, penologists, or advertising agencies may be employed as agents of the various parties; confusions may arise as to just whose agent the expert is. The following discussion of the three main roles intends only to point out controversial areas of value questions. Readers are referred to separate articles on particular means of behavior control for problems concerning their functions in the various roles.

Self-control. Uses of technology to control oneself seem to be the simplest to evaluate. Assuming everything is aboveboard and the technologies are employed competently, it would seem that this use of behavior control is in fact an enabler or extension of a person's own freedom. The behavior control technician represents the person to be controlled, acting where the person cannot act for himself. But the issue is more complex.

Consider behavior control of self aimed principally at proximate pleasure, for instance, through the use of alcohol or psychedelic drugs. Does this pursuit of pleasure detract from a person's social responsibilities? How is pleasure-seeking to be regarded as a part of human life? What are the costs of the pleasure to the person? To others? In the long or short run? Whose concern is it to see that these questions are answered? Are there rights of society to limit a person's pursuit of pleasure? What are the rights of neighbors in this regard? These questions have a special twist when the pleasure is sought through technological means that the society sanctions.

Most self-control behavior technology aims not at immediate pleasure but at making possible various activities; the activities may be pleasurable or worthwhile in themselves or they may be instrumentally valuable. Some behavior control seeks to enhance activities beyond their normal range; amphetamines, psychoanalysis, self-realization therapies, and the methods of athletic trainers do this. Special value questions here have to do with the luxury of spending scarce resources on enhancement, particularly those which in medicine are developed and earmarked for therapeutic purposes, that is, for bringing people up to normal. (Psychiatrists who practice psychoanalysis on essentially normal people are frequently criticized in this regard.)

There are many ways in which people can be "less than normal," but relative to behavior control they fall into three principal classes.

Bad behavior. The first class includes those people whose below-normal behavior is "bad," and who engage in it out of their own choice and responsibility, i.e., the *immoral* people. (Some thinkers argue that if determinism is true there are no people in this class, and that all behavior is either pathological or the result of ill-education.) Although behavior control techniques can be employed to "normalize" bad behavior, the roles do not make this a case of self-control because the self chooses something different; rather it is a matter of *social control* (to be treated in the next section). The second and third classes of deviation downward from the normal are pathology and ill-education respectively.

Pathology. Behavior control is called "therapy" when the behavior it alters is thought of as pathological. Although the therapist is acting as the patient's agent in the therapeutic relationship, he frequently takes a larger role in defining the patient's interest than agents would in other self-control situations. In therapy a patient is supposed to approve the appealing normal behavior and employ the therapist as his agent; the roles are those of the self control model. But if the patient does *not* want to get well, he is either viewed as immoral—wherein the sanctions of social control are employed to make him take his medicine (there are legal procedures for setting aside the requirements of informed consent)—or as "sick in the head" so that the diseased organ is the one that would have to give consent. It is crucial to note that in the last case, where the disease includes not wanting to get well (in severe depression, for example) the therapeutic relationship is reinterpreted. Either it is shifted from the self-control system to that of social control, where the person is treated for the good of the group, or the concept of a proxy is used to provide an analogy with self-control. Some of the moral problems of involuntary commitment and treatment arise because therapists are thought to carry many powers that would be justified in a straightforward self-control role-system (because the patient himself wants them) over into a social control system in which those powers are not

justified, or into a mere analogy with self-control.

Protection of personal integrity in a self-control system rests on some form of consent; in the medical therapeutic situation this has been codified in some countries into laws of informed consent. But consent is what cannot be given if the patient's below-normal character includes not wanting to be normal. If forcibly treated under the role-system of social control, then his integrity must be protected by the due process justifying actions within that role-system, principally those laws legitimating authorities that act with the authority of the society; these laws are not easily applied to therapeutic situations.

Ill-education. It is very difficult to define the difference between pathology and ill-education, but the difference is crucial to the authority of medical psychotherapists. By ill-education is meant a range of below-normal states running from bad socialization, deficient early experience, and lack of normal skills to lack of normal character development and lack of normal knowledge. In contrast to a pathology, for which the patient is not held responsible, a matter of ill-education is more complex regarding responsibility. An infant or young child is not held responsible for its education; as it matures it is held more and more responsible, until finally there is responsibility for having the behavioral abilities normal for the adult group. Furthermore, in many cases an adult is held responsible for remedial work to correct a deficiency for which someone else was responsible when he was a child.

Educators who wield behavioral technologies have a different kind of authority from that usually accorded therapists. Because most early education is not planned but simply results from the sociophysical environment, its authority is noticed only in the breach—for instance, when someone suggests a radical alteration in the family structure. Where authority is deliberately vested in an educator for planned education at an early stage in a person's life, for instance, in a schoolteacher or a government regulating the paideic (*paideia*—a harmonious physical, mental, and cultural development) effects of a community, it is done so usually on a social control model, e.g., "children must be educated because democracy requires an educated citizenry." But the justification of democracy's intent to legitimize education as a social demand is that people should assume control over their own education within the limits of certain social demands. As children grow, educators cease to derive their authority from the social control system and begin to derive it as agents of the student in a self-control system.

Both mental health experts and educators may distort the self-control model in yet another way. By virtue of their expertise they help the person define what his goals are, in accord with which he will be controlled. In varying degrees, psychology has defined mental health for our culture, and therapists make this specific for their patients. (Some clinical psychologists deal with clients only on a contract basis in which the client sets the goals; but even in these rare cases the behavioral technology shapes the goals it is supposed to serve.) Similarly in education, the educator cannot tell the student what he will learn in advance without giving away the content. In both the mental health field and in education, the therapeutic agent not only performs the will of the controlled person, but helps shape it. Self-control is partially a myth as a model for these situations, although the usual protection from abuse—consent—derives from that model.

Besides questions of efficiency and the right of a person to determine his own behavior (and get help in behaving that way), the basic value questions in the self-control role-system are the extent to which the behavior agent should set the goals for the sake of which the behavior is controlled, and the extent to which his authority to alter behavior derives from the person controlled or from the society.

Social control. The social control model is that in which an individual or group is controlled in the alleged interest of the larger society. Insofar as the controlled person is a member of the society he has interests that are served by the very process that controls his more personal interests; so the professional thief has his own property protected by the laws that make his profession a difficult one. But the society would not allege that its control is for the benefit in particular of the controlled person; it is not therapy or education.

The general moral problems connected with social control are, of course, those of politics. What rights does a society have as against its members, and vice versa? How does a society authorize particular agents to express and serve its interests? What are the procedures for challenge by dissidents? What are the protections of due process?

Medicine, of reasonable necessity, is sometimes practiced in institutions designed for or greatly facilitating social control, for instance, prisons, the military, or mental hospitals. Over and above the problem of misplaced therapeutic authority discussed above, there are other problems regarding medicine in these institutions.

One problem is the abuse of the therapeutic ideal by smuggling in the goals of the institution as if they were therapeutic. For instance, a prison or mental hospital may have a special interest in inmate docility, and treatments of disease may be chosen for their special sedative side effects. A soldier in the military may be given short-range treatments that return him quickly to action even though his alternatives are therapeutically far better in the long run. This is not to say that the social interest in docility or a useful fighter is unwarranted; but the decision that it is warranted, and the authority to control the behavior, ought to come through the due process of social control, not merely reflecting the private social views of the treating physician or institution.

A second problem is that some of the new medical technologies of behavior control, such as psychotropic drugs, psychosurgery, electroshock and ESB, as well as behavior conditioning techniques, can be used as adjuncts or alternatives to more traditional technologies of social behavior control such as prisons, fines, and so forth. Given the unhappy state of prisons, for instance, behavior control technologies are frequently suggested as alternatives to incarceration. But penology is confused enough as it is, vacillating among goals of punishment, social protection, and rehabilitation. Psychosurgery or mandatory tranquilization offers similar ambiguities regarding punishment, protection, and rehabilitation, but without the tradition of legal remedies and personal integrity possible (if not likely) in prisons. The concern to civilize these technologies is of utmost importance to the physicians who are required to use them not as healers but as agents of the society.

The education of newborn and older infants and young children is one of the areas where new understanding is making possible new control. Long before the Greek conception of *paideia*, societies understood that babies become people because of social conditions; but only recently has there been much understanding of how and why this works. José Delgado has pointed out that behavior control technologies connected with education now require asking, "What do we want man to be?" Whatever answers are given, the existence of the new technologies, and those in prospect, means that education will not be what it was before, innocent as that was, even if no decision is made by anyone.

Other-control. Other-control is the situation in which one party is controlled by another in the interest of the controlling party. The evil genius hypnotizing politicians or innocent maidens to do his will is a familiar bogeyman. Yet hardly any of the new biomedical technologies involving hardware has added a new dimension to this role, save when an agent in the self-control or social control systems begins to act on his own account.

New psychological knowledge is a different story, however. Motivational research provides sellers with powers to increase people's appetites for their products. Government policy reflects, in part, anticipations of psychological effect. Private citizens try to control one another with techniques learned from psychology. The principal ethical dimension of the new technologies used in this context is duplicity. In the old techniques, for instance bribery, the taker of the bribe, whose behavior was modified accordingly, knew what was going on. Even flattery was an obvious technique to observers. But a person now can be moved to buy a car or elect a President by manipulation of anxieties he does not even know he has.

The development of new powers with which one party can control another should not lead to the assumption that such control is always wrong. People generally approve certain kinds of such control in defense of property, for instance, or one's living environment, or in the management of certain social contexts. Western societies generally have legitimated certain forms of other-control by one or both of two protections of the controlled individual. One, derivative from the self-control system, suggests that other-control is legitimate if the controlled person consents to a situation in which he knows he might be controlled—let the buyer beware. The other, derivative from the social control systems, legitimates other-control if both the controlled and the controlling parties occupy social roles that the society approves for the control, for instance children and parents in a family.

Right of access

To say that behavior control provides new powers that must be civilized states only half the problem, and it casts an ambience of danger over the control enterprise. The other half of the problem is to provide access to the new powers for those who might value or profit from them. If a "happiness pill" were invented with more acceptable side effects than heroin or LSD, why should the unhappy be deprived of it? If there are treatments for psychopathology, how can the sick get them? If there are means to educate, why should anyone be deprived? Of course nearly all the issues discussed in previous paragraphs constitute partial answers to those "Why" questions. There is nevertheless a powerful argument that the scruples about moral civilization that have characterized much of the behavior control debate (and are represented above) in fact are the expression of a favored intellectual and social class that does not need behavior control. There are people who do need it.

Why is it that the public discussion so frequently tips the scales in favor of considering dangers of technology rather than its promises? Some would argue that it is because there is a natural momentum to the development of technology and that moral intervention most frequently takes the form of a brake. Others would argue that human life is naturally untechnological and that new technologies must prove themselves before wide employment is permissible. Whatever the reasons, clearly a formulation of rights of access to new technologies is an essential counterbalance to rights of protection from their abuse.

ROBERT NEVILLE

[Directly related to this article is the companion article on FREEDOM AND BEHAVIOR CONTROL. *This article will find application in the entries* BEHAVIORAL THERAPIES; DRUG USE; DYNAMIC THERAPIES; ELECTRICAL STIMULATION OF THE BRAIN; ELECTROCONVULSIVE THERAPY; HYPNOSIS; PSYCHOSURGERY; PSYCHOPHARMACOLOGY; *and* SELF-REALIZATION THERAPIES. *For discussion of related ideas see the entries:* ALCOHOL, USE OF; BEHAVIORISM; GENETIC ASPECTS OF HUMAN BEHAVIOR; INSTITUTIONALIZATION; MENTAL HEALTH SERVICES, *article on* SOCIAL INSTITUTIONS OF MENTAL HEALTH; POPULATION POLICY PROPOSALS, *articles on* GOVERNMENTAL INCENTIVES, SOCIAL CHANGE PROPOSALS, COMPULSORY POPULATION CONTROL PROGRAMS, *and* GENETIC IMPLICATIONS OF POPULATION CONTROL; PRISON-

ERS; PSYCHOPHARMACOLOGY; SEX THERAPY AND SEX RESEARCH; *and* VIOLENCE AND THERAPY. *See also:* COMMUNICATION, BIOMEDICAL, *article on* MEDIA AND MEDICINE; FREE WILL AND DETERMINISM; INFORMED CONSENT IN THE THERAPEUTIC RELATIONSHIP; *and* MENTAL HEALTH THERAPIES.]

BIBLIOGRAPHY

BANDURA, ALBERT. *Principles of Behavior Modification.* New York: Holt, Rinehart & Winston, 1969.

"Behavior Control in Prisons." *Hastings Center Report* 5, no. 1 (1975), pp. 16–48.

BERTALANFFY, LUDWIG VON. *Robots, Men and Minds: Psychology in the Modern World.* New York: George Braziller, 1967.

BIRDWHISTELL, RAY L. *Kinesics and Context: Essays on Body Motion Communication.* Philadelphia: University of Pennsylvania Press, 1970.

COMSTOCK, GEORGE A.; MURRAY, JOHN P.; and RUBENSTEIN, ELI A., eds. *Television and Social Behavior.* 5 vols. Rockville, Md.: National Institute of Mental Health, 1972.

DELGADO, JOSÉ. *Physical Control of the Mind.* New York: Harper & Row, 1969.

GAYLIN, WILLARD; MEISTER, JOEL; and NEVILLE, ROBERT, eds. *Operating on the Mind.* New York: Basic Books, 1975.

GOFFMAN, ERVING. *Asylums.* Garden City, N.Y.: Doubleday, 1961.

KITTRIE, NICHOLAS. *The Right to be Different: Deviance and Enforced Therapy.* Baltimore: Johns Hopkins Press, 1971.

KLERMAN, GERALD L. "Psychotropic Hedonism vs. Pharmacological Calvinism." *Hastings Center Report* 2, no. 4 (1972), pp. 1–3.

KOESTLER, ARTHUR. *The Ghost in the Machine.* New York: Macmillan Co., 1967.

LONDON, PERRY. *Behavior Control.* New York: Harper & Row, 1969.

NEVILLE, ROBERT. *The Cosmology of Freedom.* New Haven: Yale University Press, 1974.

———. "The Limits of Freedom and Technologies of Behavior Control." *Human Context* 4 (1972): 433–446.

SCHWITZGEBEL, RALPH K. *Development and Legal Regulation of Coercive Behavior Modification Techniques with Offenders.* U.S. Public Health Service Publication no. 2067. Chevy Chase, Md.: National Institute of Mental Health, Center for Studies of Crime and Delinquency, 1971.

SIEGLER, MIRIAM, and OSMOND, HUMPHRY. *Models of Madness, Models of Medicine.* New York: Macmillan Publishing Co., 1974.

SKINNER, B. F. *Walden Two.* New York: Macmillan Co., 1948.

"Symposium: Psychosurgery." *Boston University Law Review* 54 (1974): 215–353.

SZASZ, THOMAS. "The Ethics of Addiction." *American Journal of Psychiatry* 128 (1971): 541–546.

ULRICH, ROGER; STACHNIK, THOMAS; and MABRY, JOHN. *Control of Human Behavior.* 2 vols. Glenview, Ill.: Scott, Foresman & Co., 1966, 1970.

VEATCH, ROBERT M. "Drugs and Competing Drug Ethics." *Hastings Center Studies* 2, no. 1 (1974), pp. 68–80.

II

FREEDOM AND BEHAVIOR CONTROL

There have been stubborn disagreements among theorists about whether behavior control can be compatible with freedom, and whether, in cases of conflict between the two, the loss of freedom can be a reasonable price to pay for the ends gained by techniques of human manipulation. The resolution of these controversies presupposes a common understanding of the concept of freedom itself, an accord that is difficult to achieve, partly because the uses of the word "free" are many and various. For example, we make both singular judgments to the effect that a particular person is free in a particular respect, and "on-balance judgments" to the effect that a given person or class of persons is free "on the whole, all things considered." Persons are sometimes said to be free from irritations, emotions, and other disliked states or circumstances, and (perhaps more commonly) free from constraints on their behavior. They are said to be free to act or free to choose, to enjoy or lack "freedom of the will" or the status of free subject or citizen. None of these usages is free of obscurities and ambiguities, and these in turn have generated conflicting philosophical accounts of the nature, limits, and value of freedom.

Free action

One leading controversy concerns the analysis of "freedom from constraint" and the relation between constraints and desires. The ancient Stoics and Epicureans claimed to be speaking for common sense when they maintained that freedom (from constraint) consists simply in the ability to do what one wants most at the time to do. An advantage of this simple account is that it provides an explanation of why we consider freedom to be a valuable thing: when one is prevented from doing what one wishes to do (constrained) or forced to do what one does not wish to do (compelled), one's desires are frustrated, and frustration is usually a very unhappy experience. Since one is rarely powerful enough to do everything one desires, and greater power is hard to come by, the Stoics and Epicureans recommended that persons modify or extinguish their desires in order to minimize the chances of frustration, thereby achieving both contentment and freedom. "Demand not that events happen as you wish but wish them to happen as they do happen, and you will get on well" (Epictetus, *The Enchiridion*, VIII).

If there is only one thing that authorities or circumstances permit a person to do at a given time, but that thing happens to be the thing he wants most to do at that time, then he can do what he wishes and hence is free, according to the Stoic–Epicurean conception. Therein lies the weakness of that conception according to its critics, for to say that circumstances permit only one action (whether desired or not is immaterial) is precisely to say that one is compelled to perform that action, and compulsion is the very opposite of freedom. One can act quite willingly under compulsion, but the willingness does not change the fact of compulsion. Freedom to act, in this second conception, requires not (or not only) that one can do what one wishes to do, but that one can do many things other than what one wishes to do. In fact, the more things a person can do—the greater his options, the more alternatives kept open for him—the freer he is, no matter what his desires happen to be. The great advantage of this account is that in no circumstances is it committed to the identification of freedom and compulsion. Its main difficulty is to explain why freedom is as valuable as most people think, how there can be value in being able to do things one does not want to do. Some writers base the value of open alternatives on the security they offer to persons whose desires might change, for all they know, in the future. Others find an intrinsic value in having options to choose among even when most of the alternatives will not seem eligible for their choice. In any case, writers in this camp insist, freedom is only one value among many. It may well conflict with contentment in some circumstances and may cause confusion, unwise decisions, and frustration. It is no aid to clarity to identify freedom with other goods or to deny that it can ever conflict with other things of value.

Another controversy concerns the sorts of things that can properly be called "constraints" in the analysis of freedom. Some would identify lack of freedom to act with inability to act, whatever the nature or source of the inability, whether it be policemen's guns and locked prison gates; poverty, sickness, or ignorance; private emotions, repressions, or scruples; laws of nature (we are not "free" to high-jump twenty feet); or laws of logic (not even God is "free" to be and not be at the same time).

On the other side, it is said that freedom is not simply the absence of *any* factor that might impede a possible action, but rather the absence of one specific kind of constraint, namely, *coercion* by human beings and its indirect inhibitory consequences. Coercion includes direct forcing, for example pushing and arm twisting, as well as threats of punishment or other evils, whether by legal authorities or by private persons. Insofar as such states as poverty, sickness, and ignorance are the consequences of coercive rules and practices, they too count as constraints on freedom.

It will not do simply to identify the lack of freedom to act with any inability to act whatever its source, for there are many things persons are unable to do even though it would be natural to say they are free to do those things. I cannot compose symphonies, speak Russian, or shoot par on a golf course because I lack the requisite talent or knowledge, not because I lack freedom. Moreover, if the source of constraints is left completely unrestricted in our account of freedom, the notion of perfect freedom will be an empty and unapproachable ideal. No matter how much our freedom is enlarged, there will still be an infinite number of things we are not free to do. Perfect freedom on the alternative account consists in the largest number of open options consistent with reasonable rules and social order, an ideal that is in principle achievable.

The free person

Sometimes people are said to be free not from some specific constraint, not to do or omit doing some specific action, but simply free *tout court*. This can mean two things of quite different kinds. The judgment that a person is free "on balance" may be a rough generalization from the various singular judgments that can be made about his freedom to do or omit doing various actions. In that case it means that he is generally free from constraints to do a great many things, that he has open alternatives among which to choose in respect to a great many areas of life. A person is free, in this sense, to the extent that he has *open options*.

The second thing that can be meant when persons are described as free *tout court* is that they are autonomous, self-governing, or independent, that they have a "sovereignty" over their own affairs. Autonomy or self-government, on the one hand, and freedom from constraint (open options), on the other, are quite distinct concepts of freedom, not reducible one to the other. Isaiah Berlin, following established usage, labels the conception of freedom as autonomy "positive freedom" and the conception of freedom as absence of constraint (open options) "negative freedom." "The answer to the question 'Who governs me?' is logically distinct from the question, 'How far does government interfere with me?' It is in this difference that the great contrast between the two concepts of negative and positive liberty, in the end, consists" (Berlin, p. 130).

Applying the political metaphor of self-government to the individual person requires a clear conception of the "boundaries" of the self that is the subject of freedom. The autonomous person is not only independent of the control of external selves, he must be firmly in control of the self that is his own. This in turn has suggested to writers from Plato on that the self must be divided into a "ruling part" and a lower nature that is subject to its authority. The language of autonomy seems to require a conception of an "inner core" self, consisting of reason, conscience, or those values that are highest in a personal hierarchy and with which a person most intimately and securely identifies himself. This inner core self must be sufficiently narrow to be contrasted with other internal elements of the wider self, which it is said to govern, such as specific desires, purposes, and affections.

Many writers have identified the "ruling part" of the self with reason (Plato; Kant). David Hume, on the other hand, in a characteristic hyperbole, argued that "reason is, and ought only to be, the slave of the passions" (Hume, p. 415). If Hume had spoken of a servant instead of a slave and endorsed a democratic conception of authorities as "public servants," his metaphor might not have been far from the mark, for then it would have permitted us to derive the authority of practical reason to regulate particular aims and desires from the interests of those particular "passions" themselves. So conceived, reason is like a traffic cop directing cars to stop and go in an orderly fashion so that they might get to their diverse destinations all the more efficiently, without traffic jams and collisions. The person whose desires lack order and structure and obey no internal regulator will be torn this way and that and fragmented hopelessly. Such a person fails to be autonomous not because of outside government but because of his failure to govern himself. He will also fail to be free on balance from constraint insofar as his constituent desires constrain one another in

internal jams and collisions. At its worst, such a condition approaches that which Emile Durkheim called "anomie," one of the leading causes of suicide (Durkheim).

Respect for a person's autonomy is respect for his unfettered voluntary choice as the sole rightful determinant of his actions except where the interests of others need protection from him. Whenever a person is compelled to act or refrain from acting on the ground that he must be protected from his own folly, his autonomy is infringed. When the state, for example, refuses to permit a citizen to do something he has chosen to do on the sole ground that his choice seems contrary to his own welfare, that citizen's autonomy is violated. If we assume that "on-balance freedom" is a constituent of a person's welfare, and we therefore refuse to permit him to trade some of his "open options" in exchange for benefits of another kind, then we have violated his autonomy for the sake of his "on-balance freedom" in the long run. Even if a person is prevented, on wholly paternalistic grounds, from selling himself into slavery in exchange, say, for a million dollars to be delivered in advance to a charity or favored cause, his voluntary choice is overruled for the sake of his future freedoms. This example shows vividly that personal autonomy and freedom as "open options" are distinct values quite capable of conflict. A perfectly autonomous person would have the "power of voluntarily disposing of his own lot in life" (Mill, p. 125), even if that involved forfeiture of most of his de facto liberty in the future.

Free will

It is possible for a person to have a great deal of freedom of action and yet not be a free person on balance. Such a person would be largely free of external coercion and thus have ample capacity to do whatever he might come to choose, but in respect to one or more large categories of action he would lack the ability to choose or not choose as he might come to wish. In that case many of his options to choose (or to will, or even to desire) are closed by internal psychological conditions even though there are no external constraints to his conduct. His freedom of action is unimpaired but he falls short of freedom on balance because, for a large range of possible choices, he lacks free will.

The clearest difference between the person who has free will with respect to a given area of choice and the man who suffers from an impaired psychological capacity (to choose, will, intend, decide, or desire) is that the former's choice would be different were he presented with what he himself acknowledged to be decisively good reasons for choosing differently, whereas the latter's intention remains fixed in the presence of excellent reasons for choosing differently. Because this crucial difference is a matter of degree, it follows that free will is a matter of degree too. Even the most confirmed alcoholic will probably choose to decline another drink if he is led to believe that it will cause his painful death, though the beliefs that it will merely make him an unsafe driver or an incompetent husband, which would move the will of a freer man, leave his intention unaltered. When a person's choices are unalterable by acknowledged good reasons for changing them (or by reasons that would be so acknowledged if the person were in a rational state), then he suffers from the sort of impaired psychological capacity that diminishes his free will. In that case his intentions can be altered, if at all, only by severe threats or "by some form of manipulation such as behavior therapy or drugs" (Glover, p. 98).

Part of the reason why "freedom to will" is an intelligible notion referring to something of great value is that persons are capable of desiring that their desires, preferences, choices, and willings be other than what they are. It is precisely this "capacity for reflective self-evaluation" that renders human beings *persons*, in contrast to the lower animals, which may have wills and purposes but no "desires of the second order" (Frankfurt, p. 7). Even though a drug addict may desire to choose not to take another dose (he may hate his addiction), he finds himself desiring, and then choosing, to take it anyway. If his addiction is complete, the option to choose to abstain, in accordance with his second-order desire, is not open to him. He cannot desire as he wants to desire, and he cannot choose as he wishes to choose. On the other hand, the person whose will is free in respect to drug-taking can choose to take drugs or choose to abstain, and if he prefers to abstain that is what he will choose to do.

There is no limit in principle to the number of higher-order desires a person might form, though in fact persons rarely have occasions to form desires above the third order (a desire to desire to will to do . . .). Typically, however, persons "identify decisively" with desires of the second order and equate their freedom with the

capacity of the inner-core self so defined to will or not will in accordance with its preferences. Free will, so conceived, is valuable to its possessor because it affords him the satisfaction of knowing that "his will is his own . . . as opposed to being estranged from one's self or being a helpless or passive bystander to the forces that move him" (ibid., p. 18).

The effects of behavior control on freedom

Primarily because it is a form of manipulation, behavior control raises philosophical perplexities about the nature and value of freedom. Manipulation is one of three ways of influencing the behavior of others and can best be understood in contrast to its alternatives. Manipulation, or "dextrous management" of another person, can be distinguished both from rational persuasion and coercion, though it has more significant similarities to the latter. We induce others to behave as we wish by rational persuasion when we offer them advice, issue reminders, present new facts, invoke common principles, in short, when we present good reasons for behaving in one way rather than another. Our advice becomes effective when the other party adopts our reasons as his own and acts accordingly. In that case our persuasion was both rational and non-coercive; it did not by force close the other's option but only gave him a reason to exercise his option in a certain way. Right up to the moment of his decision, it was up to him alone whether to decide one way or the other.

Coercion is a blunter and more visible way of influencing another person's behavior. We can close one of his options by force (twisting his arm, dragging, pushing, clubbing), by expropriating the necessary means to act (money, tools, weapons), by creating physical barriers (walls, moats, stakes), or by intimidation (threats of death, mayhem, or legal punishment). Typically, of course, coercion is employed to close one or more of a person's options and thereby diminish his freedom of action. But coercion can also be used to open up some of a person's options (against his will) in which case the person is, in Rousseau's phrase, "forced to be free" (Rousseau, p. 64). Rousseau meant that a person's misinformed choices and irrational desires could be put down by external force in support of his true inner-core self, the rational will that rightly governs him. To be forced to do what one's rational will would choose to do if liberated, he argued, is to be forced into true freedom for one's real self.

Isaiah Berlin, on the other hand, speaks for many twentieth-century philosophers when he characterizes this conception as a "monstrous impersonation, which consists in equating what X would choose if he were something he is not, or at least not yet, with what X actually seeks and chooses" (Berlin, p. 133).

There are, however, less paradoxical applications of the idea of forcing someone to be freer on balance than he is or than he wants to be. It is possible to have the area of one's freedom to act enlarged by force, and, when this happens, some of one's options are closed by a coercive act that at the same time causes many more options, or options of greater importance, to open. Thus a person might be dragged struggling and kicking over the border from a cruel police state into a liberal democracy. He may have resisted out of ignorance or because he genuinely preferred tyranny to freedom. Not every one appreciates having open options and the difficult burden of having always to choose for oneself what one shall do. But, whatever a person's motives for resisting the expansion of his options, the condition so described is one of greater freedom of action. It is important to note, however, that, benign as our motives might be, insofar as we force a person against his will into a condition he did not choose, we undermine his status as a person in rightful control of his own life. We may be right when we tell him that greater freedom of action is for his own good in the long run, but we nevertheless violate his autonomy if we force our conception of his own good upon him.

Manipulation of another person characteristically works directly upon his beliefs, motives, and psychological capacities and effects change neither by means of rational persuasion nor by means of external hindrances, prods, and deprivations. Some forms of manipulation, for example extortion and aversion therapy, employ threats or something very like threats and are thus properly located near the vague boundary between coercion and manipulation. Certain forms of psychotherapy that bring the patient greater insight into his own motives through such techniques as self-revelation, free association, and suggestion are very near the equally vague border between manipulation and rational persuasion. One more clearly defined category of manipulation includes the many modes of nonrational persuasion: stimulation of stereotyped emotional responses; propaganda; posthypnotic suggestion; subliminal advertising;

salesmanship that subtly associates a product with a social status or a desired state (for example, sexual attractiveness) with which it has no actual connection; and indoctrination by appeal to authority, emphatic reiteration, even the "hypnopaedic sleep teaching" of *Brave New World*. Another category includes the various techniques of behavior control: psychosurgery, electric stimulation of the brain, psychotropic drugs, and aversive conditioning. These techniques can be employed either to close or to open a person's options, either with or without his voluntary consent. Each of these four combinations has its own effect on freedom.

Where manipulative techniques are used to open a person's options with his voluntary consent, there is an enlargement of freedom and no violation of autonomy; hence, this is the least troublesome category. For example, suppose a person so suffers from claustrophobia that he cannot bring himself to enter any small confined place, not even the closet where his guests have left their coats. Suppose a therapist proposes a series of treatments designed gradually to increase his tolerance through conditioning and hypnosis. The patient consents to the treatments, fully understanding the theories on which they are based and the risks they might involve. As a consequence his phobia is destroyed and he now has one kind of option he did not have before, namely to choose to enter or not to enter confined places as he pleases. Indirectly, many other options are also opened up. It is now open to him, for example, to enter elevators, to work in photographic dark rooms, or to become a cloakroom attendant.

Another patient might consent in a fully voluntary way to manipulative behavior control designed to close one of his options and thereby open up many others. An alcoholic, for example, may voluntarily take a drug that will make him violently ill if he should ingest as little as a half ounce of alcohol in a two-week period, thus effectively shutting off his option to accept drinks. As a consequence, many other options far more valuable to him are now opened, and he can function in the world once more. He was "manipulated into his freedom," to be sure, but his own consent to the treatment made him a party to it, so that it became a form of self-manipulation as morally innocuous as setting an alarm clock before retiring and the many other "tricks" free men play on themselves.

In other cases, persons freely consent to manipulative treatment designed to close some of their options where there is either a certainty or a high risk that this loss of freedom will *not* be compensated by a greater gain in freedom on balance. A person who suffers from uncontrollable rages or chronic suicidal depression may well elect to undergo psychosurgery knowing full well that the technique is inexact and may not have its intended effects, and also that there is a substantial risk that the treatment may restore him to tranquility at the cost of his becoming a passively docile vegetable, unable to initiate any projects or enterprises of his own. The risks may seem reasonable to him and unreasonable to those with authority over him, or he might actually have a considered preference for vegetative docility over his present intolerable condition, a preference that seems reasonable to him but unreasonable to those who have authority over him. The question these cases pose for social policy is a troublesome one: should such persons be permitted to consent to treatment that is likely to diminish their freedom by restricting their future options irrevocably, for the sake of a good that they have come to value more than their freedom? On the assumption that consent *can* be fully voluntary in such circumstances, it would be to respect an individual's own choice to permit him his dangerous manipulative treatment, and it would violate his autonomy to deny it for what *we* take to be his "own good." An autonomous being has the right to make even unreasonable decisions determining his own lot in life, providing only that his decisions are genuinely voluntary (hence truly his own), and do not injure or limit the freedom of others.

The most odious kind of case is the manipulation of a person without his consent (even without his knowledge) in order to close many of his options to choose as he pleases in the future. Patients or prisoners (the two are easily confused in totalitarian countries) can be drugged, put under total anesthesia, and then made to undergo lobotomies or other surgical manipulations or mutilations of the brain. Psychotropic drugs used in small quantities and electric stimulation of the brain for shorter periods have less severe effects and are revocable, but when imposed on a person without his consent or, worse, without his knowledge, they are hardly distinguishable on moral grounds from assault and battery. The situation is not affected morally by the motives of the controller. Whether he be kindly and benevolent or malicious and cynical, the effect of his actions

is drastically to diminish freedom of choice and to violate personal autonomy. The case is complicated morally, however, when the patient, having lost his competence to govern himself and his capacity, therefore, to grant his voluntary consent, has no autonomy left to violate. In such cases, a person can be made no worse in respect to freedom and autonomy than he already is, and behavior control may reduce his pain and anxiety and promote the convenience of those who must govern him. Respect for personal autonomy, however, requires that the benefit of every doubt be given to the patient, that every effort be made to improve his lot without irrevocable destruction of his capacity to govern himself.

The final kind of case is perhaps the most troublesome. That is where manipulative techniques are used to open a person's options and thus increase his freedom on balance, but without his consent. Here indeed a person is "manipulated into freedom," not with his own connivance, but without his knowledge, and perhaps even against his will. Being involuntarily suffered, such treatment is necessarily a violation of a person's right to be his own master and to make the choices himself that vitally affect his future. It therefore abridges his freedom in one sense (autonomy), while expanding it in another (by opening options). Where interests of third parties are not involved, every person's moral right to govern himself surely outweighs the "right" of benevolent intermeddlers to manipulate him for his own advantage, whether that advantage consist of health, wealth, contentment, or freedom. At the very most, a man's options to choose can be opened for him by manipulation to which he has not consented, only to protect others from harm at his hands.

The value of freedom

It is worth reemphasizing that freedom is only one of the good things in life, for many writers have claimed that any putative freedom that can conflict with such other undoubted goods as contentment and fulfillment of desire cannot be "true freedom" at all. As one among many values, freedom must sometimes be sacrificed or compromised in cases of unavoidable conflict. B. F. Skinner, in his provocative book *Beyond Freedom and Dignity*, has argued that freedom (and dignity too) are vastly overrated and that the value placed on them by misguided humanitarians has been one of the major obstacles to human progress. Our physical technology, he maintains, has created as many problems for mankind as it has solved, and what is needed now is a highly developed "technology of behavior." Birth control devices, for example, will not solve the population problem unless human beings in overcrowded countries can be induced to use them; pollution-control devices and recycling techniques will not protect the environment unless industrialists and consumers change their attitudes toward them; policemen and prison officials will fight a losing battle against crime until the motives, characters, and opportunities of the criminals themselves are changed. What is required to solve these problems, in short, is more effective control of human behavior. The partisans of freedom and dignity, Skinner argues, consider all kinds of control by some persons over others exploitative and inconsistent with freedom. Skinner, on the other hand, considers only certain forms of coercive control objectionable; he would minimize or eliminate if possible the use of "aversive stimuli" to control others, that is, harmful or disagreeable reinforcers that human organisms naturally "turn away from." Nonaversive controls, however, are morally unobjectionable according to Skinner, even though incompatible with freedom and dignity as those terms are commonly interpreted.

Skinner is perhaps most persuasive when he applies his thesis to the problem of criminal punishment. The current system leaves people "free" to decide whether to obey the law or risk punishment; therefore they get credit for their law abidingness and blame and punishment for exercising their freedom of choice in the wrong way. In either case, they can take responsibility for what they do and thus maintain their dignity. People who are unable to choose to behave badly cannot take credit for their goodness, and indeed, in a world in which everyone behaved well because he had no option of behaving badly, there would be no goodness of character to take credit for. On the other hand, in such a world there would be no crime. And no victims of crime. The problem, writes Skinner, "is not to induce people to be good but to behave well" (p. 70). This result can be achieved most economically by creating circumstances in which crime is not likely to occur or in which it can have no point or profit; in providing acceptable outlets for aggressive energies and other means of sublimation; or finally, if all else fails, resorting to "hormones . . . to change sexual behavior, surgery (as in lobotomy) to control violence,

tranquilizers to control aggression" (ibid., p. 68).

There is considerable plausibility in Skinner's contention that freedom and dignity are often overvalued to the detriment of social progress. Gun-control legislation, which would make certain kinds of firearms inaccessible to most people, has been opposed, for example, on the grounds that the credible threat of severe punishment for misuse of weapons would be almost as effective in preventing crime, and more consistent with human freedom. A similar principle is involved when the construction of highway overpasses as a way of obviating collisions at dangerous intersections is rejected in favor of heavier penalties for negligent and reckless driving. The latter policy would leave people "free" to behave or misbehave and punish those autonomous agents who exercise their freedom in the wrong way, as if that would be compensation for the lives and limbs of their victims. On the other hand, few protested when exact change became mandatory on public buses in New York and Washington, so that bus drivers no longer carried money to attract hold-up men. Almost overnight, bus robberies ceased once and for all, and the need for deterrent punishment vanished. These are examples of "engineering the environment" to destroy the occasions for criminal conduct, at the cost (obviously minor) of closing options to choose antisocial conduct and depriving good people of credit and bad people of blame. If all occasions for crime could be thus eliminated, the elaborate ritual complex of sin, punishment, and remorse would vanish as well, a consequence Skinner would not regret.

Similarly, some of the forms of *human* engineering, to which Skinner would resort in the end, if reliable, might seem to be good bargains even at the expense of freedom and dignity. If conditioning or psychosurgery could prevent "vicious criminals" from ever choosing to commit wantonly violent attacks on others, without at the same time increasing their own vulnerability to such attacks (unlike the crude techniques depicted in Anthony Burgess's novel, *A Clockwork Orange*) it would be difficult to appreciate the objections to their use, especially when consented to by the criminal.

Even if the prisoner's consent is not fully voluntary (since his alternative is continued incarceration) or if the operation is performed or the treatment imposed against his will, the invasion of his autonomy would probably seem to Skinner (though many or most writers disagree) to be a more economical and humane method of protecting his potential victims than a continuation of his punitive confinement.

But even if that assessment of the relative weights of efficiency and humanity against autonomy in an extreme case is correct, it does not imply what Skinner seems to say, that personal autonomy, freedom of action, and freedom of choice are only minor or trivial values. To appreciate this point one need only consider Aldous Huxley's imaginary society in *Brave New World*, where most wants are gratified instantly, anxiety and depression are eliminated, and crime and violence are unknown. All the people (with the exception of a few aberrant dissidents who are sent into a very pleasant exile) are perfectly content, even though many of the values that we readers, looking in from the outside, regard as essential to a good life, are missing. In some respect, freedom of action in *Brave New World* is enlarged: ". . . you're so conditioned that you can't help doing what you ought to do. And what you ought to do is on the whole so pleasant, so many of the natural impulses are allowed free play, that there really aren't any temptations to resist" (Huxley, p. 185). But on balance freedom to act is severely diminished, for persons are not permitted to travel where they will, read whatever they might choose, express any of a wide range of opinions, and so on. The closed options, of course, do not trouble or frustrate the happy citizens of *Brave New World* in the slightest, for they do not want to do, and could not choose to do, anything but what they can do. Since they are unable to will in accordance with any "second-order desires" other than the ones they have been conditioned to have, they lack open options to choose, or "free will" in the sense discussed above. But that doesn't trouble or frustrate them either, because they *can* will as they want to will, even though they *cannot* will other than as they do. Nor do they enjoy personal autonomy, the rightful power to make on their own the decisions that will determine their own lot in life. Yet the citizens of *Brave New World* are content, even without much freedom. Insofar as we readers find this picture both convincing and repugnant, Huxley's didactic novel proves to us that we do not value freedom merely as a means to contentment, but attribute to it an independent value of its own.

Deriving and explaining the distinctive value of freedom is one of the great unfinished tasks of philosophy. If the one thing we all value as an end in itself is happiness, and if we can get happiness without freedom, how in that case can freedom be of any further value to those who lack it? *Brave New World* provides some suggestive clues. The contented, brain-washed automata in that fictitious land, being incapable of concern or affection for one another, or original thought, or high ambition, are so alien that we hardly recognize them as members of our own species. It may be a truism that all men desire happiness, but the happiness they desire is a recognizably *human* happiness, and the contentment that does not presuppose freedom fails to satisfy that description.

JOEL FEINBERG

[*Directly related to this article is the companion article,* ETHICAL ANALYSIS. *This article will find application in the entries* BEHAVIORAL THERAPIES; DRUG USE; DYNAMIC THERAPIES; ELECTRICAL STIMULATION OF THE BRAIN; HYPNOSIS; ELECTROCONVULSIVE THERAPY; PSYCHOSURGERY; PSYCHOPHARMACOLOGY; *and* SELF-REALIZATION THERAPIES. *For further discussion of topics mentioned in this article, see the entries:* ALCOHOL, USE OF; ENVIRONMENTAL ETHICS, *articles on* QUESTIONS OF SOCIAL JUSTICE, *and* THE PROBLEM OF GROWTH; FREE WILL AND DETERMINISM; PATERNALISM; PERSON; PRISONERS; SUICIDE; *and* TECHNOLOGY. *Also directly related are the entries* BEHAVIORISM; GENETIC ASPECTS OF HUMAN BEHAVIOR; GENETIC CONSTITUTION AND ENVIRONMENTAL CONDITIONING; INSTITUTIONALIZATION; *and* SEXUAL BEHAVIOR. *See also:* MENTAL HEALTH THERAPIES; RESEARCH, BEHAVIORAL; TRUTH-TELLING; *and* VIOLENCE AND THERAPY.]

BIBLIOGRAPHY

BENN, STANLEY I., and WEINSTEIN, WILLIAM L. "Being 194–211.
Free to Act, and Being a Free Man." *Mind* 80 (1971):
BERLIN, SIR ISAIAH. *Four Essays on Liberty.* London: Oxford University Press, 1969.
BURGESS, ANTHONY. *A Clockwork Orange.* New York: W. W. Norton, 1963.
DURKHEIM, EMILE. *Suicide.* Translated by John A. Spaulding and George Simpson. New York: Free Press, 1951, pp. 241–276.
EPICTETUS. *The Enchiridion* (A.D. 138). Translated by Thomas W. Higginson. New York: Liberal Arts Press, 1948.
FEINBERG, JOEL. "The Idea of a Free Man." *Educational Judgments.* Edited by James F. Doyle. London: Routledge & Kegan Paul, 1973, pp. 143–169.
FRANKFURT, HARRY G. "Freedom of the Will and the Concept of a Person." *Journal of Philosophy* 68 (1971): 5–20.
GLOVER, JONATHAN. *Responsibility.* International Library of Philosophy and Scientific Method. London: Routledge & Kegan Paul; New York: Humanities Press, 1970.
HUME, DAVID. *A Treatise of Human Nature* (1739–1740). Oxford: Clarendon Press, 1888 and 1941.

Huxley, Aldous. *Brave New World* (1932). Harmondsworth, England: Penguin Books, 1955.

Kant, Immanuel. *Fundamental Principles of the Metaphysic of Morals* (1785). Translated by Thomas K. Abbott. New York: Liberal Arts Press, 1949.

Mill, John Stuart. *On Liberty* (1859). New York: Liberal Arts Press, 1956.

Rousseau, Jean-Jacques. *The Social Contract* (1762). Translated by Maurice Cranston. Harmondsworth, England: Penguin Books, 1968.

Skinner, B. F. *Beyond Freedom and Dignity*. New York: Alfred A. Knopf, 1971.

BEHAVIOR MODIFICATION

See Behavior Control; Behaviorism, *article on* History of behavioral psychology; Behavioral Therapies; Research, Behavioral.

BEHAVIORAL GENETICS

See Genetic Aspects of Human Behavior.

BEHAVIORAL RESEARCH

See Research, Behavioral.

BEHAVIORAL THERAPIES

This entry is related to, but distinct from, the previous entry on Behavior Control. *This entry raises the ethical issues created by the practices of behavioristic therapies, such as the freedom of the therapist–client relationship and questions concerning the mechanistic approach to training and curing.*

People who make decisions about the behavior of others—parents, educators, legislators, judges—rarely refer to the psychological laboratory for verification of their notions of human behavior. Intuition, common sense, and nonscientific writings may seem to offer more immediate and relevant answers to human problems. However, a science of human behavior has recently become available. Principles developed largely in experimental animal learning laboratories have been utilized by behavioral psychologists and therapists to modify socially relevant human behaviors.

Two areas of animal learning have contributed to the behavioral therapies: classical or Pavlovian conditioning and operant conditioning. Pavlovian conditioning presents the following model. When food (an unconditioned stimulus) is given to a dog, it salivates (an unconditioned response); after food has been repeatedly presented following the ringing of a bell (a conditioned stimulus) the dog will salivate (a conditioned response) when only the bell is rung. The conditioned response will eventually cease to occur (extinguish) if the conditioned stimulus is no longer paired with the unconditioned stimulus. Classical conditioning affects only the performance or nonperformance of innate behaviors. Perhaps the most well-known application of these principles is desensitization by reciprocal inhibition, a technique used primarily with phobic individuals. Aversion therapy for problems of alcoholism or sexual deviation is also based on a classical conditioning model. The term "behavior therapy" is often used to describe therapeutic techniques at least loosely based on classical conditioning (Franks).

Operant conditioning emphasizes the relationship between a response and environmental events that closely follow it in time. Consequent environmental events that result in an increase in response frequency are classified as reinforcing events. Those resulting in a decrease in response frequency are classified as punishing events. If a dog is given a piece of popcorn every time it whines and the rate of whining increases, the popcorn would be called a reinforcer. If the popcorn were later withheld, the rate of whining would decrease (extinguish). Operant principles have been used both to increase the frequency of some behaviors such as positive statements in job interviews, studying in college, or cleaning one's room, and to decrease the frequency of other behaviors such as hallucinatory speaking, littering, or overeating. The special advantage of operant conditioning is that behaviors never previously emitted can be taught by reinforcing each component approximation of the target behavior. The term "behavior analysis" is often given to therapeutic procedures based on operant conditioning.

The early methodological behaviorists stressed that all human learning could be understood in terms of observable environmental events and observable responses (Craighead, Kazdin, and Mahoney). Now behavior therapists in social learning (e.g., Bandura, 1974) argue that much behavior is a response to environmental stimuli mediated through the intervention of thoughts that predict consequences; the behavior is partially a reaction to those predictions. Behavior analysts, on the other hand, argue that thoughts and feelings are observable responses even though they are observable only to the person who experiences them. Thoughts and feelings, like other response classes, may be modified by altering their consequences (Skinner, 1953). Both behavior therapists and behavior analysts deal with cognitive processes (Bandura, 1969, pp. 564 ff.; Craighead, Kazdin, and Mahoney, pp. 1–34; Rimm and Masters, pp. 416 ff.). This fact is not widely understood by nonbehaviorists, who may consequently tend to label behavior therapies as mechanistic.

Behavior therapy as a generic term is frequently used to encompass all therapeutic techniques based on either the classical or the operant animal learning literature. The techniques may differ in the extent to which they are theoretical rather than empirical, but all aspire to an empirical basis. Behavior therapy is part of a broad spectrum of treatment strategies within psychology and psychiatry whose emphases vary widely, e.g., existential therapy, gestalt therapy, client-centered therapy, and psychoanalysis (Craighead, Kazdin, and Mahoney, pp. 93 ff.).

Historical review

The principles of behavior therapy have been used unsystematically since the beginning of time, but their systematic application is relatively new. Although the first systematic applications of learning principles to human behavior occurred in the 1920s, psychotherapeutic procedures derived from the medical model, which located the cause of behavior inside the individual (e.g., in a conflict between the id and ego), rather than in environmental events, predominated. In the 1950s three events seem to have occasioned the rapid development of behavioral treatment procedures: (1) a questioning of the effectiveness of psychotherapeutic techniques based on the medical model (Eysenck); (2) the development of systematic desensitization procedures (Wolpe); and (3) the analysis of social problems in terms of the principles of operant conditioning (Skinner, 1953). Initially, behavior analysts worked with populations that had largely been ignored by traditional psychotherapists, those labeled retarded or psychotic. Substantial success was reported both with individual programming (e.g., language) and group programming (e.g., token economies) with those populations. Behavior therapists at first worked largely with client populations previously handled by traditional psychotherapists. Later, therapists in both areas expanded their treatment efforts to other populations and problems with a consequent blurring of the distinctions between the two. Recent be-

havioral textbooks list (1) the following problem areas: anxiety, depression, sexual deviation, social skills, alcoholism and drug abuse, obesity, smoking, and marital problems; (2) the following settings: classrooms, mental hospitals, medical hospitals, institutions for the retarded, prisons, and experimental communities; and (3) the following procedures: desensitization, modeling, assertive training, contingency management, self-control, extinction, positive control, aversive control, and cognitive methods (Craighead, Kazdin, and Mahoney; Rimm and Masters; Bandura, 1969).

Controversial issues related to behavior therapy

Mechanism. The attention to behavior rather than personality and intrapsychic processes may appear mechanistic or at least nonhumanistic. Behavioral psychologists do not find it useful to characterize a client as schizophrenic, delinquent, or defensive. Instead they describe salient high- or low-frequency responses emitted by the client, which were reinforced or punished by the environment. Similarly the behaviorally trained teacher or parent will not characterize a child as good or bad but will indicate that particular responses were well executed or not.

The distinction between reinforcing and punishing a response rather than a person is important. When reinforcement occurs a response increases in frequency. Procedures for reinforcing a whole person do not exist. Punishment is operating if a response followed immediately by an environmental event decreases in frequency. A mother may turn off the television for five minutes (time-out from television) every time her children bicker. If bickering decreases she has punished that response. Procedures for punishing a whole person do not exist.

Misapprehensions. Retributive punishment is directed toward the whole person. It would not be defined as punishment by behaviorists since in retributive punishment the punishing event is not necessarily contingent on a response (but may be contingent on having inadequate legal defense) and is rarely documented to decrease the frequency of the response (as attested by high recidivism rates).

The term "punishment" in the context of the judicial system is not synonymous with the same term in a behavioral context. Nonbehaviorists have tended to assume mistakenly that prison terms, solitary confinement, and other isolation procedures in prisons and hospitals for the retarded and mentally disturbed were always behavioral procedures. Thinkers who believe that people always should be treated as persons may in fact defend retributive punishment for its "human" orientation, arguing that behavioral punishment "dehumanizes" people by recognizing them only as sets of conditioned responses. Their opponents may argue that isolated conditioned responses are the only aspects of a person that society has a right to change because only such isolated behaviors can be examined and judged in a socially equitable way; society, they may argue, has no right to a whole person. Behavioral procedures have also been erroneously associated with various surgical techniques and with the use of psychoactive drugs. To be categorized as behavioral, a procedure must be based on the laws of learning as they have been discovered in the basic science laboratory (National Association).

Although there is nothing new in the attempts of one or more persons to change the behaviors of other persons, deliberate planning of behavior change based on established principles of behavior can seem ominous. If such planning also includes the introduction of extraneous or arbitrary reinforcing stimuli such as giving candies to schoolchildren contingent upon the completion of assignments, some long-held values about learning for its own sake seem violated. Nonbehaviorists may think that natural reinforcers ought to be sufficient. The behaviorist would argue that if certain appropriate responses are lacking in a person then whatever natural reinforcers may be available have clearly been ineffective in establishing the target responses. Additional, arbitrary reinforcers may be temporarily needed to strengthen responding so that the individual can begin to come into contact with any natural consequences that may exist in the situation. All too often society's natural consequences are the unpleasant things that happen to persons who do not exhibit the appropriate behaviors.

Problems created by treatment effectiveness. It is important to remember that the classification of environmental events is based on the direction of the behavior change. There are no events that are always reinforcing or always punishing. If a priori definitions of punishers and reinforcers are used, behavior change may be in unexpected directions. A teacher may think that reprimanding a student for breaking classroom rules is punishing. If the student continues to break the rules, an alternative explanation, locating the cause of rule-breaking in the moral character of the student instead of the consequent environmental events, may be made. The more appropriate analysis would be that teacher attention (even though delivered in what would be subjectively perceived as a negative manner) was functioning as a reinforcer, thereby increasing the frequency of the behavior it followed.

It is incorrect to suggest that a behavioral principle did not work in the above instance. Rather, the situation was analyzed incorrectly and a nonpunishing event was chosen to follow upon the behavior. If an appropriate analysis is made and if a demonstrated consequent event is available the probability of a change in behavior is very high. Furthermore, that change would be publicly demonstrable. A behaviorist insists upon replicate intervention strategies as well as direct and quantifiable observations of the behavior before, during, and after treatment.

The documented success of behavior therapy and the potential associated with that success have occasioned ethical concern about the choice of particular target responses as well as about who will make those choices. The concern becomes especially evident when the values of the client, the client's agent, the therapist, and society at large are not consonant. For example, early behavioral interventions in elementary classrooms dealt with the reduction of disruptive behavior (Winett and Winkler). Decreasing the disruptive behavior was not always accompanied by an increase in on-task behavior, and therefore not consonant with the values of all concerned. Subsequent behavioral projects in elementary classrooms have targeted responses such as task completion rather than disruptive behavior. A similar but unresolved problem lies in the selection of the target response when the overall problem relates to the sexual identity of the client.

While these two areas have received considerable attention, almost every therapeutic intervention involves problems related to the choice of the target response and its ultimate frequency of occurrence. How many chores should a teenager be expected to do around the house, how much eye contact should a nonassertive person develop, how many pleasant statements should a husband make to his wife, how many laps in the exercise yard should the prisoner run?

These issues in behavior therapy are particularly appropriate if the client is a resident of an institution for the retarded, for the psychotic, or for prisoners. Such clients are often less knowledgeable about available treatment choices, and target behaviors are often defined by someone other than the client (ward aides object to incontinence or self-destructive behavior). The behaviorists employed by institutions may be reinforced for producing client behavior that furthers institutional goals rather than client interests (Stolz, Wienckowski, and Brown).

Behavior therapies and the institutionalized

The U.S. courts abandoned their hands-off policy toward the care and treatment of the institutionalized in the mid-1960s. While changes in the behavior of residents as a result of token economies and other behavioral procedures were well documented, it became clear that abuses had also occurred (Wexler), sometimes as a result of institutional practices unrelated to treatment and sometimes as a result of behavioral or other treatment procedures ("Viewpoints"; Budd and Baer; National Association, pp. 1–6; Martin; Wexler). Judicial decisions that have affected the activities of behavioral psychologists in institutions are discussed below.

The treatment procedures selected for any institutionalized patient must be the least restrictive of the treatment alternatives available, e.g., *Covington* v. *Harris* (Budd and Baer); for example, giving a client tokens for social interactions may be more restrictive than asking him to self-monitor those behaviors (both behavioral procedures), but less restrictive than electroconvulsive therapy (a nonbehavioral procedure). It is unclear if the courts would declare a more restrictive treatment that was quickly successful to be less or more restrictive than a less restrictive treatment that took longer.

The courts have also proscribed the use of some aversive procedures, e.g., nausea-induction in *Knecht* v. *Gillman* ("Viewpoints," p. 63), physical restraint in *Wyatt* v. *Stickney* and seclusion in *Inmates of Boy's Training School* v. *Affleck* and *Morales* v. *Turman* (Budd and Baer). Such procedures had in the past been used by both behavioral and nonbehavioral psychologists. When less restrictive aversive procedures are unavoidable, e.g., time-out, their use may be monitored by a human rights review board composed of institutional employees, parents, lawyers, community residents, and behavior analysts.

Prior notice must be given to the client before a treatment program is begun and an opportunity for a hearing must be made available. The

risks, benefits, and other consequences must be explained (Stolz in Wood, p. 246; "Viewpoints," pp. 91–92; Budd and Baer, pp. 229–233) so that the resident can make an informed consent. The possibility of an institutionalized person giving consent independent of coercion may be questioned, e.g., *Kaimowitz* v. *Michigan Department of Mental Health* ("Viewpoints," p. 59), especially if there is a likelihood that release from the institution is in any way contingent upon participation in the treatment. Behavioral analyses of responses and contingent consequences involved in consent and coercion have introduced the notion of degrees of consent and coercion (ibid., p. 81) in terms of sets of alternative responses or choices available to the client (Goldiamond, pp. 54–62). The legal and behavioral aspects of consent involve many conflicting assumptions about the fundamental variables controlling behavior. Traditionally, freedom has implied absence of aversive control by powerful persons. The behaviorist's stress on the importance of immediate positive consequences in controlling responses seems to violate some long-held ideas of freedom, e.g., being able to consent freely. A number of alternative choices may be planned in an apparently free manner yet the pattern of choices may be readily related to prior positive consequences for particular choices (ibid.). The present notion that freedom exists if aversive controls are absent may change with understanding of the principles of positive reinforcement.

Another issue for behavior analysis in institutions is the relationship between noncontingent reinforcement and the notion of absolute rights. The courts have made a distinction between absolute rights and contingent rights, i.e., those privileges which shall be available freely and those which may be made available only following some specific response. The list of absolute rights includes, in part, visits and telephone calls, meals in dining rooms, wearing of personal clothing, adequate physical space, and comfortable beds, e.g., *Wyatt* v. *Stickney* (Budd and Baer). "The crux of the problem, from the point of view of behavior modification, is that the items and activities that are emerging as absolute rights are the very same items and activities that the behavioral psychologists would employ as reinforcers—that is, as 'contingent rights'" (Wexler, p. 11); e.g., a patient might have been required to brush his hair and wash his face before being allowed into the dining room for breakfast. If self-grooming is to remain a target behavior, then some other reinforcer must be found. Absolute rights may not be entirely eliminated as reinforcers, since they can vary in frequency, duration, or kind. The duration of visiting hours, the number of telephone calls per day, or being served a preferred softboiled egg instead of the ordinary hardboiled egg could conceivably be made contingent. Absolute rights do not exhaust the possibilities for reinforcers, but alternatives are often either beyond the financial means of institutional budgets or not functionally reinforcing stimuli for institutionalized persons, e.g., the arts, theater, and travel.

The problem goes beyond that stated by Wexler as quoted above. If a reinforcing event is presented without regard to what the client is doing, whichever response happens to be occurring just before the reinforcer is presented is likely to be increased. A reinforcer will have an effect on a response whether or not anyone explicitly intended an effect. Accidental contingencies are as effective as planned contingencies. Meals as absolute rights in institutions may simply increase the frequency of sitting and staring when they could serve to increase more adaptive behaviors. The guarantee of absolute rights guarantees an ignorance of which response(s) will be reinforced and eliminates the requirement for institutionalized persons to do anything in order to receive food, medical care, and other needs. Although society may ultimately decide this requirement is wrong, that policy sharply differentiates the institutionalized from the noninstitutionalized persons who must usually work consistently to earn absolute rights for themselves.

The recipients of bountiful help are rather in the position of those who live in a benign climate or possess great wealth. They are not strongly deprived or aversively stimulated and, hence, not subject to certain kinds of reinforcement. . . . But such people do not simply do nothing; instead, they come under the control of lesser reinforcers [Skinner, 1975, p. 626].

The "lesser" reinforcers associated with leisure are less likely to be art, music, literature, and science than sweets, alcohol, tobacco, or television. In an institution, alternative reinforcers are not available. The residents have nothing to do. "They may be reinforced for mild troublemaking, and if possible they escape, but otherwise we say their behavior tends to be marked by boredom, abulia . . . and apathy" (ibid., p.

630). Helping someone has traditionally meant giving them free reinforcers. A greater help may be in providing simple contingencies between useful responses and available reinforcers.

The courts have recognized that "the mere characterization of an act as 'treatment' does not insure that the client will benefit," e.g., *Knecht v. Gillman* ("Viewpoints," p. 64). Time-out from reinforcement has not been prohibited by the courts although seclusion has (Budd and Baer). This important distinction by the courts between procedures that have been demonstrated to change behavior and those that have not suggests that the courts may soon specify that the right to treatment implies the right to effective treatment. The effectiveness of treatment procedures may be demonstrated in a number of ways. Quantifiable changes in client behavior may be made public. Questionnaires that solicit the satisfaction or dissatisfaction of persons who eventually will judge the effectiveness of the treatment (parents, teachers, judges, clients) provide important information to the therapist (Wood, pp. 131–157). Public specification of target dates for accomplishing certain treatment goals further protect clients.

Implications beyond the institutions

The decisions reached by the courts regarding behavior analysis and the institutionalized have implications for the entire society. Nonbehavioral views of human nature have held that entities such as a free will or rational mind direct behavior. Our laws were designed to control the behavior of persons possessing such entities. The model of behavior implicit in our legal system and the principles stated explicitly in the analysis of behavior are at odds. An example of a resulting problem is in the issue of the right to privacy in one's own home. Parents are permitted to raise their children in almost any way they see fit. However, it is now known that attention of any sort is a powerful reinforcing stimulus for many young children. It is also known that parents and older siblings are likely to attend to children when they misbehave and to ignore them when they behave appropriately. These child-raising procedures increase the frequency of the very responses parents wish to eliminate. This paradigm is so common that most behavioral interventions involve little more than shifting the usual consequences for desired responses to undesired responses and vice versa. It may be unethical to permit parents to raise their own children without providing parent-training programs that make the consequences of the above situation explicit.

Another ethical issue becomes immediately apparent. If parents were trained to teach the responses they desired in their children, how many parents would find it more reinforcing to teach responses that would be in the long run more useful for their children, and how many would find it more reinforcing to produce responses that were in the short run more useful to themselves? That at least some parents would prefer to reinforce rapid obedience and long periods of quiet at the expense of discussion and exploration seems reasonably high (Winett and Winkler). The rights of children to treatment (in this case the opportunity to learn the more useful behaviors) seem to conflict with the rights of the parents to privacy in child-raising (Martin, pp. 134–136).

The continued success of behavioral treatment strategies has encouraged behaviorists to think beyond the treatment of the individual to that of the entire social system in which individuals would collectively plan and arrange consequences for responses in every aspect of social living. Currently accepted social customs involved in childrearing, religious beliefs, economic and political theory, and rational philosophy would inevitably be seriously questioned. Whatever subsequent changes in behavior patterns might eventuate would be based upon an objective analysis of the relationships among response frequencies and environmental consequences.

KENNETH E. LLOYD AND
MARGARET E. LLOYD

[*For further discussion of topics mentioned in this article, see the entries:* BEHAVIOR CONTROL; *and* BEHAVIORISM. *Other relevant material may be found under* INFORMED CONSENT IN MENTAL HEALTH; INFORMED CONSENT IN THE THERAPEUTIC RELATIONSHIP; INSTITUTIONALIZATION; MENTAL HEALTH THERAPIES; PRISONERS; PRIVACY; *and* RESEARCH, BEHAVIORAL.]

BIBLIOGRAPHY

BANDURA, ALBERT. "Behavior Therapy and the Models of Man." *American Psychologist* 29 (1974): 859–869.
————. *Principles of Behavior Modification*. New York: Holt, Rinehart & Winston, 1969.
BUDD, KAREN S., and BAER, DONALD M. "Behavior Modification and the Law: Implications of Recent Judicial Decisions." *Journal of Psychiatry and Law* 4 (1976): 171–244.
CRAIGHEAD, W. EDWARD; KAZDIN, ALAN E.; and MAHONEY, MICHAEL J. *Behavior Modification: Principles, Issues, and Applications*. Boston: Houghton Mifflin, 1976.
EYSENCK, H. J. "The Effects of Psychotherapy: An Evaluation." *Journal of Consulting Psychology* 16 (1952): 319–324.
FRANKS, CYRIL M., ed. *Behavior Therapy: Appraisal and Status*. McGraw-Hill Series in Psychology. New York: 1969.
GOLDIAMOND, ISRAEL. "Toward a Constructional Approach to Social Problems: Ethical and Constitutional Issues Raised by Applied Behavioral Analysis." *Behaviorism* 2 (1974): 1–84.
MARTIN, REED. *Legal Challenges to Behavior Modification: Trends in Schools, Corrections, and Mental Health*. Champaign, Ill.: Research Press, 1975.
National Association for Retarded Children, Research Advisory Committee, Joint Task Force. *Guidelines for the Use of Behavioral Procedures in State Programs for Retarded Persons*. Assembled by the Florida Division of Retardation and the Department of Psychology of the Florida State University. Monograph no. 1. 1975. 73 pp. Pamphlet available from the National Association for Retarded Children, 2709 Ave. E East. Arlington, Texas, 76011.
RIMM, DAVID C., and MASTERS, JOHN C. *Behavior Therapy: Techniques and Empirical Findings*. New York: Academic Press, 1974.
SKINNER, B. F. "The Ethics of Helping People." *Criminal Law Bulletin* 11 (1975): 623–636.
————. *Science and Human Behavior*. New York: Macmillan Co., 1953.
STOLZ, STEPHANIE B.; WIENCKOWSKI, LOUIS A.; and BROWN, BERTRAM S. "Behavior Modification: A Perspective on Critical Issues." *American Psychologist* 30 (1975): 1027–1048.
"Viewpoints on Behavioral Issues in Closed Institutions." *Arizona Law Review* 17 (1975): 1–143. Special issue.
WEXLER, DAVID B. "Token and Taboo: Behavior Modification, Token Economies, and the Law." *California Law Review* 61 (1973): 81–109. Reprint. *Behaviorism* 1, no. 2 (1973), pp. 1–24.
WINETT, RICHARD A., and WINKLER, ROBIN C. "Current Behavior Modification in the Classroom: Be Still, Be Quiet, Be Docile." *Journal of Applied Behavior Analysis* 5 (1972): 499–504.
WOLPE, JOSEPH. *Psychotherapy by Reciprocal Inhibition*. Stanford: Stanford University Press, 1958.
WOOD, W. SCOTT, ed. *Issues in Evaluating Behavior Modification*. Proceedings, First Drake Conference on Professional Issues in Behavior Analysis, 1974. Champaign, Ill.: Research Press, 1975, pp. 1–264.
Wyatt v. Stickney. 325 F. Supp. 781 (M.D. Ala. 1971). 334 F. Supp. 1341 (M.D. Ala. 1971). 344 F. Supp. 373 (M.D. Ala. 1972). 344 F. Supp. 387 (M.D. Ala. 1972). Appeal docketed sub nom. Wyatt v. Aderholt. 503 F. 2d 1305 (5th Cir. 1974).

BEHAVIORISM

This entry offers a set of theories that are relevant for understanding the conceptual background of the previous two entries. It accomplishes this in two articles—one that traces the history of the various schools of behavioral psychology and the issues of ethical interest under the title HISTORY OF BEHAVIORAL PSYCHOLOGY, *and the other,* PHILOSOPHICAL ANALYSIS, *which discusses the philosophical and ethical implications of behavioristic schools of thought.*

I
HISTORY OF BEHAVIORAL PSYCHOLOGY

Origins of behaviorism

Unlike many other events in the history of science, the origin of behaviorism can be readily pinpointed. In 1913 John B. Watson published an article, "Psychology as the Behaviorist Views It," in which the tenets, methods, and objectives of behaviorism were presented. In that article and in several later publications, Watson introduced a new theoretical framework in psychology that stood in contrast to the then prevailing conceptualizations in method, substance, and objective. In method, Watson proposed a sharp break from introspection or disciplined self-observation as the basic avenue of data-gathering in psychology in favor of recording the overtly observable behavior of organisms. In substance, he redefined the subject matter of psychology from the study of the contents of the mind to the investigation of behavior. In reference to objectives, he stressed prediction and control of behavior over its explanation and understanding for its own sake.

The impact of this triple shift in emphasis was to redirect the efforts of psychologists from the search for the general laws that govern the functioning of the average adult mind to the study of subjects and organisms that could not sidetrack the investigator by their spontaneous or elicited introspective reports, i.e., animals and young children. Research with animals, especially white rats, came to occupy a prominent place in behavioral psychology, on the assumption that the principles underlying human behavior could be discovered by experimenting with animal subjects. Such differences as existed between animals and humans were thought to be quantitative and not qualitative. Thus, animals could be observed and the observations extended to humans. The research strategy inaugurated by Watson and followed by many prominent behaviorists to the present day involved the investigation of simple responses in order to proceed from these studies to more complex behavior. Watson was centrally concerned with the conditions that caused behavior to change, i.e., with learning, and saw human as well as animal activity in a constant flux, ever subject to modification by the environment. His belief in the malleability of human as well as animal behavior was pronounced and is well expressed in the following quotation:

Give me a dozen healthy infants, well-formed, and my own personal world to bring them up in and I'll guarantee to take any one at random and train him to become any type of specialist I might select—doctor, artist, merchant-chief and, yes, even beggar-man and thief, regardless of his talents, penchants, tendencies, abilities, vocations, and race of his ancestors [Watson, 1930, p. 82].

Anyone could, in short, become anything, and the task of behavioristic psychology was to uncover and specify the conditions under which this would be possible—not by means of the utopian experiment proposed in the passage above, but by a laborious program of systematic experiments, for the most part with animals.

Antecedents of behaviorism

Although behavioral psychology represented a radical break with the concepts and operations of psychology in the early twentieth century, its advent did not occur in a conceptual void. Two influences in particular deserve to be pointed out. Edward L. Thorndike's experimental studies on learning in cats by means of trial and error and his formulation of the law of effect represented an important antecedent to behaviorism. The law of effect postulated that responses followed by satisfaction and pleasure tend to be repeated; responses followed by discomfort are less likely to occur (Thorndike).

Another important development took place in Russia, where I. P. Pavlov demonstrated a type of learning that came to be known as classical or Pavlovian conditioning. In Pavlov's laboratory, animals came to respond to a previously neutral stimulus, such as the sound of a bell or metronome, with behavior formerly elicited by the presentation of meat powder, i.e., by salivation. In Pavlov's terminology, the buzzer was the conditioned stimulus and salivation in response to it, the conditioned reflex; meat powder served as the unconditioned stimulus (Pavlov). These experiments and similar, although independently conceived studies by Pavlov's countryman, Bechterev (1913), provided, together with Thorndike's work, an empirical foundation for the program of investigations on learning that Watson envisaged.

Comprehensive learning theories

Watson participated only in the early stages of the investigation. It fell to others to propose and develop comprehensive theories of learning. Notable in this respect were the contributions of Hull, Tolman, and Guthrie.

Hull's effort was an ambitious attempt to develop a hypothetico-deductive theory of learning composed of a set of assumptions and theorems. He proceeded from observations of rote learning in animal species, particularly rats, and extended them to the entire range of human behavior. By the time of his death his effort was not yet complete, but the basic principles on which the theoretical structure was to rest were enunciated. In a simplified form, Hull viewed all behavior as a function of habit and drive, which stood in a multiplicative relationship. It follows then that both habit and drive are necessary for a specific response to occur. All behavior is thought to be at the service of drive reduction; the organism forever tends toward a tensionless state (Hull, 1943, 1952).

Hull's great opponent was Tolman, who stressed the purposeful character of learning even in subhuman species. The rat's behavior in a maze was determined by hypotheses or a cognitive map. Proceeding from this view, a distinction was drawn between latent learning, as accumulation of experience, and its manifestation in overt behavior (Tolman). This theme reverberates in a number of recent formulations concerning the nature of learning.

In a different way, Guthrie drew a sharp distinction between learning and performance. All learning, he held, occurs in one trial, but many trials are necessary to tie the various learned responses together and to cause them to occur in the course of one act (Guthrie).

These global explanations of learning attracted both adherents and controversy, but fascination with such explanatory structures dwindled after their originators' deaths. At the time of this writing (1976), there are few psychologists who identify themselves as followers of Hull, Tolman, or Guthrie, even though specific features of their contributions continue to inspire theoretical elaboration and empirical research.

Recent developments

From the vantage point of the 1970s it can be said that behaviorism as a current of conceptualization has been tremendously successful. With the exception of a few dissenting voices (Miller; Vexliard), there is broad agreement in current psychology textbooks and other writings that psychology is the science of behavior. The concept of behavior, however, has been broadened beyond the glandular secretions and muscular contractions to which Watson restricted this term. Behavior has come to encompass speech, thought, feeling, and perception, and the range of psychologists who call themselves behaviorists has greatly expanded. Thus, there are cognitive behaviorists (e.g., Boneau; Mahoney). Strictures against the study of private internal states have been greatly loosened. Proposals for reintroduction of introspection as a method of psychology have been heard (Radford), even though there are few, if any, psychologists who would return it to the prominent place that it occupied before Watson.

Throughout all of these developments, the central figure in the mainstream of behaviorism has been B. F. Skinner. In marked contrast to Hull, he has eschewed construction of formal theories in order to concentrate on the specification of the conditions necessary for the occurrence of a response. His approach has been empirical, inductive, and minimally burdened with inference. His focus has been on the study of the operant response by means of which the organism alters, or acts upon, its environment. He has held throughout four decades that the contingencies for such responses can be found in the external environment and that operant responses are maintained and shaped by externally mediated reinforcement. The control and prediction of a response has been Skinner's central concern; any reference to internal states, subjective or physiological, is unnecessary to that end. Like Watson, Skinner is articulately deterministic. Since all behavior is under the control of its consequences, Skinner's focus in his more speculative writings (1948, 1972) has been on developing more rational and efficient ways of controlling behavior. This has taken him into the area of social design and the formulations of policies that would control behavior in the economic, political, and social areas following principles developed in his laboratory.

Social impact of behaviorism

The last two decades have been characterized by the expansion of behaviorism beyond the confines of laboratory research. Prominent among developments in that direction is behavior modification, which represents the application of behavioral principles, notably of classical conditioning and operant learning, to the changing of maladaptive or disturbed behavior (Bandura; Eysenck; Goldfried and Davison; Wolpe). These developments have had highly beneficial and promising results (Mahoney, Kazdin, and Lesswing), although there continues to be controversy concerning the scope of applications of the techniques and their relationships to their original laboratory models of learning (London, 1972). The techniques of behavior modification have expanded to include modeling or imitation (Bandura) as well as self-observation and self-control (Goldfried and Merbaum; Mahoney). The methods of behavior modification have been applied outside of hospital and clinic settings in schools (Klein, Hapkiewicz, and Roden; Harris; O'Leary and Drabman), correctional institutions (Stolz, Wienckowski, and Brown), and a variety of other real-life environments (Tharp and Wetzel).

The effectiveness of behavior modification techniques has sparked criticisms and apprehensions, many of which had been anticipated in earlier critical reactions to behaviorism and its major exponents (Koestler; Rogers and Skinner; Bertalanffy). Since behavior modification involves the exercise of power and control, the old Platonic question has been raised: Who will control the controllers? The answer the behaviorists provide is that the behavior modifier is not to be thought of as an external agent, unilaterally impinging upon the objects of his techniques. Rather, as Skinner (1972) and others (Goldfried and Davison) have asserted, he who reinforces is reinforced by the recipients of reinforcement. It has been demonstrated that experimental control produces countercontrol by the subjects of the experiment (Ulrich).

Other objections to behavioral techniques have concerned the use of painful and aversive means to modify behavior (Goldfried and Davison; Stolz, Wienckowski, and Brown) and the application of behavior modification techniques to involuntary subjects in correctional institutions (Stolz, Wienckowski, and Brown), schools (ibid.), and other settings. The consensus among recent writers on this subject (London, 1969; Mahoney, Kazdin, and Lesswing; Stolz, Wienckowski, and Brown) is that safeguards must be carefully applied and that the interests of the individual whose behavior is being modified have priority over institutional or social

preferences. Finally, questions have been raised concerning the ethical propriety of modifying such deviant behavior as homosexuality, especially in the absence of techniques for helping homosexuals develop and maintain their homosexual potential (Goldfried and Davison). While most practitioners of behavior modification would agree that these techniques can be legitimately applied only to consenting clients and only with a minimum of discomfort or pain, this does not exhaust the subtlety and complexity of ethical issues that have been raised. Some of them remain unresolved at the time of this writing.

JURIS G. DRAGUNS

[*Directly related are the entries* BEHAVIOR CONTROL; BEHAVIORAL THERAPIES; *and* RESEARCH, BEHAVIORAL. *Also directly related is the other article in this entry,* PHILOSOPHICAL ANALYSIS.]

BIBLIOGRAPHY

BANDURA, ALBERT. *Principles of Behavior Modification.* New York: Holt, Rinehart & Winston, 1969.

BECHTEREV, VLADIMIR MICHAILOVITCH. *General Principles of Human Reflexology* 4th ed. (1928). Translated by Emma Murphy and William Murphy. New York: International Publishers, 1932. Reprint. Classics in Psychology. Edited by Howard Gardner and Judith Kreiger Gardner. New York: Arno Press, 1973.

BERTALANFFY, LUDWIG VON. *Robots, Men and Minds: Psychology in the Modern World.* New York: G. Braziller, 1967.

BONEAU, C. ALAN. "Paradigm Regained? Cognitive Behaviorism Restated." *American Psychologist* 29 (1974): 297–309.

CHAPLIN, JAMES PATRICK, and KRAWIEC, THEOPHILE STANLEY. *Systems and Theories of Psychology.* 3d ed. New York: Holt, Rinehart & Winston, 1974.

EYSENCK, HANS JURGEN, ed. *Behavior Therapy and the Neuroses: Readings in Modern Methods of Treatment Derived from Learning Theory.* Oxford: Pergamon Press, 1960.

GOLDFRIED, MARVIN R., and DAVISON, G. C. *Clinical Behavior Therapy.* New York: Holt, Rinehart & Winston, 1976.

———, and MERBAUM, MICHAEL, eds. *Behavior Change through Self-Control.* New York: Holt, Rinehart & Winston, 1973.

GUTHRIE, EDWIN RAY. *The Psychology of Learning.* Rev. ed. Harper Psychology series. New York: Harper, 1952. Reprint. Gloucester, Mass.: Peter Smith, 1960.

HARRIS, MARY B., ed. *Classroom Uses of Behavior Modification.* Columbus, Ohio: Merrill, 1972.

HULL, CLARK LEONARD. *A Behavior System: An Introduction to Behavior Theory Concerning the Individual Organism.* New Haven: Yale University Press, 1952. Science edition. New York: John Wiley & Sons, 1964.

———. *Principles of Behavior: An Introduction to Behavior Theory.* New York: Appleton-Century-Crofts, 1943.

KLEIN, ROGER D.; HAPKIEWICZ, WALTER G.; and RODEN, AUBREY H., eds. *Behavior Modification in Educational Settings.* Springfield, Ill.: Charles C Thomas, 1973.

KOESTLER, ARTHUR. *The Ghost in the Machine.* New York: Macmillan Co., 1968.

LONDON, PERRY. *Behavior Control.* New York: Harper & Row, 1969.

————. "The End of Ideology in Behavior Modification." *American Psychologist* 27 (1972): 913–920.

MAHONEY, MICHAEL J. *Cognition and Behavior Modification.* Cambridge, Mass.: Ballinger, 1974.

————; KAZDIN, ALAN E.; and LESSWING, NORMAN J. "Behavior Modification: Illusion or Deliverance?" *Annual Review of Behavioral Therapy: Theory and Practice, Vol. 2.* Edited by Cyril M. Franks and Terence Wilson. New York: Brunner-Mazel, 1974, pp. 11–40.

MILLER, GEORGE A. *Psychology: The Science of Mental Life.* New York: Harper & Row, 1962.

O'LEARY, K. DANIEL, and DRABMAN, RONALD. "Token Reinforcement Programs in the Classroom: A Review." *Psychological Bulletin* 75 (1971): 379–398.

PAVLOV, I. P. *Conditioned Reflexes: An Investigation of the Physiological Activity of the Cerebral Cortex.* Translated and edited by G. V. Anrep. London: Oxford University Press, 1927.

RACHLIN, HOWARD. *Introduction to Modern Behaviorism.* San Francisco: W. H. Freeman & Co., 1970.

RADFORD, JOHN. "Reflections on Introspection." *American Psychologist* 29 (1974): 245–261.

ROGERS, CARL R., and SKINNER, B. F. "Some Issues Concerning the Control of Human Behavior: A Symposium." *Science* 124 (1956): 1057–1066.

SKINNER, B. F. *About Behaviorism.* New York: Alfred A. Knopf, 1974.

————. *The Behavior of Organisms: An Experimental Analysis.* The Century Psychology Series. Edited by R. M. Elliott. New York: Appleton-Century Co., 1938.

————. *Beyond Freedom and Dignity.* New York: Alfred A. Knopf, 1972.

————. *Contingencies of Reinforcement: A Theoretical Analysis.* The Century Psychology Series. New York: Appleton-Century-Crofts, 1968.

————. *Science and Human Behavior.* New York: Free Press; London: Collier-Macmillan, 1953.

————. *Walden Two.* New York: Macmillan Co., 1948.

STOLZ, STEPHANIE B.; WIENCKOWSKI, LOUIS A.; and BROWN, BERTRAM S. "Behavior Modification: A Perspective on Critical Issues." *American Psychologist* 30 (1975): 1027–1048.

THARP, RONARD G., and WETZEL, RALPH J. *Behavior Modification in the Natural Environment.* New York: Academic Press, 1969.

THORNDIKE, EDWARD L. "Animal Intelligence." *Psychological Review, Monograph Supplements* 2, no. 4 (Whole no. 8) (1898), pp. 1–109.

TOLMAN, EDWARD CHACE. *Purposive Behavior in Animals and Man.* The Century Psychology Series. Edited by Richard M. Elliott. New York: Century Co., 1932.

ULRICH, ROGER. "Behavior Control and Public Concern." *Psychological Record* 17 (1967): 229–334.

VEXLIARD, ALEXANDRE. *La Psychologie n'est pas une science du comportement.* Ankara: Ankara University, 1967.

WATSON, JOHN BROADUS. *Behavior: An Introduction to Comparative Psychology.* New York: Henry Holt & Co., 1914.

————. *Behaviorism.* 2d ed. New York: W. W. Norton & Co., 1930. 1st ed. 1925.

————. "Psychology as the Behaviorist Views It." *Psychological Review* 20 (1913): 158–177.

————. *Psychology from the Standpoint of a Behaviorist.* Philadelphia: J. B. Lippincott & Co., 1919.

WOLPE, JOSEPH. *Psychotherapy by Reciprocal Inhibition.* Stanford: Stanford University Press, 1958.

II
PHILOSOPHICAL ANALYSIS

Behaviorism is often thought to be a doctrine on the truth or falsity of which a great deal is at stake for ethics generally and for bioethics in particular. For the account that we give of such concepts as those of a person, of the relationship between a person and his actions, of a motive, and so on, will all clearly be affected by our beliefs about the success or failure of behaviorist claims. Yet there is an initial difficulty.

Behaviorism is not one single doctrine, but a cluster of doctrines, not all mutually compatible, which derive from a single project, that of understanding mental activities, states, events, and processes as a species of physical behavior. The arguments in favor of behaviorism are often, although not always, negative in form. Their proponents wish to deny some particular thesis about the mental and sometimes seem to take this denial as providing positive support for behaviorism. Yet what is denied is at least as various as what is asserted: Descartes's dualism, James's stream of consciousness, and the introspective techniques of Wundt and Titchener have all been targets for behaviorist attack. But such doctrines clearly do not all stand or fall together. Debates over behaviorism have therefore been of very different kinds, and we need to discriminate a number of separate, if related, debates in each of which a distinctive behaviorist thesis has been asserted. In all these debates considerations quite independent of the arguments for or against behaviorism have intruded and behaviorism has therefore acquired a set of associated beliefs, which have been its allies historically, but the strength of whose connection with behaviorism is not always clear.

Overt behavior

First it has been contended by methodological behaviorists that only overt behavior is available for investigation by the methods of natural science. The view of natural science presupposed is one according to which experimental evidence enables us to link by means of a lawlike generalization some type of antecedent observable state of affairs with some type of consequent observable state of affairs. J. B. Watson, who introduced this version of behaviorism into psychology, linked his general thesis to a particular view of learning according to which a learned response is always and only produced by a stimulus with which it has become associated through conditioning. The conditioned reflex was taken as the paradigm for the explanation of human behavior. In the course of Watson's own intellectual development two further tendencies became associated with his behaviorism: One was an emphasis on peripheral nervous mechanisms rather than on the brain in the explanation of behavior, and the other was an extreme version of the view that environment, and not heredity, molds behavior.

In the writings of some of Watson's successors, most notably Clark L. Hull, the view taken of the canons of natural science is self-consciously derived from the philosophy of science of the Vienna Circle. Edward C. Tolman had developed Watson's approach so that the task of the psychological theorist became that of specifying the intervening variables by which stimulus and response were linked. Hull attempted to set out a completely general theory of this kind in hypothetico-deductive form. The influence of P. W. Bridgman's operationalism on this project was crucial. No concept is to be admitted into Hull's theory which cannot be specified in terms of experimental manipulation. But this attempt at methodological rigor accompanies a curiously speculative bent. Hull's central thesis—derived from Thorndike's Law of Effect—was that, if a response to some stimulus is followed by a reduction in some biological drive, the tendency for that stimulus to produce that response will be strengthened. The result is that, just as Watson was self-indulgent in allowing himself to invoke speculative peripheral mechanisms, so Hull is self-indulgent in invoking and indeed inventing not only peripheral mechanisms, but also whatever biological drives are required by his theory.

There are two other central weaknesses in Hull's approach. One derives from his attempt to generalize from very limited experimental evidence; the other is carried over from the weaknesses of the positivist philosophy, which dominated his view of science. The positivist ban on the introduction of unobservables into scientific theories was at one time based on a thesis about meaning formulated by Friedrich Waismann in 1930: The meaning of a statement *is* the method of its verification. When it became clear that it was quite implausible to suppose that statements about electrons or about heat were equivalent in meaning to statements about trails in Wilson cloud chambers or about mercury in thermometers, the whole relationship of evidence to meaning was put in question, and no cogent philosophical account of that relationship from which a clear ban on unobservable entities can be derived has ever been elaborated since. Moreover, such studies as those which experimental psychologists have made of afterimages depend on reports of private experience without violating any of the conditions of a valid experiment, as that is understood by most contemporary philosophers of science. Operationalism is nowadays a doctrine usually held by psychologists and not by philosophers.

Yet these considerations are not conclusive against Hull's type of theory; but its merits, if any, must now be derived from its explanatory power and not from its logical form. One merit was certainly claimed for it. Hull seemed able to give quantitative formulation to increases in strength of association, and so seemed able to produce a number of hypotheses precise enough to be falsified or corrected. But nothing in his work in fact passes beyond the speculative and the programmatic; and in any case this feature of Hull's work has no necessary connection with and provides no particular support for his behaviorism.

There is therefore no good reason to accept the behaviorist thesis when it is formulated as the methodological contention that only overt behavior can be studied by scientific methods. The same is true of the stronger metaphysical thesis that a belief in mental activities, states, events, and processes is a belief in a set of mythological nonexistent items. Watson sometimes allowed his rhetoric to betray him into what appeared to be this position, and he was in fact rash enough to deny the occurrence of images. But no psychological behaviorist since Watson has ever seriously held this position, although it has been imputed to some behaviorists by their critics.

Inner states or events

The second important debate is a philosophical one. It has been argued by Gilbert Ryle that those expressions in ordinary language which have been construed as naming inner mental states or events do in fact name patterns of behavior or dispositions to behave in particular ways. Ryle does argue that some expressions taken to name inner occurrences name nothing at all—"volition" is a prime example. But such expressions are on his account barren technical terms invented by confused theorists; they are not part of the ordinary language of transactions between agents. The target of Ryle's attack is Cartesian dualism, what he calls the myth of the ghost in the machine. Ryle does not argue in *The Concept of Mind* that there are no inner events or states. But he says, for example, that it is logically improper to speak of observing or witnessing sensations or feelings, although we certainly do have twinges and pains, chills of disquiet, and tugs of commiseration. However, in experiencing these an agent never merely reports a private occurrence of an event only discernible by him; there is no privileged access to his own consciousness by each agent, and if by "consciousness" we were to mean that to which we have privileged access, as some philosophers have claimed, then there is no such thing as consciousness. It was this denial which led to Ryle being sometimes misread as simply denying the occurrence of inner events or states.

Ryle's philosophical behaviorism is less extreme than that propounded by B. A. Farrell. Farrell takes it that words such as "consciousness" and "experience" have been displaced from their traditional role in our language by the advances of experimental psychology. Experimental psychology teaches us that everything that needs to be said or can be said about color discrimination, for example, can be expressed in terms of behavior and dispositions to behave. Ordinary language has not yet reflected this advance, but in Farrell's view if Western societies assimilate what psychology has to teach it is possible that the notion of "experience" will come to be treated as embodying a delusion.

One of the defects in Ryle's account is that it seems to make the philosophical views presupposed by ordinary language normative for philosophy and immune from scientific criticism of the type that Farrell envisages. One of the defects of Farrell's account is that he does not seem to notice that the experimental psychology which he cites is not in fact a philosophically neutral, scientifically authoritative source. For the experimental psychology on which he relied was itself the product of a particular philosophical standpoint and it was this standpoint and not the experimental findings of the psychologists which entailed behaviorism. Since restrictions were placed by behaviorists on counting as a valid part of any experiment any feature of it which did not conform to behaviorist canons, it was scarcely surprising and not very impressive that reports of such experiments revealed nothing contrary to behaviorism. Farrell allows that in using the reports of experimental human subjects as evidence—as many psychologists do—we are going beyond what behaviorism required, but he insists that we always could dispense with such reports. We use them merely as a matter of convenience.

Accounting for human actions

The most important criticism of the philosophical grounds for behaviorism advanced so far concerns its account of human actions. For a behaviorist of Hull's kind an action is in the end no more than a highly complex set of bodily movements. Hull did not deny the reality of purposive acts, or wish to exclude the use of such concepts as those of intelligence, insight, or intention. He aspired rather to justify the use of such concepts by deducing them from what he took to be more elementary objective primary principles. But he certainly believed that ultimately statements about intentional action could be analyzed into statements about overt behavior. It has been the contention of a number of philosophers that this is not possible, that statements about actions are in no way reducible to statements about bodily movements. It is certainly the case that the truth conditions of statements about actions differ from the truth conditions of the corresponding statements about bodily movements. "He paid his debts" can be true if any one out of the following set of statements is true: "He handed over various pieces of metal and paper," "He wrote his name on a certain document," "He said certain words under certain conditions." That is to say, one and the same action may be given effect in a number of very different bodily movements. Equally one and the same set of bodily movements may be the bearer of a number of different actions: That "He wrote his name" is true can satisfy a truth condition necessary for "He signed a check," "He applied for a passport" or "He tested his fountain pen." It follows that statements about human action are never logically equivalent to statements about observable human movement.

To identify an action we must be able to say what intention was expressed in the behavior in question and not merely what behavior was enacted. The issue over behaviorism then becomes the question of whether we can or cannot give an adequate behaviorist account of the concept of intention, or perhaps whether we can find an alternative way to specify the differences between different actions embodied in similar or the same sets of bodily movements which will satisfy behaviorist criteria, so that all references to intentionality may be eliminated from our discourse. This behaviorist program is characteristically defined as an attempt to replace intentional sentences such as "He applied for a passport" and "He tested his fountain pen" by conjunctions of nonintentional sentences which conjoin categorical statements about an agent's behavior with hypothetical statements about how such an agent would behave in a range of other situations. It is by reference to these sets of hypotheticals that the behaviorist hopes to match the discriminations that are ordinarily made by references to intention.

About this program two remarks need to be made. The first is that even its achievement would not be enough to show that nothing important in the meaning of intentional sentences had been omitted in their replacement by nonintentional sentences. The second is that this program has never been carried through satisfactorily even for one single example by any of the philosophers who have propounded it. A crucial argument against the very possibility of carrying through such a program is that the relevant sets of hypotheticals could never be adequately specified, except by ending the list of hypotheticals with some such phrase as *"and so on"*; and that the only way to delimit the class of hypotheticals intended would be by reference to that very intentional sentence which the program aspired to eliminate. But this argument has never yet been set out by any critic of behaviorism in a form sufficiently cogent to convince behaviorists.

B. F. Skinner

Unlike Ryle, most contemporary behaviorists agree with their critics in allowing that ordinary language, at least in its most plausible interpretation, is antibehaviorist. The conclusion drawn by B. F. Skinner is that ordinary language is therefore almost irremediably superstitious. Skinner has no wish to deny either that behaviorism cannot represent itself as giving the meaning of what we ordinarily say about mind or that there are indeed inner states, events, and processes. What he contends is that no reference to the inner has any place in a scientific explanation of the production of behavior. What Skinner offers positively is a program for a science of overt behavior, a program whose achievement

would make the use of our ordinary sentences about actions intellectually unjustifiable. If Skinner is right, the whole philosophical debate is largely beside the point.

Skinner's position differs in two important respects from that of his psychological predecessors. First, the model of the conditioned reflex is completely abandoned. Skinner does not envisage each piece of behavior by an organism as a response to a stimulus. Instead he sees a great deal of spontaneous behavior by organisms, behavior that is gradually modified insofar as it produces either agreeable or disagreeable consequences. This process of *operant conditioning* by positive and negative reinforcements shapes behavior in such a way that complex patterns are built up out of simple movements. Some schedules of reinforcement are more effective than others; positive reinforcement is generally more effective than negative. Because all behavior is the outcome either of biological factors or of the contingencies of the environment or of both, the study of the inner, of mental states, is usually completely irrelevant to the causal explanation of behavior (and at best might provide us with suggestive clues to the presence of dispositions to behave in certain ways).

Secondly, Skinner believes that experimental psychology should abjure any reliance on neurophysiological explanations. The *only* factors to be appealed to are changes in the environment and changes in the subsequent behavior of the organism. The only defensible way of studying the causal relationship between these two types of change is an experimental method which does not make use of anything but the observation of overt behavior. Reports of experimental subjects are to be excluded, if possible, as a source of error and observations undisciplined by experimental conditions can only mislead us. Skinner himself invented a new type of experimental environment where variation in environment could be strictly controlled, the so-called Skinner box. His work on pigeons provided a model for subsequent work, which has extended outside the laboratory to human behavior in programmed learning and in producing changes in the behavior of retardates, the mentally ill, and delinquents.

The principal criticisms to be made of Skinner's theory are three. First, it has been argued by Noam Chomsky that when Skinner extends his thesis to the explanation of language-using behavior his position becomes speculative and unfalsifiable. In particular he argues that the use of such expressions as "stimulus," "response," and "reinforcement," when they are detached from their application in narrowly experimental contexts, becomes vague and arbitrary. Moreover, Skinner and Chomsky differ over the place of rules in the production of human behavior. Skinner's position is—and given his behaviorism must be—that rules can play no part in the explanation of behavior; to say that behavior accords with a rule is to speak only of a regularity that has been produced by environmental contingencies, whereas for Chomsky the rules of a grammar play a key part in the explanation of linguistic competence.

Second, Skinner's methodological canons are such that his experiments could produce no evidence that would provide counterexamples to his own fundamental position. Hence Skinner's position can be progressively confirmed, but it cannot be refuted, or rather it can be refuted only by the use of procedures that Skinner disallows. This makes rational debate between those who agree with and those who disagree with Skinner difficult. Where complex behavior outside the laboratory is concerned, that of delinquents for example, there exists no established method for deciding on the truth or falsity of a Skinnerian interpretation, as against that of rival theorists such as Freudians; hence, perhaps, the observable fact that controversy over Skinner's positions is notably sterile.

Third, there is a paradox at the heart of Skinner's behaviorism. One dominant reason for adopting behaviorism in psychology, which Skinner shares with many of his predecessors, has been the belief that only thus can psychology be scientific. We have already seen that a necessary requirement for vindicating any behaviorism is the elimination of intentional language from the description of behavior. But the concept of science invoked by behaviorists is itself an intentional, and indeed normative, concept; to prescribe the methods of science is to invite us to be guided by one type of reason and intention rather than another, to deliberate in certain ways and to frame our purposes in accordance with our deliberations. Without such a concept of science (and to eliminate intentionality from our language would be to abolish that concept) we would have no way of justifying any one set of methodological procedures, including those of behaviorism, rather than another. Skinner thus seems simultaneously committed both to the retention and to the elimination of inten-

tional language. His commitment to science is in conflict with his commitment to behaviorism. Hull avoided this paradox only by adopting the logically untenable position that intentional concepts and statements can somehow be logically derived from nonintentional concepts and statements. No one has yet shown that there is any way of formulating a behaviorism that does not fall victim either to the fallacy in Hull's position or to the paradox in Skinner's.

Conclusion

Both critics and protagonists of each of the behaviorisms so far formulated have often thought that the moral implications of asserting or denying behaviorism are easily spelled out. B. F. Skinner, for example, has suggested that traditional concepts of freedom and dignity ought not to survive in the light of his behaviorist findings. But if Skinner's behaviorism were true and all intentional language were inappropriate, it is difficult to see that there would be any place for *any* moral view, including Skinner's own. For any morality clearly requires an ability to follow some rules and precepts just because they are reasonably held to be the correct rules and precepts; and such an ability cannot be described except in terms of reason-governed intentions and purposes.

Clearly no such radical consequence follows from either Ryle's or Hull's behaviorism. But less immediate consequences of their views might be important for ethics in general and for bioethics in particular. Could any behaviorist analysis yield an adequate account of an agent's responsibility? The answer is that we do not know, simply because no behaviorist analysis has ever been adequately carried through. It is just because the force and grounds of behaviorist contentions themselves still remain unclear that the moral implications of behaviorism also remain unclear.

ALASDAIR MACINTYRE

[*Directly related are the entries* BEHAVIORAL THERAPIES; FREE WILL AND DETERMINISM; MIND–BODY PROBLEM; *and* REDUCTIONISM. *See also:* BEHAVIOR CONTROL; BIOLOGY, PHILOSOPHY OF; EMBODIMENT; GENETIC ASPECTS OF HUMAN BEHAVIOR; *and* GENETIC CONSTITUTION AND ENVIRONMENTAL CONDITIONING.]

BIBLIOGRAPHY

CHOMSKY, NOAM. "A Review of B. F. Skinner's *Verbal Behavior.*" *The Structure of Language.* Edited by Jerry A. Fodor and Jerrold J. Katz. Englewood Cliffs, N.J.: Prentice-Hall, 1966, pp. 547–578.

FARRELL, B. A. "Experience." *The Philosophy of Mind.* Edited by Vere Claiborne Chappell. Englewood Cliffs, N.J.: Prentice-Hall, 1962, pp. 23–48.

GOLDMAN, ALVIN I. *A Theory of Human Action.* Englewood Cliffs, N.J.: Prentice-Hall, 1970.

HAMLYN, D. W. "Behavior." *The Philosophy of Mind.* Edited by Vere Claiborne Chappell. Englewood Cliffs, N.J.: Prentice-Hall, 1962, pp. 60–73.

HULL, CLARK L. *Principles of Behavior: An Introduction to Behavior Theory.* New York: Appleton-Century, 1943.

KOCH, SIGMUND. "Psychology and Emerging Conceptions of Knowledge as Unitary." *Behaviorism and Phenomenology.* Edited by T. W. Wann. Chicago: University of Chicago Press, 1964, pp. 1–41.

RYLE, GILBERT. *The Concept of Mind.* London: Hutchinson, 1949.

SKINNER, B. F. *About Behaviorism.* New York: A. Knopf, 1974.

———. *Beyond Freedom and Dignity.* New York: A. Knopf, 1971.

———. *Cumulative Record: A Selection of Papers.* 3d ed. New York: Appleton-Century-Crofts, 1972.

———. *Science and Human Behavior.* New York: Macmillan, 1953.

———. *Verbal Behavior.* New York: Appleton-Century-Crofts, 1957.

TOLMAN, EDWARD CHACE. *Purposive Behavior in Animals and Men.* London, New York: Century, 1932.

WATSON, JOHN BROADUS. "Psychology as the Behaviorist Views It." *Readings in the History of Psychology.* Edited by Wayne Dennis. New York: Appleton-Century-Crofts, 1948, pp. 457–471.

BENEFIT-HARM CALCULUS

See RISK; TECHNOLOGY, *article on* TECHNOLOGY ASSESSMENT.

BEREAVEMENT

See DEATH; DEATH, ATTITUDES TOWARD; PASTORAL MINISTRY.

BIOETHICS

Introduction

An Encyclopedia of Bioethics—or of Psychology or Religion or any special field of knowledge —need not have an entry on the very title of the work itself. The present encyclopedia is an extensive, almost exhaustive, collection of those issues and topics thought to be part of or directly relevant to bioethics. Yet beyond the scope of all these articles perhaps some questions will remain for the inquisitive reader—such questions as: How is bioethics related to ethics? Where does medical ethics fit in? Does bioethics have special problems or special principles? Is bioethics related to scientific facts in a way ordinary ethics is not? These, and related questions, will constitute the focus of this article.

It would be inappropriate at this point to define "bioethics" in the sense of setting limits to what should and should not count as bioethics. Rather this article, in dealing with the questions mentioned, will aim at provoking reflection on the nature of bioethics. Such reflection is not necessary for "doing" bioethics, that is, for understanding or working through issues within bioethics. It is intended for the inquisitive who are seeking a conceptual grasp of the field itself —an overview of what it is up to and of its relations with other, but similar, concerns. This article will be a guided tour through some of the questions, tensions, alternatives, and arguments that surround the concept of bioethics but would not necessarily arise in the course of pursuing issues *within* bioethics.

Fitting the object of our focus into its natural landscape is a helpful first step. The varieties of factors giving rise to concerns labeled "bioethics" have involved two main factors: increased capability and knowledge. Being capable of something (keeping a dying patient alive, discovering fetal characteristics before birth, transplanting body organs, etc.) forces the question, "Ought we to do it?"—a question irrelevant to practice so long as we are not capable of doing it. Increased knowledge, insofar as it discovers unforeseen consequences of our actions (spray cans and the ozone layer, nuclear energy plants and perinatal development, etc.), forces moral decisions we had not anticipated. Moreover, increased capability and knowledge can bring more benefits, which in turn raises the problem of their fair distribution. This mixture is then ignited by a general, culturewide emphasis on individual rights. Additionally, increased knowledge has led to specialization, producing "the expert" into whose hands we have entrusted everything. He alone, we thought, had the necessary competence. Supposedly these were just technical, factual matters that we had relinquished to the expert. The economist, the highway engineer, the energy expert, the diplomat, the financial wizard, the doctor—they all knew best. But we eventually came to realize that *values*, unbeknownst even to the experts, were being unwittingly employed in ostensibly factual equations. The resultant decisions greatly affect our quality of life.

The preceding paragraph is merely a reminder of the context that has given emphasis to a discipline called "bioethics." It is mentioned only to reinforce our seeing bioethics as a natural response to new dilemmas, increased knowledge, and threatened rights—rather than as at bottom a new discovery of basic principles or derivations therefrom. Also, in putting bioethics into perspective, we are reminded that it is part of a general move toward ferreting out values that had been camouflaged by factuality and clarifying rights to which we had been blinded by the glare of the unquestioned "common good." All this ties in with the position that, by and large, will be taken in this article—namely, that bioethics is not a new set of principles or maneuvers, but the same old ethics being applied to a particular realm of concerns.

Some preliminary metaethical points

Given what was just said about the position to be taken in this article, it would seem that one's metaethical views would remain undisturbed. That is, what constitutes one's view of the "same old ethics"—whether it be subjectivism, emotivism, cognitivism, intuitionism, or some other—is simply carried over to the biomedical arena. This article cannot deal with what *ethics* is, but only with what bioethics is in relation to whatever "ethics" is taken to be.

However, it may be both helpful and fair to state with (precarious) brevity the general orientation toward ethics assumed in this article. To that end three aspects of this view should be mentioned: (1) It is an ethics based on rationality; (2) it is primarily an avoidance of causing evil or a prevention of evil rather than a promoting of good; and (3) its basic rules are applicable to all people, at all times and places, equally (Gert). There are few, if any, goods that we can all agree on. There are, however, a small number of evils that all rational people would want to avoid (unless they had a reason not to—such as that it would avoid an even greater evil, or would benefit someone else). Death, pain, or loss of freedom, opportunity, and pleasure would be evils to be avoided. In short, a rational person does not want harm to himself or to others for whom he is concerned, and therefore the rules most likely to be advocated by all rational people are those which proscribe behavior harmful to others (ibid.).

It is clarifying to distinguish the dedication to and achievement of some good from the avoidance of evils. The former may comprise a "philosophy of life" or a "guide to living," but the latter seems to be what has been essential to ethics. What is one person's good might not be

another's, and it might be disastrous for the former to believe himself "morally obligated" to promote that good. Some "goods" or "values" that individuals have claimed (such as domination of others, racial purity, etc.) are downright immoral. They could not be labeled as immoral if morality simply meant acting in accord with one's own principles or promoting one's own values. Furthermore, if morality were "promoting good," we could not fulfill the criteria of being moral toward all people at all times equally. So we would, by definition, be "immoral" toward most people most of the time. At most we can only avoid causing evil to all people at all times equally.

This has not been an effort to defend a position, but only to describe vaguely an orientation, in hopes of helping the reader relate to, uncover problems in, or discount various points in, all that follows. The article's aim is to explore the nature of bioethics, to push and probe, to bring issues, angles, and possibilities to light. Basically, the strategy for accomplishing this will be to take a position and then subject it to challenges and counterchallenges. No winner will be declared, but at least most of the points will have been examined. Finally, some overall considerations and relationships will be elaborated.

A first approximation: medical ethics

The issues will be more manageable if we approach "bioethics" by first examining the more limited case of medical ethics. It is a particular instance of the same position that will be taken with respect to bioethics. The basic point can be made and questioned in this more limited arena, and then expanded to the sphere of bioethics. (It should be noted that the distinction between "moral" and "ethical" will not be rigorously adhered to in this article.)

Medical ethics is a special kind of ethics only insofar as it relates to a particular realm of facts and concerns and not because it embodies or appeals to some special moral principles or methodology. It is applied ethics. It consists of the same moral principles and rules that we would appeal to, and argue for, in ordinary circumstances. It is just that in medical ethics these familiar moral rules are being applied to situations peculiar to the medical world. We have only to scratch the surface of medical ethics and we break through to the issues of "standard" ethics as we have always known them. Of course, understanding the facts, distinctions, relationships, and concepts of the world of medicine in order to apply these "ordinary" moral rules is an immense task. But it is precisely that task which primarily comprises medical ethics.

"Do not kill" is a moral rule. It would not be this rule itself that would be challenged or justified within medical ethics. Nor would medical ethics as such be concerned with articulating and defending criteria for exceptions to the rule. Rather medical ethics prepares the ground for the constructions of ordinary ethics. Is withdrawing lifesaving therapy an instance of killing? Is the refusal to initiate a life-support system an instance of killing? Are we killing one when we give the limited lifesaving facilities to another instead? We are not questioning whether we should kill or not; we accept that "ordinary" moral rule. What we are questioning is whether, in these special and difficult situations, our action is appropriately labeled "killing." If we decided these were instances of killing, we would probably take the next step: deliberating whether they were justifiable exceptions to the moral rule, "Do not kill." In considering the nature of exceptions and their justification, we would in effect be back in "ordinary" ethics. But in examining the medical details for distinctions, relationships, implications, and the like in order to apply the criteria for exceptions, we would be doing medical ethics. That is, we are preparing the ground for the "application" of ethics.

We might see the same points with issues less weighty than that of killing. For example, "Do not deceive" is a moral rule of ordinary ethics (or so it might be argued). But what constitutes deceiving in the medical realm? This again calls for a careful understanding of what goes on in that realm and perhaps for subtle distinctions and conceptual analyses in order to determine when deceiving is really taking place. And, again, intimate knowledge of these particulars would be important in determining when exceptions to the rule are justified.

This clean distinction between ethics, on the one hand, and the world of medicine, on the other, smudges a bit upon closer inspection, though not enough to invalidate the basic point. Two factors are responsible for blurring the demarcation. First, in what has been called "preparing the ground" (i.e., classifying, drawing distinctions, sorting out causes and effects, uncovering implicit values in the medical realm) there may very well be an ethics-laden element. How one views ethics—its point, methods, justification, etc.—may influence how one prepares

the factual and conceptual ground to receive the moral rules. There could conceivably be a prejudice in arranging the data for moral deliberation—a familiar phenomenon whenever data and theory are wed.

Second, problems arise within medicine as a result of unusual capabilities and circumstances that were not in view as morality was forged. These in turn put pressure on ethics to answer questions for which it was not designed or to refashion itself in order to answer those questions. If refashioning occurred in the face of these special circumstances, would not the result be what is truly medical ethics and not simply ordinary ethics applied to special circumstances? Very likely, but it is not at all clear that such refashioning has been necessary. However, it is a possibility to which the reader should remain alert. The situation seems analogous to that of the implied rights and powers of the Constitution. Do these implications, having been drawn out and articulated to meet special circumstances, really comprise a new constitution, or are they simply applications of the "old" Constitution to new circumstances?

Challenges to this view of medical ethics

Before going on to expand the limited case of medical ethics to the more general instance of bioethics, there are questions that ought to be posed concerning the preceding view of medical ethics.

Proliferation of kinds of ethics. A sort of *reductio ad absurdum* might go like this: If every area where ethics is applied gets its own name, we will have a proliferation of "kinds" of ethics beyond compare. There will be "baker ethics," "banker ethics," "barber ethics," "bartender ethics," "bicycler ethics," and on and on.

But this does not seem to be a good argument against the view presented, simply because what purports to be *absurdum* is not so absurd after all. All the different realms of activity do in fact have ethical concerns. (Indeed, physicians frequently wonder why *they* are singled out for ethical emphasis instead of car mechanics and myriad others!) What sounds silly, of course, is that each would have its own name. That we do not in fact have separate names for the infinite variety of activities where ethics is applicable can be explained in other ways. Most of these activities are more easily understood, present few conceptual difficulties, do not encounter unique situations that strain ordinary ethics, and are not intimately and deeply involved with human life, death, and well-being. Hence they are not highlighted with names of their own. Notice that some instances of naming ethics for particular areas of concern do not strike us as odd at all: "environmental ethics," "business ethics," "legal ethics," "political ethics." The labels both express and reinforce any focus on concerns that hold for us considerable importance, interest, and complexity.

Actually the *reductio ad absurdum* could be turned on the very position it purports to be defending, namely, that medical ethics is a special kind of ethics, with its own principles, rules, and methods. By extension this might suggest that every area of concern and activity has its own ethical principles—butcher, baker, candlestick maker, and everybody else. This would make a farce of ethics, which at the very least should be the same for all of us.

Why should ethics not change?   Another critical challenge to the position taken on medical ethics could be stated this way: If new knowledge is so rapidly increasing in medicine (and other fields) how can the ethics *not* change? We now understand matters differently and different situations obtain, so why shouldn't the ethics change?

To respond to this question requires that a distinction be drawn between basic and derived moral rules (Gert, p. 67). Basic moral rules would not be culturally relative; they would be those we would find applicable to all persons at all times and places. (It is not being argued here that there are such, but only that such a distinction is clarifying.) These basic moral rules would have to be general in not referring to particular beliefs, practices, or institutions. For example, "Do not be unfaithful to your spouse" would not be a basic rule, since it counts on the institution of marriage, which may not be a universal phenomenon. However, "Do not cheat" might well be a basic moral rule, independent of particular cultures and its institutions. What actions constitute cheating in a culture will depend upon the beliefs, expectations, and institutions of that culture. What remains universal is "Do not cheat"; what actions are seen as cheating will, of course, vary with understandings, practices, and contexts.

A derived moral rule would be one that was implied by a basic moral rule in conjunction with a particular practice or institution. Thus, "Do not cheat" plus the institution of marriage may yield a derived moral rule such as, "Do not be unfaithful to your spouse." Similarly, "Do not

kill" (or "Do not cause pain," or some such) plus the existence of cars and highways may elicit the derived moral rule, "Do not drive while drunk." This could not be a basic moral rule because cars and, perhaps, intoxicating beverages did not exist in every place and time.

The relevance of this for medical ethics is that new knowledge and practices may indeed yield new *derived* moral rules (what some may call "middle principles"), though not necessarily new *basic* moral rules. Suppose that the essence of the basic moral rules were that they proscribed causing harm. What constitutes harm and what procedures and substances are seen as causing harm may change from one discovery to another, so that what one is specifically admonished not to do may vary, though the basic rule "Do no harm" remains unchanged. We now avoid giving extra oxygen to neonates, because we have discovered the bad consequences; we are now beginning to question the advice not to impose discipline on children, because of the results. In all cases the goal remains the same, namely, to avoid causing harm; only our view of the means to that end has changed. ("Avoiding harm" is used throughout this article to suggest the general focus of the ethical theory assumed herein. But it is only very roughly accurate; it is neither necessary nor sufficient for an act's morality.)

The point of Van Rensselaer Potter's *Bioethics* can best be seen within the context of derived rules. Potter's 1971 book must have made one of the first uses of the term "bioethics," making comment on it here appropriate. His use of the term is entirely different from this article's position, though the thesis of his book is quite consistent with what is said here. For him, bioethics is the enterprise of utilizing the biological sciences for improving the quality of life. It also helps us formulate our goals by helping us better understand the nature of man and the world. It is the "science for survival"; it helps write prescriptions for "happy and productive lives" (Potter).

It seems odd to call applied science "ethics." Much of science has been used to advise us on improving the quality of life, but we have not been tempted to call it "ethics." Such science is seen as a means to an end, and both means and ends might be subject to moral appraisal. In the terms of this article, science does help with the formulation of *derived* moral rules. That is, given that we already have general moral rules proscribing harm to one another, science may help fill in that list of actions which will in fact lead to harm.

But Potter also says that we can use science to formulate our goals by better understanding the nature of man and the world. What can this mean? Again, it really seems to be dealing with means. The biosciences might tell us what some or even all persons in fact find deeply satisfying, or that nuclear pollution can cause cancer. But it still does not tell us whether we are obligated to promote another's satisfaction, or have a right to our own satisfaction, or whether the benefits of nuclear power outweigh its lethal detriment. In short, it seems odd to call such an enterprise "ethics," though this in no way demeans the great importance of scientific knowledge for carrying out our purposes and achieving fulfillment.

Traditional meaning of medical ethics.   The last challenge is an appeal to what has been traditionally meant by "medical ethics." This has included an extensive range of admonitions varying with culture, time, and type of medicine, and dealing with demeanor, rebates for referrals, decorum in consultations, soliciting another's patient, rumor mongering about other doctors, advertising, and endless other behavioral possibilities within medicine. There is no denying that this is largely what has been known in the past as "medical ethics." But does this traditional view of medical ethics invalidate the view of medical ethics taken in this article? The answer is probably that it partly does and partly does not. That is, traditional medical ethics is such a conglomeration of things that some aspects fall in nicely with the view espoused here, and some do not. But staking claim to the term "medical ethics" is not the goal; understanding is. What follows is an attempt to sort out several strands within traditional medical ethics and to put them in perspective from an ethical point of view. The upshot will be that one strand supports the espoused view, another is consistent with it, and a third is irrelevant to it.

The strand that confirms the view expressed here is that which is attentive to the harm that can be done others. Urging the physicians to keep confidences, to comfort patients when therapy is no longer effective, and not to insult one another might be seen as a translation of general morality into the medical context. These, and many such rules, can be seen as tailoring the general rules of morality, which are binding on us all, to specific situations within medicine. The object, as in general morality, is (very

roughly) to avoid causing harm to individuals and to the community at large (e.g., by a general breakdown of trust).

Consistent with the stated view is that strand which announces what the physician's "duty" is; such as, "Consider the well-being of the patient above all else," or "Do not have sex with patients," or even those imperatives guiding referrals or pharmaceutical rebates. A strong case could be made for the rule "Do your duty" as being a basic moral rule, which as such would hold for all people in all times and places (Gert, pp. 121–125). Of course the duties themselves of different people in their various roles (as mother, as neighbor, as airline pilot, as lawyer, etc.) vary immensely, but what remains the same is the responsibility for doing your duty, whatever it is (so long as it is consistent with the other moral rules). In essence the justification for such a rule is that we all, by arbitrary decision or tradition, come to count on each other's doing his duty. We organize our lives around this expectation. Failure to fulfill one's role causes harm to all who had depended on its being performed. So it is a rule that we all would endorse and urge others to follow, inasmuch as noncompliance hurts us all. Again, what the specific duties are is by no means universal; they could easily vary from one community to another. But whatever they are, we all urge that they be done, because it is important for our functioning that we be able to depend on their performance.

A great deal of medical ethics can be seen as an effort to decide and make explicit what these duties are or should be for physicians. Of course, there is nothing universal about the particulars arrived at, and they fluctuate according to different society structures, differing views of medicine, health, and cure, and different capabilities. The important thing is that they be explicit so that society knows what to expect and that they be consistent with the other moral rules. Indeed, many of the delineated duties are best seen simply as rational social arrangements. However lofty and solemn they may sound, they are at bottom a spelling out of "promises," shaped by abilities, needs, traditions, and expectations. They could be quite other than they are and still be good, so long as they made explicit what could be expected by patients. This interpretation fits nicely with our tendency to refer to these matters as medical "etiquette" rather than "morals." That tendency bespeaks our realization that these matters are of a different order from morality. Yet, as these last two paragraphs have attempted to show, these "social arrangements" are the spelling out of something that is itself a basic moral rule, namely, "Do your duty."

The third strand distinguishable in codes of medical ethics seems not to be concerned with ethics, according to the position taken in this article. The strictures, "Keep heads clear and hands steady," "Be humble," and "Give respect and gratitude to teachers" sound like tactical advice. Rather than admonishing one not to cause this or that kind of harm, these sayings are recommending how one's life might be enriched and how one might even promote happiness in others. In the ethical view assumed (rightly or wrongly) in this article, these statements are more a "guide to life" than morality; but it is important to observe that other views of ethics might regard them as pertaining to the essence of morality.

In this category one might also place those admonitions that are really self-serving—which protect the physician and his guild and which promote medicine as a profession. These elements are best regarded as strategical advice. Examples are here being avoided because they are individually open to a variety of interpretations, and this is not the place to argue for one or another interpretation, but only to establish this classification. An instance would be the restriction against advertising: Though it seems primarily self-serving, a case might be made for its protecting the public.

Because "medical ethics" has meant such a variety of things, and because our ethical concerns with medicine often lead us beyond issues of medicine narrowly defined, another term might be useful. "Bioethics" is a good candidate. This term offers the advantage (1) of suggesting a much wider concern than simply rules of behavior for a particular guild, and (2) of connoting more broadly both the ethics and the science–technology out of which the issues grow.

Bioethics

The plan has been to examine medical ethics prior to dealing with "bioethics." One reason for this approach was that the same stance would be taken with respect to both, namely, that both are instances of ordinary morality applied to new areas of concern. Another reason was the expectation that, if medical ethics is understood as a more particularized case of ethical concern, the expansion to the more general case of bioethics will be easier. Furthermore, the variables unique to each are thereby kept separate, facilitating clarity.

The proposition that "medical ethics" is basically just ordinary ethics applied to the realm of medicine may be vague, but is not very surprising. On the other hand, it may seem more surprising to say that bioethics is just ordinary ethics applied to the "bio-realm," yet that is what will be held, if only to force the relevant issues into the open.

"Bio-realm" obviously designates a much more inclusive universe of concerns than does "medical realm." The impetus for ethical reflection in areas connected with the biological sciences seems to have been biology's startling capabilities both actual and projected, and the consequent implications for humankind. Though capabilities in the physical sciences and in technology have had similar disconcerting implications and have generated some ethical and societal reflections, it seems to have been recent biomedical developments that have precipitated the major ethical concerns which we group under "bioethics." The ripeness of the times for moral sensitivities was no doubt a contributing factor; civil rights, environmental issues, and population problems were high in the general consciousness. In any case, "bioethics" became the focal point, and subsequently many science-technology-society issues became its concern. This has resulted in a conglomeration that almost defies characterization. The field is more likely defined de facto in terms of its issues than by any shared essence or scientific perspective. (It should be noted that there is an issue of values-in-science that is not being raised in this article. It concerns whether and how value judgments encroach on science, influencing—according to some—the problem selection, observation, reasoning processes, and drawing of conclusions. These values are as frequently aesthetic, political, and social as ethical, and the matter has a literature of its own that predates the recent emphasis on bioethics.)

Assuming that bioethics is just ordinary ethics applied to a specialized area of concern, it becomes a matter of interest to determine whether problems arise in this special area that *in principle* are not amenable to traditional ethics. Whether or not they do cannot be settled here, but identifying and examining the pressures and tensions can be instructive. What is at issue is whether this new field of bioethics will have to develop new ethical principles (not just "derived rules" as discussed earlier) in order to deal with the problems confronting it. What follows should be seen as challenges to traditional ethics, brought on by new developments in the biological sciences. Their success as challenges will not be decided here, inasmuch as that would require a depth study of traditional ethics far beyond the scope of this article. Furthermore, the challenges themselves are too new to have their full complications and implications drawn and assessed. Nevertheless, what follows should elicit some underlying issues and suggest to the reader still other possible challenges.

Concerning what is "naturally given." The basic point of this challenge can be quickly seen, though it is not at all clear that it can be sustained under careful scrutiny. It is this: The "naturally given" seems, rightly or wrongly, to influence moral considerations, generally by constituting the inviolable starting point, the point of departure for ethical deliberations. Now, if we are able to tamper biologically with the very framework within which ethical deliberations make sense, then it would seem that more basic ethical principles must be formulated to guide us in how and what may be tampered with. But this point needs considerable elaboration. It is helpful to look at this from the perspectives of individual ethics and social ethics.

Individual ethics. In individual ethics, when two people encounter each other, the "natural" makeup of each constitutes the given, the point of departure for moral behavior. The preferences, aversions, anger, temperament, etc., of each must be worked with and around by the other. These characteristics constitute the inviolable sphere of the self and the zone of privacy, and, in effect, litigation takes place among these givens. Each person tries not to harm the other unduly, given the other's temperament, aversions, and such characteristics. But what if these personal characteristics could be changed, either before birth, during childhood, or now? What if we could cause a person to have less of a · temper or preferences that would coincide with ours? As it is now, we start with complete persons as given—as completed units that barter, bargain, give and take, fashioning a symbiotic relationship that may restrain or require certain behavior but leaves the basic units or persons intact. However, with new capabilities we could perhaps alter "that" person before we even encounter him as a person.

What would guide our decision as to whether and how we would change this other? Currently, we are guided by rationality, that is, by those principles of behavior we can both agree on, being willing to follow them and have them followed with respect to us. But what criteria could we use if we were involved in changing the very makeup of the other? One answer might be: only with the consent of the other. If so, there is no challenge to standard ethics. Once again it is treating the whole person that confronts us as a given; it is not really altering that given until *after* the encounter, and then with that person's permission.

Changing a person without his consent is certainly wrong, and ordinary ethics would find it so. But we can make our problem tougher by casting doubt on the quality of consent (that the "consenter" is not really informed, that he is not in the right frame of mind, etc.). That is, reasons can of course be found for doing something against someone's expressed desire whether the act would be clearly a harm or a benefit. But even this does not necessarily force us beyond the ken of ordinary ethics, inasmuch as it is similar to problems we have had all along.

Tampering with personality characteristics prior to birth may push the problem further. There would be no ethical difficulty correcting a physical defect known to be painful or disabling to the eventual person. But what would justify changing—or refusing to change—the emotions, attitudes, or capabilities of the eventual person? The issue is no longer one of simply avoiding the causing of evil (a principle we would expect all rational beings to advocate) or even one of preventing evil. Rather this has to do with creating a good, and hence it is beyond the scope of ethics (as assumed in this article), which is essentially an avoidance of evils. Here we would not just be avoiding the causing of an evil to some given; we would be *creating* the given. Whereas we might expect universal agreement on what evils to proscribe, rational persons can and do differ widely on what things are good. Hence the problem: What criteria could be appealed to in the cases of whether and how to tamper with the endowments of eventual persons? On an individual basis there seem to be no guidelines and no possibility of there ever being any. It seems that guidelines could be framed only in terms of social goals. So the temptation would be to allow the "natural lottery" to continue; the randomness seems more fair in the absence of universal agreement on what would constitute a good person.

There may be promise of finding relevant

ethical guidelines embedded in our raising children, which is, in a sense, creating the eventual person. Yet raising children is also largely fashioned by social goals rather than by ethical imperatives. That is, in molding children we go far beyond merely what morality requires. Furthermore, in raising children as distinguished from juggling genes, it is generally assumed that our influence is not irreversible. If so, this would be a morally significant difference between the two.

Social ethics. New capabilities of altering what is "naturally given" might raise problems in the area of social ethics as well. The matter of just distribution may come up in a way it never has before. Perhaps society will no longer be willing to rely on the "natural lottery" of talents, dispositions, capabilities, etc., if these variables could be "evened" up before birth. It might be argued that justice would require an equal distribution of talent if that should become possible. Is some new principle of justice required? Or would it simply call for a decision as to the general social desirability of having so many similar and equal characteristics and talents? Yet, if these characteristics make a difference in the advantages one has in society, justice may well require us to make the characteristics equal. (Of course, the most likely solution would be not to make them all alike, but to stop allowing these characteristics to make a difference in one's obtaining rewards and status in society!)

It may be that this problem is no different from any other problem of justice. That is, we have believed justice required an evening up of talents and opportunities, insofar as this is possible with special training. Perhaps there is no difference in principle between balancing the disparities before and after birth. This does not make figuring the moral policy any easier, but it would indicate that it was the same old problem we have always had, and not something peculiar to new technological capabilities.

However, there are slight differences between the tampering before birth and the compensating endeavors after birth, and perhaps someone could argue that the differences are morally relevant. Before birth the mutation of talents, dispositions, and abilities is "artificial," that is, it is induced. After birth it takes some effort of that person to overcome his shortcomings; opportunity would be equal, but results would vary with the effort put forth, which seems intuitively fairer than "magically" making them all equal *in utero.*

Another difference between the two cases which might be seen as morally relevant is the matter of consent. Initiating change after birth at least might have some form of consent from the person himself or from his duly determined proxy.

Similarly some might see a morally relevant difference in the implicit employment of a standard or norm in the case following birth. Justice has seemed to require that corrective help be available to those who fall short in mental, physical, or dispositional ability. But to do this, what is "normal" in each category must be established. Then the obligation is to bring them up to normal, though there seems to be no obligation to help the already normal to rise above normal (or, at least, the below normal seem to have priority on the resources for improvement). Presumably, with the before-birth case, the magical equalizing injections would maximize each attribute rather than recognize norms. But it is not clear how this could be seen as a morally relevant difference of the before-birth case, such that it presents a challenge different in kind from the case following birth. There may be a question as to whether justice requires equal magical potions (and consequently unequal results) or unequal potions (in order to obtain equal results). But that is a frequent dilemma of justice. Furthermore, the postpartum case is probably *more* difficult, since it involves priorities (e.g., Which should be first, the neediest or the most promising?).

Perhaps the issue of distribution deserves further comment. Does the "new biology" (recent biomedical discoveries and technology, current and envisioned) in any sense challenge the "old" concepts of justice such that new basic principles must be articulated? This might be thought to be so in the case of our current practices of awarding certain benefits according to accomplishments and abilities. If those accomplishments and abilities which justified the awards were *themselves* induced by biologic tampering, then by what criteria would we determine who was to receive the benefits of biologic tampering? In short, if we can "artificially" create those merits in virtue of which certain benefits are bestowed, then how do we decide who should receive this merit-making magic (Shapiro)?

Yet it is not clear that this is different in principle from the ordinary problems of distributive justice. Education and training given to everyone equally have become the basis for subsequent rewards. Of course, it might be argued that natural ability and effort are what is being rewarded. But even in the case of biologic tampering, effort would be relevant. So in any case it is not obvious that the "new biology" presses on us any problem of just distribution that we have not had in principle all along. Whether to award goods on the basis of effort, worth, need, or desert continues to be a basic question. These operate within the context of social ideology, which no doubt helps determine what gets emphasized. And if biotechnology enabled us to make everyone the same in all admirable respects (courage, ability, endurance, etc.) it would be arguments from boredom or versatility in evolution or some such social ideal that would lead us to distribute the goods differently.

The scope of morality.   Another conceivable challenge might be voiced: Do the new developments in biological knowledge and technology expose as inadequate the compass of traditional ethics? Specifically, can traditional ethics handle obligations and rights in borderline cases (fetuses, the severely retarded, the totally senile) or among those living things normally outside the sphere of morality (animals, plants, streams)? The thrust of the challenge is that because of increased knowledge new capabilities and the resultant heightened sensitivities, we now see that rights must exist where traditional ethics had never envisioned them.

This cannot be done with the precision one would like. The concept of rights is a huge area. Furthermore, the variety of views on rights is compatible with a variety of ethical theories. But what can be done here is to sketch the general kind of reflection that might be stimulated by "the new biology" with respect to the inadequacy of the "old morality," and then to sketch a reply, arguing that no changes are necessitated, provided we understand rights in a certain way.

There has been a general raising of consciousness concerning the world around us. The intimate interrelationship of humankind with the environment, the interdependence of all living things, and the cumulative effect of any disruption of this balance are matters keenly impressed on us of late. Much of this results from the explosion of knowledge, particularly in the biological fields. It coincides as well with social and political movements that direct attention to environment, conservation, and appropriate lifestyles. The upshot has been pressure to reconsider the scope of moral rights and obligations, specifically whether they should be extended to include plants and animals. It is not enough,

the argument goes, to have laws protecting trees and animals from various abuses; rather, we must think of them as having rights of their own, because this alone will give the necessary edge to their defenses, shifting the burden of proof to the proper contestant. With the prima facie right to noninterference anchored firmly in the living thing itself, the challenger would have to show why he should be allowed to harm it, rather than the "defendant's" having to show why not. In short, we would assume that one could not infringe on a tree or an animal without producing adequate reasons, instead of our assuming that these things may be freely infringed upon unless there are adequate reasons to the contrary.

Sensitivity to the plight of animals is not new, but there is a recent surge of concern that appears to be part of the general bioethics movement. Perhaps it is the great empathy for the voiceless oppressed (fetuses and minorities), perhaps it is increased awareness of all suffering, or perhaps it is the scientific eroding of essential differences between man and some animals, but whatever it is, it is being expressed in an effort to include animals within the moral realm (Regan and Singer).

The move to protect the environment is well known. What is not so well known is the possibility and need that elements of the environment have basic rights. One author argues thoroughly and convincingly that natural objects (such as trees and streams) have rights to life and health (Stone). Without the "discovery" of such rights, the abuse of these natural objects can be stopped only if detrimental effects to a human's health or livelihood can be shown. However, if a natural object's right to life and health were acknowledged, evidence of possible harm simply to it would suffice for enjoining the abuse. Stone argues that no amount of rules or laws protecting the object in question are ever equivalent to acknowledging *the right* of that object to health and life. The right has connotations, force, and presumption never embodied completely in a set of rules.

The preceding considerations, though only roughly sketched, may represent a thrust that will significantly alter traditional ethics in scope, if not in substance. These basic intuitions appear to put a stress on the framework of ethics which may force a change whereby bioethics will be essentially different from ethics. However, there are other ways of understanding the matter that, if correct, would obviate the need for basic revision. What follows is one such possibility. Like all else in this article, it is not a detailed argument, though it is a hint of one. Its role here is to suggest that the situation does not necessarily require a new ethics but that the old, adequately understood, can apply to the developing new circumstances.

The suggestion to be made could be called the concept of "bestowed rights." It builds on what is taken to be the purpose of morality, which in turn establishes the scope of morality. If an essential characteristic of a rational person is that he will avoid harm to himself (unless he has a reason not to), then we would expect that the community of rational persons would work to articulate and advocate a morality. That is, they would attempt to formulate rules and procedures to which they could all subscribe in order to settle their differences and otherwise avoid a life that would be "poor, nasty, brutish and short." Thus the rational person's instigating incentive for formulating and advocating moral rules is the avoiding of harm to himself and to others he cares about. As such, morality is a kind of agreement for mutual benefit, and rationality (avoiding of harm to oneself) is the foundation (Gert). Rationality may not compel one to be moral, but it would compel one to urge that *others* be moral. Furthermore, many things and ideas might motivate one to be moral, other than simply avoiding harm to oneself. It is just that avoidance of harm is the one motivation we can count on all rational persons sharing. This motivation has a purchase on those who can be responsible for their actions and who can realize that they are able to harm others and that others can harm them. All others unable to be gripped by this sanction are outside the community of moral agents.

This however does not mean that all others—the senile, the severely retarded, infants, fetuses, the insane—are without rights, but it does mean that the source of their rights is quite different. This is where the "bestowed right" becomes relevant. Those excluded from the moral community by virtue of their inability to act and plan responsibly and their inability to appreciate the force of the sanction at the base of morality are still significant members of society. The moral community has an interest in protecting them: We ourselves might one day be in their position; we may have an emotional attachment to them; many of us have a "natural sympathy" with all forms of life; we could all become brutalized and consequently suffer if we failed to respect these

other lives. Therefore, rights are bestowed on beings outside the community of moral agents. These are extremely important rights, though their foundation is different from those within (Clouser, 1976; Green). This interpretation seems to be more realistic with respect to where *in fact* the sanctions lie and would help arguments for and against rights to focus on the appropriate grounds.

Fetuses, animals, and trees cannot act responsibly or express their interests and desires, nor can they threaten us with retaliation. There is no basis for them to "claim" rights. On the other hand, it would be terribly shortsighted of us not to ascribe rights to them, or bestow rights on them, to avoid long-range harm to ourselves. When neither their interest, nor desire, nor consent can be solicited, what other argument (other than the long-range good of humankind) could ultimately be made for infringing on what would be a basic right of any of these nonrational beings? The point is that no matter what we postulate as to the "basic rights" of these nonrational beings, our ultimate criterion for honoring the rights will be in terms of the long-range good of humankind.

The point of all this has not been the argument itself, but rather to show that bioethics is not necessarily a new ethics: It might still be seen as the old ethics being applied to new circumstances.

Other possible challenges. The matter of obligations to future generations is almost always included in any listing of bioethical issues, and yet it is not clearly a new issue. It is in fact a good example of what is probably the heart of bioethics, namely, an old issue that is exacerbated by new discoveries. For a long time we have been able to affect subsequent generations, but only recently have we been able to do it and realize it so vividly. So it is not new and different in principle, though its resolution may be more urgent. All attempts to deal with it have been attempts to draw out the implications of traditional morality, for example, by pointing out that the nature of obligation is always future oriented, or that the nature of a rule is timeless, or that from a moral perspective (whether that of the "ideal observer," the "rational man," or those "behind the veil of ignorance") all persons who are or ever will be must be regarded as contemporaneous.

In short, bioethics would seem to be the response of traditional ethics to particular stresses and urgencies that have emerged by virtue of new discoveries and technology. Ethics is pressed, not to find new principles or foundations, but to squeeze out all the relevant implications from the ones it already has. This, of course, does not solve every problem nor even necessarily narrow down the options significantly. Even after the ethical criteria are met, many alternatives may remain, thus requiring criteria other than morality for settling on a single line of action (Clouser, 1975).

This general theme is encountered time and again. The hackneyed example of the respirator, or of any life-extending apparatus, makes the same point. With new technology we are forced to make certain decisions with a regularity and urgency we had not faced before. This does not call for new ethical principles, but new applications of the old. Our concern for not harming a person and for honoring his wishes remains the same; we ponder only how to express it in these particular circumstances.

A similar case is the prevalent matter of behavior control. We have always been able to control some behavior, but new techniques make such control easier, quicker, and more certain, and have made moral clarity on the issue immensely more urgent. Again, the basic admonition not to interfere with a person's freedom without his consent still stands. But the new circumstances and capabilities drive us to more precision on what constitutes freedom, autonomy, and consent, in order to apply the basic rule. Sometimes it is clear that interference with freedom leads to even greater freedom (e.g., compulsory education); sometimes it is not clear whether meaningful consent is being given (e.g., Does the person *really* know the consequences and alternatives?); sometimes it is not clear whether the "real" self is speaking (e.g., the person before or after the mood-elevator, the shock treatment, or the hemodialysis). Furthermore, much of the concern (as is fairly typical of bioethical issues) has not been over *whether* to restrict the use of these new technologies, but *how*. That is, it is often clear when it is moral and when it is immoral to use these techniques of behavior control, but the problem comes in formulating a general policy that can make and incorporate the distinctions and subtleties necessary to capitalize on the worthy uses without risking the misuses.

Bioethics, science, and public policy

The position taken in this article has been that the revelations and capabilities mediated by science create an urgency for moral guidance but do not require a new morality, revised in its basic principles. What is required is analysis of the new circumstances and their pivotal concepts, so that the applications and implications of the "old" morality might be clearly seen. Additionally, ethics itself may be pressed to yield clarity and distinctions it had not heretofore manifested. But it would be odd to call this a "new" morality. We are more likely to see it as a further uncovering, exploration, and articulation of the old, simply because we think of morality as applying to all persons at all places and times. Morality is not invented or legislated; at most it is "discovered," that is, it is an unpacking, explication, and articulation of our deepest intuitions about what we ought and ought not to do. Of course new "derived rules" (as explained earlier) will emerge, as certain lines of action are discovered to lead to certain results that conflict with basic moral rules. It is in this role that the empirical sciences become very important. Spelling out the cause-and-effect relationships makes clearer where restraints should be imposed, so as to be in accord with the basic moral rules. The facts of sociology, biology, psychology, medicine, and other sciences are crucial in determining the outcome of various acts and policies, apart from which their morality generally cannot be judged. Analyses of pivotal concepts within these sciences (whether done by philosophers or scientists) are also crucial in determining morality: Has a person's "freedom" in fact been curtailed? Is he appropriately labeled "sick"? Was he acting "freely"? Can he really be said to have been "deceived"? And with this kind of conceptual analysis and figuring of consequences lies most of the work of bioethics. The remainder lies with probing the foundations of ethics for implications that relate more exactly to the novel predicaments characteristic of "the new biology."

Bioethics appears to have no essence that would mark it off. Rather it seems to be individuated by a de facto list of issues, extended and interrelated by "family resemblances." The initial set of dilemmas was no doubt introduced by biological discoveries, real and foretold. But we gradually became familiar with a wider list of issues: genetic engineering (cloning, in vitro fertilization, eugenics, etc.), allocation of limited health resources, obligations to future generations, environmental health and pollution, population control, abortion, euthanasia, behavior control (behavior modification, drugs, psychosurgery), human experimentation, organ transplantation, etc. By no means were all these forced on us by new discoveries; most have been around for a long time. Historical and sociological factors in addition to the moral urgency of new knowledge and capabilities contributed greatly to the coagulation of issues distinguishing itself from ordinary ethics. The result has been a considerable focusing on a set of issues, marked by urgency and importance.

Consequently, a common thread joining all the issues is hard to find. Invariably an article or book dealing with bioethics will mention quickly the "new biology" and the "new technology," and then immediately cite examples, namely, an enumeration of those issues which simply as a matter of fact are labeled "bioethics." Yet the conglomeration is not completely haphazard: Business ethics is not included, nor is economic ethics, nor diplomatic ethics. On the other hand, it is difficult to articulate a common essence that unifies the conglomerate. The core and impetus of the de facto list was no doubt concern over the technology of control of man's body, mind, and quality of life. The more such dramatic possibilities were highlighted and the more we became attuned to the issues, we began seeing similar, albeit less dramatic, instances all around us: Not only does the psychosurgeon alter our person, but so do parents, educators, and social systems; not only does the neonatologist determine quality of life, but so does the Highway Commission. Until we saw the grosser possibilities we were not sensitive to the subtler forces already at work. And thus the list grew. Perhaps an original criterion was that the issue have an obvious biological component, which affects coming into or going out of life, the nature of a person, or the quality of life. This of course directly or indirectly included almost everything. And so it must, to extend from the economics of feeding the world to paternalism in the doctor–patient relationship, from cultural determinations of illness and death to a tree's claim of a right to life! Adding to this the relevant data from law, sociology, psychology, biology, philosophy, theology, and other fields results in a vast network of issues categorized roughly as "bioethics." The aim of it all should not be lost in the vastness: to decide how humankind ought to act in the biomedical realm affecting birth, death, human nature, and the quality of life.

In this context, and as a concluding observation, the matter of public policy should be put in perspective. Much of what is compressed under the umbrella of "bioethics" is really concerned with public policy—that is, with the legislation, policies, and guidelines that should be enacted with respect to all these issues. It is helpful to see this as distinct from ethics per se. Though many views of ethics exist (and this is not the place to thrash out the differences) the assumption of this article has been, very roughly, that ethics concerns those prohibitions all rational persons would urge everyone to obey in an effort to avoid those evils on which they all agree. Specifically, disregarding these prohibitions in order to "promote good" would be regarded as immoral (unless, of course, they met criteria for justifiable exceptions).

However, on a societal level the matter is different. It is not a matter of one individual's deciding on his own how to treat another. Rather, if there is a democratically arrived at consensus that a certain good must be promoted (say, education or welfare), though it means causing some harm (taxation and some loss of freedom), it is morally acceptable. It is at this level that much of what is called "bioethics" is taking place. Whereas individual morality is primarily a system of restraints, society-wide policy is on a level where promotion of goods is a moral option. Here the question becomes "What goods ought to be promoted?" or, contrariwise, "Which goods ought to be restrained (e.g., scientific research)?" Priorities, values, and goods are at center stage, where they must be weighed, balanced, and compared. The sciences and humanities are highly relevant in analyzing and prognosticating and in otherwise assisting a pluralistic society to settle on goods to be promoted. This level and direction of discussion accounts for a large portion of what comes to be called "bioethics," although, on the ethical theory assumed in this article, it is not really ethics so much as value theory and political theory.

But there is a still higher level at which significant bioethical analysis is done. When a society promotes various goods, inevitably some moral rules are broken with respect to some individuals (depriving them of something, a sacrifice necessary to support the "common good"). Which rules are broken with respect to whom becomes an important consideration in determining the justifiability of the goals or goods fixed upon. This determination is the jurisdiction of justice, the ethics pertaining to the societal level. And insofar as this has to do with the distribution of benefits and burdens relating to biomedical issues, it is a crucial part of bio-ethics.

K. DANNER CLOUSER

[*Directly related are the entries* ACTING AND RE-FRAINING; ETHICS; FUTURE GENERATIONS, OBLI-GATIONS TO; HEALTH CARE; JUSTICE; LIFE; MEDI-CAL PROFESSION; RATIONING OF MEDICAL TREAT-MENT; *and* SCIENCE: ETHICAL IMPLICATIONS. *See also:* ANIMAL EXPERIMENTATION; BEHAVIOR CON-TROL; DEATH AND DYING: EUTHANASIA AND SUS-TAINING LIFE; ENVIRONMENTAL ETHICS; GENETIC CONSTITUTION AND ENVIRONMENTAL CONDITION-ING; INFORMED CONSENT IN HUMAN RESEARCH; INFORMED CONSENT IN THE THERAPEUTIC RELA-TIONSHIP; POPULATION ETHICS: ELEMENTS OF THE FIELD; *and* PSYCHOSURGERY.]

BIBLIOGRAPHY

BLACKSTONE, WILLIAM T., ed. *Philosophy and Environ-mental Crisis*. Athens: University of Georgia Press, 1971.
BROADIE, ALEXANDER, and PYBUS, ELIZABETH M. "Kant's Treatment of Animals." *Philosophy* 49 (1974): 375–382.
CALLAHAN, DANIEL. "Bioethics as a Discipline." *The Hastings Center Studies* 1, no. 1 (1973), pp. 66–73.
CLOUSER, K. DANNER. "Bioethics: Some Reflections and Exhortations." *Monist* 60, no. 1 (1977), pp. 47–61. This issue is devoted to bioethics.
————. "Medical Ethics: Some Uses, Abuses and Limi-tations." *New England Journal of Medicine* 293 (1975): 384–387.
————. "Some Things Medical Ethics Is Not." *Journal of the American Medical Association* 223 (1973): 787–789.
————. "What Is Medical Ethics?" *Annals of Internal Medicine* 80 (1974): 657–660.
FEINBERG, JOEL. "The Rights of Animals and Unborn Generations." Blackstone, *Philosophy and Environ-mental Crisis*, pp. 43–68.
FOX, RENÉE C. "Ethical and Existential Developments in Contemporaneous American Medicine: Their Im-plications for Culture and Society." *Milbank Memo-rial Fund Quarterly* 52 (1974): 445–483. Bibliog-raphy.
GERT, BERNARD. *The Moral Rules: A New Rational Foundation for Morality*. New York: Harper & Row, 1970.
GREEN, RONALD M. "Conferred Rights and the Fetus." *Journal of Religious Ethics* 2, no. 1 (1974), pp. 55–75.
HARDIN, GARRETT; STORR, ANTHONY; LEISS, WILLIAM; and SHEPARD, PAUL. "Rights: Human and Nonhu-man." *The North American Review*, Winter 1974, pp. 14–42. A collection of papers.
KASS, LEON R. "The New Biology: What Price Relieving Man's Estate?" *Science* 174 (1971): 779–788.
KING, LESTER SNOW. "Development of Medical Ethics." *New England Journal of Medicine* 258 (1958): 480–486.
PASSMORE, JOHN. "The Treatment of Animals." *Journal of the History of Ideas* 36 (1975): 195–218.

POTTER, VAN RENSSELAER. *Bioethics: Bridge to the Fu-ture*. Prentice-Hall Biological Science Series. Edited by Carl P. Swanson. Englewood Cliffs, N.J.: 1971.
REGAN, TOM, and SINGER, PETER, eds. *Animal Rights and Human Obligations*. Englewood Cliffs, N.J.: Prentice-Hall, 1976.
SHAPIRO, MICHAEL H. "Who Merits Merit? Problems in Distributive Justice and Utility Posed by the New Biology." *Southern California Law Review* 48 (1974): 318–370.
SINGER, PETER. *Animal Liberation: A New Ethics for Our Treatment of Animals*. New York: New York Review, Random House, 1975.
STONE, CHRISTOPHER D. "Should Trees Have Standing? —Toward Legal Rights for Natural Objects." *South-ern California Law Review* 45 (1972): 450–501.
VEATCH, ROBERT M. "Medical Ethics: Professional or Universal?" *Harvard Theological Review* 65 (1972): 531–559.

BIOETHICS AS A DISCIPLINE

See MEDICAL ETHICS, HISTORY OF, *section on* EUROPE AND THE AMERICAS, *the six articles on* CONTEMPORARY PERIOD: THE TWENTIETH CEN-TURY, *especially the article on* NORTH AMERICA IN THE TWENTIETH CENTURY. *See also* MEDICAL ETHICS EDUCATION; *and* BIOETHICS.

BIOHAZARDS

See RISK; RESEARCH POLICY, BIOMEDICAL; GENETICS AND THE LAW; TECHNOLOGY, *article on* TECHNOLOGY AND THE LAW.

BIOLOGICAL WARFARE

See WARFARE, *article on* BIOMEDICAL SCIENCE AND WAR.

BIOLOGY, PHILOSOPHY OF

The philosophy of biology refers to the sys-tematic investigation of biology from the stand-point of its fundamental assumptions, proposi-tions, and theories as well as its methodology. In its wider sense the philosophy of biology includes issues related to speculative metaphysics (e.g., the philosophy of Henri Bergson), evolutionary ethics (as initially proposed by Darwin in *The Descent of Man*), and biologically founded social philosophy (e.g., "the self-reproducing society" of Julian Huxley). Within the narrower sense of the term, the philosophy of biology concerns it-self with the logical status of biological theory—in particular with the issue of the reduction of such theory to that of physics and chemistry. This article will concern itself first with the more limited view of the philosophy of biology insofar as it bears on the ethics of the life sciences, medicine, and health care.

The problem of reduction

The question of whether or not biology can be reduced to physics can be viewed in several ways. From the viewpoint of bioethics, the issue of reduction bears significantly on such issues as the sanctity of life or the uniqueness of living things. In controversies dealing with euthanasia, abortion, and genetic engineering, arguments will often cleave along lines separating those who believe that living systems are ultimately complex physical organizations from those who hold that living systems embody certain organizational features not found in the inanimate world and, which, thereby, render them unique. The response to biological reductionism can take numerous forms, including theological. The work of Teilhard de Chardin, for instance, represents an effort to indicate the uniqueness of man by incorporating him into an overall cosmological evolutionary process. At the same time, Teilhard de Chardin holds that science is aptly suited to deal with living phenomena, thereby avoiding the criticism that such a view of man is prima facie nonscientific.

It is clear from the outset that biological systems are markedly different in their behavior from nonbiological or inanimate ones, although such entities as crystals and viruses seem to share certain important characteristics with living systems. On both a macro- and a microscopic level biologists deal with a class of entities that are, for the most part, clearly delineated from the rest of the physical world. To the extent that mitochondria, membranes, and genes are not rocks, stars, and water, biology may be regarded as not reducible to physics.

In a somewhat more interesting sense, biological terminology may be regarded as autonomous with respect to physics in that its theories and propositions are phrased in a vocabulary not derived from the physical sciences. Thus, genetics and evolutionary theory are systematic attempts to order certain phenomena regarding individual "organisms" and multiple "species" in terms not borrowed, derived from, or defined in terms of physical science. Insofar as the initial goals of these two biological theories are concerned, what is contained within other scientific theories has no formal bearing on the integrity of these intrinsically biological points of view. In a restricted sense there seems to be no need to use any terminology or scientific law outside their respective self-defined domains when describing biological events. The question remains, though, as to the ultimate theoretical possibility of stating the terms and propositions of biology in the language of physics. That is, whether or not the science of biology is able to describe its own phenomena by using an indigenously biological, theoretical, and descriptive vocabulary is quite independent of the issue as to whether or not the laws of biology are ultimately statable in terms of those of physics.

Biology can be viewed as a series of empirical or descriptive generalizations having neither the universality of physical laws nor the capacity to be incorporated into a comprehensive theory dealing with its extensive domain. There are two ways out of this minimal characterization of biology. The first is to deny any difference in kind between physical and biological laws. The second way explores critically the theoretical possibility of the reduction of biological to physical theory.

This second point of view is that of organismic biology and general systems theory. Rather than assert that biology is totally reducible to physics either theoretically or methodologically, or that biology should not enjoy the same respect as physics with regard to its status as a science, such men as Ludwig von Bertalanffy and E. S. Russell claim that biology has its own conceptual structure distinct from that of physics. The domain of biology is distinct and different enough to warrant its having unique principles not derivable or transferable from physical science. Thus, they claim that the organization of living systems is hierarchical and so different from inanimate modes of organization that the laws of physics cannot apply adequately in an attempt to explain fully the workings of living things. As von Bertalanffy claims, the organizational principles applying to the ordering of living systems are to be derived from general systems theory and not from physics.

The issue concerning the reducibility of biology to physics and chemistry has both historical and logical dimensions; that is, the arguments for or against reduction can proceed by asserting that history is on one side or the other. Classically, this is the position of the mechanists contra the vitalists (both of whose positions are defined below), who assert that the history of biological research clearly proves that vitalism is a dead issue. History, for the mechanists, seems to obviate any need to provide a formal argument that definitively dismisses vitalism as a viable theory of living systems. On the other hand, history is never definitive with respect to the open texture of science, and there is little doubt that a need exists for a formal demonstration that one or the other position or neither is correct. In this regard certain logical features of vitalism, mechanism, and holism or organismic biology will be considered briefly at this point.

Mechanism, vitalism, and holism

Mechanism. To view a living system "mechanically" may involve more than one sense. There are at least three different meanings to be ascribed to the concept of mechanism insofar as it applies to the nature of biological entities:

1. "Mechanical explanation" refers to the kind of explanation that is based entirely on the laws and theories of the science of mechanics.
2. "Physicochemical" refers to the statements constituting mechanical explanation that utilize the terms and concepts of physics and chemistry.
3. "Causal explanation" in biology states that all propositions describing a living system gain their intelligibility by being subsumed under at least one causal law.

It should be stated that classical mechanics is often touted as more than it is. For instance, it is clear that this branch of physics is insufficient to serve as a foundation for physics as a whole. Similarly, its extension to the realm of biology becomes even more problematical in this light. Also, while mechanics in a more general sense does not in itself constitute an ethical position, it does have ethical implications. This is the view of Jacques Loeb, who, in the period just prior to the First World War, asserted in his book *The Mechanistic Conception of Life* that the "riddle of life" whose solution lies in the principles of mechanics bears directly on the ethical principles upon which our lives ought to be run. The view of life as essentially mechanical influences conceptions of life and death, the autonomy of the individual, and the problem of free will.

Vitalism. Opposed to the mechanistic view is the philosophy of vitalism, which for the most part is largely abandoned in contemporary biological theory, although, historically, vitalism seemed to offer a bridge to ethics (e.g., Bergson's *élan vital*). In its least sophisticated form it asserts that the matter out of which living things are constituted is qualitatively different from in-animate matter. With the development of biochemistry and the occurrence of such events as the synthesis of urea by Wohler in the nineteenth century and, more recently, the unraveling of the alpha helical structure of DNA, this "substantive" view of vitalism is unsupportable. A somewhat more sophisticated view offered by the biologist Hans Driesch is, in essence, an entelechy theory, i.e., a theory of the organism which asserts that living systems operate in accordance with mechanistic principles up to a point and then require the guidance of an immaterial vital force in order for certain processes to occur—in particular, adaptation and repair. As a theory of explanation, the entelechy is an explanatory deus ex machina that is employed when traditional explanatory prowess is exhausted. Clearly, anyone at all sympathetic to the tenets of logical positivism would be unalterably opposed to such a viewpoint since Driesch's entelechy could have no empirical referent whereby propositions containing the term could be either verified or refuted. The vitalist position, then, served as an ideal target for Moritz Schlick, who attacked it quite clearly from the point of view of logical positivism by showing that it violated the verifiability principle upon which that entire philosophical school was built. For Schlick, ethics was reduced to the psychological expression of the emotions.

Driesch, however, felt that his argument for an entelechy also was an argument for the existence of a soul. This latter point is part of a broad metaphysical system Driesch erected around his considerations about the nature of life. Thus, individual responsibility and the personal awareness of a sense of obligation is derived from a suprapersonal wholeness that is continually evolving toward a goal which is unknown to each individual. Driesch's endowment of material man with a soul constitutes an aspect of his metaphysics in which the individual is seen to have an evolving spiritual dimension.

What mechanical explanation is to mechanism, teleology is to vitalism. That is, explanation in terms of end-points, goals, and the like is viewed as being most naturally fitted to the vitalist's position. An important point, however, is that a subscription to a teleological explanatory point of view does not necessarily commit one to the more severe ontological position of vitalism. Hence, while the vitalism–mechanism debate is essentially resolved in favor of the former, its heir is, in part, the debate over whether or not teleological explanation as well as teleological phrases have any place in rigorous scientific discourse and whether they are capable of being or ought to be translated into linguistic forms congruent with mechanical explanation.

Holism. A resolution of the vitalism–mechanism controversy has implications for bioethics in that such a solution necessarily commits itself to a view of the organism (and possibly the self) wherein certain ethical considerations concerning the uniqueness of the living system may be suggested. Such a resolution is offered by the concept of holism. Holism asserts that the organization of biological systems is what distinguishes them from nonliving systems, and hence, in a manner of speaking, the whole of the living system is greater than the sum of its parts. That is, the propositions constituting an explanation of all of the physical and chemical components of the living system cannot, by their very nature, suffice to elaborate the intrinsically biological or living character of the organism. Specific organizing principles, which, as von Bertalanffy holds, derive from general systems theory, are necessary if the living system is to be understood in its uniqueness and distinctness from the rest of the natural world. In particular, the organism is viewed as a certain sort of hierarchical organization whose individuality is a function of such a mode of constituency. Organisms, from this point of view, are multilayered and complex phenomena the explanation of which requires specific principles specifying the character of the hierarchy. This position has considerable appeal to many biologists and is sometimes associated with the not unproblematic and broader metaphysical concept of emergentism, which, by the way, can be viewed as a methodological principle rather than a more speculative metaphysical one. Emergentism holds that the properties of such hierarchically arranged systems cannot be predicted through an elucidation of the parts of that system. For example, the consistency, taste, and color of water is not deducible from an examination of the properties of hydrogen and oxygen alone. The property of water is seen as an emergent one with respect to the properties of its individual constituents. With organisms, then, their properties are a function of their complex organization, and a mechanical explanation of the various constituents of the organism cannot suffice to specify the peculiar emergent traits that are manifest as a result of this organization. An objection to holism, or organismic biology as it is called by some, is that organizational principles are involved in nonliving systems also, so that the concept of hierarchical organization of even a highly complex form does not suffice as a logical principle whereby living and nonliving systems are distinguished from one another.

Just as with mechanism and vitalism, holism too can be seen to have implications for ethics. The organismic biologist bases his argument for biological uniqueness not upon the existence of a vital principle but upon principles of organization to which science is more congenial. Hence it is possible, from the perspective of the holist, to argue for individuality and the uniqueness of life as does Driesch, and at the same time not abandon sound scientific principles. Furthermore, mechanism is not viewed as the only way to be scientific in these matters. Given such a position, issues such as free will and moral responsibility may take on somewhat different perspectives. The idea of free will may be reconcilable with that of the material basis of life since the organizing relations that characterize the living system are such as to render it unique, with the possibility that this uniqueness entails human freedom.

In broad view, then, each point of view concerning reductionism, mechanism, and vitalism carries with it certain ethical considerations. Mechanism denies the existence of a soul, whereas vitalism proposes it. The reductionist may (but not necessarily) argue on the basis of his position that free will is illusory. The vitalist or organismic biologist will argue to the contrary. Hence, such technical considerations in the philosophy of biology bear directly on bioethical considerations, to which we now turn.

Biology and ethics

There are two broad ways in which ethics can intersect with biological science such that philosophically and biologically interesting questions are raised. The first has to do with man's intervention in what have been traditionally regarded as natural processes of which man is, to a greater or lesser extent, a part. The second concerns itself with the possibility of developing explicit ethical or metaethical points of view from various parts of biology, usually those areas related to the theory of evolution. These two areas will be considered in turn.

Intervention in natural processes. For the greater part of his history man has looked upon natural processes, both biological and physical, as happenings over which he had little or no control. Disease, evolutionary trends, mutations, and the like were not regarded as susceptible to the willful or even the inadvertent actions of human beings. Whatever occurred in the natural world, living or nonliving, was—except for that small realm in which man had some influence—regarded as the product of natural, i.e., non-human forces. With the growth of biological methodology and modern medicine (e.g., the germ theory of disease), the vision of man as a largely passive recipient of the whims of nature began to decline. Thus, concerns about man's willful and accidental intervention in the sphere of natural processes has grown enormously in the twentieth century. Along with this concern have come ethical considerations that bear directly on these issues. This instance of ethical reflection constitutes not a new view of ethics or metaethics but rather a new sphere for those modes of ethical inquiry already in vogue.

As examples of these new concerns and the questions of priority that are raised, two illustrations having to do with willful and inadvertent human intrusion into natural processes can be offered here. The first is the question of the moral responsibility of those individuals who are engaged in efforts to synthesize living organisms and quasi-living systems such as viruses. As the emergentists point out, it is virtually impossible to predict the possible pathological potential of any successfully synthesized organism for the human race. It is a real possibility, for instance, that a severely pathogenic virus could be synthesized for which no treatment is known and which could wipe out large portions if not all of the world's population. Is the growth of biological knowledge in this domain worth the risks entailed in this example? On the other hand, one could argue, such research might result in the elimination of most of man's diseases. Thus, the possibility of an epidemic is countered by the possibility of an opposite practical consequence of the research. The legislation of such decisions as to whether or not to pursue a certain line of inquiry in the biological sciences constitutes an area in which ethical considerations can have the profoundest consequences.

In the case of inadvertent intrusion into natural processes, the issue is often raised with respect to ecological considerations. A chemical plant may produce valuable products for industry and society at large but may, at the same time, pollute the river that is adjacent to it. In this case there are at least two considerations to be raised. First, one must ask what priorities are to be held and in what order they will be embraced. If, for example, the public desires a clean river more than a particular chemical, then through any number of social and political processes, the plant may be compelled to close its operations. This case is not unlike the last one stated, in that a question of priorities is raised and specific ethical considerations can be brought to bear on the problem in an effort to resolve it. The second consideration, however, is rather more problematic in that it raises the issue of man's responsibility both to other living things (in this case, the fish and plants in the river) and to other natural entities (the river and its environs). How far does the right to life extend, for instance? What is the value of natural beauty in the hierarchy of values individuals construct for themselves in order to run their lives? Is it morally defensible to extinguish a species of wildlife because of certain human needs or desires? These are questions that biology, as it has grown, raises in the minds of philosophers, politicians, and the general citizenry.

Evolution and ethics.   An interesting point of intersection of ethics and biology is seen in the development of specific ethical or metaethical points of view based upon the theory of evolution. The work of C. H. Waddington and Sir Julian Huxley serve as examples in this context. What has been called evolutionary ethics consists in the building of ethical theories or systems from the framework of evolutionary theory. Biologists, more than philosophers, have been drawn to this form of theorizing. They see in it an external source of values for mankind. Evolutionary order can, say the evolutionary ethicists, serve to provide a hierarchy of values, a process for legislating between good and evil, and a theory about the moral roots of human nature. It is certainly an optimistic point of view but one that has not had the enthusiastic endorsement of many philosophers. The main reason is that the later philosophers have traditionally held the opinion that such an approach to ethics involves the "naturalistic fallacy." This fallacy, whose explication lies initially in the work of Hume and which was analyzed in twentieth-century philosophy by G. E. Moore, points out the logically illicit deduction of an evaluative statement, moral or otherwise, from solely descriptive statements about the world. The extraction of value statements from descriptive ones is precisely the naturalistic fallacy of evolutionary ethics, according to its philosophical critics. While there has been some weakening of the role that the naturalistic fallacy has played in some ethical works of the mid-twentieth century, its deeply rooted place in the minds of many moral philosophers disposes many critics to discount those who seek to derive an ethical theory or a theory of ethics from the theory of evolution. Thus, those moral principles based upon the patterns and processes of evolutionary phenomena may have to await more hospitable times when philosophers are not as ill-disposed to such theorizing or else find another base of justification.

A newer approach to the issues of bioethics and evolution is to be found in the work of Edward O. Wilson on sociobiology. Wilson takes it as a major task of his to explain altruism, a trait not readily explainable in terms of traditional evolutionary theory. By changing the focus of concern from that of the organism to that of the gene, Wilson is able to develop his theory of altruism along highly creative lines. From the perspective of bioethics, he is involved in the nature/nurture controversy (siding more with the nature theorists) and issues related to social Darwinism. Whether Wilson's approach to ethics via examination of genetically influenced or determined behaviors is ultimately successful remains to be seen. As a movement in bioethical theory, however, it is the most recent and, perhaps, the most significant one in the latter part of the twentieth century. How successful this approach is to meeting the above-mentioned criticisms leveled against other bioethical theories will, in part, determine the ultimate impact of the point of view it puts forth.

IRWIN SAVODNIK

[*Directly related are the entries* ENVIRONMENTAL ETHICS, *article on* QUESTIONS OF SOCIAL JUSTICE; EVOLUTION; MEDICINE, PHILOSOPHY OF; *and* REDUCTIONISM. *For discussion of related ideas, see the entries:* ENVIRONMENT AND MAN, *article on* WESTERN THOUGHT; FREE WILL AND DETERMINISM; *and* MIND–BODY PROBLEM. *Other relevant material may be found under* ETHICS, *article on* NATURALISM; *and* SCIENCE: ETHICAL IMPLICATIONS.]

BIBLIOGRAPHY

AYALA, FRANCISCO JOSÉ, and DOBZHANSKY, THEODOSIUS, eds. *Studies in the Philosophy of Biology: Reduction and Related Problems.* Berkeley: University of California Press, 1975.
BECKNER, MORTON. *The Biological Way of Thought.* Berkeley: University of California Press, 1968.
BERTALANFFY, LUDWIG VON. *Modern Theories of Development: An Introduction to Theoretical Biology.* Translated by J. H. Woodger. New York: Harper & Row, 1962.
———. *Problems of Life: An Evaluation of Modern Biological Thought.* New York: John Wiley & Sons, 1952.
BLUM, HAROLD FRANCIS. *Time's Arrow and Evolution.* Princeton: Princeton University Press, 1951.
CANFIELD, JOHN V., ed. *Purpose in Nature.* Contemporary Perspectives in Philosophy Series. Englewood Cliffs, N.J.: Prentice-Hall, 1966.
FLEW, ANTONY GARRARD NEWTON. *Evolutionary Ethics.* New Studies in Ethics, vol. 8, no. 6. New York: St. Martin's Press; London: Macmillan & Co., 1967.
GRENE, MARJORIE GLICKSMAN, and MENDELSOHN, EVERETT, eds. *Topics in the Philosophy of Biology.* Boston Studies in the Philosophy of Science, vol. 27. Synthese Library, vol. 84. Boston: D. Reidel, 1975.
HALDANE, J. S. *Mechanism, Life and Personality: An Examination of the Mechanistic Theory of Life and Mind.* London: John Murray, 1921; New York: E. P. Dutton & Co., 1923. Reprint. Westport, Conn.: Greenwood Press, 1973.
HEMPEL, CARL GUSTAV. *Aspects of Scientific Explanation, and Other Essays in the Philosophy of Science.* New York: Free Press; London: Collier-Macmillan, 1965.
HULL, DAVID L. *Philosophy of Biological Science.* Prentice-Hall Foundations of Philosophy Series. Englewood Cliffs, N.J.: 1974.
HUXLEY, JULIAN SORELL. *Evolutionary Ethics.* Romanes Lecture. London: Oxford University Press, 1943.
HUXLEY, THOMAS HENRY. *Evolution and Ethics and Other Essays.* Huxley's Collected Essays, vol. 9. New York: D. Appleton & Co., 1929.
LOEB, JACQUES. *The Mechanistic Conception of Life.* Edited by Donald Fleming. Cambridge: Belknap Press, Harvard University Press, 1964.
MUNSON, RONALD, ed. *Man and Nature: Philosophical Issues in Biology.* A Delta Book. New York: Dell Publishing Co., 1971.
NAGEL, ERNEST. *The Structure of Science: Problems in the Logic of Scientific Explanation.* New York: Harcourt, Brace & World, 1961.
RUSE, MICHAEL. *Philosophy of Biology.* London: Hutchinson, 1973.
SCHAFFNER, KENNETH F. "Theories and Explanations in Biology." *Journal of the History of Biology* 2 (1969): 19–33.
———. "The Watson–Crick Model and Reductionism." *British Journal for the Philosophy of Science* 20 (1969): 325–348.
SCRIVEN, MICHAEL. "Explanation in the Biological Sciences." *Journal of the History of Biology* 2 (1969): 187–198.
SIMON, MICHAEL A. *The Matter of Life: Philosophical Problems of Biology.* New Haven: Yale University Press, 1971.
SIMPSON, GEORGE GAYLORD. *The Meaning of Evolution: A Study of the History of Life and of Its Significance for Man.* New Haven: Yale University Press, 1967.
WILSON, EDWARD OSBORNE. *Sociobiology: The New Synthesis.* Cambridge: Belknap Press, Harvard University Press, 1975.
WOODGER, JOSEPH HENRY. *Biological Principles: A Critical Study.* Reissued, with a new Introduction. International Library of Psychology, Philosophy and Scientific Method. London: Routledge & Kegan Paul; New York: Humanities Press, 1967.

BIOMEDICAL RESEARCH

See RESEARCH, BIOMEDICAL; HUMAN EXPERIMENTATION; ANIMAL EXPERIMENTATION; RESEARCH POLICY, BIOMEDICAL.

BIRTH CONTROL

See CONTRACEPTION.

BIRTH DEFECTS

See FETAL–MATERNAL RELATIONSHIP; GENETIC DIAGNOSIS AND COUNSELING; GENETIC SCREENING; INFANTS; LIFE, *article on* QUALITY OF LIFE; PRENATAL DIAGNOSIS. *See also* MENTALLY HANDICAPPED.

BLOOD TRANSFUSION

The procedure

The process called blood transfusion is the introduction of whole blood or blood derivatives directly into the body's circulatory system. Transfusion replenishes depleted blood volume as in cases of hemorrhage, burns, injuries to blood vessels, and shock during surgery, or corrects blood disorders as in anemia, leukemia, hemophilia, and immune deficiencies.

Current clinical practice benefits from techniques for separating and storing blood derivatives developed during the past thirty years. Any of the cellular components of blood (white, red, and platelet cells), plasma alone, or various plasma proteins may now be used to respond to specific clinical needs.

Efforts to meet the demand for blood must deal with the constraints of short storage life, safety limits for repeated donations, and exclusion of some potential donors to protect recipients from blood transmissible diseases, notably, serum hepatitis (Mollison).

Ethical problems

Transfusion generates three sets of ethical problems: religio-cultural attitudes toward blood, social organization for securing blood, and maintenance of professional standards.

Attitudes toward blood. Confronted by cultural traditions not deeply affected by the scientific world view, donor recruitment programs must often overcome beliefs about evils resulting from the drawing of blood, e.g., impotence, infertility, general weakness, susceptibility to witchcraft, or guilt or sacrilege (League of Red Cross Societies, p. 8). In such circumstances,

transfusion becomes involved in ethical problems of resolving conflicts in cross-cultural values. Issues of power, coercion, independence, and individual and cultural dignity enter into the task of securing needed blood supplies.

Attitudes also affect the receiving of transfusions. Cultural values may oppose the mingling of racially different blood, e.g., in South Africa and the Southern United States (Titmuss, p. 193). Blood service policies are thus drawn into large ethical issues of interracial justice and equality. On religious grounds, Jehovah's Witnesses oppose any transfusion as being a use of blood forbidden by God (Farr, p. 44). Refusal of transfusion for racial or religious reasons raises two sets of problems rooted in personal autonomy and religious liberty: first, refusal by an adult for himself; second, refusal by an adult responsible for a dependent person, such as a child or unconscious spouse.

Social organization of blood supply. Questions of distributive justice and social solidarity enter into the evaluation of blood supply systems, of which there are two basic approaches: voluntary unpaid donors and quid pro quo. In the latter, blood may be exchanged for cash, social rewards, fringe benefits, or security regarding transfusions for self or family (Titmuss, pp. 75 ff.).

If equitable distribution of burdens and benefits is taken as the norm, cash systems appear to be the least just. Here the poor and derelict become the major suppliers of blood, since the motivational appeal addresses their economic situation most directly. Yet they are the least able to afford blood when they need it, because the cost of commercially purchased blood is from five to fifteen times higher than blood supplied through voluntary unpaid donor systems (ibid., pp. 205 ff.).

Other quid pro quo systems appeal especially to the working and lower middle class. The base of appeal is broader than cash systems, the spread of the burden more equitable, and added costs, if any, less than those of cash systems. However, the widest spread of the burden is achieved in voluntary unpaid donor systems. These also generate the least cost in the process of supplying blood and keep the benefit of blood transfusion most widely accessible (ibid., pp. 120 ff.).

Unpaid systems produce blood supplies of higher quality than cash systems. Despite improvement of tests for discovering blood transmissible hepatitis (Mollison, pp. 603 ff.), blood supply systems must rely heavily on donors' testimony that they are not infected. However, in cash systems the major suppliers come from populations noted for high incidence of hepatitis and have a conflict of interest in revealing a fact that would disqualify them from selling blood. Studies indicate that post-transfusion hepatitis rates are much higher when blood from commercial banks is used.

Blood supply systems give rise to the issue of social solidarity, because the giving of blood is an important means of promoting community consciousness and altruism (Titmuss, pp. 237 ff.). In voluntary unpaid systems, blood is literally a gift of oneself for the benefit of unknown neighbors. Giving the gift in the knowledge that there are many other such givers helps create confidence in one's community. Quid pro quo systems counteract these values. They tend to atomize individuals in private worlds of self-interest by closing off this opportunity for the expression of altruism and community consciousness.

Professional standards. The traditional norm of medical ethics, "Do no harm," dictates that, in the handling, processing, and administration of blood and blood products, great care must be taken to avoid injury to recipients resulting from human and computer errors in blood group identification, screening for contaminated blood, cross-matching, labeling, and patient identification. Similar care must be taken to protect donors from excessive giving of blood, infection, and various postdonation hazards (Mollison, pp. 2–10).

The same norm, at the level of social policy, requires concern about commercial methods for supplying blood. Both the International Red Cross and the World Health Organization have recommended voluntary unpaid donor systems as preferable for protection against blood transmissible diseases (Bowley, p. 16).

MICHAEL J. GARLAND

[*Directly related are the entries* HEALTH CARE, *articles on* RIGHT TO HEALTH-CARE SERVICES *and* THEORIES OF JUSTICE AND HEALTH CARE; ORGAN DONATION; ORGAN TRANSPLANTATION, *article on* SOCIOCULTURAL ASPECTS (*for the concept of gift*); RATIONING OF MEDICAL TREATMENT; *and* RIGHT TO REFUSE MEDICAL CARE. *See also:* PROTESTANTISM, *article on* DOMINANT HEALTH CONCERNS IN PROTESTANTISM; *and* RACISM.]

BIBLIOGRAPHY

BOWLEY, C. C.; GOLDSMITH, K. L. G.; and MAYCOCK, W. D'A., eds. *Blood Transfusion: A Guide to the Formation and Operation of a Transfusion Service.* Geneva: World Health Organization, 1971.

FARR, ALFRED D. *God, Blood and Society.* Aberdeen, S. Dak.: Impulse Publications, 1972.

League of Red Cross Societies. *IIIrd Red Cross International Seminar on Blood Transfusion: Blood Donor Motivation and Training of Auxiliary Personnel for Blood Transfusion Centers.* Medico-Social Documentation no. 27. Geneva: League of Red Cross Societies, 1965.

MOLLISON, PATRICK L. *Blood Transfusion in Clinical Medicine.* 5th ed. Oxford: Blackwell Scientific Publications, 1972.

TITMUSS, RICHARD M. *The Gift Relationship: From Human Blood to Social Policy.* New York: Random House, 1971.

BRAIN DEATH

See DEATH, DEFINITION AND DETERMINATION OF, *article on* CRITERIA FOR DEATH.

BRITAIN

See MEDICAL ETHICS, HISTORY OF, *section on* EUROPE AND THE AMERICAS, *articles on* MEDIEVAL EUROPE: FOURTH TO SIXTEENTH CENTURY; INTRODUCTION TO THE MODERN PERIOD IN EUROPE AND THE AMERICAS; BRITAIN AND THE UNITED STATES IN THE EIGHTEENTH CENTURY; BRITAIN IN THE NINETEENTH CENTURY; *and* BRITAIN IN THE TWENTIETH CENTURY.

BUDDHISM

Buddhist teaching: a model on the pattern of pathology

The Buddha endeavored to heal diseases of the mind. He was often called "the Great Physician" or "the King of Physicians." The outline of an important Buddhist teaching called "the Four Noble Truths" was made according to the pattern of pathology (*nidāna*) of ancient India. Why are we afflicted by suffering in our worldly existence? Why are we involved in the round of transmigration? The Buddha's inquiry into the cause of worldly suffering or afflictions proceeded on a practical, psychological level, and he discovered that the real cause of human suffering is ignorant craving or blind desire (*tṛṣṇā*). He then showed human beings that the right and effective way to deliverance from suffering is by the cessation of such craving.

The Buddha is then called a physician metaphorically. Just as a doctor must know the diagnosis of the different kinds of disease (Jolly), and must know their causes (*Vinaya, Mahāvagga* VI, 14, 1–5), and the antidotes and remedies to cure them, and must be able to apply them ("Greater Discourse"), so also the Buddha taught the Four Noble Truths, in order to indicate the range of "suffering," its "origin," its "cessation," and the "way" which leads to its cessation. According to this doctrine, if we can get rid of the cause of suffering, we shall be able to attain deliverance, comparable to the healing of a disease.

The Buddha's general opinion about the problems of ethics is typically expressed in the doctrine of the following "Four Noble Truths" (Jolly):

1. "The Noble Truth concerning suffering or afflictions. Birth, decay, disease, death, union with the unpleasant, separation from the pleasant, and any craving that is unsatisfied are forms of suffering. In brief, suffering springs from instinctive attachment, that is, the conditions of individuality." Very much of this truth is comparable to the diagnosis of diseases.

2. "The Noble Truth concerning the origin of suffering. It is the craving, comparable to thirst, that causes the renewal of the process that is accompanied by sensual delights, and seeks satisfaction, now here, now there, that is to say, the craving for the gratification of the senses, or the craving for existence, or the craving for non-existence." Our craving is so strong and blind that it was compared by the Buddha to thirst. When we are thirsty, we cannot help desiring water, forgetting everything else. In the same way our craving compels us to seek objects. This truth is comparable to knowing the causes of diseases.

3. Next, the healing of diseases should be sought. "The Noble Truth concerning the cessation of suffering. It is the vanishing of afflictions so that no passion remains. It is the giving up, the getting rid of, the emancipation from, the harboring no longer of this craving or thirst." The word "cessation" (*nirodha*) originally and etymologically meant "control." To control this craving thirst is truly the ideal state.

4. Finally, the means for healing should be made clear. "The Noble Truth shows the way that leads to cessation of suffering. It is the Noble Eightfold Path which consists of right views, right aspirations, right speech, right conduct, right mode of livelihood, right effort, right mindfulness, and right concentration."

These eight are comparable to remedies of an illness. The Path pointed out by Gautama is called the Noble Path; the truths enumerated are called the Noble Truths. They permit full elaboration by his followers. All the items of the Noble Fourfold Truths were commented upon in full detail by later expositors.

In Mahāyāna Buddhism medical science (*cikitsā-vidyā*) was one of the five sciences which should be learned, the other four being metaphysics (*adhyātma-vidyā*), logic (*hetu-vidyā*), science of language (*sabda-vidyā*), and technology (*silpakarmasthāna-vidyā*).

Health care

Despite the medical model that can be seen to underlie the Buddha's teaching, early Buddhism discouraged monks from engaging in medical care because at that time medical science was considered a sort of worldly pursuit, classified with magic and sorcery.

"Let a monk not apply himself to practicing [the hymns of] the Āthabbaṇa [the Atharvaveda], to [the interpretation of] sleep and signs, nor to astrology; let not my follower [a Buddhist monk] devote himself to [interpreting] the cry of birds, to causing impregnation, nor to [the art of] medicine [*tikicchā*; literally, 'treatment of diseases']" (*Suttanipāta*). But to help the sick was regarded as a virtue. A scripture of early Buddhism tells the following story. In the days of the Buddha, a sick brother was once neglected by the other members of the monastery. The Buddha washed him and tended him with his own hands, saying afterward to the negligent monks, who would have been eager enough to serve him, "Whosoever would wait upon me, let him wait upon the sick." He claims his oneness with humanity so that service to the sick or the destitute is in reality rendered to himself (*Vinaya, Mahāvagga* VIII, 26).

Subsequently, Buddhist orders established medical institutions. For example, monasteries of early Buddhism had halls for the sick monks. During the reign of King Aśoka (third century B.C.), a man greatly influenced by the compassionate spirit of Buddhism, hospitals were established for sick humans as well as for sick animals. This antedated anything similar in the West and animal clinics (*pinjpols*) are found to this day in Western India (Bhandarkar).

In his Rock Edict II, King Aśoka tells us that in his own dominions as well as in those of neighboring potentates, he established two kinds of medical treatment, one relating to humans and the other to animals. And he further informs us that medical herbs, roots, and fruits, whenever lacking or in short supply, were imported and planted everywhere. After Aśoka's reign hospitals were institutionalized in ancient India.

From the records of the eighteenth century it is quite clear that in two states, Mahārāṣṭra and Gujarāt, kings and chiefs frequently arranged for free medical help to be given to the needy and indigent; as a consequence, the physician was often rewarded with grants of rent-free land in a village, and in some cases the purpose of the grants was expressly stated to be the growing of medicinal herbs on the land.

The care of the sick was recognized as a duty and a meritorious act in all Buddhist countries and is recommended by the example of Buddha himself. The *Mahāvaṃsa*, a chronicle of Ceylon, repeatedly asserts that kings founded hospitals and distributed medicines. The Buddhist king Buddhadāsa of Ceylon (fourth century A.D.) cured patients, appointed doctors and provided them some compensation, established asylums, and wrote a medical work entitled *Sāratthasaṅgaha* (Turnour). A certain doctor named Caraka is said to have been the personal doctor of the Buddhist king Kaniska (second century A.D.).

After Buddhism was introduced into China sometime in the first century A.D., Buddhists engaged in a great many altruistic activities in accordance with the ideal of "Compassion." Ever since Shih-lo (A.D. 329?), of the later Chao period, the inculcation of Buddhist teachings became widespread. The social work of the Buddhist priests was especially noticeable in its medical treatment and relief of the poor. In the Eastern Chin period (A.D. 317–420), Fo-t'uch'eng, Fa-k'uang, K'o-lo-chieh, An-hui of Loyang, and Tan-tao of Lo-ching-shan helped people obtain medical attention and care. In the T'ang dynasty (618–907), the system of temple hospitals was established, and institutions for the poor, the sick, and the orphaned were built. Buddhist priests endeavored to build bridges, plant trees, dig wells, and construct rest houses.

Prince Shōtoku (574–622), the founder of Japanese Buddhism, established Shitennōji Temple in 587 in what is now the city of Ōsaka, and this temple was renowned for its creative undertaking of the relief of suffering people. The temple was laid out in four main divisions: Kyōden-in, the great central hall or religious sanctuary proper, used for training in Buddhist discipline and in aesthetic and scholarly pursuits; Hiden-in, a hall where the poor could obtain relief; Ryōbyō-in, a hospital or clinic where the sick could receive treatment without charge; and Seyaku-in, a dispensary where medical herbs were collected, refined, and distributed free of charge. It is not clear whether Prince Shōtoku established an animal hospital there, but judging by the name, the Kyōden-in (which means "institution based on respect for existent beings") was aimed at promoting the happiness and welfare of all living beings, human and animal alike. Moreover, according to the *Nihongi*, Shōtoku and other members of the imperial family, as well as officials of the court, used to set aside fixed days for the purpose of gathering medicinal herbs, and the court is known to have shown special consideration to the needy, whether living alone, destitute, or aged.

Empress Kōmyō (eighth century) engaged in philanthropic activities. Legend has it that in the public bathing room she washed and tended a leprous beggar covered with loathsome sores, who suddenly revealed himself as the Buddha Akṣobhya.

Later, the priest Ninshō (1217–1303) began such social welfare works as caring for the suffering and the sick. He dedicated his whole life to the service of others and was even criticized by his master, Eison: "He overdid benevolence." Although it was a breach of customary discipline to dig ponds or wells or to give medicine and clothing to the sick or to collect money for them, Ninshō never let himself be deterred from doing any of these things.

In Cambodia an inscription of Jayavarman VII (A.D. 1185?) reveals that there were 102 hospitals in his kingdom. He evidently expended much care and money on them. One is led to suppose that Buddhism took a more active part than Brahmanism in such works of charity (Eliot).

Medical science as revealed in Buddhist literature

The Bower manuscripts are the oldest extant works of Buddhist influence. The manuscripts, which were found in a Buddhist cairn in Kashgar (China), were probably written by immigrants from India about A.D. 450. The sixth and seventh texts of the Bower manuscripts often refer to Buddha, Tathāgata, Bhagavat, and synonyms of Buddha (Jolly). The texts describe types of early medical treatment.

In a scripture entitled "Nine Causes of Unexpected Early Death" the reader is warned against overeating, eating wrong foods, and disregarding Buddhist precepts. The ways in which one should console a seriously sick person at death are also explained.

The Chinese Buddhist pilgrim I-tsing (671–695) gives a detailed description of the Indian medicine of his time, including symptoms of bodily illness, rules for giving medicine, medical treatment and the use of herbs, rules for diagnosis, and fasting to cure disease (I-tsing). Contents of medicines are not specified. In ancient India the urine of cows was used as medicine, attributable to the general tendency in India to worship cows, and Buddhists were no exception. In Japan this custom was never followed. Medicines obtainable by killing animals were disliked because of the traditional ideal of not injuring any living beings. But nowadays these medicines are tolerated in Japan because of the persistence of the idea of Shinshu Pure Land Buddhism, which tolerates killing of animals in case of necessity but with the feeling of sinfulness.

Vajrayāna, a school of Mahāyāna, which developed after the fifth century A.D. in India, incorporated various forms of popular beliefs prevalent among common people. Wherever there is any reference to diseases and treatment in Vajrayāna scriptures, the usual course recommended is the recitation of spells (*dhāraṇīs*).

Ancient China and Japan have left a large number of medical texts which have not yet been explored and it has not as yet been ascertained to what extent they have been influenced by Buddhism.

Mutilation and suicide

In Buddhism mutilation of any sort of the human body was abhorred and discouraged. It was assumed that legal punishment should be limited to imprisonment, confiscation, scolding, and so on; but capital punishment and mutilation should not be inflicted upon criminals. The aim of legal punishment is to save one from evils and to make a man of good character. This ideal was advocated in Buddhist sacred books.

Buddhism does not necessarily prohibit suicide, but according to Buddhist sacred texts suicide is meaningless, for by resorting to suicide one cannot save oneself from the miserable condition of mundane existence (or transmigration); karma (actions) are supposed to accompany a person who has committed suicide even after his death. The shocking cases of self-immolation by Buddhist monks in order to protest against the policy of the ruling class, as took place in Vietnam in recent times, were not based upon any tenet of Buddhist teachings. This kind of action is not encouraged in any Buddhist teaching. No Japanese Buddhist priest committed suicide in order to protest either in wartime or during the American occupation. In China and Japan there were some rare cases in the past when disciplined Buddhist monks committed suicide, immolating themselves by starvation resulting from rigorous spiritual practices. They were respected. Some of them by way of repentence or redemption redeemed their own sins or crimes, even for murders committed while young. But such self-immolation was quite exceptional and has no scriptural approval.

HAJIME NAKAMURA

[*For further discussion of topics mentioned in this article, see the entries:* HOSPITALS; PAIN AND SUFFERING; *and* SUICIDE. *Also directly related are the entries* ENVIRONMENT AND MAN, *article on* EASTERN THOUGHT; MEDICAL ETHICS, HISTORY OF, *section on* SOUTH AND EAST ASIA, *articles on* PREREPUBLICAN CHINA, CONTEMPORARY CHINA, JAPAN THROUGH THE NINETEENTH CENTURY, TRADITIONAL PROFESSIONAL ETHICS IN JAPANESE MEDICINE, *and* CONTEMPORARY JAPAN: MEDICAL ETHICS AND LEGAL MEDICINE. *Compare:* CONFUCIANISM; HINDUISM; *and* TAOISM. *See* APPENDIX, SECTION I, FIVE COMMANDMENTS AND TEN REQUIREMENTS.]

BIBLIOGRAPHY

BAGCHI, PRABODH CHANDRA. "New Materials for the Study of the *Kāśyapasaṃhitā* in Chinese." *Indian Culture* 9 (1942?): 53–64. Cf. *Taishō*, no. 1385.
———. "New Materials for the Study of the *Kumāratantra* of Rāvaṇa." *Indian Culture* 7 (1940?): 269–286. A translation of *Taishō*, no. 1330, also known as *Rāvaṇakumāra-tantra*.
BHANDARKAR, DEVADATTA RAMAKRISHNA. *Asoka.* The Carmichael Lectures, 1923. Calcutta: University of Calcutta, 1925. 3d ed., rev. 1955, pp. 167–168.
The Book of the Discipline (*Vinaya-Pitaka*). 6 vols. Vol. 4: (*Mahāvagga*) [The Great Division]. Translated by Isaline Blew Horner. Sacred Books of the Buddhists, vol. 14. London: Luzac & Co., 1951.
Le Canon bouddhique en Chine: Les Traducteurs et les traductions. Translated by Prabodh Chandra Bagchi. 2 vols. Sino-Indica: Publication de l'Université de Calcutta, vols. 1, 4. Paris: P. Geuthner, 1927–1928, vol. 1, pp. 302–303. Cf. *Taishō*, no. 793.

"Channa." *The Book of the Kindred Sayings (Sanyutta-nikāya) or Grouped Suttas.* 5 pts. Pt. 4: *The Saḷāyatana Book (Salāyatana Vagga).* Translated by F. L. Woodward. Pali Text Society Translation series, no. 14. London: Routledge & Kegan Paul, 1972, text iv, 55; XXXV, II, 4, sec. 87(4); pp. 30–33. Ways of consoling a seriously ill person on his deathbed. *Saṃyutta* or *Sanyutta* is the Pali recension of *Saṃyukta.*

Eliot, Charles Norton Edgecumbe. *Hinduism and Buddhism: An Historical Sketch.* 3 vols. London: E. Arnold & Co., 1921; Routledge & Kegan Paul, 1954–1957; New York: Barnes & Noble, 1954, vol. 3, p. 124.

"Greater Discourse on the Lion's Roar (Mahāsīhanāda-sutta)." *The Collection of the Middle Length Sayings (Majjhima-Nikāya).* Translated by Isaline Blew Horner. 3 vols. Vol. 1: *The First Fifty Discourses (Mūlapaṇṇāsa).* Pali Text Society Translation series, no. 29. London: Luzac & Co., 1954, chap. 12, pp. 108–110. *Mahāsīhanāda-sutta* I, 82–83. *Majjhima* is the Pali recension of the *Madhyama.*

I-tsing. *A Record of the Buddhist Religion as Practised in India and the Malay Archipelago, A.D. 671–695.* Translated by Junjirō Takakusu. Oxford: Clarendon Press, 1896, pp. 126–140. For the theory of the four humors, see p. 130. The standard romanization for the author's name is I-ching.

Jolly, Julius. *Medicin.* Strassburg: K. J. Trübner, 1901, pp. 14–15.

Sen, Satiranjan. "Two Medical Texts in Chinese Translation." *Visva-Bharati Annals* 1 (1945): 70–75. Cf. *Suśruta, Sūtrasthāna* XIV, 34–35; XXIV, 8.

Suttanipāta, Tuvatakasutta, v. 927. "The Sutta-nipāta: A Collection of Discourses, Being One of the Canonical Books of the Buddhists." Translated from the Pâli by V. Fausböll. *The Sacred Books of the East.* Edited by F. Max Müller. Oxford: Oxford University Press, 1881; Delhi: Motilal Banarsidass, 1965, vol. 10, pt. 2, sec. 14:13, p. 176.

Suśruta, Sūtrasthāna I, 24; I, 37; XXI, 3–4.

Taishō Shinshū Daizōkyo [Taisho Edition of the Tripiṭaka in Chinese]. Edited by Junjirō Takakusu, K. Watanabe, and G. Ono. 100 vols. Tokyo: 1929–. Sometimes called the *Taishō Tripiṭaka.* Some interesting portions on medicine are: *Ekottaragāma-sūtra;* Chinese version, vols. 44, 50, 31; *Taishō,* vol. 2, pp. 776, 811, 670. *Samyuktāgama-sutta;* Chinese version, no. 684 and vol. 41, no. 1122; *Taishō,* vol. 2, p. 186, pp. 297c–298b. Also: *Taishō,* vol. 17, pp. 591, 747; vol. 2, p. 883ab. *Rāvaṇakumāra-tantra; Taishō,* no. 1330, see Bagchi, "New Materials for *Kumāratantra." Kaśyapa-ṛṣi-prokta-strīcikitsā-sūtra; Taishō,* no. 1385, see Bagchi, "New Materials for *Kāśyapesaṃhitā." Bhaisaj-yarāja-sūtra; Fo shuo fo yi wang king; Taishō,* no. 793, see *Canon Bouddhique en Chine.* Also: *Taishō,* nos. 1059, 1060.

Turnour, George, ed. and trans. *The Mahāwanso in Roman Characters with the Translation Subjoined; And an Introductory Essay on Páli Buddhistical Literature: In Two Volumes. Vol. 1 Containing the First Thirty Eight Chapters.* Ceylon: Cotta Church Mission Press, 1837, pp. 243–245. Only one volume published. Translation reprinted, with notes and emendations, and completed by L. C. Wijesiṇha, Colomba: G. J. A. Skeen, 1889. *Mahāwanso* is a varient of *Mahāvamsa* or *Mahāvansa,* attributed to Mahanama, 5th century.

Vinaya, Mahāvagga VIII, 26. *Book of Discipline,* vol. 4, pp. 431–434.

Vinaya, Mahāvagga VI, 14, 1–5. *Book of Discipline,* vol. 4, pp. 278–279. See also *Vinaya, Mahāvagga* VIII, 1f, *Book of Discipline,* vol. 4, p. 379f.

Warder, A. K. *Indian Buddhism.* Delhi: Motilal Banarsidass, 1970. Contains a bibliography and guide to texts.

BURIAL
See CADAVERS.

C

CADAVERS

I. GENERAL ETHICAL CONCERNS
                            Christian A. Hovde
II. JEWISH PERSPECTIVES   *Walter S. Wurzburger*

I
GENERAL ETHICAL CONCERNS

Several questions arise in thinking about the disposal and use of the human cadaver. The following article, after a brief reflection on the significance of the human cadaver, centers on autopsy, the use of cadavers as a source of organic tissue, experimentation on fetal cadavers, and burial and cremation.

The significance of the body

Like other animal bodies the human body is a combination of highly organized cell populations mutually dependent upon each other and, in proper combination, forming something more than the cell populations themselves. Unlike other animal bodies the human body is *human,* that is, it participates in the dignity of the human person. Even after death the human cadaver reminds us that once there was present in our midst a human person, a being like ourselves, sharing in our dignity and value.

For this reason civilized people have always been outraged at cannibalism and at the desecration of the dead. The cadavers of human persons are not, as Homer sings, to be the feast of birds nor are they to be considered as commercial property, a point brought out in a legal decision in Rhode Island in 1872 when the court declared: "There is a duty imposed by the universal feelings of mankind to be discharged by someone towards the dead; a duty, and we may say a right, to protect from violation; and a duty on the part of others to abstain from violation" (*Pierce* v. *Swan Point Cemetery*, 10 R.I. 227 [1872].

It is not that the human cadaver is something of inherent value, for it will soon decay unless measures are taken to prevent this. Rather it is that the human cadaver is a symbol of the human person, a reminder to us of our life together as a community of persons. As a symbol, the human cadaver demands respect from the living.

Autopsy

Autopsy procedures are routinely used in medical institutions today. For reasons of public health and safety, the bodies of those who have died without benefit of medical aid or in whom the cause of death is not immediately apparent are subjected to autopsy carried out in order to discover the cause of death and to establish where possible the responsible agent of that death.

Those who see no symbolic value in the human cadaver find few problems with autopsy other than the aesthetic ones having to do with mutilation. But for those who believe that the human cadaver still possesses human significance some problems are raised. Even if one grants that the common good of the entire community can be served by an autopsy, one wants to secure that good and at the same time to protect the cadaver from violation, to prevent this symbol from being used inhumanly. Thus those who, for religious or humanistic reasons, regard the human cadaver with respect, while permitting autopsy for valid reasons, insist that tissues thus examined be restored to the cadaver before burial.

Historically the first major impetus for autopsies was provided when Frederick II, emperor of the Holy Roman Empire, instructed physicians studying at Salerno or Naples to spend at least one year in the study of anatomy. The imperial edict was given about A.D. 1240 (Corner; Packard). This was followed by edicts from Pope Sixtus IV, A.D. 1414–1484, and Pope Clement VI, A.D. 1478–1534, permitting the opening of the human body for dissection (Lassek, p. 74). Christian theologians, in commenting on these edicts, expressed the belief that such dissection of the human cadaver could be done with proper respect for the dead, so long as the organs were restored to the body prior to burial.

On an individual level, emotional reactions to the prospect of postmortem desecration or mutilation of one's own body or that of someone cared for very often influences the way in which a person responds to the possibility of autopsy. Most people will acknowledge intellectually that something worthwhile may be discovered through the use of autopsy procedures. But to many, the feeling of guilt over their failure to protect that body during the last hours of life produces a rejection of autopsy in order to protect it after death. Although such feelings can be overcome and often are, the clash produces pain, uncertainty, and conflict of interest. Coupled with the emotional response is an idea that has some support in past history. In earlier years, bodies used for dissection or autopsy were obtained from the ranks of malefactors, disreputable people, paupers, or unclaimed persons (ibid., p. 73). In the United States cadavers have at times been obtained by criminal means through grave robbing and murder, and such desecration of the body contributed to the pejorative attitude of very many people toward autopsy and medical school dissection.

Since medical science cannot afford to be ignorant of the detailed structure and functioning of the human body, especially in the teaching of new physicians, dissection of the body must be undertaken. The Uniform Anatomical Gift Acts enacted in most of the states in the United States have provided a more acceptable and uniform method of providing cadavers or body parts (ibid., p. 254; Luyties, 1969). These acts make it mandatory that an unclaimed body be reported by hospital or morgue authorities to a centrally located office and prepared for use

there. When there is need for cadaver material, the body is turned over on the request of the laboratory or medical school. Bodies may also be obtained from a second category of persons. Those who wish to do so may make, prior to their own deaths, an arrangement with the authorities of the central office or society to release their own bodies for this purpose. Similar instructions may be included in their wills. However, responsibility for carrying out those arrangements rests with the surviving relatives and friends, who, if they have not known about and come to terms with the wishes of the deceased person, may object and refuse to comply.

By far the greatest number of cadavers are still obtained from among those in long-term hospitals who die without known relatives or friends to claim the body. In some places where the act has not been legislated or where it is not enforced, there is a tendency for those in the undertaking business to claim the body because of the availability of money for burial expense provided by third-party payers.

A favorable public opinion with respect to this new way of providing cadavers for dissection is created by public relations activities of medical schools and pathological societies in educating the public to the need for bodies in teaching and biomedical research. In most cases, the arrangements can also specify the final disposition of the unused or remaining cadaveric products following the termination of dissection or experimental procedures. These can be returned either to a relative or to some organization for burial, or be cremated followed by disposition of the ashes.

Organ transplants and other uses of the cadaver

While the most common medical use of the cadaver is autopsy, bodies in increasingly large number are used as the source of tissues or organs for transplant into other living bodies to replace damaged and nonfunctioning tissues. Pathological societies and organizations set up to encourage donation and to receive parts of bodies provide these parts to hospitals on call. As in the case of cadaver donation, arrangements can be made either by the donor or by relatives to give specific tissues or organs for specific purposes.

The donation of and use of body tissues for transplantation are accepted more widely and easily than is total body dissection. This is due in part to the good public relations efforts of such organizations as the Kidney Foundation, several groups concerned with eyesight, and the surgeons and medical organizations dealing with cardiac replacement. It is also due to the fact that only small parts of the body are removed such as corneas and lenses of the eye, one or both kidneys, pieces of bone, and skin. The immediate benefit of these removals is easily seen and can be justified on the basis of aiding the recovery of function and/or survival of another, usually genetically close, human being.

The widely acknowledged value of using cadaveric organs as transplant tissue that can enable living persons in need of such tissue to live has caused those, primarily in the Judaic and Christian traditions, who respect the body of the dead as symbolic of the human person and his dignity, to rethink their attitudes toward the use of cadaveric materials. Earlier it was noted that permission for autopsies was given on the supposition that the tissues examined would be restored to the cadaver prior to final interment. This, obviously, cannot be done when such tissues are used for transplant purposes. Yet those who at one and the same time believe that it is right to use the cadaver for such purposes and that the cadaver requires human respect hold that these two attitudes are by no means necessarily incompatible.

In the case of heart transplant and less stringently with kidney transplant, several technical problems occur. The organ must be removed as close to the time of death as possible in order to ensure proper function of the organ after transplant. This has required in the recent past the use of donors whose brain function has been determined to have ceased. This criterion has been used as the determinant of the state of life or death. Automatic breathing and continued heartbeat, parts of the classic signs of vitality, have lost much of their significance, in favor of signs of brain activity and function. This problem is discussed elsewhere in this encyclopedia in greater detail, but it should be pointed out here that the question of when death actually occurs is of great importance to medical, moral, and ethical authorities, not to mention the donor and his relatives.

The cadaver is also used as the base for the study of embalming and preservation of the body after death. The study of the anatomy of the body by artists in the past was extremely important not only for accurate representation of the body but also in the efforts to obtain permission from secular and religious authorities for dissec-

tion. Both aspects of this material are discussed in detail by Lassek (pp. 38–104).

In the process of continuing medical education and research, cadavers are often used by physicians and researchers whose concern is the more efficient solution of a surgical problem or the development of devices to visualize internal body parts more clearly.

Research on fetal cadavers

There is increasing need felt by the medical profession for examination and experimentation upon fetal tissue in order to obtain information leading to better care and better understanding of disease processes and normal development of the human being.

One of the major problems associated with use of the fetal cadaver is related to the religious and secular views on the value of the human fetus and the respect due to it. Although abortion practices are widely accepted by public and legal institutions as well as by private persons, there is a commonly accepted principle that respect is due to the human fetus. Consequently, we find today policies that place some restrictions on research with human fetuses. There continues to be ethical debate concerning the relevance of such factors as viability, whether a decision has been taken to abort the fetus, whether the abortion is in fact being performed or has been performed, etc.

Public policy on fetal research in Great Britain follows the guidelines proposed by the "Peel Committee Report" in 1972. The committee recommended that no harmful research be performed on the fetus *in utero* and that research on the previable fetus outside the uterus be conducted only when it promises to provide scientific information that cannot be secured in any other way. Research on the dead fetus or on tissues from dead fetuses was permitted by the committee, provided that applicable provisions of the Anatomy Acts of 1832 and 1871 and the Human Tissue Act of 1961 were observed (Great Britain).

In the United States, national policy on fetal research has been established by two sets of federal regulation. The first set, proposed in November 1973 and published in August 1974, was developed by an interagency group within the Department of Health, Education, and Welfare. This set of regulations prohibited nontherapeutic research on the fetus *in utero* in anticipation of abortion but allowed research on the "abortus," provided that such research did not terminate the heartbeat or respiration of the aborted fetus. Research involving the dead fetus was permitted if conducted "in accordance with any applicable State or local laws regarding autopsy" (U.S., DHEW, 1974, p. 30654).

A second set of regulations for fetal research was promulgated by the Assistant Secretary for Health in 1975; several amendments to the regulations followed in early 1977. These revised guidelines were based upon an intensive examination of the fetal research issue undertaken by the National Commission for the Protection of Human Subjects of Biomedical and Behavioral Research, an interdisciplinary public body established by the Congress and appointed by the Secretary of Health, Education, and Welfare. The National Commission solicited testimony on the medical, ethical, and legal aspects of fetal research prior to publishing a detailed report on the issue (National Commission). The commission's recommendations, accepted and translated into regulations, required equal treatment for all fetuses *in utero*, without respect to the mother's intention to carry the fetus to term or to have it aborted. Some types of research on the living but clearly nonviable fetus during or following induced abortion were permitted, but only on condition that the research would not alter the duration of fetal life. Research on the dead fetus was permitted, provided that it was conducted in accordance with "any applicable State or local laws regarding such activities" (U.S., DHEW, 1975, pp. 33529–33530; U.S., DHEW, 1977, p. 2793).

Burial and cremation

The two most commonly used methods of final disposal of a human cadaver are burial and cremation (Lassek, p. 17). Entombment was seen in China and Egypt as a method of protection of the body for its eventual reuse by the spirit following a period of purification and/or trial. Mummification and embalming were used to preserve the tissues of the body so that they could be activated upon the entry of the spirit.

With the advent of Judaism and Christianity, the indissoluble relationship of body and soul was emphasized. Christianity also taught the resurrection of the body for life eternal.

Burial of the cadaver in the earth provides the most direct and simple way of returning all parts of the body to the substance of the earth and is therefore the method of choice for those who strictly hold these beliefs. Anything that inter-feres with the dissolution processes of the body should be avoided. For this reason, embalming is ill thought of in Jewish tradition, although it is permitted when the law requires it for transport of the body over long distances. It is also seen as possible mutilation of the body, which is strictly forbidden in Jewish tradition. Christian thought and practice agree with the Judaic thought, although they have avoided the strict interpretation Jews have used.

In the United States Christian burial rites have changed or varied from place to place depending upon technical skills and materials present, and they have also been strongly influenced by the rise of the undertaking business. In primitive or poor areas, embalming, extended viewing of the body, and elaborate coffins and vaults to contain the coffin were not used. In more affluent or technologically sophisticated regions, with the support of professionals in the field, more and more of the above are found. The question being raised about these practices is whether they provide the proper marks of respect for the deceased person consistent with his or her religious belief, or whether in some cases they are designed more for the survivors than the needs of the deceased. There is no question that modern thought concerning mourning and grief supports the need for rites in which the realization of separation and loss can begin and gain expression, but it is also true that many modern mortuary practices appear antithetical to religious concepts of the real significance of the body.

Cremation was used in China for long periods as a normal method of disposal of the cadaver. Its use in the Western world has not been a standard part or an alternative to burial until relatively recently. That may be due in part to the feeling that burning the body essentially damages it and may inflict anguish upon the soul or spirit. Jewish tradition forbids cremation as mutilation, and, according to Lannin, Orthodox Jews are not permitted to use funeral or memorial rites nor may they bury ashes of a cremated person in a Jewish cemetery for this reason (Lamm).

Christian philosophy has followed the same outline with regard to the return of the entire body to the earth, and for many Roman Catholics and conservative Protestants cremation was seen as an interference with the natural process of dissolution of the body providing unity with the earth. That opinion has changed gradually with the changes in total popular opinion as well as with a greater appreciation of the total physical environment, including the earth, in which the body is found.

Cremation has been adopted by some advocates of ecology as being a more acceptable social policy, preserving cemetery lands for other uses and reducing costs in the disposition of the body.

Conclusion

There is a great deal of evidence that all organized groups of people have struggled both with the concrete problem of the disposition of cadaver material and with the meaning of the cadaver to the deceased person and to the group or society. The cadaver has been feared for the possibilities of what it might become as an agent of evil or unsatisfied spirits; it has been respected for what it has been in the past as the physical representation of the person; and it has been treated with wonder for what it represents in the scheme of creation. Primitive man as well as modern man recognized the physical attributes of the cadaver; it has been the nonphysical, and the relationships between the two, that have puzzled and bedeviled them. Perhaps the worst solution to the problem has been the tendency to ignore the cadaver, for that produces a degradation of all life. The best solution may be the attitude that dictates respect and protection from embarrassment for the helpless and the stranger in our midst.

CHRISTIAN A. HOVDE

[*Directly related are the entries* DEATH, DEFINITION AND DETERMINATION OF, *article on* CRITERIA FOR DEATH; FETAL RESEARCH; HEART TRANSPLANTATION; KIDNEY DIALYSIS AND TRANSPLANTATION; ORGAN DONATION; *and* ORGAN TRANSPLANTATION. *For discussion of related ideas, see the entries:* EMBODIMENT; *and* PERSON.]

BIBLIOGRAPHY

CORNER, GEORGE W. "The Rise of Medicine at Salerno in the Twelfth Century." *Annals of Medical History* n.s. 3 (1931): 1–16.

Doe v. Bolton. 410 U.S. 179. 35 L. Ed. 2d 201. 93 S. Ct. 739 (1973).

FRAZER, JAMES GEORGE. *The Golden Bough: A Study in Magic and Religion.* Vol. 1: abr. ed. New York: Macmillan Co., 1951.

GREENWALD, YEKUTIEL YEHUDAH. *Ko bo 'al avelut* [Compendium of laws about mourning]. 2 vols. New York: Feldheim Publishing Co., 5716[1955].

Great Britain, Department of Health and Social Security, Scottish Home and Health Department, Welsh Office. *The Use of Fetuses and Fetal Material for Research:* *Report of Advisory Group.* London: Her Majesty's Stationery Office, 1972. The Peel Committee report.

HOMER. *Iliad.* Translated by Samuel Butler in *The Great Books of the Western World.* Edited by Robert Maynard Hutchins. Vol 4: *The Iliad of Homer and the Odyssey.* Chicago: Encyclopaedia Britannica, 1952.

JAKOBOVITS, IMMANUEL. *Jewish Medical Ethics: A Comparative and Historical Study of the Jewish Religious Attitude to Medicine and Its Practice.* New York: Bloch Publishing Co., 1962. 2d ed. 1975.

LAMM, MAURICE. *The Jewish Way in Death and Mourning.* New York: Jonathan David Publishers, 1969.

LASSEK, ARTHUR MARVEL. *Human Dissection: Its Drama and Struggle.* Springfield, Ill.: Charles C Thomas, 1958.

LIEBES, YITZCHAK ISAAC. "Be'inyan hashtalat eivarim" [Regarding the transplantation of organs]. *Noam,* vol. 14. Edited by Mosheh Shelomoh Hasher. Jerusalem: Torah Shelemah Institute, 5731[1970], pp. 28–111.

LUYTIES, FREDERIC A. "Suggested Revisions to Clarify the Uncertain Impact of Section Seven of the Uniform Anatomical Gift Act on Determinations of Death." *Arizona Law Review* 11 (1969): 749–769.

MOORE, GEORGE FOOT. *History of Religions.* 1 vol. only. International Theological Library. New York: Charles Scribner's Sons, 1913, vol. 1.

National Commission for the Protection of Human Subjects of Biomedical and Behavioral Research. *Report and Recommendations: Research on the Fetus.* DHEW Publication no. (OS) 76–127. Washington: Department of Health, Education, and Welfare, 1975.

PACKARD, FRANCIS R. "History of the School of Salernum." *The School of Salernum: Regimen Sanitatis Salernitanum.* Edited by John Harrington. New York: Paul B. Hoeber, 1920. Reprint. New York: Augustus M. Kelley, 1970.

Roe v. Wade. 410 U.S. 113. 35 L. Ed. 2d 147. 93 S. Ct. 705 (1973).

SHILOH, AILON, and SELAVAN, IDA COHEN, eds. *Ethnic Groups of America: Their Morbidity, Mortality, and Behavior Disorders.* Vol. 1: *The Jews.* Springfield, Ill.: Charles C Thomas, 1973.

SOPHOCLES. *Antigone.* Translated by Richard C. Jebb in *Great Books of the Western World.* Edited by Robert Maynard Hutchins. Vol. 5: *Aeschylus, Sophocles, Euripides, Aristophanes.* Chicago: Encyclopaedia Britannica, 1952.

United States; Department of Health, Education, and Welfare; Office of the Secretary. "Protection of Human Subjects: Fetuses, Pregnant Women, and In Vitro Fertilization." *Federal Register* 40 (1975): 33526–33551.

———; Department of Health, Education, and Welfare; Office of the Secretary. "Protection of Human Subjects: Proposed Amendments Concerning Fetuses, Pregnant Women, and In Vitro Fertilization." *Federal Register* 42 (1977): 2792–2793.

———; Department of Health, Education, and Welfare; Office of the Secretary. "Protection of Human Subjects: Proposed Policy." *Federal Register* 39 (1974): 30648–30657.

II
JEWISH PERSPECTIVES

Jewish religious thought emphasizes the unique status of human beings as bearers of the divine image. It is this conception which provides the matrix for a variety of regulations governing the treatment of human cadavers.

Sanctity is attributed to the total human personality, not merely to selected elements or aspects. A radical dualism that relegates the body to the realm of imperfection or evil while assigning the soul to the domain of goodness or divinity is totally alien to Judaism. Hence, the physical remains of man, the bearer of the divine image, must not be degraded. A person has only limited rights to his body: One must not dispose of one's body in a manner that violates its dignity.

A human cadaver belongs neither to the heirs nor to society at large. Its inviolability is guarded by stringent prohibitions against deriving any form of benefit from the use of a human corpse. Mutilating or disfiguring a cadaver constitutes a grievous offense, unless circumstances demand it for the enhancement of the dignity of the deceased or for the saving of human life.

Judaism does not merely frown upon outright desecration of the physical remains, but calls for avoidance of even the appearance of insensitivity to the departed. Lest one be guilty of "scoffing at the poor," the Halakhah (Jewish law) prohibits eating or drinking in the presence of a corpse. Even the performance of religious rituals, unless specifically intended to honor or benefit the deceased, would be regarded as a source of embarrassment to the dead who can no longer participate in such activities (Greenwald, p. 35).

Respect for the dead also imposes the obligation to take positive action to protect their dignity. Traditional Jewish law stipulates that the human cadaver must not be left unattended. Interment should take place on the day of death before sunset, unless postponement would significantly enhance respect for the deceased. Burial serves a twofold purpose: (1) removal of a decomposing body eliminates a source of degradation of human dignity; (2) interment is viewed as helpful in attaining atonement for the deceased (Arieli, p. 83). Even explicit instructions of a deceased not to be interred must be disregarded (Greenwald, p. 53). Cremation is strictly forbidden by traditional Jewish law. Embalming is also frowned upon unless necessary to comply with the wish of a deceased to be buried at a particular site.

While Judaism demands respect for a corpse, it does not attribute to it any special sanctity that did not belong to it in life. In fact, separated from the soul, the body is viewed as a source of spiritual impurity. Anyone coming into contact with a human cadaver is disqualified from entering the site of the ancient Temple in Jerusalem or from performing a number of religious rituals until the impurity has been removed by special rites of purification. A Kohen, a member of the priestly tribe and a descendant of the original priest, Aaron, is prohibited from being in the same area or having contact with human cadavers except in the case of the burial of a member of the immediate family.

These restrictions create numerous problems for Orthodox Jews. There are serious questions, for example, whether it is permissible for a member of the priestly tribe to receive cadaver transplants (Liebes, pp. 64–70). Much attention is given to the consideration of the conditions that would permit a physician who is a member of the priestly tribe to attend to a dying patient.

Orthodox Jewish law presents other impediments to medical practice and research. Dissection of cadavers violates the injunction against disfiguring the dead. According to prevailing opinion of orthodox scholars, autopsies can be condoned only when there are indications that the information accruing from them may be of immediate value in saving the life of another individual. Thus postmortem dissections are indicated when an experimental drug or surgical procedure was utilized and the autopsy is likely to shed some light on the merits of the treatment. Similarly, when death was caused by contagious disease or genetic disorder, autopsies are warranted for the purpose of instituting prophylactic treatment or helping with genetic counseling. Most rabbinic authorities also permit postmortem dissections for forensic purposes when mandated by law. But in all cases where autopsies are indicated, they must be limited to the special areas where relevant information may be obtained. Following the examination, all organs must be returned for burial (Tendler, pp. 58–60).

Of late, with the growing utilization of organ transplants, insistence upon the inviolability of the cadaver has created new difficulties. Militating against cadaver transplants are (1) the prohibition against dissection, (2) the prohibition against deriving any benefit from the use of the human corpse, and (3) the obligation to bury the complete remains. Most authorities, however, sanction the removal and use of the cornea when consent has been given by the deceased, since restoration of eyesight is considered a life-saving act, and in addition, the prohibition against the use of external tissue is less stringent than that against the use of organs (Jakobovits, pp. 285–286). Some authorities permit the transplant of organs, provided they are needed for the preservation of life and that explicit permission has been given by the donor or his family (Liebes, p. 62).

WALTER S. WURZBURGER

[*Directly related are the entries on* JUDAISM *and* RELIGIOUS DIRECTIVES IN MEDICAL ETHICS, *article on* JEWISH CODES AND GUIDELINES. *For discussion of related ideas, see the entries:* ORGAN DONATION, *article on* ETHICAL ISSUES; *and* ORGAN TRANSPLANTATION, *article on* ETHICAL PRINCIPLES.]

BIBLIOGRAPHY

ARIELI, YITZCHAK. "Baayat nituchei meitim" [The Problem of Autopsies]. *Noam,* vol. 6. Edited by Mosheh Shelomoh Kasher. Jerusalem: Torah Shelemah Institute, 5723 [1962], pp. 82–103.

FEINSTEIN, MOSHEH [MOSES]. *Igrot Mosheh* [Epistles of Moses]. 5 vols. Vol. 2: *Yoreh deah.* New York: M. Feinstein, 1973.

GREENWALD, YEKUTIEL YEHUDAH. *Kol bo al avelut* [Compendium of Laws about Mourning]. New York: Feldheim Publishing Co., 5716 [1955].

JAKOBOVITS, IMMANUEL. *Jewish Medical Ethics: A Comparative and Historical Study of the Jewish Religious Attitude to Medicine and Its Practice.* New York: Bloch Publishing Co., 1959. New ed., 1975.

LAMM, MAURICE. *The Jewish Way in Death and Mourning.* New York: Jonathan David Co., 1969.

LIEBES, YITZCHAK ISAAC. "Be'inyan hashtalat eivarim" [Regarding the Transplanting of Organs]. *Noam,* vol. 14. Edited by Mosheh Shelomoh Kasher. Jerusalem: Torah Shelemah Institute, 5731 [1970], pp. 28–111.

RABINOVITCH, NACHUM L. "What is the Halakhah for Organ Transplants?" *Tradition* 9, no. 4 (1968), pp. 20–27.

ROSNER, FRED. *Modern Medicine and Jewish Law.* Studies in Toral Judaism, vol. 13. Edited by Leon D. Stitskin. New York: Yeshiva University, Department of Special Publications, 1972.

TENDLER, M. D., ed. *Medical Ethics: A Compendium of Jewish Moral, Ethical and Religious Principles in Medical Practice.* 5th ed. New York: Federation of Jewish Philanthropies, Committee on Religious Affairs, 1975.

CANADA

See MEDICAL ETHICS, HISTORY OF, *section on* EUROPE AND THE AMERICAS, *articles on* NORTH AMERICA: SEVENTEENTH TO NINETEENTH CENTURY; *and* NORTH AMERICA IN THE TWENTIETH CENTURY.

CARE

This entry deals with the value implications of the concept of care as it is used in various biomedical settings and as it affects the physician–patient relationship and the direction of health-related activities.

The ambiguity of "care"

Care and medicine have become closely identified, if not synonymous, in the minds of many. For example, medicine, nursing, and other health-related activities are often referred to as "caring professions." Or "care" is used to indicate that someone is receiving medical aid, e.g.: "She is getting the best care possible." But it is not clear why we associate medicine with care except as we think of both care and medicine as appropriate responses to people in distress.

On analysis, care proves to be an extremely ambiguous notion. We sometimes use "care" to indicate an attitude, feeling, or state of mind about a person or state of circumstance—"I really care for Judy," or "Everyone ought to care for the outdoors." To say that I care for X is, therefore, very similar to saying I like X, except "to care" may denote a stronger intention "to pay particular attention to."

"Care" is also used in a manner that does not involve any attitude, but rather is a correlative to someone's having a certain skill. For example, we say that a mechanic cares for our car not because he likes our car, but because he possesses a technical ability that is necessary to be able to repair a car. He cares for our car because we have established a particular relationship with him, namely, we pay him for his service.

Both senses of care require further specification to determine for what or how one ought to care. "Care" is a context-dependent term, i.e., it carries no particular meaning apart from the context in which it is used. Thus to say that "we ought to care about X or Y" does little more than to remind us that certain kinds of attitudes or skills are appropriate in certain contexts. "Care," like the word "good," is a notion that is incomplete because its significance depends on further specification in relation to particular roles, principles, expectations, or institutions (Kovesi, p. 124).

The reason "care" seems so appropriate to medical and health-related activities is that these activities involve both senses of care. For example, the doctor is expected to care for his patients because he has a responsibility to have a positive attitude toward securing their well-being. But doctors are also expected to have the skills that give them the ability to "take care" of their patients beyond simply "caring" for them. But as I will suggest below, it is by no means clear how these senses of care are interrelated or specified in contemporary medicine.

Moral ambiguity of "medical care"

The identification of medicine with care seems to be based on the assumption that we owe it to someone to pay special attention to them because they are in particular need or trouble. However, when used in this manner the moral force of care is ambiguous. For it is not clear if care as an attitude and care as a skill are both required and, if they are, on what grounds. For example, we normally think that it is a good thing to care for people in need, but we do not generally assume that it is a moral obligation to do so; that someone may know how to repair cars does not mean that he is obligated to repair our car. Do the skills that doctors possess mean that they are morally obligated to care, and if so, why?

Hans Mayeroff has suggested that to care for someone, "I must know many things. I must know, for example, who the other is, what his powers and limitation are" (Mayeroff, p. 13). But in the case of injury or illness we normally assume that the need to maintain basic physical integrity clearly sets the context for the kind of care appropriate. Moreover, because physical need is prerequisite for all other activities we assume that if persons with such need can be helped they should be helped. Thus, while we have no obligation to help some to have a better running car than others, we may feel we should care for them through the office of medicine if it is necessary to maintain their physical existence.

Thus the language of "care" when used in a medical context may assume that, because doctors have the training and skill to care for our physical integrity, they have an obligation to care for those in distress. Care and medicine are closely identified because many of the skills associated with medicine are correlative or even necessary for our most basic human needs. But it does not follow from our assumption that medicine is such a basic form of care that doctors are morally required to provide their service. Such a conclusion must be based on further argument that involves issues that cannot be settled simply by determining whether medicine is or is not a way to "care." Moreover, even if it

can be shown that it is a good thing to try to care for someone through the means of medicine, it does not follow that we always ought to do so by these means.

It may well be that we should care for the injured or the ill, but it is by no means clear that medicine offers the best or only way to care for them. Whether the "care" that medicine can provide should be provided will depend on the kind and extent of the medical skill that has been developed. For example, are we required to provide all the "medical care" that is technically possible to someone suffering from kidney disease? Such questions are not meant to deny that medicine may be a basic form of care, but they do make clear that, even if that is the case, whether such care should be provided remains open to decision by doctor and patient.

Paul Ramsey, however, has argued that "care" is not meant to provide a basis for judgment for specific actions in the medical context. Rather, "care" is the "source of all particular obligations and one's court of final appeal for deciding the features of actions and practices that makes what we do right or wrong in any context" (Ramsey, 1976, p. 47). Ramsey suggests that this sense of care generates basic rules of practice that embody the physician's commitment to the "preciousness of life." Indeed, it is Ramsey's contention that such an ethics of care provides the basis for a professional ethic that consists in: "(1) rules constitutive of medical care, e.g. the consent requirement, the prohibition of direct killing, and randomizing life-and-death decisions to insure equality of access to sparse resources, which are always binding; (2) directives to cure and save life which true care sometimes suspends and replaces by comfort and dignity for the dying; (3) balancing situational decisions, such as to operate or not to operate, or to use this or that research protocol" (ibid., p. 51). However, as we shall see below, many doubt if "care" in itself can generate the kind of ethic Ramsey thinks it implies.

Medical care as personal care

The emphasis on care as a morally significant notion for medicine often serves as a way to stress that patients have needs that are other than "strictly medical." It is not enough for physicians to provide the best technological care available; they also have a responsibility to treat the patient as a "whole person" (Menninger). The demand for a more humane practice of medicine is not a call for the physician to be personally concerned about the patient over and above what he or she can do for the patient medically, but rather it is to remind physicians that their responsibility is to treat not a disease or a medical problem but the person who is subject to the disease or injury. In other words, care and compassion for the patient are not just something nice for the physician to have beyond his responsibilities as a physician, but such personal care is an integral component for the practice of good clinical medicine.

To care in this manner means that the physician must have the capacity to share in the pain and anguish of those who seek help from him. It means that the physician must "have some understanding of what sickness means to another person, together with a readiness to help and to see the situation as the patient does. Compassion demands that the physician be so disposed that his every action and word will be rooted in respect for the person he is serving" (Pellegrino, p. 1289). Such care should not be confused with pity, condescension, or paternalism. Rather it is to respect the uniqueness of each patient by helping the patient to make those choices that are best for him or her.

Though most assume the physician should "care" in this compassionate or personal manner, the matter is not quite as straightforward as it seems. For, while few deny the medical importance of empathy for the physician's treatment of the patient, it cannot be forgotten that competent care is equally important. "Which would you rather have—warm, compassionate care to usher you into the next world, or cool scientific care to pull you back to this one?" (Greenberg, pp. 205–206.) It is, of course, hoped that this rhetorical question does not present a genuine alternative, since good medicine should combine both (Cassell, 1975, p. 2). The problem for doctors and patients alike is "how the priceless personal equation can be retained in the face of the constantly expanding arsenal of knowledge and inexorable trend toward mass production in medicine no less than in other fields. For, to be true to his calling, a doctor must always complement his expertise with his understanding and view the patient as a whole person rather than merely the sum of his symptoms" (Greenberg, p. 206).

It is important to note, however, that what it means for anyone to care for the "whole person" remains ambiguous. The problem of the kind of personal care the physician should give the patient is not just occasioned by the increasingly sophisticated technology or the demand of justice to try to extend the physician's skill to as many as possible. But it is not clear that care of the "whole person" simply means to treat patients with empathy or compassion. Indeed, it may well be that to treat someone impersonally is a way of caring, especially if we remember that respect is an important aspect of all care. For, if respect is missing, the physician's concern for the patient, even with the best will, can too easily become paternalistic manipulation. For example, the respect due the patient may perhaps mean that the physician must allow the patient not to choose to be "cared" for medically. Open-heart surgery may help many, but that does not mean that the physician has grounds for urging all his patients to undergo such surgery.

Care and the primacy of the patient's interest

The importance of understanding "care" in terms of respect is the basis of Paul Ramsey's suggestion that "care" is the term that best expresses "the ultimate requirement or standard or warrant binding in all cases upon the helping and healing profession" (Ramsey, 1973, p. 20). That the physician must "care" does not mean just that the patient should be given personal care, but that the physician has a commitment to each individual patient that is not and cannot be overridden by any other consideration. Care or respect for the patient, therefore, carries the substantive commitment that no patient should be cared for as a means for the betterment of others without his or her consent. In the language of normative ethics this means that the requirement of the physician to care for each individual patient is a basic deontological commitment that cannot be overridden by any considerations including teleological ones, e.g., the physician must continue to give care to the aged even though by ignoring them he might be able to serve more patients. Such a commitment sets the primary task of medical ethics, according to Ramsey, which is to reconcile the welfare of the individual with the welfare of mankind when both must be served (Ramsey, 1970, p. xiv).

Even if it is generally accepted that a physician may have an overriding commitment to each patient in his care, medicine and its practitioners face issues that such a commitment does not resolve. Such grounds make problematic the commitment of public health medicine to "care" for a "patient" that may be a city, state, or country. For example, does the commitment to care for the individual patient mean physicians should not recommend everyone be inoculated against an illness because they know that a few will die from the inoculation itself?

The commitment to care for the individual patient is certainly an important and perhaps even crucial commitment for medical ethics. The problem is that such a commitment, in itself, is not sufficient to show how we should care in such complex matters as the just allocation of scarce medical resources (Fried, 1970, pp. 183–207). Nor is it sufficient to determine the ethical guidelines as to how we should think about the use of statistical lives, random clinical trials, and the risks that are inherent in the development and practice of normal medicine. Because of these kinds of problems some argue that the kind of "care" offered by medicine cannot be limited to the needs of the individual patient.

Even if "care" is so limited, many questions remain unanswered about what form such "care" should take. For it is often unclear what it means for the doctor to act or to refrain from acting in the patient's interest. The definition of the patient's "interest" that is important to guide the physician depends on the definition of health, which is itself in need of clarification. "The concept of good health implies a concept of the good life, and the goodness of life includes a large number of other factors besides simply its length" (Fried, 1974, p. 150). But without a more detailed or concrete sense of what those "factors" should be, and what kind of particular responsibility medicine has for sustaining and enhancing them, there can be little consensus about what kind of "care" the physician is obligated to give the patient. Indeed, some have recently argued that there is no readily apparent moral position or philosophy that can provide the moral direction that medicine necessarily requires (MacIntyre, pp. 97–111).

It is often assumed that for a physician to care for a patient means that he should try to cure the patient. To confuse care with cure often results in the cruel abandonment of the dying, as we assume we can no longer care for them if we cannot cure them. Moreover, it may be that some patients are subjected to attempts to cure them in a manner that is antithetical to caring for them. For example, to encourage some patients to undergo surgery that only sustains but does not enhance their lives may be incompatible with care. Ironically the technological power of modern medicine raises the question whether it is not often the best way to care for the patient by refraining from doing what medically we have the skill and power to do. This kind of issue makes many decisions in neonatal care today particularly agonizing (Hauerwas, pp. 222–236).

The problem of the relation between caring and curing is perhaps most clearly, but by no means exclusively, illustrated in relation to how we deal with the dying. For example, even though Ramsey argues that medical care as a moral institution can never act directly to take the life of a terminal patient, there comes a time when to respect life means *only* to care for the dying. This means we must be ready to be with the dying, to comfort them, to assure we will not desert them, but at the same time we will not oppose their death. This means that the requirement to care and to save life is not always to be applied strictly in medical practice. "Care never ceases; yet care, never ceasing, has no duty to do the impossible or useless" (Ramsey, 1973, p. 24; 1970, pp. 124–132).

Ramsey, therefore, seems to indicate that the "care" that is incumbent on doctors does not involve simply their medical skills, but the moral skill to be present with those who are suffering. However, it is not clear why the doctor's role involves such a skill. To be sure, communities should provide someone to "only care for the dying," but there is no reason to think the doctor has any different obligation from those of any of us in this respect. It may be, however, that because of their experience in dealing with the sick and the dying doctors have learned better how to care for them, that is, to be with them, better than most of us.

Care, respect, and truth-telling

If care is not equivalent to cure, then the question of what kind of care is due the patient remains open. While no general notion of "care" can be given to account for every kind of medical context, it is clear that a fundamental respect for the patient is required in all medical care. This is often difficult in the medical context because the patient's helplessness and suffering often seem to require that the independence of the patient be qualified in order to "help" the patient. But the inequity of power in such helping situations should but remind us that care for another must be done in a manner that his integrity is not violated (Mayeroff, p. 17; Nelson, pp. 29–30). To care for another is to help him maintain or establish an independent existence, which means to help him care for something or someone else. It also means to help the person to care for himself and become responsive to his own need to care and be responsible for his life (Mayeroff, pp. 10–11).

Charles Fried, therefore, suggests that, whatever else care may involve, it must provide the conditions for the maintenance of the patient's lucidity, autonomy, fidelity, and humanity (1974, pp. 101–104). Lucidity requires that the patient know all the relevant details about the situation in which he finds himself. Autonomy means that, even if a patient is fully informed but does not wish to undergo the therapy recommended by the physician, he cannot be forced to do so. For a person's autonomy to be respected requires that he be allowed to dispose himself according to the life plan and conception he has chosen.

Fidelity requires that we meet the justified expectations that develop from our dealing with one another. Such expectations are often not articulated, but they are not any less significant because they are implicit. Not to meet such expectations is a form of deceit of which lying is but the most dramatic example. The notion of humanity, while admittedly vague, requires that a person should be treated in a manner that does justice to his particular wishes and desires. A person may have no right to be treated affirmatively, but once we are in a significant relationship, our wants, needs, and vulnerabilities should not be ignored. Simply being treated honestly and with autonomy is not sufficient. We should also be noticed (ibid., p. 103).

Assumed in this account of "care" is the importance of telling the patient the truth about his condition. For to withhold the truth is to fail to respect his status as a moral agent capable of being lucid, autonomous, and faithful. Put positively, to care for a patient means that he is to be treated in a manner that assumes that he or she is capable of acting in a morally responsible way. Concretely this means that the simple fact that we are dying does not release us from being held morally responsible for how we die. Moreover, if the patient is unwilling to know the truth about his condition, that does not mean his family or the physician has the right to withhold the truth. However, the importance of the patient's knowing the truth does not mean that he or she must be told the truth bluntly or without feeling. Rather, part of what it means to be truthful in the context of medical ethics is that the truth be spoken to a patient in a skillful, kind, and caring manner.

Conclusion

Care often appears to be a more important regulative notion for determining the moral basis and direction of health-related activities than is morally justified. Care, however, is a significant notion that reminds us that medicine serves as one of the ways we can help others maintain basic physical and psychological integrity. Moreover, care directs our attention to the concrete patient in need without subjecting him or her to manipulation for the good of others. However, it is important that the care given the patient be based on the respect due each of us, well or ill, for otherwise our attempts to care can lead to sentimental or paternalistic perversions.

STANLEY HAUERWAS

[*For further discussion of topics mentioned in this article, see the entries:* CHRONIC CARE; HEALTH CARE; INFORMED CONSENT IN THE THERAPEUTIC RELATIONSHIP; PATERNALISM; PERSON; RIGHTS; THERAPEUTIC RELATIONSHIP; *and* TRUTH-TELLING. *For discussion of related ideas, see the entries:* ACTING AND REFRAINING; HEALTH AS AN OBLIGATION; HEALTH AND DISEASE; MEDICAL MALPRACTICE; *and* RATIONING OF MEDICAL TREATMENT.]

BIBLIOGRAPHY

CASSELL, ERIC. *The Healer's Art: A New Approach to the Doctor–Patient Relationship.* New York: J. B. Lippincott Co., 1976.

———. "Preliminary Explorations of Thinking in Medicine." *Ethics in Science and Medicine* 2 (1975): 1–12.

FRIED, CHARLES. *An Anatomy of Values: Problems of Personal and Social Choice.* Cambridge: Harvard University Press, 1970.

———. *Medical Experimentation: Personal Integrity and Social Policy.* Clinical Studies, A North-Holland Frontier Series, vol. 5. Edited by A. G. Bearn, D. A. K. Black, and H. H. Hyatt. New York: 1974.

GREENBERG, SELIG. *The Quality of Mercy: A Report on the Critical Condition of Hospital and Medical Care in America.* New York: Atheneum, 1971.

HAUERWAS, STANLEY. "The Demands and Limits of Care: Ethical Reflections on the Moral Dilemma of Neonatal Intensive Care." *American Journal of the Medical Sciences* 269 (1975): 22–236.

KOVESI, JULIUS. *Moral Notions.* Studies in Philosophical Psychology. Edited by R. F. Holland. New York: Humanities Press, 1967.

MacINTYRE, ALASDAIR. "How Virtues Become Vices: Values, Medicine and Social Context." *Evaluation and Explanation in the Biomedical Sciences: Proceedings of the First Trans-Disciplinary Symposium on Philosophy and Medicine, Held at Galveston, May 9–11, 1974.* Edited by H. Tristram Engelhardt, Jr. and Stuart F. Spicker. *Philosophy and Medicine,* vol. 1. Dordrecht-Holland and Boston: D. Reidel Publishing Co., 1975.

MAYEROFF, MILTON. *On Caring*. World Perspectives, vol. 43. Edited by Ruth Nanda Anshen. New York: Harper & Row, 1971.

MENNINGER, W. WALTER. " 'Caring' as Part of Health Care Quality." *Journal of the American Medical Association* 234 (1975): 836–837.

NELSON, JAMES BRUCE. *Human Medicine: Ethical Perspectives on New Medical Issues*. Minneapolis: Augsburg Publishing House, 1973.

PELLEGRINO, EDMUND D. "Educating the Humanist Physician: An Ancient Ideal Reconsidered." *Journal of the American Medical Association* 227 (1974): 1288–1294.

RAMSEY, PAUL. "Conceptual Foundations for an Ethics of Medical Care: A Response." *Ethics and Health Policy*. Edited by Robert M. Veatch and Roy Branson. Cambridge: Ballinger Publishing Co., 1976, pp. 35–55.

————. "The Nature of Medical Ethics." *The Teaching of Medical Ethics: National Conference on the Teaching of Medical Ethics Sponsored by the Institute of Society, Ethics and the Life Sciences and Columbia University, College of Physicians and Surgeons, June 1–3, 1972*. Edited by Robert M. Veatch, Willard Gaylin, and Councilman Morgan. Hastings-on-Hudson, N.Y.: Hastings Center Publication, 1973, pp. 14–28.

————. *The Patient as Person: Explorations in Medical Ethics*. The Hyman Beecher Lectures, 1969. New Haven: Yale University Press, 1970.

CATHOLIC ETHICS

See ROMAN CATHOLICISM.

CATHOLIC HOSPITALS

See RELIGIOUS DIRECTIVES IN MEDICAL ETHICS, *article on* ROMAN CATHOLIC DIRECTIVES; ROMAN CATHOLICISM; HOSPITALS.

CERTIFICATION OF DEATH

See DEATH, DEFINITION AND DETERMINATION OF, *article on* LEGAL ASPECTS OF PRONOUNCING DEATH.

CHAPLAINS

See PASTORAL MINISTRY.

CHEMICAL WARFARE

See WARFARE.

CHILD ABUSE

See CHILDREN AND BIOMEDICINE; *and* INFANTS, *articles on* ETHICAL PERSPECTIVES ON THE CARE OF INFANTS *and* PUBLIC POLICY AND PROCEDURAL QUESTIONS.

CHILDBIRTH

See WOMEN AND BIOMEDICINE, *article on* WOMEN AS PATIENTS AND EXPERIMENTAL SUBJECTS.

CHILDREN AND BIOMEDICINE

Introduction: definitions and scope

The definition of the child is elusive; dictionaries give the following meanings of the term: "unborn or recently born," "a young person," or simply, "a son or daughter of human parents." In medicine childhood is generally defined as the "period between infancy and puberty" (Stedman). In law, a "child of tender age" is any "progeny . . . less than 14 years" (Black), but state statutes vary.

The boundary between fetus and infant is a shifting one, and ethical issues affecting fetuses are of obvious relevance to the well-being of postnatal children. The boundary between childhood and adulthood is still harder to define; it is less distinct biologically and spans a broad range of psychological and social characteristics. Definitions are even more arbitrary at this end of the scale, and, as with the fetal boundary, the definition may have profound implications for the health and well-being of a particular child.

The drawing of lines based strictly on age—whether between childhood and adulthood, embryo and fetus, fetus and child—can be seen as arbitrary, for this criterion implies that an organism passes in an instant from one status to another. Boundaries may be necessary as guides, to warn us when a significant transition may be occurring, but in an individual case it would be advisable to avoid decisions based on such strict status criteria.

A second definitional problem involves the proper scope of "medical-ethical" concerns. A child's right to health cannot be separated from his nutrition, social status, and education. A consideration of medical-ethical issues concerning children cannot be complete if it confines itself to such classic problems as experimentation and transplantation, which directly affect a minute percentage of the population, while ignoring ethical issues affecting the physical and emotional health of many more children. Such problems—including malnutrition, child abuse, custody proceedings, and citizenship rights in general—can only be mentioned in passing. This article will be confined to general considerations in the therapeutic and experimental relationships.

Finally, there are medical-ethical issues—such as the allocation of scarce resources, management of the terminally ill, and the boundary between research and innovative care—that are not peculiar to children but are compounded in the pediatric setting. The central complicating factor for the child is his inability, presumed or real, to speak for himself, leaving him both vulnerable to adult perceptions of his best interest and powerless against competing adult self-interests.

Historical aspects

"The history of childhood is a nightmare from which we have only recently begun to awaken" (DeMause). While DeMause's prose might be considered lurid by some, there is ample documentation of the lowly status of children throughout history. Even Ariès, who argues that the child's plight is becoming worse and not better, asserts that childhood was only "discovered" around the thirteenth century in the Christian era (Ariès).

The documented history of child abuse and infanticide provides dramatic evidence (DeMause; Langer). It is likely that "a very large percentage of the children born prior to the eighteenth century were what would today be termed battered children" (DeMause). It is not until 1690 that one can discover a biography of a child who has not been beaten, and in one Western European country eighty percent of the parents still admit to beating their children, thirty-five percent with canes (ibid.).

The widespread tolerance of infanticide has been easier to document. It has long been used as a means of population control and continues to be accepted in some underdeveloped cultures (Langer). From ancient times until the twentieth century the low status of infants and children made such practices commonplace. In seventeenth-century China thousands of babies were thrown on the streets like refuse each day, and in nineteenth-century London, Paris, and St. Petersburg the public "foundling homes" were admitting up to 5,000 infants annually for a more socially acceptable death sentence. Even where laws existed they were seldom enforced, so that in Disraeli's London infanticide flourished and the "police seemed to think no more of finding a dead child than of finding a dead dog or cat" (ibid.).

By the end of the nineteenth century, in response to exposés in the press and pressure from the medical societies, England had begun to tighten and enforce protective statutes. The early American colonies were apparently more solicitous, although by 1826 the laws of New York would still not allow state intervention with parents who grossly abused their children (Radbill). In 1838 the Pennsylvania Supreme Court invoked the doctrine of *parens patriae* for superseding parental authority. In the mid-twentieth century social acceptance of active killing of normal children had all but disappeared from Western societies, but passive euthanasia of infants with birth defects is still openly practiced in England and the United States (Duff and Campbell; Lorber).

The child and health care

The recent trend in the United States is for increasing state intervention on behalf of the child's health. Statutes on child abuse, now in effect in every state of the United States (Paulsen), encourage or require physicians and others to report suspicions to appropriate authorities, with civil or criminal penalties for failing to do so. In some jurisdictions a child may sue his parent for a negligence tort (*Emery* v. *Emery*), a principle generally denied earlier in this century. The juvenile court system—a well-intentioned attempt to protect children from hazards of the criminal justice system—was, in the mid-1970s, under pressure from judicial decisions requiring that children be given equal status in matters such as right to counsel, cross-examination, and protection from self-incrimination (In re *Gault*).

Concurrent with these legislative and judicial reactions to gross abuse has been a trend for state involvement in positive, preventive measures affecting the health of children. Compulsory immunization and fluoridation have been upheld not only for the protection of the community but as being in the interest of individual children (*Cude* v. *State; Mannus* v. *State*). Nearly all U.S. states require screening of newborns for phenylketonuria (National Research Council), a rare and preventable cause of mental retardation, and most states have enacted laws enabling minors to seek medical care without parental consent under specified circumstances, particularly when venereal disease is involved (Hofman and Pilpel).

Some see these trends as an excessive swing of the pendulum. The granting to young adolescents of full rights to medical care may undermine a parent's authority to affect the child's behavior, and may perhaps widen the gulf between parent and child, depriving the latter of a potentially valuable counselor. The winning of such rights, in this view, can be a pyrrhic victory for some children who become unintentionally isolated. In some states a child of *any* age may receive treatment for venereal disease without parental knowledge or consent (Wisconsin Statutes). To illustrate the undesirable consequences, consider an eleven-year-old girl who sought treatment for gonorrhea. She insisted that the treating physician promise not to inform her parents. Because of the reporting requirement, a public health nurse conducted an inquiry and discovered that the child was being repeatedly sexually assaulted after school by a sixteen-year-old neighbor prior to the parents' arrival from work. The nurse felt that the pledge of confidentiality by the doctor bound her to conceal the facts from the parents. It later became apparent that, with modest encouragement, the child was able to discuss this with her parents and enlist their support. While the statute enabling the physician to treat the child did not require him to exclude the parents, a narrow concept of the "rights" of the child may have led the health professionals to become involved in a drama that did not serve the child's best interests.

In the area of child abuse, it is also argued that excessively broad notions of neglect permit or encourage premature or inappropriate state intervention. Abuse is often not defined (Paulsen) and, particularly when extended to include emotional injury, may be used by zealous physicians or social workers to intervene punitively in families where there is either no clear abuse, or where a custody change may be more harmful than an admittedly unsatisfactory home situation (Goldstein, Freud, and Solnit).

Implicit in all deprivations of equal status for children is the notion that it is permissible for an adult to substitute his judgment for that of the child (Dworkin; Schrag), based on the assumptions that the adult has the best interests of the child at heart, and that he or she is better qualified than the child to make decisions in the child's interest. While these assumptions are true enough to gain acceptance as general principles, the exceptions are sufficiently common to arouse concern (Fost; McCollum and Schwartz; Robertson and Fost). This concern over paternalism applies to purely therapeutic as well as experimental interventions. It is not clear, for example, that a parent who advocates passive euthanasia for a newborn with Down's syndrome and intestinal obstruction is primarily seeking relief for the child rather than himself

(Gustafson). Nor is it always clear that such parents have any meaningful information to support the contention that death is more advantageous to the child than life. Similarly, a parent who initiates a behavior modification program for his child's bed-wetting may be primarily seeking relief of his own annoyance and might have difficulty establishing that the benefit–risk ratio of the behavior program is more advantageous to the child than continuation of the symptom.

While the limitations of substituted judgment by parents can be argued in the traditional therapeutic setting, it is in the area of experimentation where the validity of such proxy consent has been most extensively discussed. This will be analyzed further in the next section.

Experimentation in children

The many and complex problems of human experimentation are compounded in the pediatric setting by four factors. First, children are not simply small adults, but are biologically different in many ways, so that knowledge acquired from adult subjects often cannot be applied to children without testing them. Moreover, the U.S. Food and Drug Administration requires that drug labeling confine recommendations to adults unless testing on children has been conducted. Second, there are many diseases that occur exclusively in children, so that advances in understanding may be absolutely dependent on the use of children (Capron; Lowe, Alexander, and Mishkin). Third, the hazards of experimentation may be greater in younger age groups. Physical injuries that might be trivial in a mature person (such as radiation of the growing portion of a long bone) can become magnified when occurring early in the developmental process. Events that may have little psychological significance for an adult, such as a short hospitalization or repeated venepunctures, may have profound detrimental effects on a child. Fourth, uncoerced informed consent, the keystone of protection of human subjects, is often unattainable from the minor.

There is broad consensus that therapeutic experimentation—nonstandard interventions that have the explicit primary intent of helping the subject to whom they are being applied—can be practiced in children without major modification of the rules that apply to experimentation in general, so long as consent from a legally authorized representative is given (Curran and Beecher; Great Britain; World Medical Association). This is not to imply that present regulation of adult experimentation is satisfactory, or that parental consent for nonexperimental therapy is without controversy. But it is in the realm of nontherapeutic experimentation where concerns are greatest. Ideally, risk, benefit, and consent should all reside in the same person. When nontherapeutic research is conducted on a child, it is the child who bears the risk, while future persons gain the possible benefits, and a third party, without risk or benefit, gives consent.

Whether or not parents can legally consent to nontherapeutic interventions on their children is unresolved. The Nuremberg Code does not mention children but implies they should be excluded as subjects by stating it is "absolutely essential . . . that the person involved should have legal capacity to give consent." The Declaration of Helsinki allows nontherapeutic studies on children with consent of the legal guardian. Current (1976) regulations of the U.S. Department of Health, Education, and Welfare (DHEW) do not distinguish between the right of the guardian to consent for nontherapeutic versus therapeutic research.

In the United States, statutory law on the subject has been nonexistent until the 1970s, and as of 1975 the specific question had never been explicitly decided in a court. A 1974 federal statute created the National Commission for the Protection of Human Subjects of Biomedical and Behavioral Research, but this body was given a strictly advisory role (Public Law 93-348). The case of Neilsen v. *Regents of University of California* raised, for the first time, the explicit question of whether a parent may volunteer a child for nontherapeutic research.

Related cases come from the field of transplantation, arising when physicians and/or parents seek to use a legally incompetent person as kidney donor for a relative. The general response of courts has been to require a finding of benefit for the donor, such as the advantages derived from future experiences with the recipient should he survive, or the avoidance of remorse due to loss of companionship or later guilt from realizing that one had failed to come to the aid of his sibling (Baron, Botsford, and Cole). In instances where the donor was incapable of experiencing such benefit because of severe mental disability or where the social contact with the sibling was not close, permission to allow the transplantation has been denied (*Lausier* v. *Pescinski;* In re *Richardson*). While many of the

cases regarding incompetent donors involved intelligent adolescents or retarded adults, the general principle of the legitimacy of proxy consent would seem applicable to children in general, and at least one appellate case did involve a seven-year-old donor (*Hart* v. *Brown*).

In contrast is the famous and much disputed case of *Bonner* v. *Moran,* in which an appellate court ruled that a skin graft taken from a fifteen-year-old boy could not be upheld unless the mother consented. One legal scholar takes the decision to imply that such parental consent would have made the procedure valid, despite the absence of a direct benefit (Curran and Beecher), but the decision as written leaves room for disagreement as to how much it can be extended to nontherapeutic experimentation (Capron).

In Great Britain the Medical Research Council has stated that "parents and guardians of minors cannot give consent on their behalf to any procedures which are of no particular benefit to them and which may carry some risk of harm," although legal precedent or authority for this is obscure (Curran and Beecher).

Proxy consent

As with other ethical issues, the already complex and unresolved problems of consent are compounded when children are involved. The assumption that parents can provide uncoerced informed consent for their children rests at least on the presumption that they can provide it for themselves. There is evidence that educated, competent adults are frequently not adequately informed to give meaningful consent (Fellner and Marshall; Fletcher; Gray), so their ability to speak for others may be questioned. The barriers may not be so much a lack of intelligence or motivation on the part of patient or physician as more complex forces such as the anxiety of illness, the intimidating milieu of the hospital, and a sense of awe, trust, and dependence on the physician—all of which may conspire to make solicitation of consent a ritual wherein few are meaningfully informed (Ingelfinger).

In addition to these general barriers to informed consent, there are aspects peculiar to the parent–child relationship that complicate the matter further. The perceived vulnerability of the child may evoke excessive anxiety, which further clouds judgment. The parent may be acting out unconscious hostile wishes against the child, particularly if he is retarded or deformed. There may be a wish to repay the physician–investigator for prior service by offering the child as a sacrifice.

Even if these obstacles were overcome, the practice of proxy consent rests on other notions under challenge: the claim that a person may *ever* consent to a nontherapeutic intervention on another (Ramsey, 1970, 1976); the assumption that adults can reliably assess what is in a child's best interest; and the faith that they are capable of acting in a person's best interest, even if it can be accurately identified. The observation that adults frequently cannot identify or act in their own best interest—as manifested by decisions ranging from smoking and drinking to marriage and financial investments—undermines these assumptions.

Two common justifications for proxy consent are the *substituted judgment* doctrine, a legal doctrine which suggests that decisions be based on what the person would be likely to do if competent (Robertson), and the ethical notion that a child can be volunteered on the basis of what he *ought* to do (McCormick).

The substituted judgment doctrine is weakened by the inability of an adult to know the child's mind. Put another way, the adult may err by being able only to imagine what a reasonable adult would do if in the situation of the child, thereby fallaciously equating adult values and preferences with those of children. An adult might gladly consent to a venepuncture, a procedure of minimal risk and annoyance, but for a child the same event could be a major psychological trauma. Presumptions of what adults would do may suffer from misperceptions of the empirical situation. One could presume that adults probably would consent to minimally hazardous nontherapeutic procedures, but in many communities they in fact do not participate, unless offered significant inducements. One implication of this might be that a minimum requirement for the use of nonconsenting children in nontherapeutic studies (assuming other objections can be overcome) would include some age-appropriate indirect benefit or reward comparable to the monetary rewards that an adult would receive.

McCormick has argued that children may be used for nontherapeutic studies to which they *ought* to consent, on the grounds that there are some sacrifices all members of the human community ought to make, and it is in their interest to do so. While there might be agreement on what sacrifices people ought to make, many would object to the recruitment of children without their consent, unless adults were also required to participate on the same grounds, unrelated to their consent.

Ramsey has taken the extreme view that proxy consent for nonbeneficial experiments in children are unethical without qualification (Ramsey, 1970). He later modified this by acknowledging that such research might be done so long as one acknowledged that he was "doing wrong for the sake of the public good" (1976). Reluctantly admitting that it might be wrong, in some circumstances, *not* to do the research, he seemed to be pointing up an aspect of all true ethical dilemmas: that they involve conflicts of two important obligations, with the inevitable consequence that something of value will be lost no matter which way the conflict is resolved.

As the child gets older—and intellectual and emotional maturity allow him increasingly to participate in decisions—some have advocated a requirement that the child consent in addition to the parent, even though the child may be legally incompetent (U.S. DHEW, National Institutes of Health). While such a practice sounds appealing, there is some evidence that a principle may be honored at the expense of the child's emotional well-being. One study concluded that children informed of the research nature of their hospitalization experienced overwhelming anxiety, due in part to fantasies aroused by their primitive notions of research (Schwartz).

Rules based on inflexible age boundaries may not serve the needs of individual persons. Many children can and should be included in discussions of their participation in research; many adults are incapable of participating meaningfully. Ideally, decisions would be based on a full consideration of the facts in each case, including the probability of discomfort and risk and the emotional and intellectual capacity for consent in each child.

Requirements for consent serve two functions: protection from unacceptable risks and respect for the autonomy of each individual. It appears that trust in consent as protection from unacceptable risks has been misplaced (Fletcher; Gray) and, in the case of young children, respecting autonomy may be impossible unless nontherapeutic research is avoided entirely. If such studies are to continue, it will be necessary to pay attention to Ramsey's reminder that it is not an unmitigated good, that something of value is being lost, and that it is possible for a subject to be "wronged without being harmed" (Ramsey, 1970).

While there is obviously no consensus on a precise formulation of rules affecting nontherapeutic research on children, the following principles would probably attract broad support: (1) Children should be used only as a last resort, when information cannot be obtained in any other way. (2) Nontherapeutic studies on children should be of minimal risk. (3) The right of the child to withdraw should be respected. (4) Proxy consent, if appropriate at all, should be based on a notion of what a competent and reasonable person would do: Whether parents will actually make such a judgment in the best interest of the child is only a matter of presumption.

NORMAN C. FOST

[*For further discussion of topics mentioned in this article, see the entries:* DEATH AND DYING: EUTHANASIA AND SUSTAINING LIFE, *articles on* ETHICAL VIEWS *and* PROFESSIONAL AND PUBLIC POLICIES; HUMAN EXPERIMENTATION; INFORMED CONSENT IN THE THERAPEUTIC RELATIONSHIP; INFORMED CONSENT IN HUMAN RESEARCH; ORGAN TRANSPLANTATION; PATERNALISM; PATIENTS' RIGHTS MOVEMENT; RATIONING OF MEDICAL TREATMENT; RIGHT TO REFUSE MEDICAL CARE; RIGHTS; *and* RISK. *For discussion of related ideas, see the entries:* ADOLESCENTS; AGING AND THE AGED, *article on* HEALTH CARE AND RESEARCH IN THE AGED; CONFIDENTIALITY; FETAL RESEARCH; *and* INFANTS. *See* APPENDIX, SECTION III, PEDIATRIC BILL OF RIGHTS.]

BIBLIOGRAPHY

"AMA Ethical Guidelines for Clinical Investigation." *Annals of Internal Medicine* 67, no. 3, pt. 2, supp. 7, appendix 5 (1967), pp. 76–77. Adopted by the House of Delegates, American Medical Association, 30 November 1966.

ARIÈS, PHILIPPE. *Centuries of Childhood: A Social History of Family Life.* Translated by Robert Baldick. New York: Vintage Books, 1965. Translation of *L'Enfant et la vie familiale sous l'Ancien Régime.*

BARON, CHARLES H; BOTSFORD, MARGOT; and COLE, GARRICK F. "Live Organ and Tissue Transplants from Minor Donors in Massachusetts." *Boston University Law Review* 55 (1975): 159–193.

BEECHER, HENRY KNOWLES. *Research and the Individual: Human Studies.* Boston: Little, Brown & Co., 1970. Contains an extensive collection of codes.

BLACK, HENRY CAMPBELL. *Black's Law Dictionary.* 4th ed. Minneapolis: West Publishing Co., 1968.

Bonner v. Moran. 126 F. 2d 121 (D.C. Cir. 1941).

CAMPBELL, A. G. M. "Infants, Children, and Informed Consent." *British Medical Journal* 3 (1974): 334–338.

CAPRON, ALEXANDER MORGAN. "Legal Considerations Affecting Clinical Pharmacological Studies in Children." *Clinical Research* 21 (1973): 141–150.

Cude v. State. 237 Ark. 927. 377 S.W. 2d 816 (1964).

CURRAN, WILLIAM J., and BEECHER, HENRY K. "Experimentation in Children." *Journal of the American Medical Association* 210 (1969): 77–83.

DeMAUSE, LLOYD. *The History of Childhood.* New York: Psychohistory Press, 1974.

DUFF, RAYMOND S., and CAMPBELL, A. G. M. "Moral and Ethical Dilemmas in the Special Care Nursery." *New England Journal of Medicine* 289 (1973): 890–894.

DWORKIN, GERALD. "Paternalism." *Morality and the Law.* Edited by Richard A. Wasserstrom. Belmont, Calif.: Wadsworth Publishing Co., 1971, pp. 107–126.

Emery v. Emery. 289 P. 2d 218 (Cal. 1955).

Federal Food, Drug, and Cosmetic Act. 21 U.S.C. sec. 301 (1962).

FELLNER, CARL H., and MARSHALL, JOHN R. "Kidney Donors—The Myth of Informed Consent." *American Journal of Psychiatry* 126 (1970): 1245–1251.

FLETCHER, JOHN. "Realities of Patient Consent to Medical Research." *Hastings Center Studies* 1, no. 1 (1973), pp. 39–49.

FOST, NORMAN C. "Ethical Problems in Pediatrics." *Current Problems in Pediatrics* 6, no. 12 (1976), pp. 1–31.

———. "How Decisions Are Made: A Physician's View." *Decision Making and the Defective Newborn: Proceedings of a Conference on Spina Bifida and Ethics.* Edited by Chester A. Swinyard. Foreword by Robert E. Cooke. Springfield, Ill.: Charles C Thomas, 1978, chap. 13, pp. 220–258. Includes discussion.

In re Gault. 387 U.S. 1. 18 L. ed. 2d 527. 87 S. Ct. 1428 (1967).

GOLDSTEIN, JOSEPH; FREUD, ANNA; and SOLNIT, ALBERT J. *Beyond the Best Interests of the Child.* New York: Free Press, 1973.

GRAY, BRADFORD H. *Human Subjects in Medical Experimentation: A Sociological Study of the Conduct and Regulation of Clinical Research.* Health, Medicine and Society Series. New York: Wiley-Interscience, 1975.

Great Britain, Medical Research Council. "Responsibility in Investigations on Human Subjects: Statement by the Medical Research Council." *Report of the Medical Research Council for the Year 1962–1963.* Cmnd. 2382. London: Her Majesty's Stationery Office, 1964, pp. 21–25.

GUSTAFSON, JAMES M. "Mongolism, Parental Desires, and the Right to Life." *Perspectives in Biology and Medicine* 16 (1973): 529–557.

Hart v. Brown. 29 Conn. Supp. 368. 289 A. 2d 386 (Super. Ct. 1972).

HELFER, RAY E., and KEMPE, C. HENRY, eds. *The Battered Child.* 2d ed. Foreword by Katherine B. Oettinger. Chicago: University of Chicago Press, 1974.

HOFMAN, ADELE D., and PILPEL, HARRIET. "The Legal Rights of Minors." *Pediatric Clinics of North America* 20 (1973): 989–1004.

INGELFINGER, FRANZ J. "Informed (But Uneducated) Consent." *New England Journal of Medicine* 287 (1972): 465–466. Editorial.

Landeros v. Flood. 50 Cal. App. 3d 115. 123 Cal. Rptr. 713 (1st D. 1975).

LANGER, WILLIAM L. "Infanticide: A Historical Survey." *History of Childhood Quarterly* 1 (1974): 353–388.

Lausier v. Pescinski. 27 Wis. 2d 4. 226 N.W. 2d 180 (1975).

LORBER, JOHN. "Selective Treatment of Myelomeningocele: To Treat or Not to Treat?" *Pediatrics* 53 (1974): 307–308. Commentary.

LOWE, CHARLES U.; ALEXANDER, DUANE; and MISHKIN, BARBARA. "Nontherapeutic Research on Children: An Ethical Dilemma." *Journal of Pediatrics* 84 (1974): 468–472.

McCOLLUM, AUDREY T., and SCHWARTZ, A. HERBERT. "Pediatric Research Hospitalization: Its Meaning to Parents." *Pediatric Research* 3 (1969): 199–204.

McCORMICK, RICHARD A. "Proxy Consent in the Experimentation Situation." *Perspectives in Biology and Medicine* 18 (1974): 2–20.

Mannus v. State. 240 Ark. 42. 398 S.W. 2d 206 (1966).

National Research Council, Committee for the Study of Inborn Errors of Metabolism. *Genetic Screening: Programs, Principles and Research.* Washington: National Academy of Sciences, 1975.

Nielsen v. Regents of the University of California. Case no. 665-049 (Super. Ct. of Cal., County of San Francisco, as amended 20 December 1973).

"Nuremberg Code, 1946–1949." Beecher, *Research and the Individual,* pp. 227–234.

PAULSEN, MONRAD G. "The Law and Abused Children." Helfer, *The Battered Child,* pp. 153–178.

"Pediatric Bill of Rights: National Association of Children's Hospitals and Related Institutions." *Law, Medicine and Forensic Science.* 2d ed. *1974 Supplement.* Edited by William J. Curran and E. Donald Shapiro. Boston: Little, Brown & Co., 1974, pp. 129–130. Adopted 24 February 1974.

Public Law 93-348. 88 Stat. 348. Title II. Protection of Human Subjects of Biomedical and Behavioral Research (12 July 1974).

RADBILL, SAMUEL X. "A History of Child Abuse and Infanticide." Helfer, *The Battered Child,* pp. 3–21.

RAMSEY, PAUL. "The Enforcement of Morals: Nontherapeutic Research on Children." *Hastings Center Report* 6, no. 4 (1976), pp. 21–30.

———. *The Patient as Person: Explorations in Medical Ethics.* New Haven: Yale University Press, 1970, p. 14.

In re Richardson. 284 So. 2d 185 (La., Ct. of App. 1973).

"The Rights of Children." *Harvard Educational Review* 43 (1973): 479–668; 44 (1974): 6–157. Special issues, pts. 1 and 2.

ROBERTSON, JOHN A. "Organ Donations by Incompetents and the Substituted Judgment Doctrine." *Columbia Law Review* 76 (1976): 48–78.

———, and FOST, NORMAN C. "Passive Euthanasia of Defective Newborns: Legal Considerations." *Journal of Pediatrics* 88 (1976): 883–889.

SCHRAG, FRANCIS. "Rights over Children." *Journal of Value Inquiry* 7 (1973): 96–105.

SCHWARTZ, A. HERBERT. "Children's Concepts of Research Hospitalization." *New England Journal of Medicine* 287 (1972): 589–592.

STEDMAN, THOMAS LATHROP. *Stedman's Medical Dictionary.* 23d ed. Baltimore: Williams & Wilkins Co., 1976.

United States; Department of Health, Education, and Welfare; National Institutes of Health. "Protection of Human Subjects." *Federal Register* 38 (1973): 31738–31749, esp. 31742. Draft additions to proposed regulations.

———; Department of Health, Education, and Welfare; Public Health Service; National Institutes of Health. *The Institutional Guide to DHEW Policy on Protection of Human Subjects.* DHEW Publication no. (NIH) 72-102. Washington: Government Printing Office, 1971.

WILKERSON, ALBERT E., ed. *The Rights of Children: Emergent Concepts in Law and Society.* Philadelphia: Temple University Press, 1973.

Wis. Stat. sec. 143.07. Venereal Disease.

World Medical Association. "Human Experimentation: Code of Ethics of the World Medical Association: Declaration of Helsinki." *British Medical Journal* 2 (1964): 177. Reprint. "Declaration of Helsinki, 1964." Beecher, *Research and the Individual,* pp. 277–279.

WORSFOLD, VICTOR L. "A Philosophical Justification of Children's Rights." *Harvard Educational Review* 44 (1974): 142–157.

CHINA

See MEDICAL ETHICS, HISTORY OF, *section on* SOUTH AND EAST ASIA, *articles on* GENERAL HISTORICAL SURVEY; PREREPUBLICAN CHINA; *and* CONTEMPORARY CHINA. *See also* BUDDHISM; CONFUCIANISM; TAOISM.

CHIROPRACTIC

See MEDICAL PROFESSION, *article on* ORGANIZED MEDICINE; ORTHODOXY IN MEDICINE.

See also APPENDIX, SECTION IV, AMERICAN CHIROPRACTIC ASSOCIATION.

CHRISTIAN SCIENCE

See PROTESTANTISM, *article on* DOMINANT HEALTH CONCERNS IN PROTESTANTISM.

CHRONIC CARE

Chronic illnesses represent an ever increasing percentage of total illness, at least in the more industrialized nations. Approximately half the U.S. population suffers from one or more chronic illnesses. High on the list are "heart conditions," arthritis, rheumatism, and impairments of back and spine (U.S., DHEW, pp. 1–4). Although afflicting many young people, chronic illnesses are highly associated with advancing age and also with low income. The rising rate of chronicity is linked with the continuing advance of medical technology, which not only contributes to the control of infectious and parasitic disease but, paradoxically, has converted formerly terminal medical conditions into debilitating chronic ones. Chronic illnesses, therefore, are now a major class of medical problems faced by patients, relatives, and health personnel. With these medical problems, a variety of ethical and "quality of life" problems are directly associated.

Properties of chronic disease. There are several general properties of chronic disease. First, it is long-term; hence, whether treatments are occasional, frequent, or virtually continuous, characteristically the disease spans many months, even years. Hospitals are oriented toward treating the acute phases of these diseases, while outpatient services are focused on the intermittent monitoring of symptoms, regimens, and disease. Neither type of institution is geared very effectively toward continuity of care or offering counsel concerning effects of the disease and its treatment on the life-styles of patient or family.

Many chronic diseases are also uncertain in prognosis, phasing of the disease, and response to treatment. These uncertainties force patients to reorganize and restrict their lives in an attempt to handle the unpredictable. Again, the issues are as much social and psychological as medical.

Chronic diseases require more focus on "relief," "comfort," and "care," since cure is problematic or impossible. Correspondingly, they involve considerable attention to minimization of symptoms and management of pain and other discomforts, as well as attention to psychological and social problems associated with anxiety, grief, disfigurement, stigma, relative immobility, and enforced or voluntary isolation.

Chronic diseases are often multiple diseases, a single chronic condition often leading to multiple chronic conditions. Persons may also suffer from two or more unrelated diseases—the older they are, or the lower in socio-economic scale, the more likely are multiple afflictions to occur. Side effects of medical treatments can lead to additional chronicity. Multiplication of diseases and symptoms implies a multiplication of management (medical, psychological, social) problems.

Chronic diseases tend to intrude upon the lives of patients and their families. Thus, reduced mobility may force changes in household arrangements, in amount and kind of work. Impairment of hands or loss of energy may result in the slowing down of household duties and even in simple routines like dressing oneself. Prescribed regimens may contribute (sometimes more than the symptoms) to embarrassment before others or to the absorption of time and energy. Work lives may be affected so that, even when the disease is not completely disabling, inroads on skill, energy, and time may interfere drastically with job requirements. Furthermore, employers often refuse to hire or rehire the chronically ill. Some diseases (epilepsy or sickle-cell disease) make it difficult (at least in the United States) for the sufferer to get jobs if his condition is known, and difficult even to obtain requisite health insurance. Another notable effect of chronic illness is its potential for causing some degree of social isolation from family, friends, and community. Reduction of mobility or energy can contribute to isolation; because of changes in appearance either the patient voluntarily withdraws from social contact or others withdraw from him.

Chronic diseases are expensive. The occurrence of crises, the long-time use of drugs, and routine monitoring all contribute toward the cost, quite aside from particular diseases that regularly or occasionally require expensive technologies. The use of ancillary services also adds to the costs. All these costs are shared differently in different countries; in the United States, burdens on patients and relatives can be considerable; continuing expenses plus potential unemployment or underemployment can reduce families to welfare recipients. Unemployment or financial drain, whether total or not, everywhere leads to marital and family disintegration, psychological impairment, damaged identities, and loss of social status.

Care for chronic disease. Proper care for chronic disease requires a variety of ancillary services. Psychological counseling or therapy may be needed to cope with the impact of the disease, symptoms, or regimen. Special educational services may be needed for ill children and their siblings. Physical therapy, occupational counseling and retraining, and even marital counseling may be necessary. (In the United States, social workers can, or could, help to manage the maze of regulations, forms, and agencies involved in financing a patient's care and in reaching specialized services and agencies.) In addition, legal and financial services may be necessary. Most needed, perhaps, is counseling from a sophisticated and compassionate third party who suggests plausible modes for managing the diverse problems that arise during the course of an illness—whether rearranging household spaces and duties, suggesting "easier to handle" types of clothing, planning strategies for managing insensitive health personnel, or obtaining results from bureaucratic health agencies.

A serious barrier to improving the care of the chronically ill is that health personnel tend implicitly to utilize an "acute disease" model, one appropriate for infectious and parasitic disease but hardly appropriate to the management of chronic diseases. The acute-care and disease-oriented model tends toward an emphasis on hospital care with the utilization of a complex medical technology—drugs, surgery, transplants, complicated machinery—and concentrates on the peak periods of the disease and the weeks immediately thereafter. Organizationally, the major rewards are generally garnered by those who are skilled at that kind of acute care. Ambulatory care seems less heroic and less important, and on the whole its practitioners receive fewer monetary and status rewards. Also, the auxiliary services tend to be underused or underdeveloped in light of the range of disease-linked but nonmedical needs of patients and their families. In short, the acute-care, disease-oriented model leads health personnel to underplay the full range of strategies and organizational arrangements that would be required in order to give more humane and more efficient extensive care.

Normalization as an ethical problem. In the largest sense, *the* problem of any chronically ill person is normalization, i.e., how to live as normally as possible despite one's illness. Society in general is not sufficiently aware of the extent of the problem. Few countries, for instance, have taken into account that even streets and public buildings are designed for normal people who have full mobility and energy. Public landscapes provide clear examples of the central issue, namely, that chronicity is much more than a medical problem. It is very much a social problem. It is also an ethical problem, one in which the family and the general public, whether they recognize the fact or not, are deeply implicated.

Unquestionably needed is a more general ethical awareness of how countries are arranged —spatially, physically, socially, financially—for citizens who are relatively free from the disabilities of chronic disease, thus rendering the struggles of the chronically ill to live satisfying lives, as close to normal as possible, poignantly difficult. They become all the more difficult through the predominantly "medical" approach to chronicity. Yet one might plausibly predict that a combination of factors—increasing rates of chronicity, increasing costs of the acute-care model, and an increased sense of the rights of consumers in many countries—will eventually contribute to improving the chances for the chronically ill to live more satisfactorily than is now possible. (Improved medical technology and practice will certainly help alleviate their suffering, but it will also inevitably add more sufferers to the population.) To be unaware of that future and feasible aim would be to compound today's relatively unwitting moral irresponsibility.

ANSELM STRAUSS AND ELIHU M. GERSON

[*Directly related is* HEALTH CARE, *article on* HUMANIZATION AND DEHUMANIZATION OF HEALTH CARE. *Other relevant material may be found under* AGING AND THE AGED, *article on* SOCIAL IMPLICATIONS OF AGING; HEALTH CARE, *articles on* RIGHT TO HEALTH-CARE SERVICES *and* THEORIES OF JUSTICE AND HEALTH CARE. *See also:* CARE; MENTAL HEALTH SERVICES; *and* RATIONING OF MEDICAL TREATMENT.]

BIBLIOGRAPHY

BENOLIEL, JEANNE QUINT. "The Developing Diabetic Identity: A Study of Family Influence." *Communicating Nursing Research: Methodological Issues.* Third WICHE Nursing Research Conference. Edited by Marjorie V. Batey. Boulder, Colo.: Western Interstate Commission for Higher Education, 1970, pp. 14–32.

CALKINS, KATHY. "Shouldering a Burden." *Omega* 3 (1972): 23–36.

DAVIS, MARCELLA Z. *Living with Multiple Sclerosis.* Springfield, Ill.: Charles C. Thomas, 1973.

DEBUSKEY, MATTHEW, ed. *The Chronically Ill Child and His Family.* Springfield, Ill.: Charles C. Thomas, 1970, pp. 196–198.

FAGERHAUGH, SHIZUKO. "Getting Around with Emphysema." *American Journal of Nursing* 73 (1973): 94–99.

FUTTERMAN, EDWARD H.; HOFFMAN, IRWIN; and SABSHIN, MELVIN. "Parental Anticipatory Mourning." *Psychosocial Aspects of Terminal Care.* Edited by Bernard Schoenberg, Arthur C. Carr, David Peretz, and Austin H. Kutscher. New York: Columbia University Press, 1972, pp. 243–272.

GUSSOW, ZACHARY, and TRACY, GEORGE. "Status, Ideology, and Adaption to Stigmatized Illness: A Study of Leprosy." *Human Organization* 27 (1968): 316–325.

LILIENFELD, ABRAHAM, and GIFFORD, ALICE, eds. *Chronic Diseases and Public Health.* Baltimore: Johns Hopkins Press, 1966.

REIF, LAURA. "Cardiacs and Normals: The Social Construction of a Disability." Ph.D. dissertation, Department of Social and Behavioral Science, University of California at San Francisco, 1975.

———. "Managing a Life with Chronic Disease." *American Journal of Nursing* 73 (1973): 261–264.

STRAUSS, ANSELM. *Chronic Disease and the Quality of Life.* St. Louis: C. V. Mosby, 1975.

United States, Department of Health, Education, and Welfare. *Chronic Conditions and Limitations of Activity and Mobility, U.S., July 1965–June 1967.* Vital Health Statistics, Data from the National Health Survey, ser. 10, no. 61. Washington: Public Health Service, Health Resources and Mental Health Administration, 1971.

CIVIL COMMITMENT

See INSTITUTIONALIZATION; MENTAL HEALTH SERVICES, *article on* SOCIAL INSTITUTIONS OF MENTAL HEALTH; INFORMED CONSENT IN MENTAL HEALTH.

CIVIL DISOBEDIENCE IN HEALTH SERVICES

Before showing how the concept of "civil disobedience" can be applied to medicine and health services, it is first necessary to introduce some order into the various casual uses of the term. Then we shall illustrate the occurrence of civil disobedience in health care in the particularly clear cases of birth control, the care of infants with drastic birth defects, Captain Levy's refusal to train members of the Special Forces, and protests by feminist health centers. These cases are merely illustrative; there are many cases of civil disobedience scattered throughout the literature of the various areas of health services. Moreover, in medicine there is much dissent that does not count technically as civil disobedience but which is, as we shall see, similar in certain respects to civil disobedience.

The meaning of civil disobedience

The concept of civil disobedience is extremely rich and diverse, not at all precise and specific. Yet much can be done to analyze and clarify the concept though not formally define it. Civil disobedience, first of all, can occur only within some structure of law, enforced by established governmental authorities, some aspect of which the person engaged in civil disobedience is trying to change. Disobedience in the context of family, church, lodge, business, university, or profession does not count as civil disobedience. Being civilly disobedient, then, consists in publicly announcing defiance of specific laws, policies, or commands of the legal structure that an individual or group believes to be either unjust or unconstitutional or both. To be defiant is not enough; the defiance must be made public since its purpose is to bring an injustice to the attention of the public and government, either for the purpose of stirring their consciences to rectify it, or to pressure them into rectifying it. The notion of civil disobedience requires not only the breaking of a law on moral grounds but also the pointing up of the disobedience for its symbolic and pressure-exerting value.

To give first an example of civil disobedience outside medicine: During the Vietnam War the burning of draft cards at public meetings in the United States was an act of civil disobedience. The men burning their draft cards were disobeying Selective Service law in protest against the government's policy of continuing the war. The law was broken because of moral objections to the war, and the disobedience was intended to bring the immorality of the war to the attention of the public and the government in the hope that government policy would be changed.

Civil disobedience in health services

The area of medicine and health services that appears to have produced the most clear-cut cases of civil disobedience has been that of birth control. In the cases, e.g., of Emma Goldman, Van Kleek Allison, Margaret Sanger, and Ethel Byrne, birth control laws were defied and attention explicitly drawn to the breaking of the law for the purposes of marshaling moral and legal support for their repeal. The classical cases of civil disobedience in the birth control movement are those of Sanger and Byrne. In 1916 these nurses directly challenged Section 1142 of the New York State Statutes, which prohibited the dissemination of birth control information and the distribution of contraceptive devices, by establishing a birth control clinic in the Brownsville area of Brooklyn. Leaflets announcing the fact were widely distributed. An immediate success, the clinic was swamped with working-class women in desperate need of advice. Byrne was found guilty of violating Section 1142 by distributing contraceptive information and devices, and Sanger was found guilty of violating the same law by conducting a clinic for such purposes, as well as for maintaining a "public nuisance." Byrne was sentenced to thirty days in the workhouse on Blackwell's Island and immediately went on a hunger strike. She was forcibly fed by prison officials. Sanger and Byrne enlisted the aid of the *New York World* to keep the attention of the public focused on Byrne's ordeal and on the just cause of birth control. Sanger was surprised in her case that the prosecutor tried so hard to prove her guilty. Of course she had violated the law; that was the point of her case! She was convicted and sentenced to thirty days in the Queens County Penitentiary, where she tried to disseminate birth control information among the inmates.

It would be a mistake to think that civil disobedience stopped after birth control had become a "respectable" movement. The dissemination of birth control information had become uncontroversial as long as the information was given only to married women. In the early 1960s William Baird witnessed the death of a young mother of eight children after an effort to abort herself with a coat hanger. Since she was unmarried she had been ineligible to receive information about birth control. Baird converted an old moving truck into a birth control information dissemination unit and used it in the poverty areas in New York City and vicinity. In 1966 he was arrested in Freehold, New Jersey, while showing a woman a diaphragm and describing its use. As a direct result of Baird's case, the New Jersey law concerning the distribution of birth control information and devices was liberalized. Baird advocated making birth control advice available to *any* unmarried women, even adolescents, and making contraceptives available in supermarkets as well as drug stores. In Massachusetts in 1967 he was convicted of the distribution of contraceptive devices to unauthorized persons. Sentenced to three months in prison, he appealed to the United States Supreme Court, which eventually sustained his plea in 1972. The Court struck down as a denial of "equal protection" to the unmarried the Massachusetts laws that forbade distributing contraceptives to unmarried persons.

The disclosures of R. S. Duff and A. G. M. Campbell in 1973 count as a courageous instance of civil disobedience in special care clinics. According to some authorities, the principle is well established both in law and ethics that physicians must use all "ordinary" means to preserve and prolong life but that the decision to apply "extraordinary" means is a matter of discretion. In the special-care nursery of the Yale–New Haven hospital, fourteen percent of 299 deaths occurred as a direct result of *withholding* treatment to infants with severe birth defects. In the words of Duff and Campbell, "After careful consideration of each of these 43 infants, parents and physicians in a group decision concluded that prognosis for meaningful life was extremely poor or hopeless,

and therefore rejected further treatment" (Duff and Campbell, p. 890). Realizing that some people may argue the law has been broken, Duff and Campbell conclude that if what they have done *is* in violation of the law, then "we believe the law should be changed"; and their publication of these case reports was made in the hope that "out of the ensuing dialogue perhaps better choices for patients and families can be made" (ibid., p. 894). Subsequent legal scholarship has made it plain that Duff and Campbell were breaking numerous laws (Robertson).

A third example of civil disobedience in medicine is the refusal by Captain Howard B. Levy, a young dermatologist, to train Special Forces medics for service in Vietnam in 1967. On moral grounds he disobeyed the direct orders of agents of the government, and on many occasions publicly stated his opposition to the war. He spent twenty-six months in prison because he believed that to obey orders would have compelled him to violate canons of medical ethics. The aidmen Levy was ordered to train were not medics in the usual sense; in addition to their medical duties, they were expected to engage in guerrilla warfare. Levy felt that his moral obligation as a physician was to train personnel in the healing arts, and only in the healing arts, but he was directed to train servicemen expected to kill and wound as well as heal. His response was civil disobedience.

A fourth and final example of civil disobedience in medicine is the action taken in 1974 by the Feminist Women's Health Center in Los Angeles. The women there made a moral protest against the action or inaction of various government agencies in supporting or at least condoning the abortion clinic of Harvey Karman. Karman's allegedly substandard medical procedures they regarded as hazardous to the health and lives of women. Their protest took the form of disobedience of laws against theft and the public distribution of what they called a "writ of mandamus," which concluded: "Having confiscated the medical equipment, supplies, and office furniture necessary to the functioning of this experimental laboratory, we order these delegated official agencies to do their duty, to cease their financial aid of Harvey Karman and to stop his activities" (Feminist).

The nature of civil disobedience in medicine can be further clarified by some examples of actions that are clearly *not* civil disobedience, though they may be mistaken as such.

In 1968, when Patrick Cardinal O'Boyle, archbishop of Washington, delivered a sermon urging absolute obedience to Pope Paul VI's encyclical barring contraception, two hundred parishioners walked out of the church in the middle of Mass ("For Birth Control"). Although this walkout was a moral protest against authority, it cannot be considered civil disobedience since it did not involve disobedience of law and defiance of governmental authority.

Neither can the strikes by physicians that have become increasingly common in the 1970s be considered civil disobedience. In general, strikes are not acts of civil disobedience both because no laws are disobeyed and because the primary goal of the strikers is personal gain. Even in cases where laws are disobeyed (e.g., laws against strikes by government employees), strikes are not normally acts of civil disobedience because they lack the crucial element of moral protest. This is not to say that a civilly disobedient strike by physicians is inconceivable. If a group of physicians in Nazi Germany, in moral protest against the callous use of human subjects in experiments, had disobeyed directives from the government to treat patients, such a strike would have been preeminently an instance of civil disobedience. However, a strike by physicians in protest against, say, rates of premiums for malpractice insurance cannot be considered protest on moral grounds and consequently cannot be regarded as civil disobedience.

Dissent in medicine

It would be possible to cite many other cases in the areas already discussed, as well as in other areas, but to multiply such cases and areas would fail to disclose the focus of much current dissent against medicine and health services in the United States. One of the reasons why physicians are not more involved in what can properly be called civil disobedience is that they have considerable power to make authoritative rules that are equivalent to established laws. Civil disobedience is traditionally a method of bringing social change that the relatively powerless must use to change the policies and laws administered by those in power, usually government officials. In the case of medicine, the physicians *are* those with the power. The common practice of physicians establishes, in a sense, the common law of medicine. There are not many laws on the books governing medical practice beyond those governing birth control and abortions. Society has traditionally given physicians great power to practice medicine as

they see fit, restricted by very few laws; so *civil* disobedience, as we have defined it, is not called for in most areas in which change, of an extremely controversial sort, is needed in medical practice. However, a great deal of current dissent against the medical establishment in the United States is clearly similar to civil disobedience. Medical practice *is* the law, so to speak, and the parallel to civil disobedience in this case is disobedience against this common law of medical practice, a common law that has become institutionalized in medical organizations that are capable of wielding powerful sanctions against dissent.

The nature of disobedience against this power structure has been manifested in numerous ways. Self-help clinics for women have sprung up across the United States. Another concrete manifestation of disobedience to the power structure is the Health Policy Advisory Center (Health-PAC) in New York City, a research and action collective. Similar groups are active in other cities. Also ghetto organizers and community groups are becoming increasingly interested in the idea of neighborhood clinics. The thrust against both the American Medical Association and the medical schools is toward participatory democracy, where the community of citizens is seen to be active in decisions about where and how health resource funds are to be allocated. Moreover, nursing schools and other paramedical groups are fighting for financial and moral independence of the AMA and the influential medical schools. Finally, the general populace has become increasingly militant against the established medical profession. The legal structure is being used extensively as a way of controlling the common law practices of the medical profession, and the increase in medical malpractice suits in recent years has been enormous.

EDWARD H. MADDEN AND PETER H. HARE

[*This article will find application in the entries* ABORTION, *article on* LEGAL ASPECTS; CONTRACEPTION; INFANTS, *article on* PUBLIC POLICY AND PROCEDURAL QUESTIONS; MEDICAL ETHICS UNDER NATIONAL SOCIALISM; *and* WARFARE. *Other relevant material may be found under* LAW AND MORALITY; MEDICAL PROFESSION; *and* ORTHODOXY IN MEDICINE.]

BIBLIOGRAPHY

American Medical Association, Judicial Council. *Opinions and Reports of the Judicial Council.* E. G. Shelley, Chairman. Chicago: 1971.
BEDAU, HUGO A., ed. *Civil Disobedience: Theory and Practice.* New York: Pegasus, 1969.

Boston Women's Health Book Collective. "Women and Health Care." *Our Bodies, Ourselves: A Book by and for Women.* New York: Simon & Schuster, 1973, pp. 236–276.

BRANSON, ROY. "The Secularization of American Medicine." *Hastings Center Studies* 1, no. 2 (1973), pp. 17–28.

COHEN, CARL. *Civil Disobedience: Conscience, Tactics, and the Law.* New York: Columbia University Press, 1971.

DIENES, C. THOMAS. *Law, Politics, and Birth Control.* Urbana: University of Illinois Press, 1972.

DUFF, RAYMOND, and CAMPBELL, A. G. M. "Moral and Ethical Dilemmas in the Special-Care Nursery." *New England Journal of Medicine* 289 (1973): 890–894.

Feminist Women's Health Center. "Writ of Mandamus." *Monthly Extract: An Irregular Periodical* 3, issue 3 (1974), p. 2.

"For Birth Control, a Mass Walkout." *Life,* 4 October 1968, pp. 30–33.

LANGER, ELINOR. "The Court-Martial of Captain Levy: Medical Ethics v. Military Law." *Science* 156 (1967): 1346–1350.

MADDEN, E. H., and HARE, P. H. "Reflections on Civil Disobedience." *Journal of Value Inquiry* 4 (1970): 81–95.

MICHAELSON, MICHAEL G. "The Coming Medical War." *Readings on Ethical and Social Issues in Biomedicine.* Edited by Richard W. Wertz. Englewood Cliffs, N.J.: Prentice-Hall, 1973, pp. 269–285.

RIBICOFF, ABRAHAM. "Medical Malpractice: the Patient vs. the Physician." *Trial, The National Legal Newsmagazine,* February–March 1970, pp. 10–13, 22.

ROBERTSON, JOHN A. "Involuntary Euthanasia of Defective Newborns: A Legal Analysis." *Stanford Law Review* 27 (1975): 213–269.

SANGER, MARGARET. *Margaret Sanger: An Autobiography.* New York: W. W. Norton & Co., 1938.

CLINICAL RESEARCH

See HUMAN EXPERIMENTATION; INFORMED CONSENT IN HUMAN RESEARCH; RESEARCH, BIOMEDICAL; RESEARCH, BEHAVIORAL; INFORMED CONSENT IN THE THERAPEUTIC RELATIONSHIP, *article on* CLINICAL ASPECTS; FETAL RESEARCH; CHILDREN AND BIOMEDICINE; AGING AND THE AGED, *article on* HEALTH CARE AND RESEARCH IN THE AGED; PRISONERS, *article on* PRISONER EXPERIMENTATION; WOMEN AND BIOMEDICINE, *article on* WOMEN AS PATIENTS AND EXPERIMENTAL SUBJECTS.

CLONING

See REPRODUCTIVE TECHNOLOGIES, *articles on* ASEXUAL HUMAN REPRODUCTION; ETHICAL ISSUES; *and* LEGAL ASPECTS; GENE THERAPY, *article on* CELL FUSION AND HYBRIDIZATION.

CODES OF MEDICAL ETHICS

I. HISTORY   *Donald Konold*
II. ETHICAL ANALYSIS   *Robert M. Veatch*

I
HISTORY

In the ethics of medicine and health care, ethical standards have been formulated for physicians in their professional duties, for persons conducting medical experiments involving human subjects, and for the various health care professions. While codes of ethics have long been regarded as the classic expression of these directives, various principles and professional rules of conduct have also been stated in the form of prayers, oaths, creeds, institutional directives, and statements of professional organizations. This historical essay is concerned with the principles and rules of conduct for the medical profession as they have been formalized in prayers, oaths, and codes. Medical prayers state a very personal commitment of the physician to his professional duty; oaths publicly pledge the new physician to uphold the recognized responsibilities of his profession; and codes provide more comprehensive standards to guide the practicing physician. Each form of ethical statement implies a moral imperative, either to be accepted by the physician personally or to be enforced by a medical organization upon its members.

Most formal statements of medical ethics have been advanced by physicians themselves. Although governments and religious groups have long prescribed some controls by law and precept on the conduct of medical practitioners, only in the last century have other groups developed ethical standards for the physician–patient relationship.

Medical prayers

The most beautiful and moving expressions of dedication to medical practice are in the form of prayers. Doctors of all ages have composed deeply moving prayers expressing gratitude for divine blessings and asking for divine inspiration in their professional conduct. The most widely acclaimed of these is the Daily Prayer of a Physician, once ascribed to the philosophical Jewish physician Moses Maimonides (1135–1204) but now believed to be the work of the eighteenth-century German Jewish physician Marcus Herz (Rosner, 1967, pp. 451–452). In the manner of most medical prayers, the Daily

Prayer asks for courage, determination and inspiration to enable the physician to develop his skills, meet his responsibilities, and heal his patients. It commits the physician to place his duty to patients above his own concerns and voices high aspirations without reference to the specific issues of medical ethics.

Oaths for physicians

In the ancient world physicians expressed their ethical concepts most often in the form of oaths, which were an integral part of the initiation ceremony for medical apprentices. Like many medical prayers, ancient oaths reflect the physician's belief that success in his profession required that he ally himself with the deity in the treatment of disease. All the ancient oaths beseech the deity to inspire physicians to fulfill their moral obligations, reward those who honor their sacred trust, and punish those who violate it.

One of the oldest of ancient oaths, a medical student's oath taken from the *Charaka Samhita* manuscript of ancient India, contains concepts which had pervaded Indian ethical thought for many centuries before their inclusion in the oath about A.D. 1 (Menon and Haberman, pp. 295–296). Pledging the medical student to live the life of an ascetic and a virtual slave of his preceptor in accordance with Indian custom for apprenticeships, the oath requires a personal sacrifice and commitment to duty from the student comparable to the physician's responsibilities to patients. By the eloquent terms of the oath the student physician is to place the patient's needs above his personal considerations, serving day and night with heart and soul; abstaining from drunkenness, crime, and adultery; and observing professional secrecy scrupulously. In sharp contrast to the medical ethics of the Western world, the Indian oath obliges the physician to deny services to enemies of his ruler, evildoers, unattended women, and those on the point of death. Ancient Indian thought condemned aid to anyone immoral, interference with the process of dying, and any circumstance that might suggest illicit sexual contact. Despite these differences, the oath of the Indian student reveals significant parallels between the medical ethics of India and those of the Western world and suggests a diffusion of ideas, probably from India to the West.

The most honored and enduring medical oath of Western civilization is the Oath of Hippocrates. Despite its renown, its origin is obscure. It is a part of the Hippocratic Collection, which was catalogued and edited by a group of Alexandrian librarians sometime after the fourth century B.C. Copies of these writings available to modern scholars, however, date from the tenth to the fifteenth century A.D. and do not preserve the original text with verbal accuracy. None of the manuscripts of this collection can be positively verified as genuine works of the great physician, and clearly the documents are the products of many contributors, with the earliest predating the latest by at least a century. Recent investigations have revealed substantial evidence that the Oath conforms closely to the teachings of Pythagoreans of the fourth century B.C. and that it was used in their rituals (Edelstein, 1943). It proclaims a more strict morality for physicians than was established by Greek law, Platonic or Aristotelian ethics, or common Greek medical practice.

The Oath of Hippocrates actually consists of two parts, the first serving as a contractual agreement between pupil and teacher and the second constituting an ethical code. The opening sentences pledge the novice physician to become an adopted member of his teacher's family, to help support his teacher and his teacher's children in case of need, and to pass on his instruction to the teacher's children free of charge. Instruction is forbidden by the Oath for any student who will not agree to this stipulation or take the same oath. Since familial bonds between teacher and pupil implied careful selection of those admitted to the family group, the covenant enabled physicians to prevent unworthy persons from entering the profession by this route.

The ethical code contained in the Oath of Hippocrates places restrictions on the medical techniques of the physician and defines his relations with his patient's family. He who takes the Oath agrees to employ dietetic means to promote recovery, to refuse to dispense poisons or abortive remedies, and to leave surgery to craftsmen trained in that art. These measures, the Oath asserts, will protect the patient from unjust treatment and preserve the purity and holiness of the physician and his art. When he visits the home of his patient, the physician is under oath not to commit acts of injustice or mischief, and to abstain from having sexual relations with women and slaves as well as men. Finally he promises to protect the secrecy, not only of professional confidences, but also of those things learned outside the profession that should not be made public.

The paternalism implicit in the Oath's instruction that the physician refuse his patient's requests in some cases and judge what confidences to keep is an important element of its legacy. The Oath's provisions contrast sharply with the standards of actual Greek medical practice, which permitted physicians to abet suicide and infanticide and to perform surgery, including lithotomy (removal of a stone from the urinary bladder). They also set a higher standard for the equal treatment of all social classes than might be expected in Greek society. Even the secrecy requirement, extending to information obtained outside the professional relationship, is exceptionally stringent. Yet these precepts, representing the thought of only a small group of medical practitioners, have outweighed all others in shaping the development of medical ethics in the modern world.

For centuries following the appearance of the Hippocratic Oath, the medical profession showed no inclination to accept it. Hellenistic physicians violated its injunctions without compunction. Then the rise of Christianity produced a new idealism which was generally in agreement with the Hippocratic ethics. Increased attention to the Oath led to modifications bringing it into more perfect harmony with Christian ideological concepts and practices. The earliest of these extant revisions, entitled From the Oath According to Hippocrates Insofar as a Christian May Swear It, substitutes a statement of Christian adoration of God for the references to Greek deities in the original Oath and replaces its covenant with a statement of teaching responsibilities in terms of Christian brotherhood, pledging the physician to teach his art to whoever wants to learn it and without any stipulation (Leake, 1927, pp. 215–218). The injunction against surgery does not appear in this version of the Oath, but no reason is known for this omission, and later Christian versions do contain it. The Oath of Asaf, from the seventh-century *Sefer Asaf* manuscripts of the oldest Hebrew medical work, reveals Hippocratic influences in its injunctions against administering poisons or abortifacient drugs, performing surgery, committing adultery and betraying professional confidences (Rosner and Muntner, pp. 318–319). Like the medieval Christian oaths, it instructs physicians to give special consideration to the poor and needy. The Oath of Hippocrates also appeared in medieval Muslim literature, where the only significant changes replaced references to Greek gods with statements in harmony with Islamic theology. The Oath in its original form was also known to Christian and Muslim scholars, of course, and it may have been taken by physicians practicing in both medieval societies.

Following the transition from medieval to modern Western civilization, the Oath of Hippocrates continued to be a model for ethical pledges by physicians. Medical schools, seeking to commit their students to the pursuit of high ethical ideals, continued a tradition begun in the Middle Ages to incorporate Hippocratic concepts in oaths for their graduates, especially the covenant's requirement for the physician to instruct his teacher's children and the ethical injunctions for secrecy and against administering harmful drugs. Oaths taken by graduates of medical schools of India, most of which have been oriented toward Western medicine since the eighteenth century, have also been modeled after the Hippocratic tradition. During the nineteenth century some medical schools in the United States required their graduates to take the Hippocratic Oath in its original form, and that continued to be a common practice in the twentieth century, despite the fact that many of the Oath's provisions were archaic.

A significant revision of the Oath of Hippocrates appeared in 1948, when the newly organized World Medical Association adopted the Declaration of Geneva (*Declaration*). The Association recommended the new oath to medical schools and practicing physicians in all nations as a pledge which would inspire doctors in the fundamental principles of medical ethics. The Declaration represents an attempt to make the original Oath fully applicable to modern conditions of medical practice and to diverse cultural, religious, and ethnic factions in the world community which the Association represents.

The Declaration of Geneva is a secular oath that contains no reference to religious tenets or loyalties. Its phraseology not only makes the Declaration more acceptable to physicians of diverse religious convictions and affiliations, but also avoids making religion a source of professional discord. By pledging physicians to uphold the honor and traditions of the medical profession, the Declaration offers a basis for professional pride and solidarity. It also appeals for medical unity by eliciting from the Hippocratic covenant obligations for the modern physician to give respect and gratitude to his teachers and to recognize his colleagues as his brothers. The family unit idealized in the original Oath has thereby been expanded to embrace the international profession.

In describing the physician's responsibilities to his patient, the Declaration of Geneva renews the Hippocratic emphasis on service but significantly modifies the Oath's specific provisions. Pledges by the Declaration's physician to make the patient's health his first consideration and to respect professional confidences are simple reiterations of basic principles in the original Oath, although an amendment of 1968 specifies that physicians should honor confidences even after the patient's death. The Oath's surgical restriction, however, is omitted from the Declaration in deference to the major role of surgery in modern medicine, and the Oath's injunction against improper behavior with women and slaves in the patient's household is redirected to the patient himself, and to more relevant social categories. The physician of the Declaration vows not to permit considerations of religion, nationality, race, party politics, or social standing to interfere with his duty to his patient. Obviously, those who conceived and adopted the Declaration found united support for a clearer condemnation of these prejudices than the original Oath provided. In sharp contrast, however, the Declaration's statement of the physician's responsibility regarding suicide, mercy killing, and abortion is carefully obscured in generalities which conceal modern controversy on these matters among physicians and laymen alike. The physician of the Declaration pledges only to maintain respect for human life from the time of conception and not to use his medical knowledge contrary to the laws of humanity.

A government-sponsored medical oath has recently appeared in the Soviet Union, where the Presidium approved the Oath of Soviet Physicians in 1971 ("The Oath"). Modeled after an oath used at the University of Moscow since 1961, the Soviet oath pledges the physician to conduct himself in accordance with Communist principles and to honor his responsibility to the Soviet government. This commitment to political creed and government is unique among medical oaths. The Soviet oath does not neglect other moral obligations, however, for it instructs the physician to honor professional secrets, constantly improve his knowledge and skill, be available always to calls for medical care or advice, and dedicate all his knowledge and strength to his professional activities. Like other recent oaths, the Soviet oath voices virtually the same ideal of humanitarian duty to individual patients that appears in the earliest medical creeds, but it also pledges the physician to serve the interests of society.

Professional codes

Physicians of the modern world have not been content with the spiritual inspiration of prayers and the moral commitments of medical oaths. The large medical institutions of urban society have required complex relationships among medical personnel who demand detailed procedures to prevent embarrassing ethical controversy and disruption of services. Lengthy treatises on medical subjects, which had enlightened physicians on ethical matters since the earliest times, were not easy to cite by paragraph and line and frequently concealed ethical instruction in needless verbiage. By reducing these essays to lists of rules, proponents of professional control produced elaborate ethical codes.

One of the earliest codes of medical ethics appeared in China, where the Oath of Hippocrates has never made a significant impression. Instead, an indigenous Chinese tradition in medical ethics developed from sixth-century origins in Sun Ssu-miao's *The Thousand Golden Prescriptions*. This tradition received clear expression in the Five Commandments and Ten Requirements listed by Ch'en Shih-kung in a seventeenth-century treatise on surgery (Lee, pp. 271–273). Along with much guidance for social intercourse, Ch'en's precepts included several ethical principles of merit. In keeping with a tradition of gratuitous medical service by physicians of independent wealth in China, the precepts instruct physicians to give equal treatment to patients of all ranks, to keep expenses modest, and to treat the poor without charge. Physicians should visit women only in the presence of an attendant, a rule that had become nearly universal by the Middle Ages, and should observe professional secrecy regarding female diseases. They should keep well informed in medicine, equip their offices fully, and prepare remedies of orthodox formulae to avoid disputes. Finally, they should be humble and not insult each other. These instructions continue to characterize Chinese medical ethics in modern times, but they have had little influence elsewhere. Although they bear some resemblance to ethical concepts in Western medicine, there is little evidence of cross fertilization.

In the West, a treatise published in 1803 by Thomas Percival, an eminent physician of Manchester, England, strongly influenced the development of codes of medical ethics (Leake, 1927, pp. 61–210). Originally prepared in 1794 to guide professional conduct relative to hospitals and other medical charities and expanded in 1803 to include physicians in general practice, *Medical Ethics; Or, A Code of Institutes and Precepts Adapted to the Professional Conduct of Physicians and Surgeons* expresses standards of morality and etiquette that were in sharp contrast to the quarrelsome conduct of British practitioners of that era. Percival's treatise places greatest emphasis on the professional relationships of physicians to one another; to hospital personnel, apothecaries, and others engaged in the treatment and care of the sick; and to the law. It advances rules for conduct that would permit physicians to treat patients properly and at the same time uphold the dignity of the profession.

In its advice to physicians to treat patients with compassion, fidelity, and humanity, and to observe secrecy warranted by circumstances, Percival's *Medical Ethics* acknowledges the Hippocratic tradition. It urges physicians to keep their heads clear and hands steady by observing the strictest temperance, to avoid the use of fraudulently advertised medicines, to publicize those remedies found to be effective, to continue to treat and comfort patients during the final stages of a fatal condition, and to consider benevolence and virtue more than wealth and rank in determining fees. It also recommends the separation of physic and surgery wherever there are enough physicians to permit the excellence in performance which accompanies specialization. Unlike the Hippocratic Oath, however, *Medical Ethics* recognizes both arts as honorable branches of the medical profession and subject alike to its ethics.

A principal concern of Percival's *Medical Ethics* is with those aspects of professional conduct governed by etiquette. It offers elaborate procedures for consultation among physicians in difficult cases and for preservation of distinctions of rank in relationships between junior and senior physicians on hospital faculties and in consultations. It cautions physicians to display respect for one another, to avoid criticism of the practice of their colleagues, to conceal professional differences from the public, and not to steal patients from one another. In justifying these procedures, Percival reasoned that criticism of the profession was usually unfounded

and always degrading both to the doctors criticized and to the profession.

In most of its provisions Percival's *Medical Ethics* suggests a modified utilitarian philosophy, calling for individual physicians to conduct themselves in a manner that would enhance public respect for the entire medical profession. Although Percival frequently voiced the Christian ideals of duty and sacrifice in his treatise, he recommended that physicians carefully control their responses to those ethical demands. Wealthy physicians should not offer gratuitous treatment to patients who can afford to pay, for that would deprive other physicians of needed means of support. Physicians should expose unprofessional conduct only to the proper medical or legal tribunals, not to the patients. Only in extreme cases of incompetence or neglect should a physician interfere in another's case, and even then he should warn the patient only when the offending doctor ignores his advice. When new methods are demanded by the failure of conventional practice, physicians should proceed only after consultation with peers and only when reason and evidence suggest a favorable result. These provisions and others make it clear that physicians should police their profession against malpractice, but limitations imposed by procedural safeguards contradict the ideal of moral responsibility exercised by the individual physician.

When the American Medical Association was organized in 1847, it adopted a Code of Ethics drawn largely from Percival's *Medical Ethics*. The Code of Ethics made no mention of etiquette for hospital staffs and barely mentioned the relations of physicians with pharmacists and courts of law, but it expanded and elaborated the principles for physicians in private practice, even to include a statement of obligations of patients and the public to physicians. The medical profession in the United States was faced with a crisis in public confidence in 1847. Medical regulations in most states had been repealed with the result that uneducated practitioners and rank imposters had begun to compete with regular physicians for patients. Exponents of the Code of Ethics hoped that the public would cooperate with doctors in establishing standards for medical practice that would prevent the worst abuses of the doctor–patient relationship and re-establish public respect for the medical profession.

In response to the American profession's experience with pretenders, the Code of Ethics contained a variety of restrictions on open competition among physicians. It branded as quacks all medical practitioners who lacked orthodox training, claimed special ability, patented instruments or medicines, used secret remedies, or criticized other practitioners. The requirement of orthodox training made outcasts of doctors who belonged to medical sects such as the Homeopaths, the Eclectics, the Thomsonians, and later the Osteopaths and Chiropractors. Since each sect claimed superior results from its form of treatment, practitioners with sectarian designations were guilty of claiming superior ability as well as handicapped by their incomplete education. Claiming that these offenses resulted from selfishness and efforts to discredit rivals, the Code of Ethics demanded that reputable physicians avoid any action that might appear as an attempt to solicit the patient of another doctor. Although these provisions united the profession against quackery, the prohibition on claims of special ability produced conflict between general practitioners and aspiring specialists. This ethical rule ceased to cause dissension only after the establishment of specialist organizations to certify the credentials of their members and after specialization won sufficient acceptance to permit physicians to restrict practice to their specialties.

The Code of Ethics provided orthodox physicians with one means of exposing those undeserving of confidence. It stated that physicians should not consult professionally with anyone who lacked a license to practice or was not in good professional standing. Since professional standing was determined by local medical societies, this provision had the effect of substituting a collective professional judgment for that of individual physicians and patients. In those cases where the patient insisted on inviting a consultant who was not approved by the local medical organization, the attending physician would have to retire from the case in order to retain his professional standing. While physicians argued that they could not fulfill their obligation to patients by admitting a right for fraudulent practitioners to advise in any capacity, their ethics required that they withdraw and thus give full charge of the case to the allegedly unqualified practitioner. Moreover, the majority of physicians found the consultation restriction a useful means for excluding many qualified doctors from association with the dominant organizations. Before 1870 regular medical so-

cieties excluded from membership and forbade consultations with female physicians and Negro physicians and, throughout the latter half of the century, with physicians who adopted a sectarian designation, even when they were certified by licensing boards. Because of mounting criticism, the consultation restriction was eliminated from the Code of Ethics in 1903, but its spirit was revived by a 1924 resolution of the American Medical Association forbidding voluntary association of its members with cultists.

In the twentieth century a number of national governments have incorporated elaborate ethical codes into legal statutes governing the medical profession, to be enforced by an official medical board. The precepts in these codes generally accord with the broader principles of the Percival tradition, but many provisions deal with problems of recent origin and reflect a modern concern for public as well as individual welfare. The new codes reveal an increased concern for the ethics of abortion, which they generally allow only in accordance with legal determination or as a therapeutic measure to save the mother's life. Most of them clearly prohibit advertising, self-serving publicity, and even indirect promotional tactics by physicians. They forbid physicians to pay or receive commissions for referral of patients, to accept pharmaceutical rebates, or to offer their services in group medical care plans under conditions that would reduce their freedom of judgment. They restrict specialists to their specialties, discourage rivalry or acrimony between specialists and general practitioners, and forbid collusion or fee splitting by specialists and general practitioners against the patient's interest. Most modern official government codes also place emphasis on professional secrecy as permitted by law; for example, the regulations for West German physicians cover ethical aspects of the physician's responsibilities for secrecy and disclosure in great detail.

Establishment of the World Medical Association in 1948 encouraged physicians to develop international standards of medical ethics. The new organization adopted an International Code of Medical Ethics in 1949, which attempted to summarize the most important principles of medical ethics ("International Code"). Since 1900, certification laws had reduced the prevalence of unqualified medical practitioners, and scientific advances had increased the effectiveness of trained physicians. By mid-century physicians were directing their attention more to the actual treatment of patients and less to the formality of relations between one another or between doctor and patient. The International Code reflects the new concerns in a shift away from the detailed regulations of the preceding one and a half centuries. In place of elaborate etiquette for consultations and other medical confrontations, it recommends only that physicians behave toward colleagues as they would have colleagues behave toward them, that they call specialists in difficult cases, and that they not entice each other's patients. It warns against the profit motive and prohibits unauthorized advertising, medical care plans that deprive the doctor of professional independence, fee splitting or rebates with or without the patient's knowledge, and refusal to treat emergency cases. It also reminds physicians of their obligation to honor professional secrecy, an obligation which continues after the death of the patient, according to an amendment to the Code adopted in 1968.

The International Code only hints at the ethical problems of abortion and euthanasia by asserting the physician's responsibility to preserve life. It does, however, warn specifically against any action that would weaken the patient's resistance without therapeutic justification. Applicable to the dying patient and experimental subject alike, this standard requires the physician to consider the patient's well-being above all else. The International Code also recognizes the need for adequate testing of innovations by urging great caution in publishing discoveries and therapeutic methods not recognized by the profession.

Using the International Code of Ethics as an example, the American Medical Association reduced its elaborate code to ten Principles of Medical Ethics in 1957 ("Ten Principles"). Most of these principles had been anticipated in the International Code, but there are a few noteworthy exceptions. Reflecting a continuing distrust of sectarian practitioners by regular physicians in the United States, the 1957 Principles warn against professional associations with unscientific practitioners. They also obligate physicians to expose the legal and ethical violations of other doctors. Instead of warning against premature publication of discoveries, the 1957 Principles urge physicians to make their attainments available to patients and colleagues. Finally, while reaffirming the principle of professional confidence, the 1957 Principles authorize physicians to violate this principle as required by law

or to advance the welfare of the individual or the community. This provision suggests more discretionary authority for the physician than do the codes of most nations and the World Medical Association, which emphasize the inviolability of professional secrecy.

Scientific advances and changing social standards in recent decades have raised ethical questions in a number of areas that are not adequately covered by existing general codes. In some instances additional guidelines have appeared to help conscientious physicians make ethical decisions. The growing popularity of organ transplantation as a surgical procedure prompted the American Medical Association to issue a supplementary statement in 1968 regarding the ethics of organ transplantation ("Ethical Guidelines"). It cautions physicians to protect the rights of both donor and recipient by informing them fully of the procedures to be used and of reasonable expectations of results, and, in the case of vital organs, to have the death of the donor certified by one or more physicians other than the recipient's attendant. It stresses the need for these procedures to be conducted only by specially qualified physicians, in adequate facilities, after alternatives have been expertly evaluated. In that same year the World Medical Association adopted the Declaration of Sydney, which proposes rather technical precautions in the determination of death of organ donors ("A Statement on Death").

The development of elaborate and costly techniques for sustaining human life in cases where death threatens has also raised questions regarding the responsibility of attending physicians. The American Medical Association attempted an answer in 1973 with a guideline for treatment of terminal illnesses ("The Physician and the Dying Patient"). The Association's statement condemns mercy killing but authorizes the physician to abide by any decision of the patient or his immediate family to discontinue extraordinary efforts to prolong life when evidence of imminent death is irrefutable. Closely related to these developments are the intense efforts of medical scientists to reach agreement on guidelines for clinical research. The accelerated pace of medical research has resulted in the appearance of numerous codes governing experimentation with human subjects.

Biomedical advances and changing social imperatives have raised a number of moral questions for which no widely accepted answers yet exist. The rapidly developing science of fertility control, including legal abortion, contraceptives, and artificial insemination, has provoked stormy moral controversy. Experiments in genetic control present issues on which it may be even more difficult to reach a moral consensus. New chemicals—antibiotics, cancer controls, mood changers—with extensive and often unknown effects beyond their therapeutic purpose, also create moral dilemmas for those who would prescribe them. Finally, the extremely high cost of much contemporary medical therapy limits its availability and creates problems of distribution, pricing, and rationing with grave moral overtones. In view of growing public concern, ethical codes of the future will undoubtedly contain guidelines for physicians who deal with these problems.

Codes from outside the profession

Some recent codes of medical ethics have been sponsored by groups that do not principally represent the medical profession: religious bodies, civil governments, and consumer groups.

Unlike other contemporary world religions, the Catholic Church has, in modern times, promulgated formal codes of medical ethics in various parts of the world, where they have generated a rather widespread social effect. They are not only considered binding on Catholics but also affect non-Catholics who are associated with Catholic health facilities.

To regulate its many hospitals in the United States, the National Conference of Catholic Bishops has adopted its own code, Ethical and Religious Directives for Catholic Health Facilities, which establishes standards of medical practice within the Catholic institutions in conformity with the moral and religious teachings of the Church. Although its statements on the subjects of secrecy, consent, organ transplantation, and terminal cases closely resemble those in other codes, it has more rigorous rules. for protection of reproductive functions. It prohibits abortion except as an unintended result of a procedure employed to protect the mother, it prohibits both male and female sterilization except in treatment of a serious pathological condition, and it prohibits artificial insemination. The firm position of the Catholic Church is being subjected to increasing scrutiny from a larger society that lacks a clear moral consensus on these matters. Meanwhile, the Church's restrictions continue to have a significant effect on the nature of medical service available to patients in communities where Catholic health institutions

are the only ones. By contrast, the Declaration of Oslo, adopted by the World Medical Association in 1970, expresses a more liberal view of abortion ("Statement on Therapeutic Abortion"). While the Declaration cautions that abortion should be performed only as a therapeutic measure and that physicians need not perform abortions against their personal convictions, it authorizes abortion in the vital interests of the mother, where the law permits. Even this statement falls short of the views of many physicians and the official opinion of the United States Supreme Court (*Roe* v. *Wade; Doe* v. *Bolton*, January 22, 1973) that, in the early stages of pregnancy, abortion is the mother's prerogative.

The modern consumer movement has also influenced the ethics of medical practice. As hospitalization has become a major consumer service, consumers have become vocal in demanding the right of patients to minimum standards of care and respect. In 1972 the American Hospital Association responded to consumer pressure and adopted a Patient's Bill of Rights, which pertains primarily to hospitals but involves physicians with several responsibilities to patients ("Statement"). By its provisions the physician is obligated to keep the hospitalized patient informed of diagnosis, treatment, and prognosis, to instruct the patient fully regarding possible consequences and alternatives before obtaining consent for medical procedures, to honor a patient's refusal to consent to treatment to the extent permitted by law, to protect the patient's right to confidentiality and privacy from physicians and staff not involved in his case, and to instruct the patient about his care requirements after discharge. These standards represent a significant departure from the traditional paternalism governing the doctor–patient relationship. The physician, who once was empowered by his ethics to be sole arbiter in deciding how to manage a case and what to tell the patient, would henceforth have to take the patient into the decision-making process and even recognize the patient's superior authority in the process. The Patient's Bill of Rights applies only to patients in hospitals, but it sets a precedent that physicians may eventually be obligated to follow in their own ethical codes.

Conclusions

The difficulties confronting professional leaders who undertake to establish ethical standards on new issues reflect the conflicts in fundamental values inherent in diverse views of medical ethics. The traditional ethics of the professional physician tends to ennoble him and to place great emphasis on the virtue of benevolence and the doctor's need to devote himself to the service of his patients. This tradition honors the individuality of the doctor–patient relationship, professional secrecy, and the physician's duty to promote the patient's welfare. In these and other matters, ethical formulations by physicians have been paternalistic, making the physician the dominant party in determining what action will best advance both the doctor's and the patient's interests. Recent codes prepared by interests outside the medical profession have advanced other philosophical tenets as foundations for medical ethics. Religion's dedication to moral rectitude has challenged the reliance by the medical profession on the benefits of medical care as a justification of ethical standards. Government-sponsored codes have given the general welfare priority over the interests of individual patients in some instances, and consumer groups have demanded more rights for patients to participate in decisions affecting their welfare. This has resulted in mounting ethical confusion as physicians become subject to competing ethical authorities with conflicting standards.

Responsibility for the development of ethical guidelines relative to the physician–patient relationship may be shifting from the physician to society as a whole. Only in those contingencies not anticipated by accepted guidelines does the responsibility for ethical criteria still remain with the individual physician, and medical societies are codifying the ethics of these moral frontiers as rapidly as consensus is being reached. Future success in the use of codes to control medical practice may well depend on an accommodation of the ethical norms of physicians with those of the larger society.

DONALD KONOLD

[*For the text of codes discussed in this article as well as other related codes, see* APPENDIX, *especially* SECTIONS I, III, *and* IV. *Directly related to this article is the companion article in this entry,* ETHICAL ANALYSIS, *as well as the article* CODES OF THE HEALTH-CARE PROFESSIONS *in the* INTRODUCTION *to the* APPENDIX. *A number of articles on the history of medical ethics are directly relevant, especially:* MEDICAL ETHICS, HISTORY OF, *section on* NEAR AND MIDDLE EAST AND AFRICA, *article on* ANCIENT NEAR EAST; *section on* SOUTH AND EAST ASIA, *articles on* INDIA *and* PREREPUBLICAN CHINA; *section on* EUROPE AND THE AMERICAS, *articles on* ANCIENT GREECE AND ROME, BRITAIN AND THE UNITED STATES IN THE EIGHTEENTH CENTURY, BRITAIN IN THE NINETEENTH CENTURY, NORTH AMERICA: SEVENTEENTH TO NINETEENTH CENTURY, *and* NORTH AMERICA IN THE TWENTIETH CENTURY. *Also directly related is the entry* RELIGIOUS DIRECTIVES IN MEDICAL ETHICS. *For further discussion of topics mentioned in this article, see the entries:* ABORTION; ADVERTISING BY MEDICAL PROFESSIONALS; CONFIDENTIALITY; DEATH AND DYING: EUTHANASIA AND SUSTAINING LIFE; DEATH, DEFINITION AND DETERMINATION OF; INFORMED CONSENT IN THE THERAPEUTIC RELATIONSHIP; LIFE; MEDICAL PROFESSION; ORGAN TRANSPLANTATION; ORTHODOXY IN MEDICINE; PATERNALISM; PATIENTS' RIGHTS MOVEMENT; RACISM; STERILIZATION; *and* SURGERY.]

BIBLIOGRAPHY

BARNS, J. W. B. "The Hippocratic Oath, An Early Text." *British Medical Journal* 2 (1964): 567. Analysis of a portion of the Hippocratic Oath found on a fragment of papyrus from the third century suggests the Oath was in use by that time.

BARTON, RICHARD THOMAS. "Sources of Medical Morals." *Journal of the American Medical Association* 193 (1965): 133–138. Barton traces two conflicting deontological traditions in medical ethics from ancient times to the present.

BURNS, CHESTER RAY. "Medical Ethics in the United States before the Civil War." Ph.D. dissertation, Johns Hopkins University, 1969. Discussion of several state and local codes and the American Medical Association code of 1847.

CHAKRAVORTY, RANES. "The Duties and Training of Physicians in Ancient India as Described in the Sushruta Samhita." *Surgery, Gynecology, and Obstetrics* 120 (1965): 1067–1070. Summary of a fifth-century Indian medical text, including a commentary on ethical duties.

Code of Medical Ethics Adopted by the American Medical Association at Philadelphia in May, 1847 and by the New York Academy of Medicine in October, 1847. New York: H. Ludwig & Co., 1848.

Declaration of Geneva, Declaration of Helsinki, Declaration of Sydney, Declaration of Oslo. New York: World Medical Association, n.d.

EDELSTEIN, LUDWIG. "The Hippocratic Oath: Text, Translation and Interpretation." *Bulletin of the History of Medicine,* supplement no. 1 (1943), pp. 1–64. Edelstein advances a highly original hypothesis regarding the origin and meaning of the Oath of Hippocrates.

———. "The Professional Ethics of the Greek Physician." *Bulletin of the History of Medicine* 30 (1956): 391–419. Edelstein traces the humanistic ideal in Greek and Roman medical ethics.

Ethical and Religious Directives for Catholic Health Facilities. Washington: U.S. Catholic Conference, Department of Health Affairs, 1971.

"Ethical Guidelines for Organ Transplantation." *Journal of the American Medical Association* 205 (1968): 341–342.

ETZIONY, M. B. *The Physician's Creed: An Anthology of Medical Prayers, Oaths and Codes of Ethics Writ-*

ten and Recited by Medical Practitioners Through the Ages. Springfield, Ill.: Charles C. Thomas, 1973. Includes editorial comments on the historical and deontological significance of each entry and a useful bibliography for topics of ethical concern.

GARCEAU, OLIVER. "Morals of Medicine: Bibliography." *Annals of the American Academy of Medicine* 363 (1966): 60–69. Comprehensive bibliography includes many references to oaths and codes, and commentaries on them.

"International Code of Medical Ethics." *World Medical Association Bulletin* I (1949): 109–111.

JAKOBOVITS, IMMANUEL. *Jewish Medical Ethics: A Comparative and Historical Study of the Jewish Religious Attitudes to Medicine and Its Practice.* 4th ed. New York: Bloch Publishing Co., 1975. Jakobovits refers to prayers and oaths as well as other documentary expressions of Jewish medical ethics.

JONES, W. H. S. *The Doctor's Oath. An Essay in the History of Medicine.* Cambridge: University Press, 1924. Contains careful analysis of problems of translation, especially helpful to interpreters of the Oath of Hippocrates, and translations of several medieval and modern adaptations of the Oath.

KING, LESTER SNOW. *The Medical World of the Eighteenth Century.* Chicago: University of Chicago Press, 1958. Chapter 8, "The Development of Medical Ethics," discusses developments in medical ethics culminating in Percival's treatise.

KONOLD, DONALD E. *A History of American Medical Ethics 1847–1912.* Madison: State Historical Society of Wisconsin, 1962. Analyzes the Code of Ethics adopted by the American Medical Association in 1847 and traces its revisions down to the present AMA code.

KUDLIEN, FRIDOLF. "Medical Ethics and Popular Ethics in Greece and Rome." *Clio Medica* 5 (1970): 91–121. Explores the traditional and practical influences on medical ethics in the classical world.

LEAKE, CHAUNCEY D. "Theories of Ethics and Medical Practice." *Journal of the American Medical Association* 208 (1969): 842–847. Survey of ethical traditions in medicine provides a background for Leake's discussion of current ethical issues and situational ethics.

————, ed. *Percival's Medical Ethics.* Baltimore: Williams and Wilkins, 1927. Percival's treatise in its entirety, as well as an introductory essay discussing the background and deontological significance of Percival's ethics and a photostat and translation of a medieval Cruciform Oath.

LEE, T'AO. "Medical Ethics in Ancient China." *Bulletin of the History of Medicine* 13 (1943): 268–277. A translation of the five commandments for physicians and summaries of other important documents are included.

LEVEY, MARTIN. "Medical Deontology in Ninth Century Islam." *Journal of the History of Medicine and Allied Sciences* 21 (1966): 358–373. Several translations of Arabic documents are included.

————. *Medical Ethics in Medieval Islam with Reference to al-Ruhawi's "Practical Ethics of the Physician."* Transactions of the American Philosophical Society, New Series 59, pt. 3. Philadelphia: American Philosophical Society, 1967. An interpretive essay introduces a complete translation of al-Ruhawi's treatise.

LEVINE, MAURICE. "The Hippocratic Oath in Modern Dress." *Journal of the Association of American Medi-* *cal Colleges* 23 (1948): 317–323. To Levine the Hippocratic Oath is essentially a statement of some of the problems of countertransference in medical practice.

MACKINNEY, LOREN C. "Medical Ethics and Etiquette in the Early Middle Ages: The Persistence of Hippocratic Ideals." *Bulletin of the History of Medicine* 26 (1952): 1–31. Manuscripts described reveal an early and widespread diffusion of Hippocratic ethical concepts in medieval Europe.

"The Medical Oath: Empty Ritual or Wellspring of Dedication?" *Spectrum,* Winter 1965–1966, pp. 6–9. Brief survey of medical oaths, illustrated with reproductions of many of them.

MENON, I. A., and HABERMAN, H. F. "The Medical Students' Oath of Ancient India." *Medical History* 14 (1970): 295–299. The oath is taken from the *Charaka Samhita,* a medical text written about A.D. 1. A commentary is included.

MUNTNER, SUSSMAN. "Hebrew Medical Ethics and the Oath of Asaph." *Journal of the American Medical Association* 205 (1968): 912–913. Muntner discusses Asaf's Oath as an integral part of a Hebrew tradition.

"The Oath of Soviet Physicians." *Journal of the American Medical Association* 217 (1971): 834.

OLIVER, JAMES H., and MAAS, PAUL L. "An Ancient Poem on the Duties of a Physician." *Bulletin of the History of Medicine* 7 (1939): 315–323. Inspirational message documents the ideal standards for medical practice in ancient Greece.

"The Physician and the Dying Patient." Report of the Judicial Council, American Medical Association, December 1973.

REDDY, D. V. SUBBA. "Medical Ethics in Ancient India." *Journal of the Indian Medical Association* 37 (1967): 287–288. Summaries of ethical concepts in the *Kasyapa Samhita* and the *Kalyana Karaka.*

ROSNER, FRED. "The Physician's Prayer Attributed to Moses Maimonides." *Bulletin of the History of Medicine* 41 (1967): 440–454. Analysis of the controversy over the prayer's authorship, including a complete English translation.

————, and MUNTNER, SUSSMAN. "The Oath of Asaph." *Annals of Internal Medicine* 63 (1965): 317–320. A complete text of the Oath of Asaph accompanies a comparison of it with the Oath of Hippocrates.

SMITHIES, F. O. "On the Origin and Development of Ethics in Medicine and the Influence of Ethical Formulae upon Medical Practice." *Annals of Clinical Medicine* 3 (1924–1925): 573–603. Concentrates on the relationship between the conduct of physicians and ethical rules.

"Statement on a Patient's Bill of Rights." *Hospitals,* February 1973, p. 41.

"A Statement on Death." *World Medical Journal* 15 (1968): 133–134. Declaration of Sydney.

"Statement on Therapeutic Abortion." *World Medical Journal* 17 (1970): 125. Declaration of Oslo.

"Ten Principles of Medical Ethics." *Journal of the American Medical Association* 164 (1957): 1119–1120.

"Zum deontologischen Gehalt ärztlicher Standesordnungen." *Arzt und Christ* 17 (1st Quarter 1971): 1–41. The ethical regulations of medicine for twelve nations and the World Medical Association, along with a useful bibliographical listing of such regulations for twenty-eight other nations.

II
ETHICAL ANALYSIS

Codes, oaths, and prayers of medical ethics have emerged over the centuries from disparate sources, representing disparate societies, time periods, organizations, and perspectives. It is not surprising that they differ significantly in style and content. This article will examine systematically the ethical content of this divergent collection of documents from the earliest to contemporary times.

Ethical languages

Before looking at substantive differences in ethical content it is important to note the different languages used in various codes of medical ethics. Some of the earliest documents take the form of an oath or pledge. The Hippocratic Oath is sworn in the first person in the name of "Apollo Physician and Asclepius and Hygieia and Panaceia." The strong construction "I will" is used throughout. The Indian Oath of Initiation appearing in the Caraka Samhita and the Oath of Asaph (the oldest Hebrew medical ethical text), on the other hand, are both written in the teacher's words, to be administered to the new initiate. The Caraka Samhita uses the command language "thou shalt," the Oath of Asaph, the imperative. Modern codes, however, have tended to use the command language, secularizing the text, and frequently use the third person. The code written by Thomas Percival at the end of the eighteenth century uses "should" and "ought" constructions. In the first principle of his code, Percival says that hospital physicians and surgeons "*should* study . . . in their deportment, so to unite tenderness with steadiness, and condescension with authority" (Leake). The third-person use of "should" and "ought" was kept in the American Medical Association's (AMA) code in 1847, which was heavily dependent upon Percival. It remains in the twentieth-century AMA codes, the International Code of Medical Ethics of the World Medical Association (WMA) (1949), and many other medical professional organizations. The WMA's Declaration of Geneva (1948, revised 1968) and the Oath of Soviet Physicians (1971) returns to the earlier first-person language where the physician begins, "I solemnly swear—."

In the mid-twentieth century, especially following the Nazi experience, the language of rules becomes the common mode of expression in many professional codes, especially codes or statements dealing with human experimenta-

tion. This is seen in the Nuremberg Code (1946), the Declaration of Helsinki (1964, revised 1975), and the International Code of Medical Ethics (1949).

What is striking is the absence from the codes of physicians and most other medical professional groups of any "rights" language. The concept of rights is fundamentally modern. It is in the recent nonprofessional codes or "bills of rights" that rights are claimed, usually on behalf of patients or other nonprofessionals. The Patient's Bill of Rights (1972), the Pediatric Bill of Rights (1974), and the Declaration of General and Specific Rights of the Mentally Retarded (1968) are all documents where rights claims dominate. The Ethical and Religious Directives for Catholic Health Facilities (1971), a document from a religious denomination drafted and issued by the Roman Catholic hierarchy of the United States, mixes the language of rights with that of obligations or duties. Occasional references to rights, sometimes for health-care consumers, but often of health-care providers, occur in other modern documents such as the codes of the American dental, nursing, and chiropractic associations. In rare cases—for example, in the codes of the American Nurses' Association (1950, revised 1976) and the American Psychological Association (1963, revised 1972)—the descriptive sentences are used with clear hortatory implications, e.g., "The nurse provides services with respect for the dignity of man."

The central ethic

Ethical analysis of the codes of medical ethics creates problems. It is unfair to expect them to be fully developed, systematic theories of medical ethics. On the other hand the codes, at least the modern ones, are normally the product of much discussion, debate, and review. These, along with the historical documents that have had lasting significance, can reasonably be expected to reflect the basic ethical views of the organizations that have endorsed them. In fact it might be argued that documents that are the product of practitioners rather than theoreticians reflect even more accurately the ethical stance of the group than do the more systematic efforts at developing theories of medical ethics. For this reason it is valuable to examine the principles that seem to be implied in them.

When one turns to the substance of the codes, especially the physician codes, one can identify what might be called a central ethical obligation, a basic principle that provides the physician with a core moral stance for resolving ethical dilemmas. A striking feature is the presence of contradictions among the codes and the controversial nature of these central ethics.

Modern Western medical ethics has reiterated the central ethic of the Hippocratic Oath into the twentieth century. In spite of the fact that the Hippocratic position was a minority ethic for Greek society, it seems to be the foundation of much modern non-Marxist, physician ethics. The core ethic of the Hippocratic Oath is the physician's pledge to do what he thinks will benefit his patient. This is repeated twice in the Oath. Following the Pythagorean tripartite division of medicine—into dietetics, pharmacology, and surgery—the physician first pledges, "I will apply dietetic measures for the benefit of the sick according to my ability and judgment." Later, with regard to entering the patient's home, he pledges, "I will come for the benefit of the sick, remaining free of all intentional injustice."

The principle that the physician's first obligation is to do what he thinks will benefit the sick person is picked up in the Declaration of Geneva, where the physician swears, "The health of my patient will be my first consideration," and in the WMA's International Code of Medical Ethics, which proclaims that "the doctor owes to his patient complete loyalty and all the resources of his science."

The controversial nature of the "patient-benefiting" ethic, which at first seems so innocuous as to be platitudinous, is seen when it is contrasted with other major ethical positions both among physician groups and in society more generally. The first characteristic of the Hippocratic ethic is that it is individualistic: It concentrates only on benefit to the patient. In contrast, classical utilitarian ethics of the tradition of Bentham, Mill, and G. E. Moore would consider such a narrow focus on consequences for the patient to be ethically unjustified. Only if there were an intermediate empirical claim—a claim that, by having physicians concern themselves only with benefits to their individual patients, the greater good of the greater number will be served in the long run—would a holder of an ethical theory concerned with net benefits in aggregate find the Hippocratic principle acceptable. There is no evidence that the Hippocratic authors or their twentieth-century counterparts had such an indirect utilitarianism in mind. Rather they seem to hold that the physician has a special ethical obligation to benefit his patient,

independently of the net consequences for others who are nonpatients. The real test comes in a case where the physician believes that one course will produce the most good in total, but another course will most benefit the patient. A physician who says he must choose the course most beneficial to the patient is faithfully following the Oath and rejecting the utilitarian alternative.

The AMA in its 1957 Principles of Medical Ethics could not accept the Hippocratic individualism. It instructs the AMA physician that "the principle objective of the medical profession is to render service to humanity [not the individual patient]." The tenth principle makes this interpretation unambiguous:

The honored ideals of the medical profession imply that the responsibilities of the physician extend not only to the individual, but also to society where these responsibilities deserve his interest and participation in activities which have the purpose of improving both the health and well-being of the individual and the community.

Here the AMA is closer to the Soviet physicians' oath than to Hippocrates'. The Soviet physician more boldly swears "to work conscientiously wherever the interests of the society will require it" and "to conduct all my actions according to the principles of the Communistic morale, to always keep in mind the high calling of the Soviet physician, and the high responsibility I have to my people and to the Soviet government."

Second, the central ethic of the Hippocratic ethic is paternalistic. The physician is to benefit his patient "according to my ability and judgment." Physicians, according to Percival, should study not only tenderness and steadiness but "condescension and authority, as to inspire the minds of their patients with gratitude, respect, and confidence" (Leake). The AMA and the 1959 British Medical Association (BMA) codes held that medical confidences could be broken if, in the judgment of the physician, it is in the patient's interest for them to be broken. Ludwig Edelstein gives a paternalistic interpretation to the Hippocratic pledge that the physician will not only benefit the sick but also "keep them from harm and injustice." Edelstein, on the question of from whom the physician is to protect the patient, addresses the arguments of some scholars that the patient is to be protected from his family, from friends, or the physician himself. He rejects those arguments, citing an axiom of Pythagorean dietetics that the bodily passions may lead one to inflict harm on himself. He concludes that the Oath means that "the physician must protect his patient from the mischief and injustice which he may inflict upon himself if his diet is not properly chosen" (Edelstein, p. 25).

Finally, one sees the controversy of the Hippocratic patient-benefiting ethic when it is contrasted with other nonconsequentialist ethical theories in which certain principles are taken to be simply inherently right-making or where certain claims are taken to be "inalienable rights." The Kantian ethical tradition, for instance, holds that one can by "pure practical" reason establish certain maxims, which one can act upon and at the same time will that they be universal laws of nature. The deontological or formalist theories of the twentieth century that follow Kant would similarly hold that certain characteristics of actions are right-making—at least when they do not conflict with or are not overridden by other prima facie duties. Such duties as truth-telling, promise keeping, justice, reparation, and gratitude appear on the list of W. D. Ross, one of the leading proponents of such a view. The limitation of morally relevant benefits to those of the patient already has a deontological quality. Holders of such views consider something morally relevant besides consequences, i.e., the one to whom the consequences accrue is also morally relevant. Holders of views in which there are certain characteristics of actions that make them inherently tend toward being right (other things being equal) or holders of the view that certain things like life, liberty, and the pursuit of happiness are "inalienable rights" would have to reject the ethic of doing what one thinks will *benefit* the patient, at least in cases where benefiting the patient will be at the expense of fulfilling prima facie duties or fulfilling basic rights of the patient, such as the right to reasonable information upon which to base consent or giving some nonpatient fair access to needed medical care.

There may be a paradox in the Hippocratic Oath. The physician is to do what he thinks will benefit the patient but is not to give a deadly drug or "use the knife, not even on sufferers from stone." What is the physician to do if he believes that giving a deadly drug or an abortifacient remedy, or using the knife will benefit his patient? Perhaps this apparent contradiction is resolved by the belief of the Pythagorean physician that such actions can never be beneficial to the patient. In that case the Oath simply spells out some rules that guide the physician in deciding what will be beneficial. Alternatively these actions are seen as inherently wrong even if they might be of benefit. If so, then the Hippocratic ethic abandons its consequentialism, at least for these cases.

Specific ethical injunctions

The strictures against abortion, euthanasia, and surgery are examples of specific injunctions that occur from time to time in the codes and oaths of medical and physician ethics. Code-by-code systematic comparison of these injunctions reveals interesting differences. The conflict among the codes on the question of confidentiality is perhaps the most dramatic. It will be taken up first, followed by several other specific injunctions.

1. Confidentiality. The Hippocratic injunction on confidentiality is sometimes taken to forbid breaking medical confidences. The text is really much more ambiguous. It says, "Whatever I may see or hear in the course of the treatment or even outside of the treatment in regard to the life of men, which on no account one must speak abroad, I will keep to myself holding such things shameful to be spoken about." The individual physician, however, is left with the question, just which things which he hears "on no account must be spoken abroad"? Possibly we are to use the "patient-benefiting" criterion for deciding when breaking the confidence is appropriate. That was the explicit principle in the British Medical Association Code in its 1959 version, which said:

It is a practitioner's obligation to observe the rule of professional secrecy by refraining from disclosing voluntarily without the consent of the patient (save with statutory sanction) to any third party information which he has learnt in his professional relationship with the patient. The complications of modern life sometimes create difficulties for the doctor in the application of this principle, and on certain occasions it may be necessary to acquiesce in some modification. Always, however, the overriding consideration must be adoption of a line of conduct that will benefit the patient, or protect his interests.

The World Medical Association's International Code of Medical Ethics (1949) and the Declaration of Geneva (1948, revised 1968) both close any such patient-benefiting loophole in the confidentiality principle. They simply require "absolute secrecy," much as did the ancient Jewish Oath of Asaph. No exception is considered even in a case where the physician has learned that his patient is about to commit mass murder. The Ethical and Religious Directives for Catholic Health Facilities (1971) are almost as blunt. They require that "professional secrecy must be carefully fulfilled not only as regards the information on the patient's charts and records but also as regards confidential matters learned in the exercise of professional duties. Moreover, the charts and records must be duly safeguarded against inspection by those who have no right to see them." The only escape might be in the interpretation of "those who have no right to see them." That qualifier has somewhat the character of the Hippocratic "which on no account one must spread abroad."

Keeping with their more social commitment to the welfare of others as well as the patient, the American Medical Association Principles (1957, revised 1971) (and the American Psychiatric Association's [1973] which are based on them) are quite explicit in providing three exceptions to the general principle of confidentiality:

A physician may not reveal the confidences entrusted to him in the course of medical attendance, or the deficiencies he may observe in the character of his patients, unless he is required to do so by law or unless it becomes necessary in order to protect the welfare of the individual or of the society.

Confidences can be broken not only when the physician thinks it will benefit the patient but also when he thinks it will benefit society or when it is required by law, e.g., informing the police of a bullet wound incurred in a crime. The ethical problem of such broad exceptions, of course, is not only the paternalism of the patient-benefiting exclusion but the potential subordination of the patient's interests and rights to the interests of the society. The Soviet oath, which one might expect to be as explicitly societal in its concerns as the AMA Principles, ambiguously pledges to "keep professional secrets."

The British Medical Association was confronted by a particularly difficult case in which the physician disclosed to the parents of a sixteen-year-old that she was taking birth-control pills. He defended the breaking of the confidence on the grounds that he thought it was for her benefit. This being explicitly permitted by the existing British Medical Association code, the General Medical Council acquitted him of the charge of unprofessional conduct. After that case the BMA in 1971 amended its confidentiality principle to provide the first recognition of the patient's right to confidence in cases where the patient and physician disagree about the proper course. The new code states:

If, in the opinion of the doctor, disclosure of confidential information to a third party seems to be in the best medical interest of the patient, it is the doctor's duty to make every effort to allow the information to be given to the third party, but where the patient refuses, that refusal must be respected.

2. Abortion. On the controversial subject of abortion, groups authoring codes have followed the ethical stance of the group subculture. The Hippocratic Oath follows the Pythagorean prohibition on abortion even though abortion was not generally considered unethical in the broader Greek culture (Edelstein, pp. 9–20). In the Oath of Asaph the early medieval Jewish medical initiate is instructed, "Do not prepare any potion that may cause a woman who has conceived in adultery to miscarry." The 1971 Ethical and Religious Directives for (U.S.) Catholic Health Facilities follow, consciously and precisely, a traditional theological explanation of official Church teaching, devoting six of its forty-three principles to the subject. Directly intended termination of pregnancy before viability is never permitted, nor is the directly intended destruction of a viable fetus. Treatments not intended to terminate a pregnancy but which nonetheless have that effect are permitted provided there is a proportionately serious pathological condition of the mother and the treatments cannot be safely postponed until after the fetus is viable.

When the cultural base of the group writing the code is very broad, the code is predictably less specific about the ethics of abortion. The Declaration of Geneva (1948, revised 1968) says, "I will maintain the utmost respect for human life from the time of conception" without directly prohibiting abortion. The WMA's International Code in its draft, but not in its finally adopted form, stated, "Therapeutic abortion may only be performed if the conscience of the doctors and the national laws permit." The American Nurses' Association (ANA), also representing individuals with a wide variety of viewpoints, also avoids direct comment. In their code revised in 1968 and in effect prior to the 1976 revision they say that "the nurse's respect for the worth and dignity of the individual human being extends throughout the entire life cycle, from *birth* to death" (italics added). The implication may be that fetal life is not included.

A 1966 statement approved by the ANA Board of Directors recognizes "the right of individuals and families to select and use such methods for family planning as are consistent with their own creed and mores," again appealing to individual conscience. Is the combined implication a tolerance of the nurse's participation in abortion? If so, what is the Catholic nurse to do, or what is the nurse who believes in the right of the individual to select methods for family planning to do if she works in a Catholic health facility? These conflicts for individuals who are simultaneously members of more than one group authoring a code need serious attention.

3. Euthanasia. An explicit obligation to preserve life is strikingly absent from the codes of ethics, both professional and public. In the light of a widely held view that the duty, or one of the duties, of the physician is to preserve life one would expect to find this duty emphasized. The only explicit reference with which we are familiar is the weak formulation in the International code (1949), which says that "a doctor must always bear in mind the obligation of preserving life." This obligation to "bear in mind" rather than explicitly attempt to preserve life is a very soft injunction, especially when it is combined with the patient-benefiting principle that an act which could "weaken physical or mental resistance of a human being may be used only in his interest."

Proscribing active killing is much more common in the codes, as might be expected from the general ethical prohibition on active killing even for mercy in many cultures and subcultures. The Hippocratic formula is, "I will neither give a deadly drug to anybody if asked for it, nor will I make a suggestion to this effect." Interpretation of this prohibition is controversial, some taking it to forbid any criminal attempt on a patient's life. That seems less likely, however, than a prohibition against assisting in suicide. While suicide, especially in the face of medical suffering, was not uncommon in ancient society, it was forbidden by the Pythagorean cult. This fact is cited by Edelstein in his defense of the hypothesis that the Hippocratic Oath is a Pythagorean document. "Acts causing another's death" were one of the few things the Indian medical student should not do at his teacher's behest according to the Caraka Samhita. The Oath of Asaph instructs the Jewish medical student to "take heed that you kill not any man with a root decoction." The prohibition against assisting in an act of killing, however, has never been extended to

apply to cooperating in withdrawal from treatment. The distinction between active killing and withdrawal of certain treatments is clear in the Ethical and Religious Directives for Catholic Health Facilities, where it is held that "the directly intended termination of any patient's life, even at his own request, is always wrong," and that "euthanasia ('mercy killing') in all its forms is forbidden." The directives go on, however, to say that "failure to supply the ordinary means of preserving life is equivalent to euthanasia. However, neither the physician nor the patient is obliged to use extraordinary means." This also makes clear that "giving a dying person sedatives or analgesics for the alleviation of pain, when such a measure is judged necessary, even though they may deprive the patient of the use of reason, or shorten his life," is not taken to be euthanasia.

The distinction between active killing and omitting treatment by medical professionals is made clearer when the rights language is used, as in A Patient's Bill of Rights (1973). That document proclaims that "the patient has the right to refuse treatment to the extent permitted by law," presumably even if the result will be the death of the patient. It is clear, however, that the authors were not saying, nor did they intend to say, that the patient has the right to demand of the physician that drugs be given that will actively hasten death. Without using rights language the AMA, in its House of Delegates meeting in December 1973, took a similar position stating that, while intentional termination of the life of one human being by another is contrary to that for which the medical profession stands, "the cessation of the employment of extraordinary means to prolong the life of the body when there is irrefutable evidence that biological death is imminent is the decision of the patient and/or his immediate family" ("The Physician and the Dying Patient," report of the Judicial Council of the AMA as adopted by the House of Delegates, 4 December 1973). This statement, of course, does not go as far as the Patient's Bill of Rights in granting the right of the patient to refuse treatment insofar as it is legally permissible. It goes much further, however, than the more paternalistic resolution adopted by the New York State Medical Society House of Delegates in February of that year, which granted "the right to die with dignity with the approval of the family physician."

4. Truth-telling. One of the most conspicuous conflicts between the patient-benefiting principle and the more deontological ethical theories is over the question of what one ought to tell a dying patient. Many of the professional codes are simply silent, presumably expecting the patient-benefiting principle to apply. The Indian oath of the Caraka Samhita is more explicit, stating, "Even knowing that the patient's span of life has come to its close, it shall not be mentioned by thee there, where if so done, it would cause shock to the patient or to others." The 1847 version of the AMA code instructs: "A physician should not be forward to make a gloomy prognostication . . . but should not fail, on proper occasions, to give to the friends of the patient timely notice of danger, when it really occurs, and even to the patient himself, if absolutely necessary." The violation of confidentiality in communicating to family or friends before informing the patient either is not noticed or is justified on patient-benefiting grounds. The grounding of the violation of any obligation to tell the truth in the patient-benefit principle is traditional in professional physician ethics. The AMA code makes the grounding explicit: "It is, therefore, a sacred duty . . . to avoid all things [that] have a tendency to discourage the patient and to depress his spirits."

Even the authors of A Patient's Bill of Rights seem to yield to the paternalistic patient-benefiting principle when it conflicts with the patient's proclaimed right to know. The Bill states that "the patient has the right to obtain from his physician complete current information concerning his diagnosis, treatment, and prognosis in terms the patient can be reasonably expected to understand." But it then qualifies this by stating that, "when it is not medically advisable to give such information to the patient, the information should be made available to the appropriate person in his behalf." The potential conflict of such an exception with the later-proclaimed right to privacy or the right to receive information necessary to give informed consent are not discussed. In any case even A Patient's Bill of Rights would be found wanting by one fully committed to a more deontological ethic in which truth-telling was at least a prima facie duty.

5. Justice in delivering health care. Many of the codes of physician and other medical ethics have some reference to the duty to deliver health care equitably. The Hippocratic Oath commits the physician to "remain free of all intentional injustice." The Greek term, *adikiē*, which is translated "injustice," has the meaning of "wrongdoing" more generally. The Hippocratic commitment to equal treatment of males and females, free and slave, in abstaining from sexual relations during a medical visit is as close as the Hippocratic text comes to a pledge to equal treatment. The commandments written by Chen Shih-Kung, a seventeenth-century Chinese physician, include a much more explicit commitment that "physicians should be ever ready to respond to any calls of patients, high or low, rich or poor." The twentieth-century Declaration of Geneva holds forth the same ideal: "I will not permit considerations of religion, nationality, race, party politics, or social standing to intervene between my duty and my patient," as does the American Nurses' Association indicative statement of the ideal: "The nurse provides services with respect for the dignity of man, unrestricted by considerations of nationality, race, creed, color, or status." Equality of access seems generally recognized as an ideal. That providing general access to professional services may directly conflict with fulfilling other ethical duties—such as the duty to do what will benefit the (present) patient—has not been explicitly addressed in the codes.

6. Rules, laws, and cases. In the mid-twentieth century a debate emerged in ethical theory between those who, like Joseph Fletcher, hold that what is right must be decided on a case-by-case basis and those who, like John Rawls in philosophy and Paul Ramsey in theology, give a more significant place to rules or law in deciding what is right ethically. It is the nature of codes of ethics that they are general statements of right and wrong kinds of acts—i.e., guidelines or sets of rules. Thus it is not surprising that, especially when dealing with specific issues such as abortion and euthanasia, they are seen as raising the problems of systems of ethics that emphasize rules.

Nevertheless, the overarching centrality of the patient-benefiting principle provides an out for the situationalist. Thus the Hippocratic Oath says with regard to confidentiality that the physician is not to disclose those things that ought not to be disclosed. The American Osteopathic Association code (1965) warns that "no code or set of rules can be framed which will particularize all ethical responsibilities of the physician in the various phases of his professional life." This commitment to the uniqueness of individual cases is typical of the strong situationalism of the medical professions in contrast with other groups and other ethical theories. It contrasts, for instance, with the governmental requirement that informed consent be obtained before a subject is used for research regardless of the uniqueness of the situation. In spite of that situationalism, however, some of the modern codes—especially those that are open to consideration of societal as well as patient interests—emphasize the necessity of obeying the law. The Osteopaths' code specifies that "the physician shall cooperate fully in complying with all laws and regulations pertaining to practice of the healing arts and protection of the public health." The AMA permits breaking confidentiality when required by law.

The ethics of professional relations

Virtually all of the professional codes—in contrast with the lay and public codes or bills of rights—devote major attention to relationships among professionals. The Hippocratic Oath begins with a covenant by which the new physician pledges "to hold him who taught me this art as equal to my parents and to live my life in partnership with him, and if he is in need of money to give him a share of mine, and to regard his offspring as equal to my brothers in male lineage and to teach them this art—if they desire to learn it—without fee and covenant." It includes a pledge to keep secrets much as any initiation ritual into a cult might. The longest of the three sections of the AMA code of 1847 is devoted to "the duties of physicians to each other and to the profession at large." Since many of the codes emerged at a point historically when the profession was separating itself from others claiming to offer treatments and cures, there is often strong language forbidding association with those not properly members of the group. The American Osteopathic Association, for instance, requires that a physician "shall practice in accordance with the body of systematized knowledge related to the healing arts and shall avoid professional association with individuals or organizations which do not practice or conduct organization affairs in accordance with such knowledge."

In terms of the sociology of the professions, it has been suggested that restraints on advertising, rules structuring the referral of patients, instructions on the ways of handling the incompetent member of the profession, or exclusion of those not properly initiated into the profession play important functions in maintaining the professional monopoly. Apart from the sociolog-

ical functions of the codes, i.e., as rationalizations for protecting professional interests, it is also pertinent to analyze them as sets of ethical obligations.

If, for purposes of ethical analysis, we presume that the function of the sections of the codes dealing with relations among professionals is to spell out what are really perceived as ethical obligations, it should still be clear that appeals are being made to specific types of underlying ethical principles. Three different kinds of ethical arguments may underlie the detailed formulations of professional obligations to other professionals. First, such duties to one's colleagues may be defended on what could be called "universal" grounds. That would be the case if the ethical principles claimed as the foundation of such intraprofessional obligations are principles generally recognized by all persons. For instance, the AMA code of 1847 states detailed rules regarding professional consultation prohibiting "exclusion from fellowship" of duly licensed practitioners, punctuality in visits of physicians when they hold consultations, and secrecy and confidentiality so that the patient will not be aware that any of the consultants did not agree. These standards for consultation, however, are defended on the grounds that "the good of the patient is the sole object in view." Although it is generally not argued, there is a presumption that rational patients should accept this underlying principle. We have seen, of course, that the principle of patient-benefit is quite controversial when put up against competing ethical principles.

A second foundation for intraprofessional duties might be a special ethic for a special group, which, in principle, nonmembers of the group would not be expected to share. The ethic of a profession is in part the ethic of fraternal loyalty, of special obligation to one's adopted brothers. This special professional ethical obligation may be seen as deriving from the professional nexus rather than from some more universal source. It is a special ethic of a special cult.

The ethic of the AMA 1847 code, as of that written by Percival, is an ethic of the gentlemanly class. The ethic is one of dignity and honor among gentlemen. According to the AMA's 1847 code, "there is no profession, from the members of which greater purity of character and a higher standard of moral excellence are required, than the medical." It introduces the discussion of duties of physicians to each other by stating that "each physician on entering the profession, as he becomes thereby entitled to all its privileges and immunities, incurs an obligation to exert his best abilities to maintain its dignity and honor, to exalt its standing, and to extend the bounds of its usefulness." The text goes on to entreat the physician to avoid "all contumelious and sarcastic remarks relative to the faculty, as a body; and while by unwearied diligence, he resorts to every honorable means of enriching the science, he should entertain a due respect for his . . . seniors who have, by their labors, brought it to the elevated condition in which he finds it."

This gentlemanly ethic of honor and purity (the Hippocratic phrase is "purity and holiness") gives rise to special ethical burdens for the medical professional that the layman cannot be expected to grasp. Professional "courtesy" (gratuitous services for practitioners, their wives, and their children) should probably be understood in these terms. "Courtesy" is an ethical expectation for members of the brotherhood.

A third possible foundation conflates the two. It could be that professional duties are defended as being in the public interest (or in some other manner consistent with a more universal ethic), but that only members of the profession can be expected to understand this to be so. Advertising, for instance, could be attacked as it is in the AMA's 1847 code as "derogatory to the dignity of the profession" and necessary to separate the profession from "the ordinary practices of empirics." The authors might well hold that it is really in the public interest that the separation be made, but also concede that only members of the profession could see the necessity of that separation.

If there are special ethical obligations for members of the profession that in principle cannot be recognized from outside the professional group, it follows that there are likely to be conflicts between the profession's formulation of its ethical obligation and the broader public's formulation. The issue is not the existence of different ethical responsibilities attaching to different roles but rather a disagreement between the profession and the broader public over what constitutes the proper behavior of the professional in his specific professional role. Even if a profession agreed that it had a special duty to preserve life or limit advertising, it is still an open question whether the public wants physicians always to act on that norm. If the professional group holds that there is a special professional source of norms, then conflict is predictable.

A specific example of such conflict involves the ethics of advertising. Many professional codes in the manner of the 1847 AMA code prohibit or restrict advertising by members of the profession. The 1957 Principles of Medical Ethics of the AMA claim that "this principle protects the public from the advertiser and salesman of medical care by establishing an easily discernible and generally recognized distinction between him and the ethical physician." While such prohibitions on advertising might be seen as the behavior of a cartel restraining price competition, it is also possible that physicians really believe that they are engaged in a service that must be radically separated from peddling medical services as a commodity. Whether the medical profession sees such advertising as unethical or not, the public may see restraint on advertising as unethical. At stake are not only two different perceptions of ways of maximizing benefits to potential patients, but also two sources of ethical norms—one from within the professional nexus and the other from the broader society.

Conclusion

The codes, oaths, prayers, and bills of rights derive from radically different contexts, representing differing professional groups, public agencies, and private lay organizations such as churches and patients' groups. It is not surprising that radically different ethical conclusions are reached and that they are based on radically different fundamental ethical theories and methods of ethical reasoning.

ROBERT M. VEATCH

[*For the text of the relevant codes, see* APPENDIX, SECTION I: GENERAL CODES FOR THE PRACTICE OF MEDICINE, SECTION III: PATIENTS' BILLS OF RIGHTS, *and* SECTION IV: CODES OF SPECIALTY HEALTH-CARE ASSOCIATIONS. *For further discussion of topics mentioned in this article, see the entries:* ABORTION; ADVERTISING BY MEDICAL PROFESSIONALS; CHILDREN AND BIOMEDICINE; CONFIDENTIALITY; CONTRACEPTION; DEATH AND DYING: EUTHANASIA AND SUSTAINING LIFE, *article on* PROFESSIONAL AND PUBLIC POLICIES; ETHICS, *articles on* RULES AND PRINCIPLES, DEONTOLOGICAL THEORIES, TELEOLOGICAL THEORIES, *and* SITUATION ETHICS; HEALTH CARE, *articles on* RIGHT

TO HEALTH-CARE SERVICES *and* THEORIES OF JUSTICE AND HEALTH CARE; HUMAN EXPERIMENTATION, *articles on* BASIC ISSUES *and* SOCIAL AND PROFESSIONAL CONTROL; INFORMED CONSENT IN HUMAN RESEARCH, *article on* ETHICAL AND LEGAL ASPECTS; INFORMED CONSENT IN THE THERAPEUTIC RELATIONSHIP, *article on* LEGAL AND ETHICAL ASPECTS; MEDICAL PROFESSION; NURSING; PATERNALISM; PATIENTS' RIGHTS MOVEMENT; RIGHT TO REFUSE MEDICAL CARE; SURGERY; *and* TRUTH-TELLING. *See also:* RELIGIOUS DIRECTIVES IN MEDICAL ETHICS.]

BIBLIOGRAPHY

[The bibliography for this article is the same as for the previous article. In the Appendix, the reader will find the texts of codes and additional bibliography of codes and commentaries on codes of ethics for the medical and other health professions.]

CODES OF THE HEALTH-CARE PROFESSIONS

See APPENDIX, INTRODUCTION, *article on* CODES OF THE HEALTH-CARE PROFESSIONS. *See also the texts of numerous codes, oaths, prayers, and statements in the* APPENDIX.

COMMISSION AND OMISSION

See ACTING AND REFRAINING; DEATH AND DYING: EUTHANASIA AND SUSTAINING LIFE; *and* TRUTH-TELLING, *article on* ETHICAL ASPECTS.

COMMUNICATION, BIOMEDICAL

The two articles in this entry, MEDIA AND MEDICINE *and* SCIENTIFIC PUBLISHING, *deal with ethical questions in communicating biomedical information in the mass media and the ethics involved in the publication of scientific findings.*

I. MEDIA AND MEDICINE   *Lois DeBakey and Selma DeBakey*

II. SCIENTIFIC PUBLISHING   *Lois DeBakey*

I
MEDIA AND MEDICINE

Historical basis of journalistic ethics

Medicine is a discipline whose direction and consequences affect the public as a whole. Since science writers, through whom the public receives much of its medical information, can have an important impact on human health and social welfare, the question of moral and ethical responsibility for the information disseminated in the mass media assumes importance. Like most other social and ethical concepts, those concerning the responsibilities of the press have changed with time. Journalistic ethics, in fact, is largely a development of the twentieth century, the very existence of a free American press having originally been interpreted as assurance that it would serve the public welfare. In the authoritarian and totalitarian systems, the press is subject to direct political control, and any ethical principles observed would be at the discretion of the government in power. A brief review of ethical developments in general journalism will help place in perspective the present status of ethics in medical reporting.

The concept of freedom of the press originated in the libertarian theory, which held that censorship abridged man's natural right of free expression and that the press operated, ultimately, in the public interest. If man had free access to information and ideas, he could presumably, as a creature of reason, find "truth" himself. Freedom of the press thus carried no guarantee of verity or ethical propriety.

In colonial America, newspapers carried heavy medicinal advertising to subsidize printing costs, and manufacturers of proprietary drugs, knowing that early settlers depended on self-medication, exploited the public press. Henry Jarvis Raymond, the founder of *The New York Times*, wrote such advertisements for a quack for fifty cents apiece (Lee). With increasing technology and urbanization in the 1830s, newspapers acquired a mass audience, and yellow journalism flourished. Scare headlines, fictitious items, and stolen pictures became commonplace; ethics was totally ignored. About mid-nineteenth century, however, there emerged a sense of social responsibility among journalists.

In the first decade of the twentieth century—an era of moral awakening—newspapers made notable ethical advances, with new standards for the editorial, advertising, and circulation departments. Regulations were also imposed by state and national legislation, with more stringent libel laws. The threat of greater governmental intervention prompted the industry to establish, voluntarily, codes of professional behavior. Many newspapers refused medical advertising that promised cures for incurable diseases or contributed to drug addiction. In 1923, the American Society of Newspaper Editors adopted a code of ethics ("Code of Ethics or Canons of Journalism"), signaling a break with the libertarian tradition. Fourteen years later, the radio broadcasters adopted their code ("Standards of Good Practice for Radio Broadcasters of the United States of America"), and fifteen years still later, in 1952, the television industry followed suit ("The Television Code of The National Association of Radio and Television Broadcasters"). Although the mass media thus acknowledged a social responsibility to act in the public interest, ethics remained largely theoretical.

Whereas other professionals with a public trust, such as physicians, lawyers, and teachers, must pass licensing examinations before they can practice, journalists are not required by law to have educational qualifications, certification, or licensure, or to take a Hippocratic-like oath. Anyone can be a journalist who can find someone to publish his material. This phenomenon is paradoxical in view of the fact that those in the mass media reach, and possibly influence, more people than any other profession does. Total journalistic objectivity is, of course, impossible, and many journalists subtly inject subjective opinions in "straight news" reporting or editorialize to some extent when they are presumably merely informing. In a television program, for example, a newsman—a nonphysician—endorsed mammography for the detection of cancer, to the consternation of those physicians who question the safety of this procedure. The newsman's defense was that the medical reporter's responsibility is not merely to transmit information, but to interpret it as well. The reliability of such interpretation, and of any medical guidance derived therefrom, by those without a medical education or a medical license, however, raises ethical questions. Sometimes opinions are conveyed nonverbally: a raised eyebrow, a skeptical frown, or a sardonic smile can often be more telling and more devastating than anything spoken. But even if journalists do not tell the public *what* to think, they do influence, by the very selection of the material disseminated, what the public thinks *about*. The need for the industry to observe ethical criteria is therefore real.

Recognizing this need, the National Association of Science Writers, in June 1960, followed the precedent established by the rest of the news industry by formulating its own code of ethics to ensure the transmission of accurate, truthful, impartial information (Cohn).

An early example of medical reporting in the American public press had obvious socioethical implications. *Publick Occurrences,* identified by some historians as the first newspaper printed in the United States, devoted two paragraphs on 25 September 1690 to "Epidemical Fevers and Agues," a public health problem of serious concern to the colonists, who had experienced the ravages of smallpox (Harris). In the following year (1691), John Dunton established the *Athenian Mercury* in England (Cormick). Questions submitted by readers regarding medicine (primarily melancholy and lunacy) and other subjects were answered by the "authorities" of the Athenian Society, a fictional board of experts. Journalistic ethics was thus hardly a consideration.

With the advent of specialization in the late nineteenth and early twentieth centuries, American scientists began to cultivate a private jargon that only their peers understood. Research became deified, and professionals considered explanations to the uninitiated unworthy of their status. The reluctance of scientists to discuss their work publicly was reinforced by the medical code of ethics prohibiting publicity and by the early emphasis on sensationalism in medical journalism. After World War I, however, the medical profession's attitude toward journalists improved, partly because a corps of professional science writers assumed greater responsibility for accuracy. With the availability of governmental research funds after World War II, scientific experimentation mushroomed, and research became a professional status symbol. About mid-twentieth century, however, an antiscience attitude emerged. Exposés like Rachel Carson's *Silent Spring* and James Watson's *The Double Helix* spurred the demands for social and ethical accountability. The retrenchment of governmental funds forced scientists to go public in an attempt to prove the social relevance of medical research.

Science writing, evolving as it did from a tradition of almost unlimited freedom and invulnerability of the press, largely ignored ethical criteria and evoked varying degrees of public umbrage and distrust. This distrust, coupled with the opposing precepts of confidentiality in medicine and disclosure in journalism, erected a barrier between the two professions that made access to reliable sources of information difficult for early medical reporters. The tendency of zealous scientists to overestimate research findings and their inexperience in explaining scientific activities in lay language also impaired competent medical reportage in the mass media.

Responsible journalism

Medical reporting in the public interest. Ethical journalism is responsible journalism. Since the effects of irresponsible medical reporting extend far beyond personalities to possible impairment of scientific progress, unjustified public hostility toward science, and application of potentially dangerous medical treatment or procedures, professional medical reporters have a responsibility to convey accurate, reliable information to the public. Journalists have helped effect a number of health reforms. Exposure by crusading journalists of the maltreatment of patients in mental hospitals spurred authorities to ameliorate the sordid conditions in psychiatric institutions. When health hazards or crises occur, the mass media can alert the public almost instantaneously. Notifying consumers of contaminated or otherwise dangerous products, alerting a community to the increasing incidence of venereal or other infectious diseases, debunking quackery, and exposing other illicit or unethical practices are all in the public interest.

Television is a powerful educational tool that can also inform the public on controversial medical subjects, including ethically questionable experimentation, abortion, passive euthanasia, birth control, drug addiction, and psychic surgery. In one documentary, for example, scientists debated the dangers of genetic engineering and recombinant DNA (deoxyribonucleic acid), discussed the implications of the methods, agreed to a self-imposed moratorium on certain types of experiments, and formulated a set of guidelines to regulate future research. Providing a balanced, comprehensible discussion of such a complex, but socially important, research activity helps the public understand the prolonged and careful deliberations that precede medical experimentation and the responsibility that the scientific community assumes for its activities.

General ethical criteria. Because lay medical journalism is relatively young, little has been published on the ethics of the discipline. Many journalists readily admit, in fact, that they have never seen a code, and of those who have, few refer to it for guidance. Rather, most follow their own judgment, which must then pass the scrutiny of an editor, producer, or other higher authority before publication. Ethical violations in medical reporting may relate to the subject matter involved, the manner in which information is obtained, or the quality of the story published. Is the subject appropriate for public dissemination? Was the information obtained without duress or bribery from a reliable, reputable source? Is the story clear, accurate, and unbiased? Transgressions may include premature or immature reports in the mass media, invasion of privacy, sensationalism, and misquotations or disclosure of "off-the-record" remarks (DeBakey, 1974). Also to be avoided is conflict of interest, in which the material disseminated is influenced by emoluments, bribery, awards, or other such considerations.

Particular ethical criteria

Attribution. Attribution is requisite in medical news stories, since credibility depends on the authority of the source. Assigning statements or opinions to "reliable" but unnamed sources, as is sometimes done in other forms of journalism, is therefore inappropriate in medical reporting. Credibility is enhanced if the credentials of the writer or speaker are unassailable. Medical information conveyed by a physician is more likely to be reliable than that provided by a journalist who has no firsthand knowledge of the subject but acts merely as a medium of transmission. The information disseminated by nonphysician columnists has, in fact, sometimes been inaccurate and, on occasion, has had to be retracted. Although medical columns have long appeared in newspapers under physicians' names, it was not until the latter half of the twentieth century that physicians began to have regular health programs on radio and television, medical ethics having previously discouraged such activities as a form of advertising. Some still question the ethical propriety, however, of a physician's dispensing advice over the airwaves while remaining in the private practice of medicine.

Verbal and visual content. The medical journalist has a responsibility to convey information in simple, clear language that is comprehensible to the reader and is socially acceptable. In addition, most newspaper, radio, and television executives impose certain ethical restrictions on language used. The latter half of the twentieth century witnessed considerable relaxation of previous standards of propriety and good taste in mass communication. Before 1936, the mass media avoided the word "syphilis," a scheduled appearance of a high public health official having been canceled because he refused to delete that word from his prepared text. The purpose and focus of a story, to a great extent, govern its ethical propriety. The names of the sexual and reproductive organs, so carefully avoided in the past, are now often seen and heard in open educational discussions in the mass media. Until the 1970s, the female breast was not shown exposed on television, but today health education films regularly show how to perform self-examination of this region. The delivery of a baby and various operations, including transplantation and vasectomy, have been shown on television, even though some viewers find the sight of blood disturbing. Permission should, of course, be obtained to photograph any patient for publication.

Ethical problems

Premature publication. The ethical medical reporter obtains his information from unimpeachable sources rather than from an unreliable informer through subterfuge, intimidation, or bribery. He honors mutually approved ground rules and release dates. Since direct financial reward for contributions to medical knowledge is rare, public recognition is a strong motive in medical research, and priority is therefore of critical import. Dissemination of new scientific information in the news media before publication in professional journals has been a subject of ethical debate and a source of contention between the professions of journalism and medicine (DeBakey, 1976). Opponents of this practice point to the false hopes that may be aroused by precipitate reporting of a medical advance that has not yet been fully tested, and some have cited alleged "breakthroughs" and "wonder" drugs that were later proved false. Proponents of prepublication argue that the public has "a right to know," and to know immediately, the results of scientific research, particularly that supported by public funds. In the rare instances in which the public health is at risk, the information should obviously be released immediately. The rush to print, however, is often motivated by competition among the news services rather than eagerness to serve the public weal. The ill effects of premature enthusiasm are well illustrated by the unfortunate experiences with krebiozen, Liefcort, thalidomide, and especially human cardiac transplantation, the circus-like publicity of which hampered sober assessment. Since peer review is intended to safeguard standards of accuracy and validity, those who bypass it to make announcements first in the uncensored mass media may be interested more in self-advancement than in the integrity of science. Some physicians and medical scientists have circumvented critical peer review by publishing books, which are then widely publicized, and favorably reviewed, in the mass media, even though their content may be censured by medical experts as scientifically invalid and even dangerous.

One source of medical news in the public press is the scientific meeting, where physicians and scientists present research results, often before their publication in professional journals. When material is presented at an open meeting, it enters the public domain, but because the oral presentation represents the speaker's intellectual property, the speaker's approval should be obtained before others record or publish it. Prepublication may, in fact, deny the speaker publication of his address in a first-rate professional journal, in which originality is highly valued. For a scientific author to be victimized in this way when he has not, himself, released his report to the press prematurely is unfair. When a speaker's visual aids are copyrighted, permission to reproduce them is, of course, legally required.

When the *Washington Post* published a story on the relation of estrogens to breast cancer three days before the original scientific article appeared in the *New England Journal of Medicine*, F. J. Ingelfinger, the *Journal*'s editor, censured the reporter for "ignoring the convention not to release news of a report scheduled to appear in a scientific journal until the official publication date of that report" (Ingelfinger). An editor's note accompanying the critical Ingelfinger letter in the *Washington Post* contended that the reporter had received an advance copy of the scientific article independently. The question Ingelfinger posed is crucial: "Did [the reporter] have the right to use for himself and his paper material that clearly belonged to others?"

Leaks may have broad implications. If it is rumored that an article soon to be published in a professional journal is favorable or unfavorable to a certain medication, the stock market can be manipulated accordingly. Some journalists have pressured editors of scientific journals to release details of such articles prematurely by threatening to publish the leaked information, accurate or not. Suppression of news may, indeed, lead to publication of misinformation, but threats and duress are incompatible with ethical journalistic conduct.

Sometimes the scientist himself releases news directly to the press. Before addressing the

British Medical Association, a scientist reportedly circulated a press release about three "test-tube babies," at least one of whom, he stated, was developing normally ("The Baby Maker," p. 58). His formal presentation, however, reportedly made no reference to this claim (ibid.). Newspapers throughout the world promptly heralded the first "test-tube babies" as a miracle of modern research, leaving the impression with many that fetuses were actually conceived in test tubes. During the storm that ensued over the "unprofessional manner" of the disclosure, the scientist refused to divulge the identity of his patients, despite an offer of $72,000 from one newspaper and $120,000 from another. Declaring himself "fed up" with the publicity, the scientist announced that he was abandoning the research. Although the bizarre may constitute news, journalists should not, as Irvine Page cautioned, present it as "proved, generalized, and accepted by fully competent critics" (Page, p. 646).

Experienced journalists sometimes recognize overly exuberant claims of medical scientists and exercise skepticism and restraint in reporting such claims. At a press conference on cancer research at the National Academy of Sciences in October 1971, for example, a scientist announced that he had detected, in the milk of women with a family history of breast cancer, virus-like particles similar to milk-borne viruses known to transmit breast tumors (Wade). Women with such a family history, said the scientist, would do well not to nurse their babies. Rather than run a scare story based on an incautious announcement, professional medical reporters posed incisive questions that elicited the proper qualifications and limitations of the study, then wrote circumspect stories indicating that a diagnostic test was not yet generally available and that evidence was inconclusive that the suspected virus causes breast cancer.

News stories sometimes make broad inferences that are unsupported by the data. Extrapolation of animal data to human beings, especially when done by nonprofessionals, is not only risky from a scientific standpoint, but may cause unnecessary panic among the people. Conjecture, when advanced, should be based on adequate knowledge of the subject involved and on sound research data. Debating a medical problem superficially in the mass media before adequate evidence has been accumulated may confuse rather than enlighten the public, which is not generally qualified to weigh the pros and cons of a controversial medical issue. The publicity surrounding the "tolbutamide debate" and the saccharin ban created panic among patients, who look to the medical authorities for guidance based on scientific resolutions, not equivocation.

Falsification of scientific data. The critical need for medical reporters to view announcements of scientific "breakthroughs" skeptically has been further dramatized in recent years by disclosures of falsification of scientific data. Most widely publicized, perhaps, was the painted-mouse incident at a well-known cancer research institution. In 1969, science writers described as a "breakthrough" the researcher's experimental work to prolong the life of skin removed for grafting. Despite consistent reports of experimental success by the researcher in overcoming transplantation rejection, others, including Nobelist Sir Peter Medawar, had been unable to reproduce the results. In 1974, artificial coloring of one of the researcher's experimental mice was disclosed, and the validity of the entire program collapsed. The falsification was ascribed to pressure exerted on the scientist to publicize positive research results. The scientist suspected of painting the mouse left the research field, but others investigating methods of culturing to solve immunologic rejection reaped the negative effects of the scandal. Despite some promising findings, the undue skepticism within the scientific community created difficulties in finding professional journals to publish the data ("Was the Painted-mouse Doctor Right?").

Premature claims and overzealousness. Particularly in cases of dubious or unconfirmed "firsts" and "breakthroughs," the reliable journalist exercises caution, regardless of the prestige of his sources. The need for such skepticism on the part of journalists is substantiated by scientists' occasional recantations. Two respected scientists, after having discovered that an undergraduate assistant had falsified letters of recommendation, published a "potential retraction" of scientific articles that were co-authored by the assistant (Dressler and Potter, "Authors' Statement," "Transfer Factor"). Interestingly, a Nobelist had hailed this work as "one of the biggest things ever to come out of the Harvard labs" ("Researchers Retract Cancer Study Report").

In some instances, the scientist's zeal for his research may create problems. In April 1973, at a press conference during a meeting of the National Academy of Sciences, a well-known scientist announced that he had almost conclusive evidence that herpes viruses cause certain types of human cancer. At a science writers' seminar one year later, however, he disclosed his inability to repeat his earlier findings, and published in a professional scientific journal an official retraction of his earlier data (Sabin).

Invasion of privacy. Among the most vehement charges leveled at the press is the invasion of privacy. Such transgressions to obtain a titillating story serve little purpose beyond satisfying perverse curiosity. Compassion and good taste are not incompatible with good journalism. Good taste, admittedly difficult to define, was likely violated by the headline "Family Refuses to Give Heart" for a story about a teenage youth who had died playing Russian roulette. Consideration for the grief of the family might properly have overridden the journalist's instinct for drama, particularly since the disclosure had little constructive value.

Traditionally inviolate is the physician–patient relationship and the confidentiality of personal information transferred therein, protection of which dates back to the Hippocratic Oath (Perr). Several developments of the twentieth century have threatened the confidentiality of medical information: third-party insurance companies, computers, and the Freedom of Information Act. Because private medical information is now accessible through data banks, the journalist should exercise scrupulous ethical judgment in selecting material for public dissemination. Apprehension that private, intimate details of one's health may find their way into ill-intentioned hands has increased since passage of the Freedom of Information Act. Of special significance is psychiatric information that a patient may not wish divulged. News of the break-in of the office of Daniel Ellsberg's psychiatrist on 3 September 1971 outraged Americans and was vigorously denounced by the press as a flagrant intrusion of the patient's privacy, but the same press doggedly probes for intimate medical information about newsworthy people.

The practice of serializing, in the press, detailed medical information about prominent persons is a relatively recent development. President Cleveland was secretly whisked on board a yacht in New York Harbor to have an operation for cancer, and the full story of Franklin Roosevelt's failing health during his presidency was withheld until long after his death. Newspapers carried detailed accounts, however, of President Eisenhower's ileitis and his heart attacks; of President Kennedy's back ailments and purported Addison's disease; of Lyndon Johnson's operation for kidney stones and his heart attacks; of the emotional problems of political figures and their families; and of the mastectomies performed on the wives of high elected officials, including the President and Vice President of the United States. The ensuing public debate about the merits of radical mastectomy versus lumpectomy and the survival statistics may have frightened and perplexed more people than it edified. Moreover, whether a reporter has a right to divulge personal information about a relative of a "public figure" when the relative seeks privacy may create an ethical dilemma.

The line between the public's "right to know" and sheer medical gossip is not always easy to draw. In the coverage of a prominent senator's radical cystectomy in a weekly news magazine, not only were details given of the precise nature of the incision, but readers were informed of the cost of the hospital room, the frequency with which he would need to empty the plastic bag he would have to wear, and the "virtually inevitable impotence" that would ensue. Some readers wrote letters to the editor to protest the invasion of privacy and to recommend greater decency and respect.

To preserve freedom of the press, our laws make it extremely difficult to collect damages for misleading, false, or deprecatory material published about a person; one must *prove* knowing or reckless falsehood, and that is not easy to do. Nevertheless, some whose medical histories have been made public are beginning to take legal action. The Duchess of Windsor, for example, sued a television channel and a newspaper for using films and a photograph of her being supported by others as she walked in her garden. The suit charged that such photography, representing her as a helpless old woman, was damaging and constituted an invasion of her private life.

Sometimes the health of a public official may be of legitimate concern to the people. During the prolonged illness of a United States Supreme Court Justice, the press unsuccessfully sought information about how the state of his health may have affected the work of the Supreme Court. If an official's health affects public business, the public is entitled to be informed.

Sensationalism. The responsible medical science writer reports the facts, both favorable and unfavorable, and avoids slanting, exaggeration, and sensationalism. The inexperienced reporter, however, cannot always distinguish the natural enthusiasm of the dedicated scientist from the exaggerated claims of the publicity seeker. If a lack of scientific training does not allow the medical reporter to evaluate a startling new discovery, he should try to authenticate the significance of the discovery before he publicizes it as a "breakthrough." One way to enhance the accuracy of a medical story is to ask a recognized authority on the subject to read it—something that many journalists are reluctant to do, even though mistakes in this field can be extremely dangerous. To help ensure accuracy in scientific programs, the British Broadcasting Company employs a committee of scientists to serve in an advisory capacity. Periodic claims of cancer "cures" carried by newspapers and popular magazines, but later proved false, have caused needless anguish to victims of the disease, as well as to their families. It is true that imminent deadlines often preclude such detailed preliminary review, but getting it right is more in the public interest than getting it first. Publicizing of dangerous weight-reduction regimens, which have been responsible for deaths of gullible laymen, certainly might have been delayed until adequately assessed.

Sometimes the dramatic nature of a medical "discovery" invites journalistic excess, as in the case of the first human heart transplantation. Almost a decade later, after a plethora of insipid articles on the heart as the seat of the soul and on other irrelevant, meretricious, and often sordid stories had thoroughly desiccated the subject of its drama, human heart transplantation was discontinued by most heart surgeons as a therapeutic procedure. Christiaan N. Barnard, who was catapulted by the press into the limelight after performing the first human heart transplantation, later condemned the news media for creating dissension within the medical profession, exploiting the public taste for the macabre, and paying relatives or friends for controversial statements (Barnard). Such hysterical medical reporting generally disrupts the normal conduct of research and interferes with rational thinking. The heart transplant frenzy, however, had at least one salutary effect: the public debate regarding its ethical implications led to their serious consideration by the medical, as well as nonmedical, communities and contributed to the development of a new and needed discipline, bioethics.

Science writer Joseph Hixson censured television for valuing the visual impact of news items over balance and good judgment. In October 1974, a New York television channel showed ear-stapling being used for treatment of obesity, alcoholism, and depression without, Hixson argued, presenting the views of opponents of the procedure or giving adequate warning of the dangers involved. Such a "gimmicky piece of arrant quackery," Hixson maintained, violates the basic principles of responsible reporting (Hixson, p. 197).

Sensationalism is often the keystone of exposés, and medical exposés became prolific and profitable in the 1960s and 1970s. Articles and books on medical malfeasance flourished, including Medicare excesses, questionable therapeutic practices, and illegal dispensing of prescription drugs. Some were based on flimsy or inadequate evidence, but writing that is slanted to convey an unsubstantiated negative view, although unethical, may not be illegal. In a nationally televised segment entitled "Ghost Surgery," a reporter elicited from a patient a denial of any foreknowledge that a senior resident physician, not the chief surgeon, was to perform his operation. The chief surgeon insisted, however, that the patient had agreed, in advance, to allow the resident (who had previously performed more than 100 similar hernia operations) to do the operation under his chief's supervision, and he speculated that the patient may have simply been confused on the first postoperative day ("Clearing a TV Ghost"). The purported method of obtaining permission to make the film in this case raises ethical questions. Network representatives were reported to have requested permission to film "the training of a surgeon," not a story about medical ethics. Gaining access for one stated purpose and focusing the film on another, particularly if it has a negative focus, not only has ethical implications, but creates distrust. In this instance, a well-known surgeon's reputation may have been damaged, even though he denied the charge of ghost surgery. Persons whose character is impugned or whose reputations are thus damaged have recourse through laws against libel (malicious written defamation) and slander (oral defamation), but intentional malice is hard to prove.

Misquotations. Garbled quotations, whether direct or indirect, may not only create dissension between the press and the subject quoted, but may even have international implications. A neurologist, protesting the accuracy of a newspaper story about his visit to the Soviet Union, objected to the headline "Soviet Brain Study

Aim Is Behavior Control," which attributed "a sinister connotation and an implication of malicious intent" to his Russian hosts. The physician denied the reporter's implication "that patients are put into hospitals in the U.S.S.R. for the primary purpose of human experimentation," which, he contended, was "not a factual report of what I said" (Fields). Fear of distortion, false emphasis, or unbecoming levity has made some medical scientists acutely wary of the press.

Controversies. An ethical reporter does not create controversy for controversy's sake or falsely attribute intellectual differences among scientists to personal rivalry. Although such stories may sell newspapers, magazines, and books, they serve little constructive purpose. Open discussion of dubious practices, on the other hand, may have beneficial effects. The wide press coverage given to the questionable ethics of the cancer experiments on aged patients at the Jewish Chronic Disease Hospital in New York and of the Tuskegee syphilis study undoubtedly contributed to the formulation of ethical guidelines for human experimentation.

Headlines. Although the journalist is usually blamed for all errors in news stories, the responsibility sometimes lies elsewhere. Among the most common complaints about newspapers is that headlines are misleading, inaccurate, or sensational. The journalist has no more control, however, over headline writers who may cheapen his story with a shocking banner than he has over editors and rewriters who may change his copy. Headlines, designed as they are to attract attention, sometimes take liberties with the truth. Since, however, many people do not read beyond the bold print, accuracy is important. The impact of jarring headlines such as these may be profound: "Studies Say Doctors Harmful to Health," "Harvard Surgeon Reports Starvation in Hospitals," "One Step Nearer to the Super Race," "Research Group Says Milk Can Be Harmful," "Jews, Italians Complain More of Pain," "The Pill Will Kill, Says Doctor." Such headlines hardly suggest a sober treatment of the subject matter. Analogous to the sensational headline is the shocking title for a television program, such as "Don't Get Sick in America," which organized medicine considered biased and designed to frighten more than inform.

Misinformation. Although television is relatively young as a journalistic medium, its power to shape public opinion and policy is widely acknowledged. That power extends beyond informational programs to entertainment and commercials. Television dramas about medicine, by projecting an idealized image of physicians, may create unrealistic expectations in patients. The fictional physician in television serials is totally self-sacrificing and devotes his full attention to a single patient at a time, often extending his ministrations to resolution of the patient's personal problems. Diagnoses and treatment are quick and certain, rarely ambiguous or equivocal as in real life. Conveying such inaccurate impressions is not in the public's best interest. Also questionable is the ethicality of certain television advertisements of over-the-counter drugs, often with testimonials by actors posing as pharmacists or other health professional surrogates. Not only have these been censured as misleading, but the safety and efficacy of some of the products have also been under attack. Some firms, in fact, have been required to withdraw therapeutic claims for products that could not be proved.

Corrections and regulations

Corrections. If each science writer maintained a file on the "major medical advances" he has reported and, after a reasonable interval, arranged follow-up interviews with the scientists who announced them, he would discover that a large proportion of the "advances" fail the test of time. Subsequent emendation of such extravagant stories would clearly show the tentative and fragmentary nature of scientific "truths." Because newspapers serve as part of our historical archives, moreover, setting the public record straight is vital. Corrections, like retractions, rarely appear in the mass media, however, and when they do, they are usually buried in an obscure place or are relegated to letters to the editor.

Feedback. The American mass media, owned by private enterprise and largely autonomous, have a responsibility to allow dissenting opinions to be published. Most newspapers, in a spirit of fairness, have a regular feature of letters to the editor, and broadcasting stations provide time for the expression of contrasting opinions. Radio and television talk shows also permit listeners to call in and voice their opinions on various matters. Permitting such feedback by the public is an ethical responsibility of the free press, for the right of free expression extends beyond the press to the people.

Self-regulation. Self-analysis and self-regulation are beneficial in any profession, and especially in a free press. The British Broadcasting

Company has a three-man commission that acts as an appellate court in evaluation of viewers' complaints about news reporting and editing. Attempts in the United States to establish a press council to investigate complaints against journalists have largely failed, most representatives of the media considering such a body unnecessary and undesirable. Newspeople view themselves as representatives of the people, but since they are self-appointed, not elected, and since they have a vested commercial interest in their product, adherence to a code of ethics is essential. Such a code is especially important for medical reporters, who disseminate information that may affect the health and lives of human beings. The most practical ethical principles that medical reporters can follow are to obtain information from reputable, reliable sources, use common sense and fair play, and treat each story honestly and accurately.

Lois DeBakey and Selma DeBakey

[*Directly related is the other article in this entry,* SCIENTIFIC PUBLISHING. *Also directly related are the entries* CONFIDENTIALITY; PRIVACY; RESEARCH, BEHAVIORAL; *and* RESEARCH, BIOMEDICAL. *For discussion of related ideas, see:* ADVERTISING BY MEDICAL PROFESSIONALS; *and* DRUG INDUSTRY AND MEDICINE. *See* APPENDIX, SECTION I, MEDICAL ETHICS: STATEMENTS OF POLICY DEFINITIONS AND RULES, BRITISH MEDICAL ASSOCIATION.]

BIBLIOGRAPHY

"The Baby Maker." *Time*, 29 July 1974, pp. 58–59.

Barnard, Christiaan N. "Medicine and the Mass Media." *American Journal of Cardiology* 30 (1972): 579–580.

"Clearing a TV Ghost." *Medical World News* 18, no. 6 (1977), p. 11.

"Code of Ethics or Canons of Journalism." Adopted by the American Society of Newspaper Editors at annual meeting in Washington, D.C., 27 April 1923. American Society of Newspaper Editors, Box 551, 1350 Sullivan Trail, Easton, Pa. 18042.

Cohn, Victor. "Science Writer Ethics." *National Association of Science Writers Newsletter* 8, no. 3 (1960), p. 11.

Cormick, Jean. "Medical Advice in Seventeenth-Century Journalism." *Journal of the American Medical Association* 224 (1973): 83–86.

DeBakey, Lois. "Medicine and the Press: Resolving the Conflicts." *Clinical Research* 22 (1974): 214–225.

———. *The Scientific Journal: Editorial Policies and Practices: Guidelines for Editors, Reviewers, and Authors.* St. Louis: C. V. Mosby Co., 1976, chap. 8, pp. 36–39.

Dressler, David, and Potter, Huntington. "Authors' Statement." *Proceedings of the National Academy of Sciences of the United States of America* 72 (1975): 409.

———. "Transfer Factor: Warning on Uncertainty of Results." *Annals of Internal Medicine* 82 (1975): 279.

Fields, William S. "Doctor Lodges Protest of Reported Interview." *Houston Chronicle*, 5 September 1971, sec. 3, p. 13. Letter to the editor.

Harris, Benjamin, pub. *Publick Occurrences Both Forreign and Domestick*, 25 September 1690, pp. 1–2. Printed in Boston by R. Pierce at the London-Coffee-House. Evans 546. *Historical Magazine* (Boston) 1 (1857): 228–231.

Hixson, Joseph. "Epilogue: The Responsibility of the Media." *The Patchwork Mouse.* Garden City, N.Y.: Anchor Press/Doubleday, 1976, pp. 183–197.

Ingelfinger, F. J. "The Case of the Hoover Paper." *New England Journal of Medicine* 295 (1976): 896–897.

Lee, James Melvin. *History of American Journalism.* Boston: Houghton Mifflin Co., 1917, pp. 225–226.

Page, Irvine H. "Science Writers, Physicians, and the Public—Ménage à Trois." *Annals of Internal Medicine* 73 (1970): 641–647.

Perr, Irwin N. "Current Trends in Confidentiality and Privileged Communications." *Journal of Legal Medicine* 1, no. 5 (1973), pp. 44–47.

"Researchers Retract Cancer Study Report: Student Forged Letters." *Houston Chronicle*, 17 December 1974, sec. 1, p. 20.

Sabin, Albert B. "Herpes Simplex-Genitalis Virus Non-virion Antigens and Their Implication in Certain Human Cancers: Unconfirmed." *Proceedings of the National Academy of Sciences of the United States of America* 71 (1974): 3248–3252.

"Standards of Good Practice for Radio Broadcasters of the United States of America." Washington: National Association of Broadcasters, 1771 N St. N.W., Washington, D.C. 20036, 1937.

"The Television Code of The National Association of Radio and Television Broadcasters." Washington: National Association of Broadcasters, 1771 N St. N.W., Washington, D.C. 20036, 1952.

Wade, Nicholas. "Scientists and the Press: Cancer Scare Story That Wasn't." *Science* 174 (1971): 679–680.

"Was the Painted-mouse Doctor Right?" *Medical World News* 18, no. 8 (1977), pp. 28, 30.

II
SCIENTIFIC PUBLISHING

The history of biomedical communication, and particularly of the biomedical journal, is intimately associated with the ethos of science —the sharing of new knowledge by a discoverer without his risking priority for his original intellectual concepts. That ethos, tacitly understood and widely accepted, is inherent in, and essential to, the very being of science. It implies honesty, mutual trust, and good faith among all those involved in the biocommunication system, including the researcher-author, editor, reviewer, publisher, reader, advertiser, speaker, listener, science reporter, and others. The ethics of biomedical communication remains largely uncodified, and the following discussion will therefore treat primarily practices that have evolved through general agreement.

Establishing priority

The inauguration of the *Journal des Scavans* in France in January 1665, and of *Philosophical Transactions* in England in March of the same year, allowed scientists for the first time to share their observations without fear of losing priority. Thereafter, the secrecy practiced by early scientists began to be replaced by disclosure. When Oldenburg, editor of *Philosophical Transactions* of the Royal Society, agreed to publish several of Robert Boyle's papers, he assured the author that the papers were "now very safe, and will be wthin [sic] this week in print" and that he therefore no longer need fear "a Philosophicall [sic] robber" (Hall and Hall, p. 291). Because of the lag between submission of a manuscript and its publication, some journals still protect authors' priority by publishing the date of receipt or acceptance in a footnote.

Before the era of professional journals, scientists used various means of protecting their intellectual property, including anagrams and sealed letters. Some scientists deposited with learned societies sealed letters, carefully dated, or, in later years, mailed themselves certified letters containing ideas or data, to be kept as proof of priority. Today, scientists establish priority more often through publication, in a conventional journal, of a letter to the editor, brief note, or abstract, which can be published more quickly than a full report, or through publication of a longer communication in a rapid-publication journal.

Despite the presumably free flow of information today, many scientists are still reluctant to disclose their work fully until they have firmly established their priority. The need for free discussion while guarding priority led to the formation of "invisible colleges," which restrict access to information to a select group. The question of ownership of information has become more complicated as its transmission has become easier.

Biocommunication ethics

Because physicians, scientists, and others who use the biomedical communication system assume that the information so stored and retrieved is honest and accurate, and because the application of that information often affects the lives of human beings, a code of biocommunication ethics is important. Some aspects of such ethics are assumed and therefore left to the integrity of individual persons, whereas others are safeguarded by guidelines designed to impose external control. These guidelines have not yet been systematized, however, as have those for the biomedical research that underlies much of the information.

Peer reviewing of manuscripts

One of the ethical guidelines in biomedical communication is validity of material published. To help ensure validity, most journal editors, with the help of expert reviewers in the subject under consideration, screen manuscripts before accepting them for publication. Two opinions are usually adequate for acceptance of a manuscript, but if one of the first two reviewers recommends rejection, most editors consider it appropriate to seek a third opinion. Papers read at professional meetings are sometimes published without benefit of peer review, particularly in society-owned or society-sponsored journals. At the base of the peer review system is the tradition of scientific skepticism, which dates back to Heraclitus and requires scientists to consider, and account for, contrary views. As in the legal system, however, the literary judges are not themselves without serious ethical responsibility (DeBakey and DeBakey, 1975), and the fact that a journal has a peer review system does not eliminate the chance for errors or bias, since reviewers, like everyone else, are subject to human frailties.

The reviewer is expected to maintain confidentiality, that is, to avoid disclosing the substance of the paper or using his privileged knowledge to the detriment of the author. Once a reviewer has certain information, it is difficult for him to suppress any ideas it may prompt for further research, but he should guard against doing anything that will deny the author his rightful priority.

Punctuality in evaluating manuscripts is another responsibility of reviewers. Delayed reviews create problems not only for authors and editors but for readers as well. Prompt publication of worthwhile information allows scientists to use the new knowledge to generate additional information or to prevent costly and time-consuming duplication of research that has already proved fruitless. If a reviewer cannot examine a manuscript within about two weeks, he should return it and so advise the editor.

Influence of authorship on reviewing. It is the scientific merit of an article that editors and reviewers are expected to evaluate—the plausibility, originality, validity, and comprehensibility of the thesis, methods, results, and conclusions—not the professional reputation, stature, nationality, or political views of the author. Many believe, however, that borderline ideas or questionable theses are more likely to be rejected if proposed by obscure scientists than by those of wide repute. Yet removal of authors' names from manuscripts before circulation to referees is not only impractical but will not erase other readily identifiable signs, such as references cited, methods used, and opinions stated.

Anonymity of reviewers. Traditionally, reviewers of manuscripts for scientific journals have been anonymous, serving as advisers to editors, who are the visible "gatekeepers" of scientific periodicals. Since most scientific reviewers serve without remuneration, they should not, it is reasoned, be exposed to importunings, rebuttals, or acrimonious communications from rejected authors. Whether or not reviewers are sometimes prejudiced in evaluating manuscripts, their anonymity has led to suspicion of dark motives in the minds of some rejected authors. Such prominent scientists as Thomas Huxley have openly expressed their distrust (Huxley, p. 141) and have objected to "psycho-political manoeuvres," such as protracted delays and demands for successive revisions, used by the reviewer while he, himself, rushes into print (Wright).

Cloaked in anonymity, some reviewers may reject a paper with such blanket condemnation as "topic inappropriate," "defective methodology," or "data weak," or they may consign the paper to oblivion with such an unsupported verdict as "ludicrous," "asinine," or "totally incompetent research." The author whose paper receives such a judgment has been peremptorily denied an opportunity to present his ideas in the journal of his choice. He may understandably feel that, just as *he* is required to provide supporting evidence for statements in his manuscript, so should editors and reviewers be expected to support their judgments. When denied a forum in scholarly journals, some authors will publish their material in book form and thus bypass peer review.

The critic who privately points out weaknesses in a manuscript is protecting the author against their public disclosure and should therefore be considered his ally rather than his adversary. The reluctance of a reviewer to sign a fully documented evaluation, even if it is negative, is puzzling. Most book reviews are signed today, and even though such critiques are made in public *after* the material has been published, few serious problems have resulted. In nine years as editor of *The New England Journal of Medicine*, Ingelfinger (p. 1372) had "never seen an abrasive or insulting word used by a reviewer who identified himself." Identification of reviewers, by promoting accountability, should foster careful documentation of criticism, which, in turn, will assist authors in improving their manuscripts and will reduce their distrust (DeBakey and DeBakey, 1975, 1976).

Editorial criteria for ethical research

Until relatively recently, editors and reviewers, in evaluating manuscripts for publication, paid little attention to ethical criteria of experimentation (DeBakey, "Ethically Questionable Data"). It was a biomedical communication that jolted the scientific community and aroused its conscience regarding the ethics of human experimentation; an exposé published in 1966 cited numerous examples of ethically questionable practices found among research reports examined (Beecher). The transplantation of the first human heart in 1967 focused further attention on the ethics of research on human subjects. The inhumane practices uncovered during the Nuremberg trials were cited for comparison, and various groups began debating ethical issues in an effort to prevent scientific zeal from infringing human rights. These discussions by scientists, clergymen, jurists, sociologists, philosophers, and others conferred new prominence on the discipline of medical ethics.

Notwithstanding disclaimers, readers usually assume that the entire contents of a journal carry the imprimatur of the editor. Aware of this assumption, most editors today examine the ethical as well as the scientific aspects of submitted material. Since most manuscripts of experimental research emanate from established scientific institutions, some editors rely heavily on mechanisms within these institutions to ensure the ethicality of the research. The Department of Health, Education, and Welfare (DHEW) has published rather stringent guidelines to encourage ethical human and animal experimentation for the many projects it sponsors (Transportation, Sale, and Handling; United States). The guidelines include the establishment of institutional review boards (IRBs) to attest to the ethicality of all experimentation under DHEW grants.

Approval by an institutional review board usually signifies only that the research protocol submitted prior to the experimentation has been adjudged to meet ethical guidelines—not that the research itself has been monitored or certified to have been ethical. The experiments being reported may differ substantially from the proposal approved, since the direction research takes must sometimes be altered during the experimentation. Because the degree of responsibility exercised by some IRBs may be rather perfunctory, some editors may require more than a simple statement of approval by the IRB. The method section of the report, for example, may be required to identify the ethical criteria observed and the mechanism by which they were met.

Ethically questionable data.   A 1955 report on human experimentation in the Netherlands advocated that medical editors reject articles based on unethical experiments (Public Health Council). The editor of *The Practitioner* similarly urged editors to deny publication to any manuscript based on ethically improper practices, even if it is an "epoch-making article" (Thomson). In 1960 the editor of *The Lancet* announced his refusal to publish material "wrongly obtained" according to professional ethics (Fox). Several years later the British Medical Research Council recommended rejection of manuscripts describing ethically dubious research (Medical Research Council). The guidelines of the Massachusetts General Hospital of 1970 also called for the suppression of unethically obtained data, in an effort to curb unacceptable practices (*Massachusetts General Hospital Human Studies*). And in the same year an editorial in *The New England Journal of Medicine* exhorted institutions to exercise responsibility in certifying the ethicality of experimentation, to relieve editors of the dilemma regarding publication of unethical material ("Ethics of Ethical Evaluation").

Readers, too, have called for stricter editorial control regarding ethical experimentation. One reader denounced editors who, by publishing certain reports, sanction harmful procedures on patients who cannot possibly benefit from those procedures (Shapiro). Another called upon editors and publishers to demand that manuscripts contain a full explanation of the method of consent used (Blumgart). And Sir John Eccles urged that publication of data derived from unethical experiments be suppressed as a means of discouraging such practices (Eccles).

Some contend that, once research is completed, it is unethical to withhold from publication any useful information so derived—a retroactive justification of means on the basis of the end. Any breaches cannot be corrected at this point, they reason, and requiring the research to be repeated under ethical circumstances, even if possible, would not only be wasteful but would also expose additional subjects to risk. Rejection of unethical data, others say, would only remove experimental improprieties from visibility, not from commission, whereas publication would promote open discussion, help resolve conflicting values, and perhaps even deter further breaches. Still others suggest that ethically questionable data be published, but only if accompanied by an editorial commenting on or questioning the ethicality of the research. In such instances, the challenged author should be permitted to respond to the criticism, they argue, for denial of such an opportunity would suppress controversy and stifle open discussion, both vital to scientific progress.

Multiple publication

Most editors will not knowingly publish material that has already appeared elsewhere, whether in a scientific or a lay periodical. Authors are therefore expected not to submit to one journal essentially the same material that has already appeared elsewhere and not to submit the same manuscript simultaneously to two or more journals in an effort to expedite publication. Although multiple publication may expand the author's bibliography, it ill serves the scientific community. Editors have, in fact, publicly reproached authors whose material they have published without realizing that it had appeared several months earlier in another journal.

Confidentiality of medical data

In case reports, authors have long identified patients by initials as well as hospital number, but some journal editors have abandoned this practice to protect the identity of patients. Some editors also require signed consent forms before they will publish photographs of patients, even when the eyes are blocked out in the illustration.

Confidentiality of the patient's medical history is widely endorsed, but the advent of the computer has increased the risks of disclosure. The threat to privacy posed by easily accessible medical information stored in a computer data bank is of concern to many who envision potential abuses. The illnesses of well-known persons, for example—including politicians—have always been of keen interest to newspeople. Physicians, allied health personnel, and hospital administrators are expected by some patients to guard against unwanted publicity. Except when legally required, medical information about a patient should not generally be released without his specific approval.

Retraction and refutation

Although retraction of published information that later proves to be erroneous would seem to be an intellectual responsibility, scientific errors are rarely disavowed by their authors or by the editors who published them. Repudiation sometimes appears in subsequently published letters or articles, but these are usually written by readers, not the original authors. Since refutation generally brings less recognition than new discoveries, fallacious ideas are often simply ignored and allowed to die painlessly.

Mutual criticism of research and publications is accepted practice among scientists. It is, in fact, considered essential and is the rationale for peer reviewing. The criticism is expected to be unprejudiced and confined to the scientist's work rather than his person. Rarely has the right of an editor to publish critical material been questioned, but an occasional author may resort to the courts over derogatory statements about his work. In 1970 a dental surgeon, Drummond-Jackson, sued the British Medical Association and the authors of a paper published in the association's official organ, the *British Medical Journal*, for defamation. The article was critical of an anesthetic technique introduced by Drummond-Jackson. At the Court of Appeal, Lord Denning reportedly said that "it would be a sorry day if scientists were to be deterred from publishing their findings for fear of libel actions. So long as they refrained from personal attacks, they should be free to criticize the systems and techniques of others. Were it otherwise, no scientific journal would be safe" ("Science in Court"). Fortunately, scientists who disagree with one another usually express their views in professional periodicals, not by bringing libel suits.

Authorship and the by-line

Because a scientist's bibliography is a weighty criterion for academic promotion, admission to prestigious professional societies, and general professional advancement, a mentor may gen-

erously include in the by-line of an article the name of a protégé who contributed little or nothing. The names of some research directors have also been routinely added to by-lines, in deference to their seniority. As a result, the by-line no longer necessarily identifies the actual writers, as it once did in the scholarly tradition.

Despite the looseness with which "author" is used today, dictionaries continue to define the term as one who originates or composes a piece of writing. Thus, authorship refers denotatively to the origin of a *literary* production, not to experimentation. By this definition, one would expect the by-line to contain the names of those who contribute substantively to the form, as well as to the content, of the report, and to display those names in descending order of magnitude of their contribution to the intellectual concepts in, and the literary exposition of, the report (DeBakey and DeBakey, 1975). Such a policy would eliminate granting authorship to a colleague who merely reads a manuscript and offers suggestions for its improvement, to a superior or subordinate who is unassociated with the project under consideration, or to a technician, resident physician, or anyone else who performs prescribed, remunerated duties. Yet the names of all such persons have appeared in by-lines. This laxity in assigning auctorial credit led Price to propose that editors refuse publication in cases in which team members are given credit because of "participation in the work reported rather than . . . specific responsibility for the publishable contribution" (Price).

Ghostwriting. A relatively recent development is for experimental or clinical researchers to turn over the preparation of the research report to a ghostwriter. But is there a place in the biosciences for the surreptitiousness intrinsic in ghostwriting? By its very designation and definition, ghostwriting involves pretense; one person publicly claims as his own the literary efforts of another (DeBakey, "Honesty in Authorship"). Since form and content, or language and thought, are difficult to separate, the ghostwritten product may also represent, at least in part, the intellectual efforts of the spectral scribe. The accolades derived from such publications may thus belong to the ghostwriter rather than to the auctorial impostor (DeBakey, "Rewriting and the By-line"). Editors often solicit editorials or articles from "experts," and others make awards, on the basis of previous publications. If those publications were ghostwritten, the basis for solicitation or recognition is fraudulent, and in a discipline dedicated to intellectual honesty and the pursuit of truth, fraudulence of any kind is inimical. Since integrity and authenticity are of the essence in the scholarship of biomedical science, phantom authorship is indefensible. If a person will pose as the author of a composition that someone else wrote, can he be relied on to report his data completely honestly? Some have suggested that ghostwriters be acknowledged by a phrase such as "as told to . . ." or "with the literary assistance of . . . ," but the commercial ring of such phraseology seems incongruous in a scholarly journal.

Editorial revision. If ghostwriting of material to be published in a learned scientific journal is unethical, what about extensive editing or rewriting? Is it appropriate for a journal editor or copy editor to rewrite an author's article before publication? How much may an editor properly alter a manuscript? It seems fair to expect the published material to represent principally the conceptual, ratiocinative, and literary efforts of those named in the by-line and insignificantly those of the editor or others (ibid.). Such slight efforts may be directed toward making the manuscript conform to the policies of the journal in citation of references, abbreviations, and similar mechanical details; remedying an occasional grammatical lapse; clarifying an ambiguous phrase; or refining an awkward syntactic structure. To go beyond that by reorganizing a paper, reconstructing tables or graphs, or recasting the entire text is tantamount to ghostwriting and is therefore to be discouraged. Those who wish to publish in scholarly journals have a responsibility to learn to write comprehensibly so as not to require extensive editorial revision of their manuscripts. If a manuscript is so poorly written as to warrant major revision, the reviser risks misinterpreting the original text and thus distorting the author's intended meaning. Even if the author is given an opportunity to approve the revision, he may overlook subtle errors in the rewritten version while focusing on major ideas.

Citation of references

Ethics requires that the ideas and the words of others be acknowledged by citation of their sources. To pad the list of references cited merely to appear scholarly is as improper as to omit essential references because of professional rivalry or opposing views. The ethical author documents statements that have not become general knowledge and that the reader may want to consult to evaluate the thesis being presented. All direct quotations should, of course, be properly acknowledged. Because "unpublished data" and "personal communication" are inaccessible to the reader, they are inappropriate in references cited, although the information and source may be referred to, when appropriate, in the text.

Advertisements

Since advertisements for medical products carry scientific information that can affect the health, welfare, and even the life of human beings, a code of advertising ethics is essential. The United States Food and Drug Administration exercises some control over advertisements for prescription drugs, but it is possible to fulfill the letter of the law while violating the spirit of the law and, as in other spheres, much therefore depends on the integrity of the manufacturer. Since advertising revenue helps support some scientific publications, the editor may be confronted with a conflict of interest in evaluating advertisements. An editor would therefore do well to provide potential advertisers with precise policies governing handling and publication of advertisements, and to adhere to these as much as possible in the selection of promotional material. Manuscripts submitted for publication that raise questions about a product advertised in a journal should not be rejected solely on that basis, but should be subjected to the same criteria for acceptance as all other manuscripts.

The pre-meeting abstract and oral presentation

Abstracts submitted to program committees for consideration for presentation at scientific meetings should contain authentic data obtained from completed, ethical research. Abstracts written before the research is undertaken, or before it is completed, and containing anticipatory results are obviously unethical. Publication of such abstracts by the sponsoring organization carries additional risks for the author who submits fictitious material.

Ratnoff and Ratnoff interpret the reporting, at a meeting, of unjustifiable risks to human experimental subjects as an endorsement by the sponsoring society (Ratnoff and Ratnoff). Society may sometimes have to wait for answers to questions, they contend, until those answers can be obtained ethically. Program committees may well inform scientists who submit ethically questionable reports that the material is unacceptable on ethical grounds. Editors must, however, be cautious about exerting undue policing pressures while guarding against unethical practices.

Conclusion

Despite the lack of a formal code of ethics in biomedical communication, certain tenets that have evolved through the years are now widely accepted in the scientific literary community. These include intellectual honesty; scientific integrity; acknowledgment of the original concepts and contributions of others; respect for the rights, and protection of the privacy, of patients and experimental subjects; unbiased evaluation of the work of colleagues; and recognition and admission of errors. Basic to this ethical code is the placement of fundamental human rights and the advancement of science above any selfish personal goals of the researcher.

LOIS DeBAKEY

[*Directly related is the other article in this entry,* MEDIA AND MEDICINE. *Also directly related is* RESEARCH, BIOMEDICAL. *For further discussion of topics mentioned in this article, see the entries:* CONFIDENTIALITY; HUMAN EXPERIMENTATION, *article on* BASIC ISSUES; INFORMED CONSENT IN HUMAN RESEARCH, *article on* ETHICAL AND LEGAL ASPECTS; MEDICAL ETHICS UNDER NATIONAL SOCIALISM; *and* PRIVACY. *Other relevant material may be found under* ADVERTISING BY MEDICAL PROFESSIONALS; DRUG INDUSTRY AND MEDICINE; HUMAN EXPERIMENTATION, *article on* SOCIAL AND PROFESSIONAL CONTROL; MEDICAL MALPRACTICE; MEDICAL PROFESSION, *article on* MEDICAL PROFESSIONALISM; *and* RESEARCH, BEHAVIORAL.]

BIBLIOGRAPHY

BEECHER, HENRY K. "Ethics and Clinical Research." *New England Journal of Medicine* 274 (1966): 1354–1360.

BLUMGART, HERRMAN L. "The Medical Framework for Viewing the Problem of Human Experimentation." *Daedalus* 98 (1969): 248–274.

DeBAKEY, LOIS. "Ethically Questionable Data: Publish or Reject?" *Clinical Research* 22 (1974): 113–121. Editorial.

————. "Honesty in Authorship." *Surgery* 75 (1974): 802–804. A letter to the editor.

————. "Rewriting and the By-line: Is the Author the Writer?" *Surgery* 75 (1974): 38–48.

————, and DeBAKEY, SELMA. "Ethics and Etiquette in Biomedical Communication." *Perspectives in Biology and Medicine* 18 (1975): 522–540.

————, and DeBAKEY, SELMA. "Impartial, Signed Reviews." *New England Journal of Medicine* 294 (1976): 564. Correspondence.

ECCLES, JOHN. "CIOMS Round Table Conference: Fourth Discussion." *Biomedical Science and the Di-*

lemma of Human Experimentation: Round Table Organized with the Assistance of Unesco and the World Health Organization. CIOMS Round Tables, no. 1. Edited by Vittorio Fattorusso. Paris: Council for International Organizations of Medical Sciences, 1967, p. 107.

"Ethics of Ethical Evaluation." *New England Journal of Medicine* 282 (1970): 449–450. Editorial.

FOX, T. F. "The Ethics of Clinical Trials." *Medico-Legal Journal* 28 (1960): 132–141.

HALL, A. RUPERT, and HALL, MARIE BOAS, eds. and trans. *The Correspondence of Henry Oldenburg.* Vol. 2: *1663–1665.* Madison: University of Wisconsin Press, 1966.

HUXLEY, LEONARD. *Life and Letters of Thomas Henry Huxley.* 2 vols. London: Macmillan & Co., 1900, vol. 1.

INGELFINGER, F. J. "Charity and Peer Review in Publication." *New England Journal of Medicine* 293 (1975): 1371–1372. Editorial.

Massachusetts General Hospital Human Studies—Guiding Principles and Procedures. 2d ed. Boston: 1970. Cited in *Experimentation with Human Beings: The Authority of the Investigator, Subject, Professions, and State in the Human Experimentation Process.* Jay Katz, with Alexander Morgan Capron, and Eleanor Swift Glass. New York: Russell Sage Foundation, 1972, p. 935.

Medical Research Council. "Responsibility in Investigations on Human Subjects: Statement by Medical Research Council." *British Medical Journal* 2 (1964): 178–180.

PRICE, DEREK J. DE SOLLA. "Ethics of Scientific Publication." *Science* 144 (1964): 655–657.

Public Health Council of the Netherlands. "Human Experimentation." *World Medical Journal* 4 (1957): 299–300.

RATNOFF, OSCAR D., and RATNOFF, MARIAN F. "Ethical Responsibilities in Clinical Investigation." *Perspectives in Biology and Medicine* 11 (1967): 82–90.

"Science in Court." *Nature* 225 (1970): 1179.

SHAPIRO, SAMUEL. "Ethical Aspects of Urethral Manipulation." *New England Journal of Medicine* 286 (1972): 1160. Correspondence.

THOMSON, WILLIAM A. R. "Editorial Responsibility in Relation to Human Experimentation." *World Medical Journal* 2 (1955): 153–154.

Transportation, Sale, and Handling of Dogs, Cats, and Certain Other Animals for Research Purposes. 7 U.S.C. § 2131 et seq. (1970), Pub. L. 89–544, 80 Stat. 350: amended by the Animal Welfare Act of 1970, Pub. L. 91–579, 84 Stat. 1560.

United States, Department of Health, Education, and Welfare; The Secretary. "Protection of Subjects: Technical Amendments." *Federal Register* 40 (1975): 11854–11858.

WRIGHT, R. DOUGLAS. "Truth and Its Keepers." *New Scientist* 45 (1970): 402–404.

CONFIDENTIALITY

Conceptual analysis

Essential elements of confidentiality. Concern about confidentiality begins when a child first experiences a desire to keep secrets as well as to share them. The desire to keep a secret is a manifestation of a developing sense of self as separate from others; the desire to share a secret stems from a need to retain or estabish intimate relationships with others (Ekstein and Caruth). A child will often keep secrets he or she believes to be embarrassing, shameful, or potentially harmful. To be willing to tell secrets to another, a child must have confidence that the other can be trusted. Other persons may, however, fail to keep the secrets entrusted to them. They may not wish to enter into an intimate relationship; they may not be trustworthy; they may believe that other factors outweigh the importance of keeping the secret; they may be tricked or forced into giving away secrets. In addition, unless a child feels that the environment is safe, for example, that no one else is listening in, he or she may be afraid to reveal secrets.

The example of childhood secrets presents in microcosm many of the elements germane to an analysis of confidentiality. It brings out that the keeping and sharing of secrets is linked to a complex set of personal attitudes, beliefs, and expectations that are intertwined with the conduct of other persons.

The adult social practice of designating certain information as confidential, like the behavior of children keeping secrets, has a twofold aim. On the one hand, it seeks to facilitate communication pertaining to intimate or other sensitive matters between persons standing in special relationships to each other. On the other hand, the practice is designed to exclude unauthorized persons from access to such information. Thus, confidentiality is essentially linked to *control* over the disclosure of and access to certain information.

To understand better the nature of confidentiality as a social practice, it is helpful to distinguish three of its aspects: subject matter, special relationships, and procedures. Sometimes attention is focused upon the subject matter—the informational content—which is confidential. For example, the use of the label "confidential" on certain documents is one familiar method to identify sensitive information. At other times the persons who respectively receive, transmit, or have access to such confidential information are the target of concern. Whether such persons stand in a special relationship which includes the authority to disclose or obtain confidential information is often at issue. For example, attorneys and physicians are designated by law as persons eligible to receive and preserve confidential communications in appropriate circum-

stances. A third important aspect of confidentiality is that of the procedures for protecting or limiting its scope. For example, locked files and soundproof rooms preserve confidentiality, while unregulated computerized records and hidden microphones violate it. These three aspects of confidentiality deal with *what* information is confidential, *who* has control over such information, and *how* confidentiality is affected by communication procedures.

Scope of confidentiality. Two essential aims (facilitating sensitive communication and excluding unauthorized persons) and three important aspects (subject matter, special relationships, and procedures) of confidentiality have been identified. Nevertheless, the boundaries of the concept of confidentiality are unclear because it is so closely tied to a cluster of concepts such as confidence, confession, trust, reliance, respect, security, intimacy, and privacy. Consider the following illustration: I may wish to keep personal information confidential to prevent exposure to ridicule or humiliation. For example, I might not want others to know of my fear of insects or certain sordid facts about my past. But I may wish to discuss my fears with or to confess such facts to a therapist or a friend. Unless I have confidence that I can trust another person to keep my secrets, I may withhold such information. Even if I believe that the person is worthy of respect and can be relied upon not to betray my confidences, I may fear that other persons or the state might seek to force or deceive the other person to obtain such information. A reasonable expectation that my communications to the other person will be protected may be a prerequisite to my disclosure of facts about myself. However, there may be circumstances in which I might choose to relinquish confidentiality or circumstances in which others might feel justified in refusing to respect my desire for confidentiality.

An explication of the many logical and contingent connections among the related concepts just mentioned would reveal both a complex and an overlapping conceptual pattern. It is difficult, therefore, to distinguish sharply and precisely define confidentiality apart from its companion concepts. As a result, one might say that the concept of confidentiality has "blurred edges" (Wittgenstein). For example, privacy and confidentiality are easily confused. Some writers define privacy as the right to control information about oneself (Fried). This suggests that privacy and confidentiality are coextensive. Other writers define privacy in terms of the right to personal autonomy and freedom. Confidentiality, in this view, is only one aspect of the right to privacy.

Just as the concept of privacy is elastic and vague, so also is the concept of confidentiality. One might define confidentiality narrowly in terms of protection of *communications* among persons in certain special relationships. But one might also define confidentiality more broadly, in terms of the right to control *information* about oneself. We are not here concerned with the appropriateness of alternative definitions of privacy and confidentiality. The examples are presented only to bring out that confusion may arise out of conflicting definitions, which imply differences in conceptual scope.

Value of confidentiality. The social practice of maintaining confidentiality provides one means to facilitate, control, and protect communications about intimate or other sensitive information. In this context confidentiality has instrumental value; it is not an end in itself. The measure of instrumental value is determined by the extent to which confidentiality contributes to achieving the desired goal. Confidentiality is more or less valuable depending upon whether other means provide better ways to accomplish the same purposes.

Like any instrument, however, confidentiality can be used for good or evil purposes. If the goal to be achieved with the aid of confidentiality is thought to be desirable—such as promoting love, friendship, or trust—then efforts to preserve confidentiality should be made. But if confidentiality is used, for example, to help perpetrate crimes, it should not be protected. In this respect the value of confidentiality is derived from the worth of the purposes that it serves.

It is uncertain whether confidentiality has intrinsic value as an end in itself. Charles Fried has argued that privacy, identified as a necessary condition for valuable forms of interpersonal intimacy—respect, love, friendship, and trust—has an intrinsic significance. If confidentiality is coextensive with privacy because both are defined in terms of control over information about oneself, then confidentiality would also be intrinsically valuable. However, others have claimed that privacy has intrinsic value because it is the foundation for a moral recognition of one's status as a person (Reiman). Accordingly, one might argue that confidentiality has value only as one means to protect privacy, not as an end in itself. A sense of self may begin with the

keeping and sharing of secrets, but the development of personhood requires a capacity to experience intimacy and care for other persons. The control and exchange of confidential information is at best only one limited aspect of privacy.

The value of confidentiality can be brought out in another way: Imagine a world without it. First assume that no information about oneself would be treated as confidential by other persons; there would be no assurance that secrets would be kept. As a result relationships among persons could not be established upon a basis of trust that humiliating or harmful information will not be disclosed. A person would naturally be very reluctant to reveal sensitive information. Relationships among persons would become fragmented and superficial; this would impair, if not undermine, certain forms of intimacy such as marriage or friendship. One can also imagine a world in which secrets are valued and persons desire to be trustworthy, but the environment does not provide an opportunity for confidentiality. In a world such as that depicted by George Orwell's *1984* (updated to include more sophisticated technological monitoring and eavesdropping devices), fear, suspicion, and insecurity would prevail even among persons of goodwill. The context of human interaction would be so threatening that no one would be able to rely on the confidentiality of interpersonal communications. Either a world in which persons do not desire to form confidential relationships or a world in which the forming of such relationships is prevented would preclude the possibility of certain desirable forms of human interaction.

Protection of confidentiality

Persistent demands for increased protection of confidentiality are challenged by equally persistent demands for limitations on confidentiality. Policymakers are frequently faced with a conflict between the need to facilitate confidential communications about sensitive matters and the need for public information to protect the safety and promote the welfare of society. The purpose of this discussion is not to propose how particular competing claims should be evaluated. Instead, it is to examine different methods for protecting confidentiality and consider factors that justify limiting its scope. For convenience reference will be made only to practice in the United States.

Restriction of information. Confidentiality is, or is thought to be, protected by conventional social practices. In American culture many persons have the attitude that all information about one's body, including medical information, is confidential; it may be disclosed to others only for very good reasons. For example, public health laws, designed to prevent unnecessary and preventable suffering, require physicians to report instances of certain communicable diseases and to warn their patients of their condition. Recently questions have arisen about the extent to which genetic information discovered in the course of a physician–patient relationship about a person is confidential. May a person with a genetic disease or defect prevent this information from being disclosed to an employer, or even to members of his or her family? Does a person's fear of loss of livelihood or a desire to avoid feeling shame about an imperfection override the possible harmful consequences to society or family members resulting from their ignorance of a genetic disease or defect? Attitudes and beliefs in this area are uncertain and varied; we lack agreement about what ethical and legal principles should apply to such cases.

The cultural attitude about confidentiality of information concerning one's body partially explains the public outcry in response to reports that the confidentiality of medical records is sometimes inadequately protected. Controversy about medical records is complicated, however, because cultural attitudes come into conflict with professional practices and policies. Medical records typically contain, in addition to factual data, reports and interpretations of patient information made by hospital personnel, institutional data, and notes made by hospital staff concerning treatment. As a result disputes sometimes occur between a hospital's and a patient's claim to ownership of the medical records. The question of ownership then becomes the crux of the issue of control over the disclosure of information contained in the records. A person may wish to prevent or permit disclosure, for example, to an employer or an insurance company, but may be restricted by hospital policy. If control of medical records is vested solely in patients, then hospitals and their staff would be reluctant to enter relevant information that they, as professionals, may wish to keep confidential. And both hospitals and patients may fear disclosure of confidential information to unauthorized or undesirable third parties, including the government, private attorneys, employers, or insurance companies.

A related problem pertaining to restriction of information arises because of the widespread use of computerized files and data banks. Health facilities, insurance companies, and government agencies have compiled complex information systems in order to facilitate the rapid retrieval of relevant information. However, such practices also pose a threat to confidentiality. Most persons are not fully aware of the extent to which personal and private information, including medical information, is vulnerable to exposure. As a result government and other administrative agencies as well as consumer organizations have sought new methods of monitoring access to and use of computerized data.

Virtue of those entrusted. Confidentiality may be adequately protected in some situations by the psychological disposition or the personal virtues of the recipients of confidential information. For example, a family member might refuse to disclose a secret to an outsider because of fidelity to the clan or because of a firm moral commitment not to reveal secrets. However, trust can be misplaced; secrets may be intentionally revealed. Sometimes confidential information is exposed because of carelessness or mistakes. Fraud and deception are also used to obtain confidential information. Thus confidentiality in interpersonal relationships is limited by inherent human weaknesses and evils.

In the context of relationships between professionals and their clients, ethical backing is typically given to the confidentiality of clients' communications by codes of professional responsibility such as the Hippocratic Oath or the American Medical Association Principles of Medical Ethics. However, the degree of protection afforded to confidential information and communications varies among professions and from country to country. These variations result from the way in which conflicts are resolved among other fundamental values as well as conflicts that arise between the claims of confidentiality and the need for public information.

The very existence of ethical codes for protection of confidentiality in the professional–client relationships reflects not only the need for guidance but also the presence of human limitations. It is all too common that professionals publicly discuss clients' confidential communications. Indeed, some believe that codes of professional responsibility have a very limited effect on the conduct of professionals. Even when codes of professional responsibility have legal backing, it is common that the codes are not strictly enforced. Part of the explanation for this is that usually professionals in the same category, such as attorneys, physicians, or psychotherapists, administer the disciplinary proceedings against their own members. As a result, only the most flagrant violations of standards of professional conduct are prosecuted.

Bills of rights. Another form of ethical support for confidentiality comes from a 1972 "Statement on a Patient's Bill of Rights" of the American Hospital Association, which has been adopted by many health facilities ("Statement"). It states in broad terms that "case discussion, consultation, examination, and treatment are confidential and should be conducted discreetly." If such documents do not become merely window dressing and are given operative force, the scope of confidentiality will at least be reinforced, if not enlarged.

Legal protections. In addition to support provided by ethical codes, confidentiality is protected by law in some states which have adopted codes of professional responsibility or established patients' rights that are legally binding on appropriate persons. Further legal recognition of confidentiality is found in standard tort law doctrines, which permit lawsuits for libel, slander, and invasion of privacy for breach of confidential communications.

Another form of protection for some confidential communications in the context of special interpersonal relationships is the statutory law of evidentiary privileges. A "privileged communication" between persons in special relationships —such as attorney–client, physician–patient, or psychotherapist–patient—is one that is protected from disclosure in a legal proceeding even though it would otherwise be relevant evidence. For example, certain communications made in confidence by patients to their physicians relevant to medical treatment may not be disclosed by the physician without the consent of the patient, or his or her legal representative after death, unless the privilege has been waived or certain exceptions apply. The reasoning that underlies the privileged communications doctrine is that disclosure by a client of personal or other sensitive information may be necessary for obtaining adequate professional services. It is important to keep in mind that the holder of the privilege is the client or patient, not the professional. However, in appropriate circumstances the professional may invoke the privilege on behalf of the patient.

A few states have enacted laws which give greater protection to confidential communica-

tions disclosed in psychotherapy. Because the revelations that occur in psychotherapy often pertain to matters of great emotional significance, a person undergoing psychotherapy feels especially vulnerable to humiliation or harm. To enable the process of psychotherapy to go forward, laws have been established to assure psychotherapeutic patients that their disclosures will be adequately protected. As we shall see more fully later, even in the psychotherapeutic setting confidentiality is not unlimited.

Confidentiality is given further legal backing as a result of the development and expansion of a limited constitutional right of privacy from governmental intrusion through opinions of the U.S. Supreme Court. In the case of *Roe* v. *Wade* (1973) the Court determined that a woman's right to privacy entitles her, with the aid of her physician, to terminate her pregnancy. In a separate concurring opinion Justice William O. Douglas emphasized that the physician–patient relationship has a conspicuous place within the right of privacy.

The U.S. Congress passed the Privacy Act of 1974, which expressly deals with the right of an individual "to safeguard individual privacy from the misuse of Federal records" and "to provide that individuals be granted access to records concerning them which are maintained by Federal agencies." Individuals are provided with the right to determine the uses made of their personal records, to correct erroneous information, and to prevent unauthorized uses of such information. One can readily see that general concern about access to, accuracy of, and use of government records will have a spillover effect on medical records. Indeed, many state legislatures in the United States favor laws similar to the federal Privacy Act which would deal, among other things, specifically with the problems connected with medical records.

The preceding discussion brings out both ethical and legal issues germane to the conflict between private interest in confidentiality and public interest in obtaining sensitive information. Although the legal literature on privacy is extensive, much less scholarly attention has been given to ethical problems related to confidentiality. There is a need for formulation, clarification, and justification of the ethical principles that can help to resolve ethical conflict and guide social practices. This is especially important in an age dominated by rapid changes in the technology of communication systems, increasing interpersonal interdependence, and expansion of governmental and institutional control over sensitive information. Problems frequently arise, and are not easily resolved, with regard to who should have control over access to and disclosure of personal information as well as sensitive information possessed by government agencies and other institutions.

Limitations on confidentiality

Throughout the previous section emphasis has been placed upon the tensions between pressure to expand the scope of confidentiality and forces that would restrict it. It should also be mentioned that some persons believe that many demands for confidentiality are excessive. For example, some legal scholars dispute the value of privileged communications laws on the grounds that such laws merely obstruct truth in the legal process. Some critics of the U.S. Supreme Court believe that individual rights of privacy have been expanded at the expense of the public need for information and social control.

However the merits of such controversies should be assessed, it is generally agreed that confidentiality is not an inalienable right. Even if a person has a moral or legal right to protection of confidential communications, this right may be waived. For example, a person might consent to the disclosure of confidential information for educational purposes, for economic gain, or personal recognition.

In other contexts, such as litigation, a person who sues for injuries suffered, for instance, in an automobile accident must allow his or her treating physician to disclose confidential information gained in the course of treatment that pertains to the alleged injury. If a choice is made to bring a lawsuit, the need for confidentiality is outweighed by the need for truth in litigation.

More difficult issues emerge when the patient-litigant has been treated by a psychotherapist for alleged emotional injuries. It is sometimes argued that because confidentiality is essential for the process of psychotherapy to be effective, confidentiality here is more critical than in other aspects of medical practice. Nevertheless, the general rule is that confidential communications, even in psychotherapy, may in certain circumstances be overridden by the need for relevant information in litigation.

Confidentiality is also limited by the need for protection of public safety. For example, the confidentiality of communications between attorneys and clients is protected if a client reveals that he or she has committed a crime in the past. But the expression of an intention to commit a crime in the future is not protected. Similar reasoning underlies public health laws. For example, a physician must report incidents of suspected cases of child abuse, even if violation of confidentiality may be required. Psychotherapists are permitted, and in some area of the United States are required, to take steps to protect the public against dangerous patients. This may not be possible without disclosure of confidential information against a patient's wishes. Such problems were confronted by the California Supreme Court in the case of *Tarasoff* v. *Regents of the University of California*, in which it was concluded:

that the public policy favoring protection of the confidential character of patient–psychotherapist communications must yield to the extent to which disclosure is essential to avert danger to others. The protective privilege ends where the public peril begins [*Tarasoff*].

WILLIAM J. WINSLADE

[*Directly related are the entries* PRIVACY; RIGHTS; THERAPEUTIC RELATIONSHIP; *and* TRUTH-TELLING. *This article will find application in the entries* GENETIC DIAGNOSIS AND COUNSELING; GENETIC SCREENING; *and* SEX THERAPY AND SEX RESEARCH, *article on* ETHICAL PERSPECTIVES. *See* APPENDIX, SECTION I, MEDICAL ETHICS: STATEMENTS OF POLICY DEFINITIONS AND RULES (BRITISH MEDICAL ASSOCIATION); SECTION III: PATIENTS' BILLS OF RIGHTS; *and* SECTION IV, *codes of the* AMERICAN NURSES' ASSOCIATION, AMERICAN OSTEOPATHIC ASSOCIATION, *and* AMERICAN PSYCHOLOGICAL ASSOCIATION.]

BIBLIOGRAPHY

DAVIDSON, HENRY A. "Professional Secrecy." *Ethical Issues in Medicine: The Role of the Physician in Today's Society.* Edited by E. Fuller Torrey. Boston: Little, Brown & Co., 1968, chap. 9, pp. 181–194.

EKSTEIN, RUDOLF, and CARUTH, ELAINE. "Keeping Secrets." *Tactics and Techniques in Psychoanalytic Therapy.* Edited by Peter L. Giovachinni. New York: Science House, 1972, chap. 10, pp. 200–215.

FRIED, CHARLES. "Privacy." *Yale Law Journal* 77 (1968): 475–493.

In re Lifschutz. 2 C.3d 415. 85 Cal. Rptr. 829. 467 P.2d 557 (1970).

"The Principles of Medical Ethics with Annotations Especially Applicable to Psychiatry (Section 9)." *American Journal of Psychiatry* 130 (1973): 1063.

The Privacy Act of 1974. Pub. L. No. 93-579. 57 U.S.C. sec. 215 (1970). 88 Stat. 1896.

REIMAN, JEFFREY H. "Privacy, Intimacy, and Personhood." *Philosophy and Public Affairs* 6 (1976): 26–44.

Roe v. Wade. 410 U.S. 113. 35 L. Ed. 2d 147. 93 S.Ct. 705 (1973).

"Statement on a Patient's Bill of Rights." *Hospitals* 47, no. 4 (1973), p. 41.

Tarasoff v. Regents of the University of California. 131 Cal. Rptr. 14, 551 P.2d 334 (1976).

WASSERSTROM, RICHARD. "Legal and Philosophical Foundations of the Right to Privacy." Los Angeles: University of California, Los Angeles, February 1976.

WIGMORE, JOHN HENRY. *Evidence in Trials at Common Law* [Wigmore on Evidence]. 10 vols. Rev. ed. by John T. McNaughton. Boston: Little, Brown & Co., 1961, vol. 8, sec. 2380–2385, pp. 818–849.

WITTGENSTEIN, LUDWIG. *Philosophical Investigations.* 3d ed. Translated by G. E. M. Anscombe. New York: Macmillan Co.; London: Blackwell, 1953.

CONFUCIANISM

The effects of Confucianism on the development of health care and medical ethics in China were manifold; thus, medical ethics was a direct outgrowth of the basic content and tendency of Confucian social theory. Decision makers of the Former Han dynasty (206 B.C.–A.D. 25) chose to recognize Confucianism (rather than any of several other social theories that were offered by philosophical schools during that time) as the most appropriate ideology to stabilize the social pattern that had emerged under their rule and to prevent social crises that might have led to social change.

Ensuing actions on the part of Confucian policymakers consequently were strictly conservative in the sense of "conserving in Chinese society the distribution pattern of resources preferred by the ruling class." Confucianists were aware that accumulation of control over potentially powerful resources by specialized groups might lead to shifts in the pattern of distribution of those resources within society, with social change as the unavoidable consequence. Countless decisions were made to prevent this from happening. Deliberate measures to destroy or erode the power bases of groups that had, indeed, managed to gather control over certain resources during times of administrative weakness were a rather constant theme of the government. Official policy toward salt merchants, financial experts, military leaders, and others reveals these efforts.

Two diametrically opposed alternatives were open to Confucian politicians: either to dilute control over potentially dangerous resources among all the people, or to concentrate all control in the hands of the government, that is, the ruling bureaucracy. The resources watched most carefully included those relating to the knowledge and practice of medicine.

In the following a distinction will be made between primary medical resources and secondary medical resources. The former include medical knowledge and skills, drugs and medical technology, and medical equipment and facilities. Secondary medical resources are defined as rewards of material or nonmaterial kind, i.e., money, gifts, prestige, social power, to be gained through medical practice. Access to secondary resources is generally achieved by a group only after having gained control over existing primary resources. The result is the emergence within society of an influential elite group, with consequences harmful to the continuity of social structure. Policy toward medical practice, therefore, followed the line determined by these premises.

Inherent in Confucianism is the appreciation of life and the desire to keep the body from untimely or unnecessary death. It is difficult, however, to assess all the corollaries of that basically positive attitude toward life. There is some indirect support for the assumption that children with certain congenital malformation were killed in prerepublican China, though few such cases have been recorded. Also, as sources indicate, abortion was frequently induced—a practice that evoked little, if any, concern among Confucian thinkers. Confucian ideology contains several values of bioethical relevance, for instance *jen* (humane benevolence) and *tz'u* (compassion). These, however, were applied at least by some dogmatists within strict socially defined limits. Thus, some Confucians argued that a medical practitioner should not follow every call he received but should only respond to requests for help by those who were suitable for social intercourse.

Mencius (372–289 B.C.), an early Confucian philosopher, commented on the universality of benevolent human nature when he pointed out that anyone who happened to see a child fall into a well would certainly rush to the scene and attempt to rescue it from drowning. Furthermore, Confucianism regarded *hsiao* (filial piety) as one of the key values necessary to maintain social stability. The duty to assist one's parents and other relatives to reach advanced age without unnecessary suffering naturally entailed providing medical care for them. The Confucian tenet stressing the role of the individual layman and his ability to assist his relatives became the focus of political efforts designed to spread control of medical resources over society as a whole in order to make the impact of medical practitioners of marginal importance if not superfluous. Time and again statements and admonitions released by concerned Confucianists asserted that possession of sufficient medical knowledge was necessary to fulfill one's obligations of filial piety.

In spite of this attempt to distribute responsibility for primary health care, social circumstances and political expediency (the nature of which is not always entirely clear) led Confucian decision makers to promulgate a variety of public health measures; the ensuing institutions had to be staffed with at least partially specialized personnel. Thus, ironically, the stimulus for the professionalization of a specifically trained group within Confucian society was a result of Confucian health policy itself. It is a moot point to what extent credit for humanitarian health-policy decisions during the imperial era can be attributed to the voluntary acts of the Confucianists and how much was forced upon them by external events. Still, the mere fact that public health solutions to impending problems were conceived and that attempts were made to put them into practice must be regarded as an achievement of the Confucian culture. Again, today's readers of classical Chinese accounts of public health measures must be cautioned, for such reports do not reveal much about the actual implementation of the programs decreed.

At the beginning of the Confucian era, now slightly more than 2,000 years ago, medical practitioners enjoyed the status of more or less renowned craftsmen. Some of them were itinerant and offered their services to the general populace; others whose skills had created sufficient fame for them would approach the rulers at the many feudal courts existing during that period (Bridgman). "Medical workers" were attached to the military and to administrative posts from Han times on. Somewhat later, better trained experts were required, and it was only natural in Confucian society that the necessary training supplement the standard education of Confucian civil servants, again as a strategy to preserve control over medical resources for the ruling class. During the early seventh century this led to the establishment of institutions for the teaching of medicine outside the imperial court. By the twelfth century, medical training in certain government institutions was restructured and became even more integrated with classical nonmedical knowledge.

Possibly as a response to the opening of such an institution under Buddhist auspices in the fifth century, one finds soon thereafter the first reports of the establishment of a hospital under secular control. The competitive character of public health policies when directed toward followers of Buddhism became even more evident in A.D. 653 when Buddhist (and also Taoist) monks and nuns were prohibited from the practice of medicine, and in A.D. 845 when all Buddhist-controlled hospitals were secularized (Needham, pp. 265, 277, 278).

After a period of weakness during which even Chinese emperors had shown commitment to the Buddhist faith, this kind of loss of control over important primary and secondary medical resources could not be tolerated by a reviving Confucian society.

From the eighth through the twelfth century a mass migration of people from northern regions to southern parts of China occurred as a result of climatic changes in the north. It is estimated that previously ninety-five percent of the Chinese population inhabited the plains of the north, which were more favorable for husbandry and agriculture; during the period of the Southern Sung dynasty (1127–1179), approximately forty-five percent of the total Chinese population lived in the south with its mountainous geography (Kracke, pp. 479–488). The population shift produced unprecedented large cities with often hundreds of thousands and, not infrequently, more than a million people crowded together. Possibly as a consequence of the living conditions in the cities, in which so many people had been uprooted from their former style of life and natural environment, a welfare program was initiated during the eleventh century which entailed the establishment of public dispensaries and state-controlled polyclinics. That system continued in operation at least until the sixteenth century, possibly even until the eighteenth century. The impact of these institutions cannot be regarded as decisive for public health at any time. The numbers of "offices" established were too small for this purpose. Furthermore there were such severe scandals surrounding them that even the Confucian chroniclers could not avoid mentioning them. Not surprisingly, in a slight modification of the official title, the public dispensaries were called by the people "offices for the welfare of the bureaucrats" (Unschuld, 1973, pp. 9–14; 1975, n. 19).

Public health programs were continued even during times of alien rule over China. Reports from the time of the Mongols (Yüan dynasty, 1206–1368), for instance, show an abundance of directions to provide medical assistance to prisoners through "medical workers," the lowest category of governmentally employed practitioners.

The foregoing reference to examples of public health policies in Imperial China may suffice to indicate that it was possible for any medical group to achieve a higher level of professionalization and thus to become socially influential. Orthodox Confucianists, however, observed these developments closely and continuously promoted what might in effect be called an anti-medical-professionalization campaign.

By the twelfth century, three distinguishable main groups were contending for control over medical resources. The first were the free-practicing physicians outside Confucianism. This group included Taoists, Buddhists, and others who practiced medicine to make a living or as a sideline when they were economically independent. Many famous physicians and medical writers belonged to the group. They should be distinguished from those favored by Confucian dogmatists, persons who used their medical abilities only to assist family members, friends in need, or during medical assignments as civil servants.

One outstanding early representative of free-practicing physicians was Sun Ssu-miao (581–682?) who possibly was the first to recognize the need of the free-practicing group for explicit medical ethics to advance in professionalization against the Confucian class. It is not surprising that many of the famous members of this group were offered official positions at the imperial court or elsewhere. This may not only be understood as an attempt by the decision makers to secure the best physicians for their own care but also to alienate them from free-practicing peers who might have gained in status by association with outstanding personalities. The second group is the Confucian class itself, whose interests have been dealt with earlier in this article. Within this group a third one emerged, composed of those Confucianists who because of either an official assignment or personal interest practiced medicine outside of their own families on behalf of clients of all kinds, often accepting money and other material rewards. The third group did not adhere to the famous saying of Confucius (551–479 B.C.): "The accomplished scholar is not a utensil!" Its strategy, carried out to gain acceptance within its own

superior group and to compete successfully with the group of the free-practicing physicians, was twofold.

In their explicit medical ethics these people on the one hand had to assure the orthodox Confucianists that their medical practice was in perfect accordance with Confucian values. On the other hand they continuously stressed that "common physicians," as non-Confucian practitioners were called officially, constituted a source of permanent evil practice. In this latter effort the group was supported, of course, by the orthodox Confucianists.

A severe blow against the social acceptance of medicine as more than just an ordinary craft resulted from some sayings of Chu Hsi (1130–1200), the leading Confucian philosopher of his time. In commenting on the ancient classic *Lun yü* ("Analects"), which supposedly comprises sayings by Confucius and his disciples, compiled by the latter, Chu Hsi made some statements regarding medicine that were bound to stigmatize all who wished to practice medicine, outside the domain of their own families, as a means of earning a living.

Confucius had originally stated: "The people in the South have a saying: 'A man without persistency cannot become a sorcerer-physician.' Good!" (Legge, vol. I, p. 272). There were at least two grammatically correct ways to interpret these words. Chu Hsi chose to separate the terms "sorcerer" and "physician" and commented: "Sorcerers communicate with demons and spirits; physicians are entrusted with matters of death and life. If such petty personnel (cannot do without persistency), how much more is this true for others!" (Chu Hsi, 1958, pp. 598–601). Elsewhere in the *Lun yü* the following remark is attributed to a disciple of Confucius: "Petty teachings certainly also contain some aspects which cannot be disregarded. But if you carry them far, you will become soiled. The noble man, therefore, does not deal with them" (Legge, vol. I, pp. 340–341). In this case Chu Hsi wrote in his commentary: " 'Petty teachings' does not mean 'strange (or: heterodox) principles'; 'petty teachings' refers to 'teachings' too, but just to 'petty' ones. These are for instance: agriculture, horticulture, medicine, divination, and all other specialized occupations" (Chu Hsi, 1965, chap. 19, p. 23a).

These two comments exerted an almost continuous influence over most of the remaining centuries of the Confucian era. They provoked many defensive criticisms by medical writers from both the group of free-practicing physicians and the group of Confucian medical practitioners. A well-known physician named Hsü Ch'un-fu, who lived around 1556 and had served as an official at the Imperial Medical Office at court for a while, questioned Chu Hsi's interpretation of Confucius's statement and argued that "sorcerer-physicians" were to be regarded as one single category of people, namely, those who would dance, pray, and offer sacrifices to avert sickness; through this sort of practice they proved not to have any knowledge of medicine and drugs. Therefore, they should not be confused with true medical practitioners.

Later, at the end of the sixteenth century, Lai Fu-yang focused on the meaning of "petty" and argued: "If one directs his medical knowledge only on his own body, this is to be regarded as 'petty'; if one spreads the application (of his medical knowledge) all over mankind, this is not to be regarded as 'petty'!" Here Lai Fu-yang attempted to reverse completely the orthodox Confucian attitude toward medical practice.

Chang Chieh-pin (fl. 1624) is a third and last example of criticism of Chu Hsi's remarks on medicine. Chang Chieh-pin was a noted medical writer who originally was in the group of free practitioners but became a close follower of the ideas of Sung-Confucian medicine, a healing system that integrated the use of drugs into medical theories of the Confucian tradition. The use of drugs had been developed mainly in Taoist traditions. Chang Chieh-pin did not dare or did not find it effective enough to voice his strong criticism of Chu Hsi's comments himself. He placed his thoughts into the mouth of a "strange man," whom he allegedly met somewhere in the wilderness. This "strange man" in conversation with Chang Chieh-pin showed an outburst of anger when the latter told him that, although medicine was to be regarded as a "petty teaching," he was still aware of the necessity to be careful in its application. The stranger then gave him an emphatic lecture on the importance and subtlety of medicine and admonished him to keep it in high esteem. Chang Chieh-pin as a result of this lecture felt extremely ashamed and noted it down so that it might not be forgotten.

Another dimension of the Confucian attitude toward medicine that was expressed in many ethical statements focused on what were called "heterodox" practices and beliefs. Orthodox or officially endorsed medicine consisted of theoretical foundations and actual treatments by means of acupuncture or other techniques, in-

cluding drugs at a later time. All of these were related to the same cosmogonic theories and philosophical concepts of nature that were also basic to the Confucian social theory.

Effective medical practice outside of those theories and philosophies might have jeopardized the validity of the Confucian paradigms as a whole and could not be tolerated. This is not surprising, for the way of life recommended by Confucian-endorsed medicine as a guarantee for physiological harmony, i.e., health, is the same way of life demanded by the Confucian social theory to maintain social order and stability. It was again Sun Ssu-miao, a leading thinker critical of the Confucian way of life, who recommended demonic medicine as an alternative. The notion inherent in this healing system was that one is constantly subject to attacks by evil demons, which may cause diseases if one doesn't protect oneself carefully enough. The consequences of this theory of disease causation for individual and social behavior were quite different from those put forth by the Confucian social theory.

The resulting ideology toward heterodox knowledge and practices was part of the overall competition between Confucianists and the followers of other social theories. Shamans, Taoists, Buddhists, and often private individuals who had taken up a healing practice on their own by using charms, prayers, or other means that were not in conformity with Confucian medicine, provided the major target for accusations of heterodox practice.

The need to advance over other groups in society competing for control of secondary resources (i.e., the material or immaterial rewards to be gained from practice) is one of the major forces behind medical progress. However, several well-documented historical examples indicate that the pace of medical progress is generally retarded when the control over primary medical resources rests in the hands of a group whose access to secondary resources is not wholly dependent on the use of these primary resources but possesses other means to maintain its control over the people.

Orthodox Confucianists constituted such a group. They attempted to control primary medical resources or to spread them all over society merely to prevent any specialized group from rising to influence and power in society. Their own power was by no means solely dependent on primary medical resources. Therefore, orthodox Confucianists had no interest as such in increasing or improving primary medical resources. In contrast the free-practicing physicians and those Confucianists who practiced medicine outside their own families appear to have been genuinely interested in improving their skills and expanding the available materia medica. The resulting antagonism manifested itself, for example, in the delineation of medical jurisdiction and in repeated admonitions to practitioners not to develop new theories but to stick to the old interpretations. This restrictive policy could not prevent the invention or importation of new primary medical resources, for example, theories, drugs, techniques, and facilities. However, it is impossible to estimate to what extent it may have impeded progress and served to preserve those archaic medical paradigms which dominated Chinese medical literature up to this century.

One of the last Confucianists to resort to this kind of argument was Li Han-chang (1821–1899), elder brother of the famous statesman Li Hung-chang (1823–1901). In the preface to a medical work of a previous century he castigated those who would originate or follow other than the classical theories and condemned those who would try their "unintelligible prescriptions" at the cost of thousands of human lives. It is not unreasonable to assume that these criticisms were meant to discourage those practitioners who were just then experiencing the initial impact of Western surgical and pharmaceutical knowledge. A subsequently increased influx of Western primary resources of many kinds into China brought on dramatic changes in the overall pattern of resource distribution. The millennia-old maxims of Confucian ideology concerning professionalization proved to be infeasible at a time when the amount and the character of primary resources available in the field of medicine and elsewhere seemed to necessitate groups of specialists to control and handle them. The Confucian social system collapsed with the revolution of 1911.

PAUL U. UNSCHULD

[For further discussion of topics mentioned in this article, see: MEDICAL ETHICS, HISTORY OF, section on SOUTH AND EAST ASIA, articles on GENERAL HISTORICAL SURVEY and PREREPUBLICAN CHINA. Also directly related are the entries BUDDHISM; DEATH, article on EASTERN THOUGHT; ENVIRONMENT AND MAN, article on EASTERN THOUGHT; and TAOISM. For discussion of related ideas, see the entries: MEDICAL PROFESSION; PUBLIC HEALTH; and RATIONING OF MEDICAL TREATMENT.]

BIBLIOGRAPHY

BRIDGMAN, R. F. "La Médecine dans la Chine antique." *Mélanges chinois et bouddhiques* 10 (1952–1955): 1–213.

CHU HSI, commentator. *Lun yü chi chu* [Commented Analects], by Confucius. 10 vols. Taipei: Chung-hua ts'ung-shu wei-yüan-hui, 1958. Translated by Pyun Yung-tai as Confucius. *Analects.* 2 vols. Seoul: Minjungsugwan, 1960.

————. *Chu-tzu ta ch'üan* [Master Chu's Complete Works]. *Ssu-pu-pei-yao*, vols. 396–406. Taipei: Chung-hua-shu-chü, 1965.

KRACKE, E. A., JR. "Sung Society: Change within Tradition." *Far Eastern Quarterly* 14 (1954–1955): 479–488.

LEGGE, JAMES. *The Chinese Classics.* Hong Kong: Hong Kong University Press, 1960.

NEEDHAM, JOSEPH R. *Clerks and Craftsmen in China and the West.* London: Cambridge University Press, 1970.

UNSCHULD, PAUL U. *Die Praxis des traditionellen chinesischen Heilsystems.* Wiesbaden: F. Steiner Verlag, 1973.

————. *Medizin und Ethik: Sozialkonflikte im China der Kaiserzeit.* Münchener ostasiatische Studien, vol. 11. Wiesbaden: F. Steiner Verlag, 1975. This monograph gives the original sources of all Chinese citations provided in this article.

CONSANGUINITY

See EUGENICS AND RELIGIOUS LAWS.

CONSENT

See INFORMED CONSENT IN HUMAN RESEARCH; INFORMED CONSENT IN MENTAL HEALTH; *and* INFORMED CONSENT IN THE THERAPEUTIC RELATIONSHIP.

CONSEQUENTIALISM

See ETHICS, *articles on* TELEOLOGICAL THEORIES *and* UTILITARIANISM.

CONTRACEPTION

Early methods

Ethical judgment on contraception presupposes the existence of contraceptive technique. Five papyri from the period 1900–1100 B.C. show that Egyptian medicine possessed prescriptions designed to prevent pregnancy (Deines, Grapow, and Westendorf). Crocodile dung figures prominently in two recipes; another stresses acacia tips, coloquintada, and dates. In each case the aim was to block or kill the male semen. Like other formulas of ancient and medieval medicine, those contraceptive compounds were subjected to insufficient experimental control to be established as truly effective; they do reveal an appreciation of the objective of preventing conception and a rational sense of the means that might achieve the objective; their existence implies the ethical acceptance of contraception by the physicians of Egypt.

Among the "Incantations and Ceremonies for Procreation," the Force Brāhamana of the *Brihad-Aranyaka Upanishad* (seventh century B.C.), is the formula, "With power, with semen, I reclaim the semen from you." It is to be said by the male during intercourse if he does not want the woman to conceive; if it is properly uttered, "she comes to be without seed." By 300 B.C. the Tantras taught that the true yogi would have the self control to have intercourse without emitting semen; Śiva was said to have had such intercourse with Pārvatī for a thousand years, until the gods interrupted them (O'Flaherty, pp. 261–262). But Tantrism was a Hindu heresy, and mainline Hinduism, by teaching that a male descendant was necessary to perform the rites to save one after death, placed an enormous value on procreation.

In the Greco-Roman world, potions are the first and most common contraceptive to be mentioned. A drink of *misy*, apparently a distillate of copper, appears as a contraceptive in *The Nature of Women* 93, a treatise of the fifth-century B.C. Hippocratic school. In the fourth century B.C., Aristotle observed that conception could be impeded by the use of cedar oil, ointment of lead, or frankincense and olive oil on the part of the woman's body where "the seed falls," (*History of Animals* 7.3, 583a). By the first century A.D., writers on pharmacology are familiar with a variety of contraceptive drinks (e.g., Dioscorides, *Materia medica* 1.135; Pliny, *Natural History* 20.51, 142–143) and with use of pessaries like the Egyptians' (e.g., Dioscorides, *Materia medica* 3.36, 136). Both Dioscorides and Pliny also list salves or ointments to be applied to the male genitals to act as spermicides. The classical world was also familiar with physiological ways of avoiding conception. The Hippocratic school had theorized that the period when a woman was most likely to be fertile was just after menstruation. The foremost of Greek gynecologists, Soranos of Ephesus, recommended avoiding this time if conception was to be avoided (Soranos 1.19.61), while he noted that conception was unlikely during menstruation or just before its onset (ibid., 1.10.36). Herodotus reported that Pisistratus, the sixth-century tyrant of Athens,

avoided having children by having intercourse with his wife "not according to custom" (*History* 1.61.1); either anal intercourse or coitus interruptus is meant.

The most celebrated report of coitus interruptus is in Genesis 38:8–10, the story of Onan who habitually spilled his seed rather than carry out his obligation to his brother's widow. This single reference to contraceptive technique by the Jews of the Old Testament may be supplemented by references in the *Babylonian Talmud* going back to at least the first century of the Christian era. Coitus interruptus is mentioned in *Yebamoth* 34b and *Niddah* 13a, pessaries in *Yebamoth* 35a and *Niddah* 32, and potions made from roots in *Shabbath* 110a–110b and *Yebamoth* 8.4.

Although references to charms and amulets as contraceptives suggest the failure to establish any single reliable contraceptive, the evidence is ample that the ancient Mediterranean world —Egyptian, Jewish, Mesopotamian, Greek, and Roman—knew enough physiology to try to have sexual intercourse without conception and enough chemistry to attempt to prevent conception. Contraceptive practices were believed to be engaged in by rulers like Pisistratus; by slaves who did not want to bear children for their captors (*Babylonian Talmud, Kethuboth* 37a), by prostitutes who did not want the inconvenience of childbearing (*Yebamoth* 35a), by women concealing adultery (Soranos 1.19.60–61), by women preserving their looks (ibid.), and by women with too many children (Pliny, *Natural History* 29.27.85). What ethical judgment was given upon it?

Ancient ethical thought

Judaism. In Jewish thought, the intense consciousness of Israel as a people, the descendants of Abraham, the elect of God, led to a strong emphasis on the good of progeny and the duty of procreation. From "Increase and multiply" spoken by God in Genesis 1:27–28 to the promise of God in Deuteronomy 7:13, "No man or woman among you shall be childless," there was divine encouragement of childbearing. Sterility was a curse; a big posterity and, by implication, a big family were blessings (Gen. 15:5, Job 42:13, 1 Kings 1:1–28). No law in the Jewish scriptures condemned contraception as such. But its emphasis on fertility disfavored the practice. What Onan did "displeased Yahweh, who killed him" (Gen. 38:10). Onan had disobeyed his father in failing to provide his brother's widow with offspring; his crime was against the family. Although his contraceptive habit was not the explicit ground of Yahweh's judgment, the story suggested that contraceptive intercourse was the way of a wicked man.

Later Jewish thought, citing the punishment of Onan, treated coitus interruptus as a serious sin. One tradition linked the loss of seed to a Messianic theme: The Son of David would not come until all the souls of the unborn were born (*Babylonian Talmud, Niddah* 13a and 13b). Jewish opinion, however, divided on the duty to propagate the race, some rabbis teaching it to be the obligation of both men and women, others only of a man, and some limiting the duty to begetting two boys or a boy and girl (*Yebamoth* 61b, 65b). Associated with the milder views on procreative duty was the recognition by some rabbis of cases where a woman might legitimately use root potions as a contraceptive (e.g., *Babylonian Talmud, Niddah* 45a; *Tosefta, Yebamoth* 8.4).

Greco-Roman world. Greek philosophy and medicine took less interest in the morality of contraception. Nothing similar to the pledge not to give abortifacients appears in the Hippocratic Oath with reference to contraceptives. Aristotle raised no moral objection to the contraceptive technique he reported in the *History of Animals*. Plato, in his *Republic* (372c), portrayed Socrates as sketching an ideal city whose inhabitants do not beget too many children "lest they fall into poverty or war"; the avoidance of conception was implied as a civic obligation.

Conception was seen as controversial in the Greco-Roman world when population was related to the security of the state. By the time of Augustus the Roman government made modest efforts to reward childbearing by the upper class (e.g., Gaius, *Institutes* 1.145, 1.194) and later even celebrated fertility among freedmen (Pliny, *Natural History* 7.13.60). Imperial Roman law attempted to regulate the sale of abortifacient and contraceptive "medicines" (e.g., Justinian, *Digesta* 48.8.3). Effective enforcement, however, probably did not occur.

A second and more powerful current against contraception in the Mediterranean world came from philosophers. The Stoics taught that the purpose of sexual intercourse was procreation. Anything else was unnatural and therefore wrong (Musonius Rufus, *Reliquiae*, sec. 63). The neo-Pythagoreans, imbued with Stoic doctrine, similarly taught that "we have intercourse not for pleasure but for the purpose of pro-

creation" (Ocellus Lucanus, *The Nature of the Universe*, sec. 44). The Essenes, according to Josephus, held the same view (Josephus, *The Jewish War* 2.120, 160). By necessary implication, these views condemned contraception.

Civic responsibility, Stoic natural law, and the authority of the gods were combined by Musonius Rufus, the first-century Roman Stoic, when he argued that the lawgivers had forbidden contraception, and he who practiced it sinned "against his ancestral gods and Zeus, protector of the family" (Musonius Rufus, "Should All Children Born Be Brought Up?", *Reliquiae*). Philo, the Alexandrian intellectual who melded classical philosophy with his Jewish heritage, appropriated the Stoic distinction between marital intercourse for procreation and intercourse for the unlawful purpose of pleasure (Philo, *Joseph* 9.43). A man acted evilly, he taught, if he married a woman known to be sterile. "Those persons," Philo added, "who make an art of quenching the life of the seed as it drops stand condemned as the enemies of nature" (*The Special Laws* 3.36).

Early Christianity. The Christian position on contraception emerged in the first century in Palestine. It represented a confluence of doctrinal elements and a response to the Mediterranean milieu. In an ethic in which love of God and love of neighbor were the great commandments (Matt. 22:40), there was a specific doctrine on sexuality, analytically reducible to five themes: the superiority of virginity (e.g., Luke 1; Luke 20:34–36); the institutional goodness of marriage (Mark 10:7–8; John 2:1–12; Eph. 5:25–33); the sacred character of sexual intercourse (1 Cor. 6:16; 1 Thess. 4:4; 1 Pet. 3:2,7); the goodness of procreation (John 16:21; 1 Tim. 2:15); and the evil of extramarital intercourse and homosexual conduct (Matt. 5:27–28; Rom. 1:24–27). In the context formed by these themes, the Christian community found a balance, permitting and rewarding a way of life in which sexual intercourse was renounced for the higher good of following the personal example of Jesus' virginity, and permitting and rewarding a way of life in which intercourse occurred in marriage. Against the Christian Gnostics, who were found within the community even in its beginnings, it was urged that there were limits to the sexual liberty of the Christian: women would be saved "through motherhood" (1 Tim. 2:15). *Pharmakeia*, i.e., abortifacient and contraceptive drugs, were denounced as sinful by St. Paul (Gal. 5:20) and by the Apocalypse (9:21, 21:8, 22:15).

As Christianity permeated the Mediterranean world, it entered a society in which women were widely regarded as objects of pleasure; prostitution, particularly of slaves, was widespread; divorce and sexual infidelity were common. Infanticide was a frequent phenomenon (e.g., Seneca, *De ira* 1.15; Suetonius, *Gaius Caligula* 5; Tacitus, *Histories* 5.5). The Christian view of contraception may be understood as in part a reaction against these societal tendencies to treat woman as a thing, to destroy the special place of marital love, and to encroach on human life. In the *Didache* or *Teaching of the Twelve Apostles* 5.2, a late first-century document, "killers of offspring, corrupters of the mold of God," were classed with murderers and adulterers, whose life is the "Way of Death." As it was difficult for even the best gynecologists to distinguish contraceptive from abortifacient potions (Soranos 1.19.60–63), so Christian moralists did not distinguish between them.

Not only reaction against society, but reaction against Gnostic trends within the Christian community fortified the Christian exclusion of contraception. The Gnostic Right asked, What was the purpose of procreation? Now that the Messiah had come, now that death was overcome, should not every Christian imitate Christ in a total self-control excluding sexual conduct? (Clement 3.12.90.) The Gnostic Left asked if Christians were not "Lords of the Sabbath," free of any Mosaic commandment including the law against adultery (Clement 2.4.30). To Right and Left, the Christian Center had an answer: Virginity was desirable, but marriage was good. Christ had superseded the law of Moses but had not abolished the law of nature. The formula of the Center adapted the teaching of the Stoics to the needs of the Christian community. The Christian law, Clement of Alexandria wrote, was for "husbands to use their wives moderately and only for the raising up of children" (Clement 3.11.71.4). To have coitus "other than to procreate children," he taught, "is to do injury to nature" (Clement, *Pedagogus* 2.10.-95.3). Responding to internal challenges, rebuking the societal evils of abortion, adultery, and prostitution, the Stoic rule adopted by the Christians excluded contraception.

Manicheanism. In the fourth century A.D., as Christianity became the state religion of the Roman Empire, it was challenged by an underground religion, Manicheanism, whose prophet

Mani had been put to death in Persia; his teachings were conveyed by a sacred scripture, and his organization had the shape of a hierarchical church. The central Manichean myth taught that human beings originated in the lustful intercourse of the princes and princesses of darkness after they had devoured the sons of the King of Light. Within humans, particles of light subsisted, which struggled to be free but remained imprisoned as long as man emulated his devilish sires and procreated. This view of the universe in which alienated lights sought to return to the Father of Light and procreation was the worst of sins, appealed to a wide variety of intelligent minds, including that of Augustine, who between the ages of eighteen and twenty-nine was a Manichee. It was a view that did not exclude sexual intercourse but did exclude procreation and favored contraception, including the practice of coitus interruptus (Augustine, *Against Faustus* 22.30), the use of contraceptive potions (Augustine, *Marriage and Concupiscence* 1.115.17), and intercourse at times believed (erroneously) to be sterile (Augustine, *The Morals of the Manichees* 18.65). Manichees may be found in conflict with Zoroastrians in midfourth-century Persia and with Catholics in mid-fourth-century Charcar, Mesopotamia (Hegemonius, *Acts of Archelaus* 16), in Bostra, Asia Minor (Titus, *Against the Manichees* 2.33, *Patrologia graeca* 18:1197), in Constantinople (John Chrysostom, Homily 62 on Matthew 17), in the Mediterranean littoral (Epiphanius, *Panarion* 66.26), and in Italy (Ambrose to Chromatius of Aquileia, Letters 50). Manicheanism may be taken as the apogee of the contraceptive mentality prior to the mid-twentieth century.

Augustine. Opposition to the Manichees by the Roman government and by the Catholic Church was intense. Beginning in 320 a series of imperial decrees outlawed them and their practices. The climax of the Catholic Church's opposition came as late as 444, when Pope Leo the Great drove the Manichees from Rome and instructed the bishops of Italy to give them no respite anywhere. But more important than this official persecution was the powerful reinforcement given in Christian ethics to the Stoic rule that marital intercourse must be procreative. For Augustine, this was the most significant difference between the morals of the Manichees and the morals of the Catholic Church, which he had now joined (*Against Faustus* 22.30). The intensity of Augustine's own reaction against Manicheanism, reenacting in the life of one man the reaction of Christianity, was of extraordinary significance for Western ethical thought. The most influential of Western moralists became a convinced enemy of contraception.

In Augustine's analysis, offspring were one of the goods of marriage, and marital intercourse, to be entirely free from sin, must have offspring in view (*The Good of Marriage* 16.18). Mere absence of procreative intent made marital intercourse venially sinful; positive prevention of procreation turns "the bridal chamber into a brothel" (*Against Faustus* 15.7). Capping his anti-Manichean stance, Augustine explained, against Pelagius, that original sin was transmitted in the act of generation, since concupiscence, that is "heat" or "the confusion of lust," always accompanied the act of intercourse (*Marriage and Concupiscence* 1.18.21). Offsetting concupiscence, so as to justify marital intercourse, was the good of offspring. Forging the synthesis in which the doctrine of original sin was tied to the defense of procreative intercourse, Augustine formulated a comprehensive anticontraceptive ethic. Husbands and wives who used "the poisons of sterility" systematically to exclude conception were "not joined in matrimony but in seduction" (ibid., 1.15.17). Reasserting the link of Christianity with the Jewish scriptures, he taught that Onan's sin was contraceptive marital intercourse, "and God killed him for it" (*Adulterous Marriages* 2.12.12). Augustine's synthesis of personal experience and reaction, Old and New Testaments, anti-Manicheanism and anti-Pelagianism, Stoic natural law, and Christian sacramental theory was to constitute the strongest ethical case against any form of contraception.

Islam. By the seventh century the ethical tradition of Islam was dominant in the Middle East and North Africa, where Christianity had once flourished. The Koran has no expressed teaching on contraception, and although Islam inherited the propopulation outlook of the Bible, the major theologians and jurists of Islam did not condemn the contraceptive measures developed by Arabic medicine. By the time ibn Sina (known to the West as Avicenna) wrote his encyclopedic *Canon of Medicine* in eleventh-century Damascus, a wide range of contraceptives was known. In his pharmacopoeia he listed a plant that acts as a spermicide, another that acts as a pessary, another that is a talisman against conception (Avicenna 2.2.163, 277, 495). In book three, under "The Prevention of

Pregnancy," suppositories, spermicides, and a single potion were listed. He carefully distinguished contraceptives from abortifacients (3.21.2.12). Like the preventive measures of the Greco-Roman world on which it drew, the Islamic panoply of techniques against conception had a variety reflecting a lack of a single certain method. Apparently because of theological disapproval, coitus interruptus was not mentioned by the medical writers.

Medieval ethical thought

Early medieval Europe. The Celtic and Germanic peoples who came to inhabit Western Europe were familiar with herbal potions designed to prevent conception. Condemnation of these means was a constant theme of the penitential literature developed under monastic auspices from the sixth through the eleventh centuries. Part of the objection to them was their association with pagan magic, but the rationale of opposition also included objection to the killing of the seed and making infecund what God made fertile. The formula owed to Caesarius of Arles, "so many conceptions prevented, so many homicides," became popular. Burchard of Worms noted that the difficulty of feeding the children was not an excuse (*Patrologia Latina* 140:972). The penitentials, picking up the rabbinic and early Christian objection, also vigorously condemned anal and oral intercourse, where of course procreation was impossible. The eighth-century legislation of Theodulphus, bishop of Orléans, included condemnation of coitus interruptus. Implicitly, a standard of natural marital intercourse was assumed. Besides classifying the contraceptive acts as sinful, the penitentials prescribed inquiry to detect them and penances to punish them.

Catharism. Beginning in the early tenth century with Bogomil of Bulgaria, a new form of Gnosticism challenged the value of procreation. Organized as a church, Bogomil's adherents spread to the Eastern Empire's capital, Constantinople, and then westward to Bosnia. By the eleventh century they had appeared in Aquitaine, at Arras, and at Monteforte. A century later they were well established in Southern France and in some of the Northern Italian cities as the Cathar Church. The troubadors of courtly love from Languedoc and Aquitaine were drenched in their ideology of "pure," i.e., nonprocreative, love. Their doctrine opposed sexual intercourse leading to procreation. The devil had given "seed to the children of this world"

(*Un Traité cathare*, ed. C. Thouzellier, p. 96). When a woman conceived, Satan resided there (*Le Traité contre les Bogomils*, eds. Puech and Vaillant, p. 345). A pregnant woman was always to be denied the Cathar sacrament of the *consolamentum* (Borst, *Die Katharer*, p. 181).

To the Orthodox of the East and the Catholics of the West, the Cathars were a reappearance of the Manichees, and they were fought with the scriptural texts favoring procreation which had combated Manicheanism. Between 1140 and 1234, the most creative period of Western Catholic canon law, the Cathars were perceived as a socioreligious threat, challenging the Catholic Church in Southern France and Northern Italy and, like the Manichees, endangering the institution of marriage and the procreation of the species. The extent of the institutional Catholic response indicated the extent of the crisis. Ecumenical councils beginning with the Second Lateran in 1139 condemned the new heretics. The Dominican order was founded to convert them. The Inquisition was used to discover them. The Fourth Lateran Council in 1215 encouraged a holy crusade against them. The Hail Mary, with its key words "Blessed are you among women, and blessed is the fruit of your womb," became a popular prayer, prescribed to counter Cathar sentiment. The canon law, drawing on Augustine in particular, was shaped to include public teaching that condemned contraception and contraceptive marriage (Gratian, *Decretum* C. 32 q. 2 c. 7 and Gregory IX, *Decretals* 5.12.5).

Medieval Europe. Western Europe after 1150 knew the full range of contraceptives set out in Avicenna's *Canon of Medicine*, which, translated into Latin, was the standard textbook of general medicine for the next five hundred years. Actual practice is difficult to ascertain, but in Chaucer's *Canterbury Tales*, three methods of contraception were set out under the Sin of Wrath, including "drynkynge veneouse herbes thurgh which she may not conceive" ("The Parson's Tale," lines 570–580). Peter de Palude noted that a husband might seek to practice coitus interruptus because he had "more children than he can feed" (*On the Sentences* 4.31.3). Catherine of Siena had a vision whose contents suggest that contraceptive acts were common among the married bourgeoisie. The fifteenth-century Franciscan, Cherubino of Siena, in *The Rule of Married Life*, a book for the laity, treated coitus interruptus as a familiar sin. The canons of the Church, the teaching of

the theologians, and inquiry in confession were directed against these practices. The contraceptive act was condemned by all articulate ethical opinion as destroying potential life, as frustrating the function of coitus, and as violating a principal purpose of marriage (e.g., Thomas Aquinas, *Evil* 15.2).

Christian doctrine, nonetheless, contained currents that ran in a counter direction. In a famous passage, St. Paul had taught, "Let the husband render to his wife what is due her, and likewise the wife to her husband" (1 Cor. 7:3). As developed by scholastic theologians, the marital debt was a duty, and the satisfaction of it was virtuous even though procreation was not the purpose (Thomas Aquinas, *On the Sentences* 4.32.1.2). Moreover, the Church permitted the sterile and those past the age of childbearing to marry, implicitly conceding that procreative purpose was not necessary for a marriage. Finally, and perhaps most importantly, the theologians taught that "the good of offspring" meant not merely their procreation but their education as rational, spiritual creatures (e.g., William of Auxerre, *Summa* 4, f.287v). The universal acceptance of religious education as a constituent element in the good of offspring was a rejection of quantity and of population for its own sake. With the emphasis on education, Western Christianity carried the possibility of a different crystallization of values in the rule on contraception.

Reformation and post-Reformation thought

Protestantism. No change, however, occurred with either of the two upheavals that shook the doctrinal unity of medieval Christendom. The Protestant leaders were as severe on matrimonial conduct as their Catholic predecessors. Martin Luther, invoking Augustine for his theology, could scarcely have been anti-Augustinian in his morality. His *German Catechism* taught that the purposes of marriage were for a husband and wife "to live together, to be fruitful, to beget children, to nourish them, and to bring them up to the glory of God" (Luther). This was standard scholastic doctrine. John Calvin was more passionate. Coitus interruptus was "doubly monstrous." To commit Onan's act was "to extinguish the hope of the race and to kill before he is born the son who was hoped for" (Calvin). Not only did the new religion offer no alternative or critique of the old on contraception; the religious rivalry that followed led to a new premium on population. In Germany, the

Low Countries, and France, serious shifts in population growth would have affected the religious composition of the country and political control. That the strength of a state lay in its numbers was now stated with Machiavellian dispassionateness by that astute political observer Giovanni Botero in *Greatness of Cities* 3.1.

Rationalism. Analogously, the second upheaval, the spread of rationalism and deism in the seventeenth and eighteenth centuries, led to no alteration in expressed ethical opinion. While the old ethic on usury and on the indissolubility of marriage was under constant criticism, no one publicly advocated contraception as ethical conduct. The absence of challenge to the Christian rule may be explained in part by the reserve that all premodern people have experienced about the mystery of sex; in part by the lack of any institutional group desiring change; in part by the outlet the European colonies afforded for population; and in part by the absence of technological improvements. One new contraceptive device, the condom, did appear in the middle of the seventeenth century, but it was neither cheaply nor efficiently produced, and it won no medical support. Coitus interruptus and potions continued to be the chief contraceptive techniques. This limited technology remained the result and the cause of ethical intransigeance.

China. In non-Western societies contraceptive practice had little impact on population. China, for example, increased its numbers from about 150 million in 1650 to 430 million in 1850 (Ho, pp. 277–278). As the population outstripped economic resources, Hung Liang Chi, "the Chinese Malthus," in 1793 wrote two essays, "Reign of Peace" and "Livelihood," which linked overpopulation to social misery (ibid., pp. 271–272). But the principal means of meeting the problem was infanticide, especially of girls. The scholar Wang Shih-to (1802–1889) did recommend the spread of drugs to sterilize women and also recommended a tax on families with more than two children, the postponement of marriage, the increase of nunneries for women, and the forbidding of remarriage to widows, but he also urged the wholesale infanticide of females (ibid., p. 274). In fact, the killing of baby girls remained a nineteenth-century practice (ibid., pp. 58–61). Milder means of control do not appear to have been widely known.

Modern developments

The first advocates. At the very end of the eighteenth century, Thomas Malthus, "the

English Hung," wrote his famous *Essay on the Principle of Population*, positing a geometrical increase in population every twenty-five years if growth were unchecked; but his solution was "moral restraint," i.e., postponement of marriage, not contraception. About the same time, Jeremy Bentham hinted at the use of "sponges" to limit the poor and so reduce the poor rates. In 1806 Jean Baptiste Étienne de Senancour in *De l'amour* recommended "precautions" for women desiring to avoid unpleasant consequences from fornication; but he was unspecific. Francis Place, the first English advocate of particular means—coitus interruptus and sponges—remained anonymous in his advocacy. In the United States the first open advocacy of the means of birth control was undertaken in 1830 by Robert Dale Owens in *Moral Physiology: or a Brief and Plain Treatise on the Population Question*. Owens recommended coitus interruptus as a well-tested French technique.

Practice in France had in fact outstripped theory in the last part of the eighteenth century. A precipitous drop in the French birthrate from 1750 to 1800 reflected its effect, "the most important fact of all [France's] history" (Sauvy, p. 13). Disaffection from Catholic belief, followed by revolutionary emancipation from ecclesiastical control, lay at the root of this shift. The age of birth control had its roots in the age of *l'homme machine*, of a clear-eyed rationalism impatient with the mysterious and convinced that nature was controllable and man perfectible. Yet it was not in obedience to any express injunction of the rationalist philosophers but in response to a silent logic and in rejection of the old spirituality that birth control spread in France.

Christian theology, Catholic and Protestant, remained adamantly opposed to contraception, and medical and governmental opinion remained hostile. Even revolutionaries were unsympathetic: Proudhon in 1858 predicted that "Malthusianism" would depopulate France as it had done the Roman Empire (*De la justice dans la révolution et dans l'église*, I, pp. 348–349). After the debacle of the Franco-Prussian war, analysts of French society and journalists joined in attacking contraception as dooming France as a great power. In England in 1877, the government prosecuted Annie Besant and Charles Bradlagh for distributing Charles Knowlton's American text on contraception, *The Fruits of Philosophy*. In the United States, the federal Comstock law, enacted in 1873, forbade the mailing or importation of contraceptives, and most American states forbade their sale or advertisement (Smith, pp. 275–277).

The acceptance of contraception in the West. By the last quarter of the nineteenth century a small number of persons were convinced that contraception was the answer to miseries attributable to "over-childbearing." A Malthusian League was formed in England in 1878 to propagate this viewpoint. Analogues followed in Germany (1889), France (1898), Bohemia (1901), Spain (1904), Brazil (1905), Belgium (1906), Cuba (1907), Switzerland (1908), Sweden (1911), Italy (1913), and the United States (1913). By the twentieth century the birth control movement was clearly a Western European–American phenomenon (Chachaut, pp. 195–213, 453). International congresses were held in Paris in 1900, in Liège in 1905, in The Hague in 1911, in Dresden in 1912, in London in 1922, and in New York in 1925. Margaret Higgins Sanger, the American apostle of birth control, brought the message to Japan in 1921 and to India in 1936.

New forms of old contraceptive methods were developed in that period of expansion. In 1880 Wilhelm Mensinger developed a diaphragm for use as a pessary. By 1935 some two hundred types of mechanical devices, either condoms or pessaries, were in use in Western societies, and a wide range of chemicals was being employed as spermicides or occlusive agents; contraception was now a substantial business (Himes, p. 321).

In the period 1880–1930, medical opinion shifted from disapproval of contraception to doubt to acceptance. The shift paralleled changes in the learned worlds of science, sociology, and economics, where the humanist arguments of the advocates of birth control won much support. As a girl Margaret Higgins had been moved by the misery and ill health caused by undesired pregnancies among the very poor (Sanger, 1938, pp. 88–90). She also saw contraception as a substitute for "the barbaric methods" of infanticide and abortion (Sanger, 1969, p. 133). The relation between population growth and war was often stressed. The Sixth International Congress in 1925 declared flatly, "Overpopulation produces war." Malthus's predictions were refined and restated. It was estimated that by 1964 the United States would have a population of 214,000,000, which could not be agriculturally supported (East, p. 167). As the solution to overpopulation, as a substitute for abortion, and as an aid to personal happiness, contraception won the support of humanist ethicists in the West.

In Belgium, Ireland, and Spain, legislation of Catholic inspiration banned the sale of contraceptives. In France basically nationalistic legislation of the 1920s was directed to the same end. In the dictatorships of Germany, Italy, and Russia, contraception was discouraged as the nations prepared for war (Noonan, pp. 410–411). But after the Second World War nationalistic opposition to contraception began to disappear in Western countries.

In the United States contraception was widely practiced and, under the leadership of the Planned Parenthood movement, encouraged as "family planning." The last vestiges of secular opposition to contraception disappeared when the United States Supreme Court in *Griswold* v. *Connecticut* declared unconstitutional Connecticut's nineteenth-century statute against the use of contraceptives and when the same court in *Eisenstadt* v. *Baird* declared unconstitutional a Massachusetts law against selling contraceptives to the unmarried. From being illegal, contraception, now seen in the context of ethical concern with overpopulation, had become governmental policy, funded in the United States by such laws as the Family Planning Services and Population Research Act of 1970. On the international level, the Population Council, founded by John D. Rockefeller III in 1952, brought American technology and know-how in contraceptive technique to a variety of Asian, African, and South American nations. The United States moved officially to do the same with the Foreign Assistance Act of 1971.

Asia and Africa. The ethical-political response to contraception in the non-Western world remained mixed. Under the impetus of the American occupation, Japan had become fully committed to contraception with the Eugenic Protection Law of 1948. In other American client-states, such as Taiwan and South Korea, successful family planning programs flourished. Some of the new African states, however, did not value contraception highly, stressing their own relative underpopulation and observing the traditional importance of large families. Other countries like Indonesia gave lip service to the ideal of family planning but did little to implement it. India, with a government dedicated to population control, became a mammoth test case. In that country, "for all but a relative few, a woman's destiny lies in her procreation; the mark of her success as a person is in her bearing thriving children" (Mandlebaum, p. 16). Partly because of Hindu emphasis on the need for a son to perform salvific rites, partly for economic reasons, partly because of conflicts between villages and classes that could be won by manpower, and partly for personal status, large families were prized, and the value of contraceptives was questioned by the people (ibid., pp. 16–33). In competition with these traditional reasons were considerations of personal health and the national interest in curtailing population growth.

In Communist China birth control was officially encouraged in the cities in the mid-1950s, but after the Great Leap Forward, Chairman Mao in May 1958 asserted that China's numbers were a national asset (Aird, p. 699). Following the Cultural Revolution of 1966–1969, however, the government gave much publicity to marital postponement and birth limitation within marriage (Tien, p. 709). Ethical argument within the ruling party attempted the reconciliation of a belief in "planned population increase" with the ideology that "the question of 'overpopulation' does not exist in China" (Chi Lung, quoted in ibid., p. 710).

Modern Judaism.   Orthodox Jewish thought had always insisted on the evil of coitus interruptus; it viewed use of a condom as an analogous practice, destructive of the semen and the normal completion of the heterosexual process, e.g., the nineteenth-century *Responsum Shevet Sofer*, n. 2 (Feldman, p. 229). In Europe even the position on the use of contraceptives by women had hardened into opposition with the rulings of Rabbi Meir Posner of eighteenth-century Danzig, Rabbi Akiva Eger of nineteenth-century Poland, and Rabbi Moses Sofer of Pressburg (died 1839) (ibid., pp. 213–218). The permissive tradition as to women, however, had been strongly upheld by Rabbi Solomon Luria (died 1573). In the twentieth century it was reasserted. The diaphragm, analyzed as a means that did not interrupt the coital act, was accepted by rabbinic authorities (ibid., pp. 227–228). When the anovulant pills were developed, they, too, fell within the range of permitted means (ibid., pp. 245–246). Merely cultural Judaism had already accepted the mores of the modern world.

Christian changes.   Christian ethicists at first had remained critical. But in 1930 a significant break in the Christian front occurred. The bishops of the Anglican church by a vote of 193 to 67 approved a cautious acceptance of "methods" other than those of sexual abstinence to avoid parenthood ("Resolutions of the Lambeth Conference"). Between that date and 1958 the major Protestant churches all publicly abandoned the absolute prohibition of contraception by married couples. Leading Protestant theologians such as Karl Barth, Jacques Ellul, and Reinhold Niebuhr also accepted contraceptive practice. By 1959, when the World Council of Churches endorsed it, the Protestant consensus in its favor was overwhelming (Fagley, pp. 195–208).

The Orthodox Churches of the East did not alter the rule they had inherited. The Catholic Church remained adamant. The national hierarchies of Belgium (1904), of Germany (1913), of France (1919), and of the United States (1920) published strong pastorals denouncing contraception in their respective countries (Noonan, pp. 419–424). The climax of this episcopal and theological opposition was the encyclical letter *Casti Connubii* issued by Pius XI on 31 December 1930. "Any use whatever of marriage," the Pope declared, "in the exercise of which the act by human effort is deprived of its natural power of procreating life, violates the law of God and nature, and those who do such a thing are stained by a grave and mortal flaw" (Pius XI, 1930).

Catholic debate.   In the late 1950s a new advance in technology offered occasion for reconsideration of the Catholic position: Progesterone pills or anovulants producing temporary sterility were developed. The first tentative essay in defense of their morality by Louis Janssens at the University of Louvain was met by a strong rebuke from Pius XII (pp. 735–736). But the theologians continued to probe, and a lay Catholic, John Rock, one of the developers of the pills, wrote *The Time Has Come* (1963) in favor of their legitimacy. John XXIII appointed a commission to investigate.

Within Catholic theology itself, the anti-Augustinian current had expanded from the base which the medieval recognition of non-procreative intercourse had afforded it. Beginning with the fifteenth-century theologian Martin Le Maistre, it had been argued that marital intercourse might without sin be for pleasure. The influential seventeenth-century theologian Tomás Sanchez, found no sin in spouses who intended "only to copulate as spouses" (*The Holy Sacrament of Matrimony* 9.8). By the end of the eighteenth century, the Catholic theological consensus no longer insisted on procreative purpose in marital intercourse; a part of the underpinning of the rule on contraception had been removed. The next step was to see a positive value in nonprocreative intercourse. The step was taken in the nineteenth century by the French Jesuit, Jean Gury, who taught that intercourse might "manifest or promote conjugal affection" (Gury, n. 688). The view became common. In the work of Herbert Doms, *Vom Sinn und Zweck der Ehe* (1935), love was shown to be central to the moral meaning of conjugal coitus. The Second Vatican Council (1963–1965) incorporated this long-matured doctrine, teaching that love "directed from person to person" was "singularly expressed and perfected by the proper work of marriage" (Second Vatican Council, sec. 49). *Casti Connubii* itself had approved marital intercourse at times when the wife would be sterile.

In the theological climate generated by the Council, a majority of the papal commission did in fact recommend the permission of contraceptive intercourse in marriage (Hoyt, pp. 76–77). The leading moral theologian on the commission, Josef Fuchs, was of the majority, and he was supported outside the commission by the equally eminent moralist Bernard Häring. Paul VI, however, decided otherwise, issuing on 25 July 1968 the encyclical letter *Humanae Vitae*, which repeated the old condemnation in familiar terms (Paul VI).

The Catholic world responded to the letter in a divided way. National episcopates such as those of England, Ireland, Italy, and the United States issued statements accepting it without reserve. Other episcopates, notably those of Belgium, Canada, France, Germany, Indonesia, and, above all, the Netherlands treated the condemnation in such a way as to permit conscientious Catholics to practice contraception (Horgan). The discussion did remain open; Paul VI's authoritative but fallible statement of Catholic doctrine had not closed debate; in practice many Catholics adopted a different rule.

Recent issues

By 1970 a new trend was visible in the United States with 2.75 million American couples of childbearing ages choosing to be sterilized, half by vasectomy and half by tubal ligation (Bumpass and Presser, p. 532). Irreversible action to produce sterility raised the question of whether commitment to contraception had not led many young persons to give up prematurely a basic human good.

The issue was also raised as to whether a strong public policy fostering contraception did not also lead to dependence on abortion when contraception failed. For example, in Japan a correlation between the use of contraceptives and the acceptance of abortion was observed (Nizard, p. 1252).

The problem of ancient medicine remained current: It was difficult to discriminate abortifacients from contraceptives. The operating principle of a popular contraceptive, the intrauterine device (IUD), was uncertain: It probably acted by preventing the nidation of a fertilized human ovum. But the solution to this problem depended not so much on ethical reflections as on refinement of the experiments testing the IUD's mode of action.

In the late 1960s it was argued that voluntary contraception, governmentally aided, would not reduce the world birthrate sufficiently, and a variety of coercive government measures were called for, chiefly by U.S. scientists. Among the proposals were Kenneth Boulding's to license the procreation of children; Paul R. Ehrlich's to add sterilants to the water supply and to make population control "the price of food aid" from the United States; and William Shockley's to sterilize all girls temporarily with reversibility allowed only on governmental approval (Berelson, pp. 1–3). These measures were opposed as unethical violations of human freedom by the mainstream of American thought (ibid., pp. 8–9).

The very advocacy of such means raised the suspicion in some quarters that government-aided contraception in the United States had a racist objective (Weisbod, p. 571). In the United States, as in India and in all countries divided into social or ethnic classes, the ethics of contraception remained tied to the ethics of group competition.

Marxist thought did not treat contraception as intrinsically evil but saw an emphasis on family planning programs as a capitalist ruse to divert attention from fundamental economic and political problems. Faithful to this Marxist viewpoint, the head of the Chinese delegation at the 1975 World Population Conference in Bucharest declared that "the primary way of solving the population problem lies in combatting the aggression and plunder of the imperialists, colonialists, and neo-colonialists, and particularly the superpowers, breaking down the unequal international economic relations" (Finkle and Crane, p. 106). At Bucharest, orthodox Marxists joined with Third World nations suspicious of the United States and with the official Vatican delegation to deemphasize contraceptive programs as the principal governmental approach to problems of population. The ethical judgment made was that contraception could not be used as a shortcut to economic and political justice.

Conclusions

Contraceptive technology has presented ethical problems for mankind almost from the beginning of recorded history. As long as the technology was weak, however, no strong pressure existed against ethical judgments unfavorable to its use. With the existence of a panoply of effective techniques, the ethical questions have shifted to the degree of governmental involvement in programs of contraception and the effect of contraception on group, class, or national security.

Contraception, however, is not mere technology in the way that, for example, bathroom plumbing is technology. By definition an act making intercourse infertile, it affects the act still expressive in all cultures of the unity of love, and it affects the transmission of life. Ethical judgment cannot be made upon it without taking into account its impact on a society's sexual morals and valuation of human life, nor without an appreciation of the demographic context, the commitment of parents to the education of the children they conceive, and the value of interpersonal human love. The weighing of these disparate elements has led to one consensus in the past and to another consensus in the present. A moralist sensitive to history will be aware that the balance now struck is not eternal.

JOHN T. NOONAN, JR.

[*For further discussion of topics mentioned in this article, see the entries:* ABORTION; INFANTS, *article on* INFANTICIDE: A PHILOSOPHICAL PERSPECTIVE; NATURAL LAW; POPULATION ETHICS: RELIGIOUS TRADITIONS; *and* POPULATION POLICY PROPOSALS. *For discussion of related ideas, see the entries:* CIVIL DISOBEDIENCE IN HEALTH SERVICES; SEXUAL ETHICS; *and* STERILIZATION.]

BIBLIOGRAPHY

[Classical sources are cited in this article with standard numerical divisions; the *Oxford Classical Dictionary* should be consulted for references to available texts and English translations.]

AIRD, JOHN S. "Review Symposium: *China's Population Struggle* by H. Yuan Tien." *Demography* 11 (1974): 695–701. A sharply critical discussion of H. Yuan Tien's *China's Population Struggle: Demographic Decisions of the People's Republic, 1949–1969.*

AUGUSTINE. "Adulterous Marriages (De incompetentibus nuptiis)." Translated by Charles T. Huegelmeyer. *Writings of Saint Augustine.* Vol. 15: *Treatises on Marriage and Other Subjects,* pp. 53–132, especially bk. 2, chap. 12, par. 12, pp. 115–117. "De conjugiis adulternis ad Pollentium." *Patrologia Latina,* vol. 40, cols. 453–486, esp. cols. 478–479.

———. *Against Faustus* 15.7. "Reply to Faustus the Manichean." *The Works of Aurelius Augustine, Bishop of Hippo: A New Translation.* Edited by Marcus Dods. Vol. 5: *Writings in Connection with the Manichean Heresy.* Translated by Richard Stothert. Edinburgh: T. & T. Clark, 1822, bk. 15, chap. 7, pp. 275–278, esp. p. 276. "Contra Faustum Manichaeum." *Patrologia Latina,* vol. 42, cols. 309–311, esp. col. 310.

———. "The Good of Marriage (De bono coniugali)." Translated by Charles T. Wilcox. *Writings of Saint Augustine.* Vol. 15: *Treatises on Marriage and Other Subjects,* pp. 1–51, esp. chap. 16, par. 18, pp. 32–33. *Patrologia Latina,* vol. 40, cols. 374–396, esp. col. 386.

———. *Marriage and Concupiscence* 1.19.21, 1.15.17. "What Is Sinless in the Use of Matrimony? What Is Attended with Venial Sin, and What with Mortal?" and "Thus Sinners Are Born of Righteous Parents, Even as Wild Olives Spring from the Olive." "On Marriage and Concupiscence." *A Select Library of the Nicene and Post-Nicene Fathers of the Christian Church.* Edited by Philip Schaff. Vol. 5: *Saint Augustine: Anti-Pelagian Writings.* Translated by Peter Holmes and Robert Ernest Wallis. Revised by Benjamin B. Warfield. New York: Christian Literature Co., 1887, bk. 1, chap. 17 [XV]; chap. 21 [XIX], pp. 270–273. "De nuptiis et concupiscentia." *Patrologia Latina,* vol. 44, bk. 1, chap. 15, sec. 17; chap. 19, sec. 21; cols. 421–422, 424–425.

———. *Writings of Saint Augustine.* Vol. 15: *Treatises on Marriage and Other Subjects.* The Fathers of the Church: A New Translation, vol. 27. Edited by Roy Joseph Deferrari. New York: 1955.

AVICENNA. *Canon medicinae.* Translated by Gerard of Cremona. Venice: Apud Juntas, 1582. The arsenal of contraceptive prescriptions known to antiquity, the Arabic world, and medieval Europe.

BEHRMAN, S. J.; CORSA, LESLIE, JR.; and FREEDMAN, RONALD, eds. *Fertility and Family Planning: A World View.* Ann Arbor: University of Michigan Press, 1969.

BERELSON, BERNARD. "Beyond Family Planning." *Studies in Family Planning,* no. 39 (February 1969), pp. 1–16. Current ethical issues.

BERGUES, HÉLÈNE; ARIÈS, PHILIPPE; HÉLIN, ÉTIENNE; HENRY, LOUIS; RIQUET, R. P. MICHEL; SAUVY, ALFRED; and SUTTER, JEAN. *La Prévention de naissances dans la famille: Ses origines dans les temps moderns.* Institut national d'études démographiques: Travaux et documents, cahier no. 35. Paris: Presses Universitaires de France, 1959. An historical account of French contraceptive practice.

BUMPASS, LARRY L., and PRESSER, HARRIET B. "Contraceptive Sterilization in the U.S.: 1965 and 1970." *Demography* 9 (1972): 531–548.

CALVIN, JOHN. *Commentarius in Genesim* 38.8–10. Translated by John King as *Commentaries on the First Book of Moses Called Genesis.* 2 vols. Grand Rapids, Mich.: Wm. B. Eerdmans Publishing Co., 1948, vol. 2, chap. 38, v. 8, p. 281.

CHACHAUT, M. *Le Mouvement du "Birth Control" dans les pays Anglo-Saxons.* Bibliothèque de l'Institut de droit comparé de Lyon, sér. centrale, vol. 32. Paris: M. Giard; Lyons: Bosefrères, M. & L. Riou, 1934. A history of the movement.

CHANDRASEKHAR, SRIPATI, ed. *Asia's Population Problems, with a Discussion of Population and Immigration in Australia.* New York: Frederick A. Praeger, 1967. Problems and issues from the perspective of a convinced family planner.

CLEMENT OF ALEXANDRIA. *Stromata* 2.4.30, 3.12.90. Bk. 2 translated as "The Stromata, or Miscellanies." *The Ante-Nicene Fathers: Translations of the Writings of the Fathers down to A.D. 325.* Edited by Alexander Roberts and James Donaldson. Revised by A. Cleveland Coxe. Vol. 2: *Fathers of the Second Century: Hermas, Tatian, Athenagoras, Theophilus, and Clement of Alexandria (Entire).* American reprint. Grand Rapids, Mich.: Wm. B. Eerdmans Publishing Co., 1956, bk. 2, chap. 4, sec. 30, pp. 349–351. Bk. 3 translated by John Ernest Leonard Oulton as "On Marriage: Miscellanies, Book III, The Text." *Alexandrian Christianity: Selected Translations of Clement and Origen.* Introduction and notes by John Ernest Leonard Oulton and Henry Chadwick. Philadelphia: Westminster Press, 1954, pp. 82–83. Oulton and Chadwick do not include book 2. Roberts and Donaldson do not translate book 3 because it is "necessarily offensive to our Christian tastes" (p. 381).

DEINES, HILDEGARD VON; GRAPOW, HERMANN; and WESTENDORF, WOLFHART. *Übersetzung der medizinischen Texte.* 2 vols. Grundriss der Medizin der alten Ägypter, no. 4. Berlin: Akademie-Verlag, 1958.

DOMS, HERBERT. *Vom Sinn und Zweck der Ehe.* Breslau: Ostdeutsche Verlagsanstalt, 1935. Translated by George Sayer as *The Meaning of Marriage.* New York: Sheed & Ward, 1939. Fundamental to modern Catholic views on the purpose of marriage.

EAST, EDWARD M. *Mankind at the Crossroads.* New York: Charles Scribner's Sons, 1923.

Eisenstadt v. Baird. 405 U.S. 438. 31 L. Ed. 2d 349. 92 S. Ct. 1029 (1972).

FAGLEY, RICHARD M. *The Population Explosion and Christian Responsibility.* New York: Oxford University Press, 1960. A review of modern Protestant positions on contraception.

Family Planning Services and Population Research Act of 1970. Pub. L. 91-572. 84 Stat. 1504. 42 U.S.C. sec. 300r.

FELDMAN, DAVID MICHAEL. *Birth Control in Jewish Ethics: Marital Relations, Contraception, and Abortion as Set Forth in the Classic Texts of Jewish Law.* New York: New York University Press, 1968. A comprehensive survey arguing that literary history, not economic-historical factors, has determined the rabbinic positions.

FINKLE, JASON L., and CRANE, BARBARA B. "The Politics of Bucharest: Population, Development, and the New International Economic Order." *Population and Development Review* 1 (1975): 87–114. The current secular debate on contraception in terms of Marxism and international politics.

GLASS, D. V., and REVELLE, ROGER, eds. *Population and Social Change.* London: Edward Arnold; New York: Crane, Russak, 1972. Focused on demographic history, this symposium is a good introduction to the relations between social contexts and contraceptive practice.

Griswold v. Connecticut. 381 U.S. 479. 14 L. Ed. 2d 510. 85 S. Ct. 1678 (1965).

GURY, JEAN. "De Matrimonio" [Marriage]. *Compendium Theologiae Moralis* [Compendium of moral theology] (1846).

HAUSER, PHILIP M., ed. *The Population Dilemma.* 2d ed. Englewood Cliffs, N.J.: Prentice-Hall, 1969. The modern "population problem."

HIMES, NORMAN EDWIN. *Medical History of Contraception.* Foreword by Robert Latou Dickinson. Preface by Alan F. Guttmacher. New York: Gamut Press, 1963. Unreliable as history due to Himes's unfamiliarity with foreign languages; useful on the modern birth control movement.

HO, PING-TI. *Studies in the Population of China, 1368–1953.* Harvard East Asian Studies, vol. 4. Cambridge: Harvard University Press, 1959. Primarily a demographic study, this touches incidentally on means of control.

HORGAN, JOHN, ed. *Humanae Vitae and the Bishops: The Encyclical and the Statements of the National Hierarchies.* Analytic Guide by Austin Flannery. Shannon: Irish University Press, 1972. A complete collection of episcopal responses to the encyclical. Text of Encyclical in English and Latin.

HOYT, ROBERT G., ed. *The Birth Control Debate.* Kansas City: National Catholic Reporter, 1968. The majority and minority reports of the papal commission on contraception.

LEE, LUKE T., and LARSON, ARTHUR, eds. *Population and Law: A Study of the Relations Between Population Problems and Law.* Leiden: A. W. Sijthoff; Durham, N.C.: Rule of Law Press, 1971. A worldwide compendium of statutes on birth control.

LUTHER, MARTIN. "Der grosse Katechismus, 1529." *Luthers Werke in Auswall.* Vol. 4: *Schriften von 1529 bis 1545.* 5th rev. ed. Edited by Otto Clemen. Berlin: Walter de Grunter & Co., 1959, p. 31–34. On the Sixth Commandment.

MACURA, MILOS. "Population Policies in Socialist Countries of Europe." *Population Studies* 28 (1974): 369–379. Eastern European governmental attitudes on contraception.

MANDLEBAUM, DAVID G. *Human Fertility in India. Social Components and Policy Perspectives.* Berkeley: University of California Press, 1974. Practice and attitudes affecting ethical judgment in India.

NIZARD, ALFRED. "Le Japon vingt ans après la loi eugénique." *Population* 25 (1970): 1236–1262. A comprehensive study of population and means of control since 1948.

NOONAN, JOHN T., JR. *Contraception: A History of Its Treatment by the Catholic Theologians and Canonists.* Cambridge: Belknap Press, Harvard University Press, 1965. The history of doctrine on contraception from its pre-Christian roots to the Second Vatican Council.

O'FLAHERTY, WENDY DONIGER. *Asceticism and Eroticism in the Mythology of Śiva.* School of Oriental and African Studies. London: Oxford University Press, 1973.

Patrologiae cursus completus: Series Graeca [Patrologia Graeca]. 161 vols. Paris: Apud Garnier Fratres, editores & J.-P. Migne successores, 1857–1894.

Patrologiae cursus completus: Series Latina [Patrologia Latina]. 221 vols. Paris: Apud Garnier Fratres, editores & J.-P. Migne successores, 1851–1894. *Supplementum.* Paris: Éditions Garnier frères, 1958–.

PAUL VI. "Humanae Vitae." *Acta Apostolicae Sedis* 60

(1968): 481–503. Translated as "Humanae Vitae (Human Life)." *Catholic Mind,* September 1968, pp. 35–48.

PIUS XI. "Casti Connubii." *Acta Apostolicae Sedis* 22 (1930): 539–592, esp. 560. Translated as "On Christian Marriage." *Catholic Mind* 29 (1931): 21–64.

PIUS XII. "Essais de solution." *Acta Apostolicae Sedis* 50 (1958): 732–737. Especially pp. 735–736. Text in French.

"Resolutions of the Lambeth Conference, 1930: II. The Life and Witness of the Christian Community: Marriage and Sex." *Report of the Lambeth Conference, 1930: Encyclical Letter from the Bishops with Resolutions and Reports.* London: Society for Promoting Christian Knowledge; New York: Macmillan Co., n.d., resolution 15, pp. 43–44.

ROCK, JOHN. *The Time Has Come: A Catholic Doctor's Proposals to End the Battle over Birth Control.* Foreword by Christian A. Herter. New York: Alfred A. Knopf, 1963.

SANGER, MARGARET. *Margaret Sanger: An Autobiography.* New York: W. W. Norton & Co., 1938.

———. *My Fight for Birth Control.* New York: Maxwell Reprint, 1969.

SAUVY, ALFRED. *La Prévention des naissances.* "Que sais-je?" Le Point des connaissances actuelles, no. 988. Paris: Presses universitaires de France, 1962. 3d ed. 1967.

Second Vatican Council. "Pastoral Constitution on the Church in the Modern World." *The Sixteen Documents of Vatican II and the Instruction on the Liturgy.* Boston: St. Paul Editions, 1962, pp. 511–625; esp. pt. 2, chap. 1, sec. 49, pp. 563–564. *Gaudium et Spes.*

SMITH, PETER. "The History and Future of the Legal Battle over Birth Control." *Cornell Law Quarterly* 49 (1963): 275–303. A survey of statutory and case law in the United States.

SORANOS [SORANUS]. *Peri gynaikeiōn pathōn* [Gynecology] 1.10.36, 1.19.60–63.

THOMAS AQUINAS. *Evil* 15.2. "Utrum omnis actus luxuriae sit peccatum mortale" [Whether all sex acts are mortal sins]. *Questiones disputatae.* 7th ed. 5 vols. Vol. 2: *De malo.* Rome: Marietti, 1942, pp. 245–250.

TIEN, H. YUAN. "Review Symposium: *China's Population Struggle* by H. Yuan Tien: Reply." *Demography* 11 (1974): 708–714. A spirited rejoinder to Aird.

WEISBOD, ROBERT G. "Birth Control and the Black American: A Matter of Genocide?" *Demography* 10 (1973): 571–590.

COST-BENEFIT ANALYSIS

See RISK; LIFE-SUPPORT SYSTEMS; TECHNOLOGY, *article on* TECHNOLOGY ASSESSMENT; LIFE, *article on* VALUE OF LIFE.

CRYOBANKING OF SPERM, OVA, AND EMBRYOS

See REPRODUCTIVE TECHNOLOGIES, *articles on* SPERM AND ZYGOTE BANKING, ETHICAL ISSUES, *and* LEGAL ASPECTS.

CRYONICS

The study of the biological effects of cold is known as cryobiology. Cryonics is a more specific term used to identify the practice of freezing human bodies in the hope of achieving suspended animation. Luyet and Gehenio in 1940 compiled the first comprehensive survey on the survival of organisms at low temperature. In 1964 an increasing volume of laboratory work on low temperature biology precipitated the founding of a new journal, *Cryobiology,* devoted exclusively to the subject. Since the mid-1960s reviews dealing with various aspects of cryobiology have been published (Meryman; Mazur; Popovic and Popovic).

Human beings, like other mammals but unlike most animal species, normally maintain their body temperature within very narrow limits. In a mammal, the decline of the body temperature is accompanied by a corresponding reduction in vital activities. Actual freezing of tissues essentially halts all life processes. States of low temperature above freezing (hypothermia) have been found useful in the preservation of isolated organs and in some surgical procedures. Segregated mammalian cells and some tissues have been frozen to very low temperatures and successfully recovered. The freezing of most cells without previous exposure to cryoprotective solutions results in their death.

The more ambitious goal of maintaining the whole body of a human or of an animal in the frozen state and eventually resuscitating it has not been attained. Nevertheless, this prospect has stimulated the organization of "cryonics" or "life extension" societies, which disseminate information about the freezing of human bodies and aid those who are interested in applying cryonic interment, rather than conventional burial or cremation, to bodies of relatives or friends.

In most cases of human cryonic preservation, the bodies are first perfused with a cryoprotective agent, usually Dimethylsulfoxide (DMSO), temporarily frozen in dry ice, and then permanently stored in liquid nitrogen at $-196°C$. Endowments must be provided so that the liquid nitrogen can be replaced periodically. Ettinger (1964, pp. 170–180) and other proponents of this cryonic interment have been forecasting its widespread application since the mid-1960s. The reason for the freezing of bodies is the anticipation of the possibility of resuscitation at some distant future date when science is greatly advanced and both the pathology that caused the death and the injury resulting from the freezing process itself can be reversed.

Possible methods of cooling

There are at present three cooling methods whereby a human body might be maintained in a reduced metabolic state for a long period: hypothermia, hibernation, and the frozen state.

Hypothermia. Hypothermia involves the cooling of the body to a temperature below normal but above freezing. This can take place when the body temperature regulating mechanisms fail, or whenever the heat production of an individual is too small to compensate for the heat loss resulting from cold exposure. Some men and women have accidentally become deeply hypothermic and have subsequently survived. However, cooling was of relatively short duration. No records of human survival following extended hypothermia (weeks or months) exist. The very low body temperatures required for long-term preservation cause injury even if the period of cooling is brief. Generally in medical usage, regional or differential hypothermia is preferred over whole body cooling. The reasons for limited survival time in deep hypothermia are still not understood, but it seems that inadequate tissue perfusion is responsible for death.

Hibernation. Hibernation, a state of greatly reduced body temperature, occurs naturally in some mammals and birds. The hibernating animal retains the capability of spontaneously rewarming to its normal level of around 37°C by a mechanism of internal heat production without absorbing heat from its environment. Hibernating animals are able to recover fully from week-long periods of profound torpor, a state in which the temperature of the entire body falls to within a few degrees of freezing, heart rate is slowed to a few beats per minute, and metabolism is depressed as much as ninety-nine percent. The physiological depressions are reversible in a hibernator when arousal takes place. It could be useful for research, for surgery, and for future space travel to be able to induce states of hibernation at will in man, but at present it cannot be done. Despite an extensive research effort, the mechanism of hibernation production is still unknown.

At present, therefore, hibernation is not a practical method of producing long-term suspended animation of man, and in any case the aging process would continue.

Freezing. Total body freezing is presumably the best method for long-term preservation of man in a state of suspended animation, if it could be technically accomplished. Cryopreservation of individual human cells and some small or thin pieces of tissue have met with considerable success. Numerous attempts to freeze adult kidneys or hearts have not produced methods allowing for subsequent survival of rewarmed organs on transplantation. The lethal effects of freezing at the mature organ level are not yet controllable, even by the introduction of cryoprotective agents.

Probably because of its complexity, the freezing of whole animals has received relatively little serious attention. The most thorough studies were conducted on golden hamsters by Smith and co-workers (Smith, pp. 199–205). Like most hibernators the hamster has a high resistance to cold injury, but even under these circumstances, full recovery of a completely frozen animal has never occurred. Attempts to "supercool" (i.e., achieve below freezing temperatures without the crystallization associated with freezing) whole mammals, thus avoiding the adverse effects of crystal formation, have also failed to provide a method for long-term preservation. According to Malinin, at present any attempts to preserve humans by freezing must be regarded as based on unfounded hopes. There is essentially no material "prospect of immortality" for those bodies frozen by the cryonic methods now employed.

Moral issues in human freezing

Moral arguments against the use of cryonic interment are based on questions of justice to immediate survivors as well as to future generations, the use of extraordinary means in attempts to extend life even briefly, and religious, sociological, and anthropological considerations. Moral implications vary depending on whether actual current practice or the use of a possible perfected technique is being considered.

Current freezing of bodies. It is argued that if resuscitation from the frozen state appears not to be possible even in the future, there is nothing to be lost by subjecting a body to freezing rather than to burial. This is not necessarily the case, however. False expectations could be encouraged, thereby delaying an acceptance of the reality of a particular death and risking adverse psychological effects on the related family. Further, the freezing and maintenance procedure is costly and would place a large burden on most families. Anxieties could be developed in those who cannot afford the procedure and whose sense of love and loyalty might encourage them to try to use the procedure as something truly desirable.

If the practice ever grew, the cumulative effect on society could be great as resources were diverted to this activity. Perhaps lower age limits would be imposed and only certain types of deaths would justify the procedure. Any exaggerated resource-consuming efforts for individuals would have to be limited by the common good.

A materialistic and, according to some, even a selfish view of human life seems inherent in this procedure, especially if it became widespread, for it would be based on the assumption that the extension of this material life is desired at almost any cost.

The philosophy favoring cryonic interment seems to be contrary to the Christian understanding of the purpose of life and the meaning of death, but Ettinger (1967) does not see this conflict. He understands cryonic interment to be an "urgent spiritual goal," a goal that can serve as an "antidote" to defections from Christianity. He proposes a vision of "supermen" greatly enriched by biological discoveries and advancing toward the material greatness envisioned by the creator himself. Ettinger sees this as an important element in the development of a Christianity that is universal and evolutionary rather than narrow and static.

If freezing of humans were perfected? If perfected, freeze preservation of a human for days or months would present the same moral questions facing any patient and doctor before a significant medical procedure. If the service is limited or the cost is very high, factors such as wishes of the patients, age, likelihood of real utility, demand on resources, etc., would contribute to the final judgment.

If perfected, preservation for extensive periods of years or decades might be defended in circumstances such as long space flights, to await medical developments, or even for purposes of historical continuity of mankind. Each situation would have to be evaluated individually. Widely applied long-term human preservation, however, would confront us with a very different set of moral questions, some of which have already been considered above in the treatment of current freezing methods.

According to Vaux (pp. 96–110), man, as a social being, must learn to die for the sake of the future. Vaux maintains we must learn that death energy is creative. We face population and ecological disaster if we disrupt the evolutionary death now in process without simultaneously disrupting birth. The success of the freezing procedure would not of itself mean that man's actual active biological life would be significantly extended, although his chronological life span would be increased. It could mean that age proportions in our population would be disrupted. Maybe our concentration on health care would be greatly emphasized. Unless there is some limit to birth rate, and death rate is at least maintained in step with this limit, the quality of life on this planet may be radically altered.

In view of the aforesaid problems involved in large scale preservation, someone or some group would have to face crucial choices about who is to be freeze-preserved, when this is to happen, and, perhaps even more important, at what point thawing and resuscitation are to take place. The possibility of population manipulation is as evident here as it would be in cases of genetic engineering. Who would make these choices? On what basis? Obviously, to avoid chaos, economic and social balance would require that humans be reintroduced into society in some planned manner. What would be the basis for this planning?

How would human freedom be affected? Would the right to die be respected? Would the consent of the individual be required before preservation? In the frozen state, where there can be no dialogue with the individual, how are rights negotiated? Is the preserved individual legally dead? What happens to his property, his family relationships? Does anyone own him?

Man's behavior is dependent on the constant interactions between himself and the surrounding objects and actions that impinge upon him. He might hope to be unchanged after a long period of preservation, but his ambience, his historical context, and his associations would be radically disrupted. What would be the effect on his own development? What would be the effect of a long cessation of biological rhythms, so essential for a balanced human existence? What subtle behavioral variation might result in an individual or a population? Long-term preservation would probably produce individuals who are out of step with the historical development of man. And, of course, it is more than likely that the preservation procedures would be at least slightly imperfect and would yield large numbers of either mentally or physically unhealthy individuals. Would society accept a moral responsibility to see that such defective persons are cared for until they die naturally? There are many other unpredictables involved, such as the effect on human motivation, expectancies, and drives, which would result from what is essentially a lack of unity and compactness in the individual life.

It must be emphasized that possible moral ramifications should not necessarily deter scientists from seriously trying to perfect preservation methods. There are clear advantages for man if such methods are available, especially for short-term emergency use. And intermediate successes, such as the successful banking of frozen organs, would have vast benefits. Moral questions become much more complex, however, when the goal of the methodology becomes a frustration of the life–death rhythm of human existence.

J. A. PANUSKA

[*For further discussion of topics mentioned in this article, see the entries:* AGING AND THE AGED, *article on* THEORIES OF AGING AND ANTI-AGING TECHNIQUES; CADAVERS, *article on* GENERAL ETHICAL CONCERNS. *Also directly related are the entries* DEATH, ATTITUDES TOWARD; DEATH, DEFINITION AND DETERMINATION OF; LIFE; *and* LIFE-SUPPORT SYSTEMS. *See also:* FUTURE GENERATIONS, OBLIGATIONS TO; HUMAN EXPERIMENTATION; *and* ORGAN TRANSPLANTATION.]

BIBLIOGRAPHY

BRYANT, CLIFTON D., and SNIZEK, WILLIAM E. "The Cryonics Movement and Frozen Immortality." *Society*, November–December 1973, pp. 56–61.

ETTINGER, ROBERT C. W. *The Prospect of Immortality.* Garden City, N.Y.: Doubleday & Co., 1964.

———. "Cryonics and the Purpose of Life." *Christian Century* 89 (1967): 1250–1253.

LUYET, BASILE JOSEPH, and GEHENIO, P. N. *Life and Death at Low Temperatures.* Normandy, Mo.: Biodynamica, 1940.

MALININ, THEODORE I. "Freezing of Human Bodies." *Journal of the American Medical Association* 221 (1972): 598.

MAZUR, PETER. "Cryobiology: The Freezing of Biological Systems." *Science* 168 (1970): 939–948.

MERYMAN, HAROLD T., ed. *Cryobiology.* New York and London: Academic Press, 1966.

POPOVIC, VOJIN, and POPOVIC, PAVA. *Hypothermia in Biology and in Medicine.* New York: Grune & Stratton, 1974.

SMITH, AUDREY U., ed. *Current Trends in Cryobiology.* New York: Plenum Press, 1970.

VAUX, KENNETH. *Biomedical Ethics.* New York: Harper & Row, 1974.

D

DEATH

Because views on the ethical issues surrounding death and dying are constantly changing, this entry offers a history of the conceptual and value perspectives on death in different cultures and philosophies as background material for the discussions of the concrete ethical issues presented in the entries on DEATH AND DYING: EUTHANASIA AND SUSTAINING LIFE, *and* DEATH, DEFINITION AND DETERMINATION OF.

I
ANTHROPOLOGICAL PERSPECTIVE

Peoples of every known human society value life and deplore its end. Each society has evolved a set of conventions for determining under what circumstances a life may be terminated. There are transcultural variations regarding the extinction of life deliberately or accidentally as well as in the perception of what constitutes natural death. While no society welcomes death, there are conditions under which a death may be intentionally invited and implemented by victim and community; death may become a social obligation. This article is confined to societies termed preindustrial, nonliterate, and non-Western.

Natural death and the desire for immortality

Hartland expresses a long-held view that there is a universal abhorrence of death and a tacit refusal to accept its inevitability (Frazer, 1913, 1927). Myths of many peoples suggest that humanity was originally immortal but was brought down to mortal status by gods angered at some human indisposition: disobedience, deception, betrayal of spirits, or violation of moral and social norms. Hocart ("Death Customs") rejects the notion that preindustrial peoples "are alleged to feel an overwhelming fear of death which prompts measures for self-protection. This is not confirmed by observation." It appears to be not so much horror of the corpse as fear of the symbolic power of spirits as well as love and reverence for the deceased and desire for immortality that motivates human ethics of death (Malinowski). This ambivalence—a reflection of the ambivalence toward the living, whether relative, leader, stranger, or friend—characterizes cults of the dead and ancestor worship and influences forms and functions of mortuary rites (Bendann).

Myths of immortality, often transmitted through tales of sick and old persons through dreams and visions, predicate the notion prevalent in many cultures that the death of a mature adult is not a natural happening but the effect of spiritual retribution, or of sorcery or witchcraft, i.e., human retribution (Frazer, 1913, 1927). Some writers insist that all preindustrial peoples hold the idea of death as unnatural, but the evidence does not support this. Simmons (pp. 217–220) found that, of forty-seven societies in his cross-cultural survey, seventeen regarded all death as unnatural, four believed it to be natural, and twenty-six "partially admitted" the possibility. Thus nearly two-thirds of these societies thought natural death to be possible, seemingly contrary to the more florid ethnological generalizations.

There appears to be a universal tendency to conceive of each person as possessing a vital substance, an élan vital, that animates his behavior and quickens his body. Sometimes the dead will be conceived to have more than a single essence. The Trobriand Islanders divide it into the *kosi* (ghost) and *baloma* (spirit), each with its own characteristics and vicissitudes (Malinowski). Frazer and Tylor felt that the wish for immortality springs from experience (especially of dreams), not intuition, and frequently results in the raising of dead ancestors to godhood in a pantheon that also includes nature spirits. The desire to live indefinitely combined with the actual hazards of life in an unpredictable environment lead easily to the notion that, but for spiritual or human trickery, each mortal would be immortal. Therefore those states that conduce toward death, such as sickness, starvation, accidents and injuries, and other misfortunes, are a consequence of natural, supernatural, and human malevolence.

All peoples attempt to protect themselves from lethal forces and events with often elaborate precautionary systems. Life at its fullest is coterminous with health and happiness (as indigenously defined). But serious illness or injury, states of decrepitude, and disabilities of age are seen as related more to death than to life. When a member of the Murngin of Australia has been "boned" (condemned to death by sorcery) his community classifies him as "half-dead" (Warner, 1958 ed.), a state that Van Gennep and Turner define as "liminal" or "betwixt and between" two conditions while being neither. Since this vulnerable state poses a threat not only to the victim but through ritual contagion to his family and clan, this hunter–gatherer community withdraws physically and psychologically, behaving as though their ill-fated colleague no longer exists. Then they subject him to a

mourning ceremony to hasten his journey to the land of the dead. Through transgression of moral norms the victim has endangered his entire group and cannot be allowed to live.

Durkheim (1965) and Hertz (1960) accepted the universality of the human belief in immortality but felt that it derives not from individual psychological need but from "the naive expression of a permanent social need. Indeed society imparts its own character of permanence to the individuals who compose it: because it feels itself immortal and wants to be so, it cannot normally believe that its members, above all those in whom it incarnates itself and with whom it identifies itself, should be fated to die" (Hertz, p. 77). Van Gennep asserted that death was the last in a series of "rites of passage," beginning with birth, that punctuate the life cycle as individuals or cohorts of individuals pass from one status and role-set to another. The implementation of these ceremonies of individual-social transformation occurs in three phases: separation, transition, and incorporation. Various points of potential crisis (birth, adolescence, marriage, death) emphasize one or another phase, but all contain some aspects of each, and frequently include subphases. In separation rituals, survivors mourn their loss, attempting thereby to adapt to bereavement by working out feelings regarding the deceased. In the transition phase the corpse is not yet completely dead (in the social and psychological sense) nor alive, and its ghost hangs about to ensure that appropriate actions have been taken by the living. Rites of incorporation occur finally in which ghost becomes transformed into spirit and a permanent inhabitant of the afterworld, though in touch with mundane affairs and influencing and controlling them through stringent moral and ethical sanctions. In death the rites of passage deal not only with the organic end of the person but with his rebirth in spiritual form (Van Gennep).

Durkheim and Hertz remark upon the fact that in most cultures there is not one but often two or more rituals connected with disposal of the dead. It takes time for the ghost of the deceased to find a comfortable place in the society's collective consciousness, since the familiar image of the dead person seems a long distance from the hazy, exalted image of the worshiped and dreaded ancestors. During this period the group recoils from the shock of bereavement and through ritual finally regains its new equilibrium. Another way to conceive of the process might be as a patterned struggle to reestablish the balance of power between the quick and the dead. Relations between the living society and its spiritual environment are patterned after its internal social relations. Not only psychological balance but a reorganization of the social structure is required.

Homicide and suicide

The first systematic theory of suicide, proposed by Durkheim (1951), had little to say about homicide, and anthropological theories concerning both have since been few (Bohannan). Durkheim suggested that the greater the integration of social groups, the lower the suicide rate, and vice versa. Social institutions are most integrated when they command the greatest loyalty. Persons lying outside the major institutions, or unable to subscribe to their values and demands, are most likely to resort to suicide. Durkheim termed such suicide "anomic." In areas of social life that remain uninstitutionalized (a measure of the "openness" of a society), where pressures to perform in certain ways are not simply inadequate, as in anomic suicide, but nonexistent as social consensuses, resort to suicide is termed by Durkheim "egoistic" and "is a concomitant of a type of social structure, not the result of social pathology." A third form of suicide, "altruistic," occurs in extremely highly integrated institutions in which the individual's adherence to cultural values overrides valuation of his own life. Like egoistic suicide, altruistic suicide is not a criterion of social malfunctioning. A fourth type, vengeance or "samsonic" suicide, which occurs when a person takes his life as a form of revenge against others, was suggested by Jeffreys.

Examples of all four types appear in ethnographic literature. Bohannan suggests that the Durkheim model of suicide could well be applied, with modifications, to homicide. Either action involves the taking of human life and is therefore threatening to any society. Indeed, suicide may be perceived as more threatening, since it symbolizes a person's decision that life in his social groups is not worth living. Suicide frequently stimulates intense emotional responses of alarm, fear, anger, outrage, and even revenge (upon the suicide's property, kin, etc.), as well as sorrow and sympathy.

"Homicide within the society is, under one set of conditions or another, legally prohibited everywhere. Likewise, it is universally recognized as a privilege-right under certain circumstances, either in self-defense against illegal, extreme assault (including sorcery) or as a sanction for certain illegal acts" (Hoebel, p. 286). Since the social subordination of women is nearly universal, it has generally been considered justifiable for husbands in preindustrial societies to kill adulterous wives. In societies where legal institutions are rudimentary, homicide may be used by strong men to achieve power, wives, property, and honor, or to avenge some real or imagined offense. Blood revenge is expected in most Eskimo tribes, except the Copper, Iglulik, and East Greenlanders (ibid., pp. 85–99), though a feuding chain reaction is avoided through certain moral substitutes: institutionalized wrestling, butting, or boxing, frequently as accompaniment to a song duel. Social catharsis may be achieved through vicarious combat. Justice may not be served, since the offender or his representative may vanquish the offended. The victor wins admiration, the loser loses rank. A single homicide may result in a feud, but a second murder by the same person transforms him into a public enemy who is then executed by a public-spirited man with community consent, thus providing another check on excessive slaughter.

Categories of homicide vary with a society's values and social organization. The Tiv of Nigeria practice "ritual" killing (to obtain anatomical items for fetishes), murder of thieves, infanticide, "accidental" killings (usually from poisoned arrows in communal hunts), killings involving sexual jealousy or adultery, and slayings because of illness believed to be caused by witches or sorcerers (Bohannan). Among the Gisu of Uganda, "*all* deaths were considered murder in that responsibility for them was laid at someone's door." However, not all such accusations were followed by revenge since frequently agreement could not be reached on the identification of the culprit (La Fontaine, pp. 94–129).

Deaths of murderer and victim in most cultures are treated somewhat differently. Even in justifiable homicide, frequently the killer must undergo rites of purification since the shedding of blood is a ritually dangerous condition. The victim may also undergo lustration, but in addition the corpse may be disposed of more quickly, perfunctorily, and with less ceremony. Among the LoDagaa (Goody, pp. 112 ff.) only other murderers may handle the corpse. The killer's bow, hung out of reach of children, is broken upon his death. Special obsequies are performed by the eldest killers. Intraclan homicides are also regarded differently from interclan ones. Anyone who has been in contact with a dead or dying killer, especially his wife, must take a special medicine to ward off harmful mystical effects. Just as all societies make a distinction among classes of persons who may be killed, so do they also with respect to categories of non-human animals. Domestic animals are differentiated from undomesticated ones, nontotemic from totemic ones, and animals considered to be in some way connected with evil are contrasted with those considered harmless, as permissible victims (ibid., pp. 116–121).

While homicides in most societies frequently occur between related or acquainted persons, *permissible* homicide generally (though not invariably) seems to coincide roughly with the degree of social and geographical distance—and therefore of difference—between killer and killed. Under conditions of deep-going political and economic change homicide may become a "way of life." In the Mayan Indian township of Teklum frequent recourse to homicide occurs under conditions of sharpened economic competition, changed political conditions (power shifting from indigenous leaders to town president), loss of leadership and esteem by curers (becoming increasingly competitive, losing control over recruitment to the role and respect for their power to vanquish witchcraft), and increased emotional insecurity due to loss of faith in the protective power of ancestral spirits and their earthly mediums (the curers). Traditional social control mechanisms operating through the curers, local officials, and others that served to limit effects of witchcraft and resort to murder to settle disputes and conflicts are critically weakened, and homicide and witchcraft accusations have increased, even though both are outlawed by national Mexican law (Nash).

The relationship between suicide and homicide is often close and complex. Among the Maria aborigines of India similar circumstances provoke homicide in one personality and suicide in another. Disputes over possession of dancing equipment lead one man to murder his betrothed, while another who has his equipment stolen kills himself rather than the thief. One person insulted by a kinsman reacts by killing himself, another by killing the offender. Some persons kill the sorcerer they believe has afflicted them, others take their own lives to break the spell. Both homicide and suicide have a high incidence, and most homicides are against fellow tribesmen, not strangers. Most murderers are men, but the sex ratio of suicides is nearly one to one (Elwin).

Some preindustrial peoples may become preoccupied with actual or threatened suicide, e.g., the Mohave Indians of California, who rarely commit murder. The Mohave myth of the origin of death is at the same time the myth of the origin of suicide. The Mohave define a broad variety of events as suicides, some actual, others symbolic, and all are bound up with Mohave social structure, religion, and mythology: (1) stillbirths, (2) death of an infant after abrupt weaning to nurse an anticipated sibling, (3) death of one or both twins in childbirth or at any time prior to marriage, (4) symbolic suicide involving incestuous marriages between kinspersons, (5) several types of vicarious suicide, (6) funeral suicides, (7) actual suicide (Devereux, 1961, pp. 286–484). The Gisu believe suicide to be evil because it is caused by conflict between men or between men and ancestors. Suicide is contagious, so a nonrelative removes the body for pay and the suicide's evil spirit is appeased through sacrifice. Because it is usually ill feeling among people that causes suicide, though impelled by the ancestors, those closest to the dead person are blamed, and so a suicide must be prevented if possible. The threat of suicide may be used to extort concessions from relatives (La Fontaine).

Various Eskimo tribes also have recourse to suicide because of old age and a feeling that the individual's social usefulness is ended, to spare families the burden of caring for an unproductive member, to terminate a condition of serious illness, from remorse or unrequited love, in the face of starvation, and for other reasons. Generally Eskimo suicide is nonritualized and quite individualistic and variable; but among the St. Lawrence Island Eskimo, patterns are more elaborate, involve more people, and provide notice to family and kin with opportunity to prevent the act. A close relative is usually asked to act as executioner, but if he refuses the individual has to take his own life or ritually appease the spirits who already anticipate his end (Leighton and Hughes).

Balikci believes Netsilik suicide is best explained as Durkheimian "egoistic" (I would say "anomic"), resulting from the isolation and alienation of individuals attempting to deal with contradictions between integrative forces of this culture (extended kin ties, cooperation, dyadic relations) and disintegrative historical and social forces (restriction of kin alignments, jealousies and hatreds born of tight family ties but weak communal ones, unpredictably harsh spiritual beings, lack of relatedness to larger social groupings).

In the period before European contact the Iroquois and Huron Indians held an ambivalent attitude toward suicide: general hostility toward suicide as a cowardly and vengeful act that would exclude the soul from a place in the land of the dead, especially toward males who killed themselves to avoid torture after capture or responsibility for misdeeds, coupled with approval of females who committed suicide out of anger, shame, and revenge against mistreatment or betrayal by spouses or lovers. After conquest and conversion the Iroquois-Huron attitude crystallized into solid opposition toward suicide as a sin, in conformity with Christian dogma. Throughout the centuries after contact "the same motives, the same methods, and similar beliefs concerning the fate of souls prevail," so that enduring suicide patterns are a diagnostic of cultural stability for this long period (Fenton).

Cannibalism and war

Some forms of killing may not always be defined as such, in particular cannibalism and war. Cannibalistic killing may spring from a number of motives both aggressive and affectionate, but it has been widespread in human history and prehistory, and under extreme conditions it has been sanctioned in Western society. Whether cannibalism can be perceived as a stage in cultural evolution, as Sagan suggests, is difficult to say, but he nevertheless concludes that cannibalism is not correlated with level of cultural or technological complexity, and in all places where it was socially and ritually approved, there were always many individuals who were repulsed and abstained.

Vayda (p. 468) notes that "war among nonliterate peoples ranges from the hit-and-run raids and ambuscades of warriors from autonomous local communities of primitive horticulturalists or hunters and gatherers to the military campaigns carried out by the armies of such state-organized societies as the old African kingdoms and the Inca empire of the New World." Warfare, of whatever degree, though it causes death, destruction, and suffering, serves a number of important regulating functions: psychological (reduction of anxiety and aggressiveness), political (settling disputes, rebelling against authority, overcoming tyranny, regulating relations with other groups), economic (control of trade routes, distribution of goods and resources, territorial expansion, taking captives as slaves), religious (taking of captives for sacrifice or ritual cannibalism), and demographic (reduction of population pressure, room for population expansion) (ibid., pp. 468–472). In war killing is morally sanctioned, and death as a warrior is culturally honored, at times even sought.

Not all anthropologists agree with Vayda's broad conception of "primitive" warfare. Some doubt seriously that the patterned feuding, blood revenge, and raids for booty, women, slaves, or scalps in small preindustrial societies represent warfare at all so much as culturally prescribed ways of settling conflicts and dissipating tensions with relatively minimal violence. Such "wars" seem mainly symbolic in character, and, with some exceptions, result in little loss of life. Wars require, these scholars assert, a high level of social, economic, and military development and a level of technology not reached by preindustrial cultures. (For arguments on both sides see Bramson and Goethals; Fried, Harris, and Murphy.) However, the question of the moral and ethical valuation by the participants themselves of such culturally patterned infliction of death on fellow humans is known incidentally and superficially. What does seem universal is that for large-scale killing of other humans their group must be defined by the killers as strange, foreign, evil, dangerous, and/or less than human.

Feticide, infanticide, and the death of children

Most human societies have discovered methods of aborting unwanted pregnancies so that feticide is very nearly universal (Devereux, 1955). Frequently the unwanted offspring is a consequence of a casual or illegitimate procreative encounter, and in the latter case the mother may be severely punished or even killed. Penalties seem less frequent and less severe for the biological father, but where children born out of wedlock are condemned by society they may receive ridicule, physical punishment, and even death should they be permitted to come to term. On the other hand, some societies may welcome and adopt such children, and, as in rural Puerto Rico (Landy), they may grow to adulthood with as much love and care as children born of legal unions. Motives for abortions vary widely among cultures and include marital discord, adultery, jealousy among co-wives, religious and magical demands or omens, survival of older siblings in times of scarcity, rape, incest (as culturally defined), and what Devereux terms "unconscious" factors. In most preindustrial societies in cases of complicated births the decision usually is to destroy the fetus in order to save the mother's life.

Infanticide, the voluntary killing of a neonate by its parents or with their consent, should be distinguished from other forms of child death, including child sacrifice (Hocart, "Infanticide"). Infanticide, so defined, is found among many Eskimo tribes but may be absent in some. A group among whom infanticide has been reported of high frequency is the Netsilik (Balikci; Freeman; Hoebel). Most frequently it is baby girls who are killed, but paradoxically by the time of adulthood the sex ratio becomes balanced again due to the high casualty rate among male hunters in the harsh environment. Balikci (pp. 147–162) concludes that, while infanticide was ecologically adaptive by reducing population size, it was socially maladaptive and "led to an imbalance in the sex ratio, an effort to keep marriageable girls within the kinship unit, and a consequent division of the community into many small, mutually suspicious, unrelated kinship groups." However, Freeman contends that the social motive of female infanticide among the Netsilik is not simply keeping down population numbers in an environment that will not sustain them but the "assertion of male dominance within the household." An adaptive advantage is the preservation of more older persons, for not only are they more productive than infants, but their accumulated knowledge increases information storage and retrieval for the group, thereby improving both its ability to control the environment and its demographic stability (Freeman).

Infanticide not only occurs in harsh environments among hunter-gatherer cultures but has been reported from many parts of the world, including the indigenous societies of Africa and Oceania and the upper classes of China, India, Greece, and Rome (Hocart, "Infanticide") for a variety of social and cultural reasons, only some of which are related to ecology or demography. One or both twins may be destroyed when they are deemed harbingers of evil, and deformed or "weak" infants may be killed in many societies either because they are doomed by religious or social dogma to a life of tragedy or herald misfortune for their families, and/or because their

economic liability is too heavy to bear for groups living on the edge of bare subsistence (ibid.).

Some cases of reported infanticide in fact seem to involve children far past infancy and ought to be more accurately classed as child murder. The death of a child from whatever cause is not regarded in many preindustrial or peasant societies with the same seriousness as the death of an adult. In rural Puerto Rico, as in many Latin countries, a small child is considered to lack full intellectual and moral capacity, to be not yet a complete person, and to exist in a state of moral purity, unblemished by the sins and corruption of adult life (Landy). The death of a child is viewed not as a calamity but as a guarantee that the child's soul will migrate directly to the company of angels, and mortuary rites are light-hearted and joyful. Among the Arapaho Indians, however, death of a child was regarded as seriously as that of an adult (Hilger). The Arapaho believed that all persons, including children, continued to live in the land of spirits after death, the only exceptions being suicides or persons who had grievously erred morally and did not become spiritually repentant. The dead child was treated as an adult and buried in the same manner, with parents slashing themselves in grief.

In a society with a high infant death rate, as the LoDagaa, children are wanted and highly valued. Paradoxically, however, when a child dies unweaned, or before the advent of a following sibling, he is assumed not to have achieved a social personality and to be not yet fully human; indeed, in this state the child represents a mystical threat to the living, a still wild being who has ventured on earth to plague its parents. Deaths of such children are greeted with consternation, and in order that they may not be reincarnated to return again and again to earth to haunt the parents they are buried quickly with scant ritual. However, after weaning a son's death is mourned with great display (Goody).

Senilicide and death of the aged

Because of the hazards of life in many subsistence economies, relatively few persons reach old age. Infant and child mortality are high, and life in early or middle adulthood may be ended suddenly and agonizingly by starvation, migration, accident, environmental cataclysm, disease, enemy assault, or sorcery. Death is a frequent and familiar guest. Where elders are respected they may also be feared for their greater knowledge and envied for superior power and privilege. Children may have more to gain than to lose by the death of a parent. The old may be seen as having lived their full measure, and as they become weakened by disease and the infirmities of age they constitute economic handicaps for younger members. In myth as in actuality attitudes toward the aged and toward their final departure carry negative as well as positive emotional valence. Still, the desire to reach mature years persists in all cultures and is reflected in beliefs and lore regarding rejuvenation; and in prayers and rituals, potions taken, counsel sought, and behavioral techniques designed to attain longevity and a place in the afterworld. The Hopi Indians pray frequently toward this goal and believe that the person who works hard and cooperatively with others, obeys his parents, and shuns conflict, trouble, and worry will achieve a ripe age (Kennard). Each individual anticipates a long term of years, but this may be interrupted by misfortune or failing to live according to Hopi ethics. When a person becomes sick and does not recover, his death is laid to his lack of strength or will to live, not to failure of the cure. Old people are expected to die soon, become increasingly disengaged from the social and religious structure, and are treated with indifference; if they persist too long they may be blamed for putting off their own demise.

The Murngin of Australia, on the other hand, venerate age. The society is rigidly age-graded with complex ceremonials marking each passage from one status to another. Women remain in a profane status throughout much of the life cycle, but men acquire degrees of sacredness, and old men are especially inviolable. They are the repositories of tribal lore and wisdom, their counsel respectfully sought, their authority dominating group decisions. The death of an older male is particularly poignant for the band as a whole, and especially his sons. Male elders stand at the apex of family, kinship, and social structure; they embody the cultural ideal and model for socialization of young males (Warner).

Older males in LoDagaa culture maintain dominance and power by clinging to wealth and social positions until they die, ensuring that their sons will work and provide for them. The death of an older man, though celebrated with full ceremony, is not a time of deep sorrow to his sons, who are waiting impatiently to inherit rights in property, women, and offices. A grandparent is provided a special burial in his own courtyard, "for it is he who has successfully established that home by producing two generations of descendants" (Goody). Since a grandparent has had a long and full existence, permanent place in the lineal social structure, and certainty of ancestorhood, "very soon after the beginning of his funeral, his joking partners begin to clown and the young women to dance, and the whole funeral is suffused with a spirit of enjoyment, rather than mourning" (ibid.).

Even societies that revere old age may desire the elderly to get on with the business of dying, so that paradoxically they may be treated with neglect and sometimes cruelty. When a nomadic group is forced to migrate, the elderly and sick are often abandoned, at times almost indifferently, but usually with some show of solicitude. Since these eventualities are traditional and anticipated by all, they are not evaded but usually accepted with equanimity by the concerned participants. Missionaries attempting to save such old persons from death frequently reported that they declined aid and confirmed their inability to be of service and the justice of their fate. Old age and infirmity may become a time of pain and travail. Simmons found that, while advanced age is a time of misery in many societies, actual abandonment is not as widespread, occurring most frequently among nomadic collectors and hunters, less so among herders and fishermen, and least in agricultural societies. Nevertheless, in societies where the elderly are honored and respected, they are more likely to prepare for their own death in a dignified, calm manner, surrounded by families and friends, treated with affection and admiration, and afforded special privileges and favors (Simmons, pp. 241–244).

What are the ecological, social, and cultural concomitants of senilicide? It seems to be positively correlated with severity of climate, residential impermanence, and irregular food supply. With increasing residential stability and food supply, real property rights, centralized authority, and codified laws, the practice tends to occur infrequently or not at all. Sympathy and respect are greatest in those cultures where the necessity seems obvious for group survival and where the elderly volunteer to die with grace and equanimity (Simmons, pp. 239–241).

Hoebel (pp. 76 ff.) attributes patterned slaughter of the elderly mainly to environmental vicissitudes and the need for group survival, but Balikci says that the reasons for senilicide (whether through the Janus-headed alternatives of homicide or suicide) are estrangement of the aged from their social networks and desperation over a now unproductive life that no longer seems worth preservation.

Implications for bioethics

This brief article points up the need to consider the bioethics of death in cross-cultural perspective. Not only are there often striking differences in the ethics of the termination of life, voluntary or involuntary, among the cultures of the world, but anthropology makes it obvious that these differences in values and practices surrounding death in any society can be understood only within the context of that society's ecological and demographic situation, social system, and cultural beliefs. Killing the sick, the infirm, and the aged may be not only an act of mercy but an economic necessity if the group is to survive, although, as I have suggested, a consistent food supply makes this form of euthanasia less probable. Infanticide poses painful ethical problems in industrialized societies but may be imperative for groups living on the edge of subsistence. As I have shown, homicide and suicide become socially sanctioned under certain cultural-historical conditions.

An anthropological view of the bioethics of death suggests that ethical judgments of the attitudes and actions regarding death in other societies require ethnographic and historical knowledge, and even so should be made with extreme caution. It also suggests that such knowledge provides a profound and essential framework in which to cope with the ethical dilemmas that confront our own society.

DAVID LANDY

[*For concepts of death in other societies and cultures, see the other articles in this entry:* EASTERN THOUGHT, WESTERN PHILOSOPHICAL THOUGHT, WESTERN RELIGIOUS THOUGHT, *and* DEATH IN THE WESTERN WORLD. *For further discussion of topics mentioned in this article, see the entries:* AGING AND THE AGED, *articles on* SOCIAL IMPLICATIONS OF AGING *and* ETHICAL IMPLICATIONS IN AGING; *and* SUICIDE. *For discussion of related ideas, see the entries* DEATH AND DYING: EUTHANASIA AND SUSTAINING LIFE, *article on* ETHICAL VIEWS; INFANTS, *articles on* ETHICAL PERSPECTIVES ON THE CARE OF INFANTS, *and* INFANTICIDE: A PHILOSOPHICAL PERSPECTIVE. *See also:* ABORTION; DEATH, ATTITUDES TOWARD; *and* LIFE.]

BIBLIOGRAPHY

BALIKCI, ASEN. *The Netsilik Eskimo.* Garden City, N.Y.: Natural History Press, 1970. Recent study of well-known Eskimo tribe, with thoughtful material on death, homicide, suicide, infanticide, and senilicide.

BENDANN, EFFIE. *Death Customs: An Analytical Study of Burial Rites.* The History of Civilization. Edited by C. K. Ogden. New York: Alfred A. Knopf; London: Kegan Paul, Trench, Trubner & Co., 1930. London: Dawsons of Pall Mall, 1969. Ann Arbor, Mich.: Gryphon Books, 1971. Useful attempt to explain cross-cultural similarities and differences in beliefs and practices regarding death.

BOHANNAN, PAUL, ed. *African Homicide and Suicide.* Princeton: Princeton University Press, 1960. Specifically referred to in this article are Bohannan's "Introduction," "Theories of Homicide and Suicide," and "Homicide Among the Tiv of Central Nigeria." Pioneering anthology of research among tribal groups in Nigeria, Uganda, Kenya, and Tanzania.

BRAMSON, LEON, and GOETHALS, GEORGE W., eds. *War: Studies from Psychology, Sociology, Anthropology.* New York: Basic Books, 1964. Relevant pieces by W. G. Sumner, R. E. Park, B. Malinowski, M. Mead, and J. Schneider.

DEVEREUX, GEORGE. *Mohave Ethnopsychiatry and Suicide: The Psychiatric Knowledge and the Psychic Disturbances of an Indian Tribe.* Bureau of American Ethnology Bulletin no. 175. Washington: Government Printing Office, 1961. Includes multifaceted analysis and rich documentation with case studies of suicide.

——. *A Study of Abortion in Primitive Societies: A Typological, Distributional, and Dynamic Analysis of the Prevention of Birth in 400 Preindustrial Societies.* New York: Julian Press, 1955. Unique, but non-statistical, cross-cultural study of 400 preindustrial societies.

DURKHEIM, EMILE. *The Elementary Forms of the Religious Life: A Study in Religious Sociology.* Translated by Joseph Ward Swain. London: George Allen & Unwin, 1950. New York: Free Press, 1965. Classic monograph purporting to show origins of religious systems reflected in those of Australian Aborigines.

——. *Suicide: A Study in Sociology.* Translated by John A. Spaulding and George Simpson. Glencoe, Ill.: Free Press, 1897, 1930, 1951. Using his own methodological principles, Durkheim analyzes suicide trends and sociological concomitants, and proposes a theory of suicide.

ELWIN, VERRIER. *Maria Murder and Suicide.* Foreword by W. V. Grigson. London: Oxford University Press, 1943, 1950. Rich data, generally well organized, occasionally marred by anachronistic comments on tribal society.

FENTON, WILLIAM NELSON. "Iroquois Suicide: A Study in the Stability of a Culture Pattern." *Anthropological Papers.* Bureau of American Ethnology Bulletin no. 128. Washington: Government Printing Office, 1941, pp. 79–137.

FRAZER, JAMES GEORGE. *The Belief in Immortality and the Worship of the Dead.* 3 vols. London: Macmillan & Co., 1913–1922. Vol. 1 contains Frazer's major ideas on the topic.

——. *Man, God, and Immortality: Thoughts on Human Progress.* New York: Macmillan Co., 1927. Excerpts from Frazer's huge corpus, with much related to death and immortality in preindustrial societies.

FREEMAN, MILTON M. R. "A Social and Ecologic Analysis of Systemic Female Infanticide among the Netsilik Eskimo." *American Anthropologist* 73 (1971): 1011–1018.

FRIED, MORTON; HARRIS, MARVIN; and MURPHY, ROBERT,

eds. *War: The Anthropology of Armed Conflict and Aggression.* Garden City, N.Y.: Natural History Press, 1968. An interesting symposium of anthropologists' views.

GOODY, JOHN RANKINE. *Death, Property and the Ancestors: A Study of the Mortuary Customs of the LoDagaa of West Africa.* Stanford: Stanford University Press; London: Tavistock Publications, 1962. Undoubtedly the finest anthropological analysis and documentation of social-cultural processes and interrelations between death and society.

HARTLAND, EDWIN SIDNEY. "Death and Disposal of the Dead." *Encyclopedia of Religion and Ethics.* 12 vols. Edited by James Hastings. New York: Charles Scribners' Sons, 1912, vol. 4, pp. 411–444. Useful anthropological analysis despite anachronisms.

HERTZ, ROBERT. *Death and the Right Hand.* Translated by Rodney and Claudia Needham. Introduction by E. E. Evans-Pritchard. Glencoe, Ill.: Free Press, 1960. Translated in part from "La Représentation collective de la mort." *Mélange de sociologie religieuse et folklore.* Paris: F. Alcan, 1928. Original appearance. *Contribution à une étude sur la réprésentation collective de la mort.* Paris: F. Alcan, n.d. Also, *L'Annee sociologique,* 1907, and *Revue philosophique,* 1909. Paris: Press Universitaires de France. Seminal essay on cultural and social forces underlying multiple funeral practices.

HILGER, M. INEZ. *Arapaho Child Life and Its Cultural Background.* Bureau of American Ethnology Bulletin no. 148. Washington: Government Printing Office, 1952. Includes beliefs and practices concerning death of children.

HOCART, ARTHUR MAURICE. "Death Customs." *Encyclopaedia of the Social Sciences.* Edited by Dewin R. A. Seligman and Alvin Johnson. New York: Macmillan Co., 1937, vol. 5, pp. 21–27.

———. "Infanticide." *Encyclopaedia of the Social Sciences.* Edited by Dewin R. A. Seligman and Alvin Johnson. New York: Macmillan Co., 1937, vol. 8, pp. 27–28.

HOEBEL, EDWARD ADAMSON. *The Law of Primitive Man: A Study in Comparative Legal Dynamics.* Harvard University Press, 1954; New York: Atheneum Publishers, 1973. Contains useful material on cultural-legal implications of homicide, suicide, etc.

"Infanticide." *The New Encyclopaedia Britannica: Micropaedia.* Chicago: Encyclopaedia Britannica, 1974, vol. 5, p. 350.

JEFFREYS, M. D. W. "Samsonic Suicides: Or Suicides of Revenge among Africans." *The Sociology of Suicide: A Selection of Readings.* Edited by Anthony Giddens. London: Frank Cass & Co., 1971, chap. 13, pp. 185–196.

KENNARD, EDWARD A. "Hopi Reactions to Death." *American Anthropologist* 39 (1937): 491–496.

LA FONTAINE, JEAN. "Homicide and Suicide among the Gisu." Bohannan, *African Homicide and Suicide,* pp. 94–129.

LANDY, DAVID. *Tropical Childhood: Cultural Transmission and Learning in a Puerto Rican Village.* Chapel Hill: University of North Carolina Press, 1959. New York: Harper & Row, 1965.

LEIGHTON, ALEXANDER H., and HUGHES, CHARLES C. "Notes on Eskimo Suicide." *The Sociology of Suicide: A Selection of Readings.* Edited by Anthony Giddens. London: Frank Cass & Co., 1971, chap. 13, pp. 158–169.

MALINOWSKI, BRONISLAW. *Magic, Science and Religion and Other Essays.* Introduction by Robert Redfield. Glencoe, Ill.: Free Press, 1948. Garden City, N.Y.: Doubleday & Co., 1954. In addition to title essay, also "Myth in Primitive Psychology" and "Baloma: the Spirits of the Dead," all apposite to the anthropology of death.

NASH, JUNE. "Death as a Way of Life: The Increasing Resort to Homicide in a Maya Indian Community." *American Anthropologist* 69 (1967): 455–470.

SAGAN, ELI. *Cannibalism: Human Aggression and Cultural Form.* Foreword by Robert N. Bellah. New York: Harper & Row, 1974. Cannibalism seen as step in cultural evolution.

SIMMONS, LEO WILLIAM. *The Role of the Aged in Primitive Society.* New Haven: Yale University Press, 1945. New York: Archon Books, 1970. Excellent cross-cultural study using Human Relations Area Files.

TURNER, VICTOR WITTER. *The Ritual Process: Structure and Anti-Structure.* Chicago: Aldine Publishing Co.; London: Routledge & K. Paul, 1969. Turner's ideas on symbolism in ritual with a focus on death and life rituals and development of Van Gennep's notion of liminality in transition states.

TYLOR, EDWARD BURNETT. *Religion in Primitive Culture.* Introduction by Paul Radin. Library of Religion and Culture. New York: Harper & Brothers, 1968. Original appearance. *Primitive Culture: Researches into the Development of Mythology, Philosophy, Religion, Art and Custom.* London: J. Murray, 1871. Reprint. New York: Gordon Press, 1974, vol. 1, chap. 11, pp. 377–453; vol. 2, chaps. 12–19, pp. 1–410. Deals mainly with Tylor's theory of animism as foundation of "primitive" religion with much on attitudes and beliefs regarding death.

VAN GENNEP, ARNOLD. *The Rites of Passage.* Translated by Monika B. Vizedom and Gabrielle L. Caffee. Introduction by Solon T. Kimball. Chicago: University of Chicago Press, 1960. Original appearance. *Les Rites de passage: Étude systematique des rites de la porte et du seuil, de l'hospitalité, de l'adoption, de la grossesse et de l'accouchement, de la naissance, de l'enfance, de la puberté, de l'initation, de l'ordination, du couronnement des fiançailles et du mariage, des funérailles, des saisons, etc.* Paris: É. Nourry, 1909. Classic essay on social and cultural functions of ceremonies of transition, including birth and death.

VAYDA, ANDREW P. "Primitive Warfare." *International Encyclopedia of the Social Sciences.* Edited by David L. Sills. New York: Macmillan Co., Free Press, 1968, vol. 16, pp. 468–472. Concentrates on functions of war, assumes it to be universal.

WARNER, WILLIAM LLOYD. *A Black Civilization: A Study of an Australian Tribe.* New York: Harper & Brothers, 1937. Rev. ed. 1958. Richly documented ethnography of the Murngin tribe, focus on religion and social structure, much on death.

II

EASTERN THOUGHT

The enigmas of dying and death have been a serious preoccupation in the philosophical and religious thought of all peoples, not least the peoples of the "East." In each of the great traditions men have sought to understand and develop appropriate responses to the reality of death as it impinges on the life of each individual human being. They have grappled with the problem of communal continuity in the face of the inevitable intrusions of death. And they have sought to identify the place and function of death in the cosmic order, however that order may be defined.

In Eastern thought, as in human thought more generally, a number of themes emerge from man's encounter with death which cut across all geographical, cultural, and social divisions. So, too, particular kinds of groups in widely different contexts share common understandings of death and its meaning; for example, some emphases are common to the warrior and ascetic elements in the poulation all across classical Asia, whereas other emphases are broadly disseminated among peasant communities. However, for our purposes it will be most appropriate to treat the subject matter in terms of three basic historical traditions—the Sinitic tradition including both its Confucian and Taoist strands, the Vedic–Hindu tradition, and the Buddhist tradition.

Death and Sinitic thought

Many commentators on Chinese thought have noted its distinctively "this-worldly" cast and the emphasis it has traditionally placed on the specifically human mode of existence. Thus it is not surprising that any premature or "unnatural" death was considered to be an aberration; according to the tradition such a death not only prevented the natural fulfillment of the individual involved but also, in so doing, produced an evil, demonic spirit, which posed a continuing threat to the peace and well-being of the community. From the time of the early Chou dynasty (ca. 1050–222 B.C.) we have clear evidence that the avoidance of such a premature death and the attainment of longevity were preeminent concerns. In the supplicatory prayers that have been preserved from this very ancient time, longevity is the boon which is sought after more commonly and more ardently than any other. Moreover, in spite of a deeply embedded popular and to some extent Confucian tendency toward fatalism concerning the timing of death (and many other things as well), the goal of longevity remained a primary focus of attention throughout all of the later periods of Chinese history. For example, in certain of the classical funerary customs of China strongly emotional expressions of mourning were considered to be completely appropriate in cases where the deceased was a younger person; on the other hand,

the appropriate response at the funeral of an individual who had attained the age of seventy or more was thought to be celebration of a life that had been lived to the full.

Among some segments of the population in China this continuing concern with the postponement of death and its effects was pushed much farther. In the period of the Shang dynasty (ca. 1500–1050 B.C.) burial remains clearly indicate the presence of the conviction that a thoroughly "this-worldly" mode of existence continued beyond the grave, at least for the elite who could follow the appropriate burial prescriptions. During the period of the early Chou dynasty a rather different extension of the conceptions concerning longevity is reflected in prayers in which men sought to escape from the ravages of old age and to postpone their death into an indefinite future. Moreover the emphases on "the preservation of the body," "long life," and "no death," which were established in these very early times, persisted as important strands throughout the subsequent history of traditional Chinese thought.

Still another dimension of the Chinese concern to avoid or to overcome the implications of death appears in specifically Taoist circles around the fourth century B.C. with the emergence (or possibly the intrusion from India) of the belief that a new, truly immortal mode of being could be attained. At first the attainment of such a radically new mode of being was associated exclusively with certain reclusive sages (*hsien*) who retired to mountain areas, practiced a highly disciplined life, and learned to live in harmony with the processes of nature and ultimately to control them. However, in subsequent centuries the belief that this new, deathless mode of being could be acquired through the transmutation of one's ordinary physical body into an indestructible subtle body became a goal avidly sought by many members of the elite, including a number of important emperors. Thus during the period of the Han dynasty (206 B.C.–A.D. 220) a widespread cult of immortality came into being in which various esoteric sacrifices, drugs, purifying diets, and the like were utilized in an effort to achieve the desired result. But it should also be noted that, as a part of this same process of popularization, the goal of true immortality soon became inextricably fused with the earlier and still persisting concern for the extension of more normal patterns of worldly and social existence.

Despite the strong emphasis the Chinese have

traditionally placed on avoiding or overcoming the implications of death, and despite the reluctance of many of the literati (including, most notably, Confucius himself) to speculate in any detail on the fate of the dead, most Chinese thought has recognized death as the inevitable dénouement of human life and has understood it as a transformation into new though still limited modes of existence. Generally speaking, in classical Chinese thought death has been viewed as the dispersion of the complex of souls (often two—one associated with the yang [male] principle and one with the yin [female] principle—but in some cases more) and body that constitutes each individual human being. Moreover the Chinese have viewed this dispersion as a process through which men are transferred into the role of an ancestor and, at the same time, enter into a postmortem existence conceived in terms of either heavenly enjoyment or the torments of hell. Certainly a man's postmortem condition as an ancestor, along with the resulting extension of the system of family reciprocity and filial piety which have traditionally been at the very core of practically every aspect of Chinese culture from the period of the earliest dynasties up to the twentieth century, represents the more ancient, the more pervasive, and the more comforting of the two conceptions. Nevertheless, it is also true that at least during the long medieval period of Chinese history large segments of the Chinese population were convinced that their death would also result in a postmortem existence in which their virtues and piety would be rewarded or (much more likely) their various sins and transgressions would be punished.

Though, as we have already suggested, most traditional Chinese believed that the souls of the individual maintained an existence after death, many of the more profound thinkers realized that the phenomena of continuation, even if it were true, constituted no final solution to the problem of death. Rather, they recognized that the various souls, like the body with which they had been associated, must sooner or later return to the natural cosmic source from which they had come. As one might expect given the basically positive attitude the Chinese have always taken toward what they have conceived to be the natural cosmic source of life (the Tao), those thinkers who reached such a conclusion seldom evaluated this final dissolution in a totally negative or morbid way. But, on the other hand, there were clearly significant differences

in the attitudes taken by various sages and traditions. For the most part the Confucians did not place great emphasis on the process, and when they did consider it they exhibited an attitude characterized more by equanimity than by enthusiasm. On the other hand, in the thought of many of the more philosophically oriented Taoists an appreciation of the process of the individual's return to the Tao was cultivated as the essence of wisdom, and its full realization was equated with the attainment of salvation.

Vedic–Hindu conceptions of death

In India, as in China, any serious discussion of traditional conceptions related to death must take account of the primacy that has consistently been given to the goal of maintaining this-worldly existence. In the Vedas, most of which were composed in the second millennium B.C. and constitute our earliest source of Indian thought, the positive value of vigorous, worldly living is strongly emphasized, and the quest for longevity through prayer and sacrifice is a predominant motif. In fact in several passages a full life of one hundred years is equated with the attainment of immortality. This same basic concern for a full life prior to death is reflected in a very different way in the later *ashrama* ideal of the orthodox Brahmanic tradition according to which each individual (at least each individual included within the true "Aryan" community constituted by the three upper castes of Hindu society) should pass through a complete cycle of adult activity in which a period of education and a period of social responsibility as a householder are followed by two periods of increasingly austere preparations for death. In addition, the mythology, ritual, and devotion of later Hinduism clearly reflect the concern for longevity; for example, in the mythic tradition there are numerous stories that give expression to the belief that old age and death can be averted and youth magically restored through various means including living in a particular holy place, the aid of a saint, an exchange of life with another mortal, or the hearing of an especially sacred text. Nevertheless, in spite of the hope that longevity might be achieved and even that the restoration of youth might occasionally be possible, most Indians have adopted a more fatalistic attitude toward the arbitrariness and unpredictability of death, often associating it with retribution for their own deeds in previous existences (karma). Moreover, throughout the long history of Indian philosophy and religion, conceptions concerning man's destiny after death have played a very significant role.

Already in Vedic times the belief that death involves a transition through which the individual takes on the role of an ancestor was firmly established; and in the later Brahmanic–Hindu tradition this belief came to be expressed in a highly elaborated series of funerary ceremonies through which the success of the transition is assured and the proper reciprocal relationships between the ancestral community and the continuing family unit are established. In addition to this ancestral role, the fate of the deceased has been perceived in a variety of other ways as well. In the earlier Vedas the dominant view seems to have been that, for those who act in accordance with the universal cosmic law (*rta*), death will constitute a transition into a realm not essentially different from the land of the living—a realm in which the individual's bodily existence, social relationships, and worldly enjoyments will be restored. In the period of the Brahmanas (commentaries on the Vedas dated ca. 950–700 B.C.) the conviction developed that through his ritual action a man could actually create for himself the postmortem "body" or "world," which he would inhabit after his death. Beyond this, some of the more profound priestly writers speculated that the various mystical correlations made in the ritual between the elements of a sacrificer's being and the elements of the sacrificial altar which he built, and between those same elements of the sacrificial altar and various aspects of the cosmos, assured the sacrificer that the "immortal" aspects of his being (his eye, his breath, etc.) would survive the decay of the gross elements of his body and rejoin the cosmic elements to which they corresponded (the sun, wind, etc.). In the context of Hinduism proper, beliefs in the possibility of a blissful postmortem existence have also been very much to the fore, but important differences from the earlier Vedic tradition are evident. For example, the great theistic sects have strongly affirmed the possibility of a heavenly afterlife, but they generally held that the attainment of such a goal is dependent not upon man's action (either moral or ritual), but rather on the grace of a preeminent deity such as Vishnu, Śiva or the Goddess. On the more popular level it has commonly been believed that those whose mind is focused on a proper thought at the moment of death will attain a heavenly rebirth; and there has been (and still is) a widespread conviction in India that a heavenly destiny is assured to anyone who dies in an appropriate holy place—notably at Benares—and especially to anyone whose ashes are purified by the sacred Ganges River.

In India, however, more somber conceptions concerning man's destiny appeared at a very early date and ultimately came to dominate much of the Hindu ethos. Even in the Vedas (especially in the fourth or Atharva Veda) there are passages affirming that death may be followed by an afterlife of suffering and torment; in the Brahmanas the possibility of a terrifying "second death" is raised; and in the much later texts of medieval Hinduism a great deal of emphasis is placed on the existence of various hells in which men suffer the results of their earthly transgressions. But it is more important to emphasize the fact that in the period which immediately followed the completion of the Brahmanas a new conception emerged in which death came to be associated with a kind of suffering that posed a more basic threat than any of the hells the Indians were able to conceive. According to this new and extremely influential conception, which came to the fore in texts known as the Upanishads (600 B.C.–?) and was later expressed in different ways in the various orthodox traditions of medieval Hindu philosophy, the core of each man's being is constituted by an indestructible soul or self (*atman*), which, through the power of ignorance and/or the desire for bodily attachment, has become entrapped in an ongoing cycle of death and rebirth. Though the structure of this cycle of transmigration is conceived in such a way that men are able to enjoy limited satisfactions (including the possibility of attaining more advantageous rebirths through proper ritual practice or moral action), existence within it is seen as devoid of any ultimate meaning and is therefore experienced as a hopeless process of indefinitely extended suffering and dying.

During the past 2,500 years, the most authoritative and esteemed sages and thinkers of classical India have viewed death in this context—that is to say, they have viewed it as *the* pervasive fact of the cosmic existence in which men are imprisoned. But these same sages and thinkers have also insisted that death, when it is viewed from a slightly different point of view, may serve as a paradigm for a truly soteriological experience of Release; it is at the point of death, they have noted, that the soul which has been dragged into the cycle of transmigration gains, for a very brief moment, a certain separation from the grosser elements of psyche and body that hold it in bondage. Thus, at this most profound level of Indian thought, death comes to serve as a prefiguration and model for various meditations and disciplines (classical yoga, devotional disciplines, tantra, etc.) through which the ties that bind man's self or soul to cosmic impermanence can be completely broken, and through which the ultimate soteriological goals of immortality and freedom can be finally and definitively attained.

Buddhist conceptions of death

Though Buddhist conceptions of death can never be truly understood apart from the Indian ethos in the last half of the first millennium B.C. within which Buddhism emerged, they are intimately bound up with a religious and philosophical perspective that cannot be interpreted simply in terms of Vedic or Hindu modes of thought. Moreover, in the process of Buddhism's establishment and development in other parts of Asia many of its specifically Indian emphases have been profoundly influenced and even transformed through their interaction with a variety of indigenous traditions.

At the more popular level, Buddhists have shared the common human concern that death be postponed as long as possible. And contrary to some stereotyped views of its strictly "otherworldly" character, Buddhism has always provided a framework within which such a goal has a limited place and has provided a variety of means for its adherents to use to achieve it. In the Buddhist perspective it was generally assumed that the deeds that one had done in one's previous lives were the primary determining factor in establishing not only the basic conditions of one's present life but also its duration (thus generating a kind of "fatalism" that has been observed in the attitudes of many Buddhist peoples); but Buddhist teaching has also affirmed that good and pious deeds done in one's present life can help not only to improve the quality of that life but also to extend its length. In addition, in practically all Buddhist traditions special forms of chanting and other "magical" practices have been developed to ward off various evil influences, including death. In the later Mahayana (Great Vehicle) phases of Buddhist history, beginning shortly after 100 B.C., proper devotion came to be recognized as an efficacious means for the attainment of many boons, including longevity; and in many esoteric Buddhist traditions, which first began to

appear about A.D. 350, longevity emerged as one of the many more mundane goals sought through the cultivation of spiritual and magical power. Perhaps the ultimate extension of this Buddhist quest for longevity was reached many centuries later in Japan, when under the influence of the esoteric Shingon school a tradition developed in which a few very determined ascetics strove to attain permanent longevity through a highly elaborate process of self-mummification.

Since very early Buddhist times the great majority of Buddhist faithful have held firmly to the belief that when death comes it leads to rebirth in one of the many heavenly realms that extend above the earth, in a favorable or unfavorable condition in the human world, or in one of the four lower worlds of suffering and woe. For a very few practitioners of the higher forms of meditation this meant rebirth in the highest heavenly realms, which corresponded to the various stages of meditational trance. But for the great majority of men the mode of rebirth was thought to be determined by the balance between a man's good and pious deeds on the one hand, and his evil or impious deeds on the other. Though great emphasis was often placed on the importance of a man's last thought before death in determining the character of his next existence, most Buddhist thinkers have been careful to make clear their view that this thought was itself the result of what the individual had believed and done during his lifetime.

Throughout Buddhist history the idea of rebirth has continued to play a crucial role, but the conceptions related to this idea have undergone a number of significant changes. At a very early point in Buddhist history the original belief that one's own good and evil deeds were the sole factor in determining the quality of one's future existence was compromised by the conception that the fate of a deceased individual might be affected by merit that had been gained through the pious deeds of a living relative and then dedicated to his benefit. Moreover, this view made an important contribution to the development of a very rich tradition of Buddhist funerary practices including various "masses" for the dead, which Chinese Buddhists developed into highly elaborate rituals. In the later, especially Mahayana, traditions devotion to a preeminent Buddha or Bodhisattva (a future Buddha who had postponed his entry into Nirvana in order to work for the salvation of all beings) replaced moral or cultic action as the dominant motif, at least as far as access to a favorable rebirth was concerned. This development was extended even farther in more recent, especially Japanese, schools of Buddhism in which the effective force in attaining a favorable rebirth has come to be seen not as the devotion itself but rather as the infinite compassion of the Buddha or Bodhisattva to whom the devotion is directed. Finally, it is important to note that in these later forms of devotional Buddhism the attainment of a paradisal rebirth in the realm of a great Buddha or Bodhisattva came to be more or less equated with the attainment of Final Release.

It is nevertheless true that most Buddhist thinkers from the time of the Buddha onward have shared the more somber attitudes toward death that characterized the views of the Upanishadic sages and the philosophers of orthodox Hinduism. That is to say, they have viewed death as a constitutive flaw that is endemic to all forms of this-worldly existence, including even those associated with the highest and most paradisal heavens. In fact, various meditational practices have been developed in order to implant this conception deeply into the consciousness of the more serious Buddhist adherents; for example, the contemplation of corpses and their decomposition has been practiced from very early Buddhist times, and contemplations that continually focus attention on the onset of one's own death have been developed by Buddhists who had close associations with the Samurai warrior tradition in Japan. What is more, Buddhists have also shared the Upanishadic and Hindu conception that death may serve as a prefiguration and model of the complete break with worldly existence which can bring Final Rest and Release (Nirvana). However, in this connection it is crucial to emphasize that, unlike other Indian and many other soteriologies, the path for the attainment of Release that the Buddhists have propounded does not depend on belief in any kind of soul or self that has suffered bondage and must regain its state of pristine purity. Quite to the contrary, it involves the conviction that any such belief is a delusion which breeds attachment and therefore results in a continuation of the ongoing cycle of rebirth, suffering, and death; or, to state the matter more positively, it is through a thoroughly appropriated insight into the truth that there is no soul or self of any kind that attachment, suffering, and death may be overcome and Release attained.

In the course of Buddhist history there have been many variations on the themes of man's bondage to death and the nature of Release. In the early tradition suffering and death are seen as the inevitable results of actions motivated by ignorance (i.e., any belief in the existence of a soul or self) and craving or attachment; the conquest of death and the attainment of Nirvana are, on the other hand, equated with the practice of an Aryan or Noble Path, which is a radically distinct mode of action motivated by wisdom (the insight into the self-less character of reality) and compassion. In the Mahayana tradition there is a significant shift in emphasis, and the basic distinction becomes primarily epistemological; through an insight into the truth that all reality is self-less and void one realizes that in the final analysis Nirvana and the cycle of transmigration (including death) are one and the same and cannot be distinguished. When this insight is fully appropriated, death is conquered and true Release is experienced. As this Mahayana perspective became established in East Asia and was gradually adapted to indigenous, particularly Taoist, modes of thought, still further changes occurred. Thus many of the most important Chinese Buddhist thinkers came to insist that the bondage of death could be finally overcome only when men awakened and recognized in themselves the Buddha-nature, which, in this new context, had come to be viewed as the true source of both individual and cosmic life. And finally, in Japan, this process of adaptation was carried to its limit in the works of Saigyo and Basho and other classical poets who attributed man's bondage to suffering and death to his rejection of the natural world. For those Japanese writers the awakening to one's own Buddha-nature and the attainment of a complete harmony with the rhythms and transformations of the natural world were two sides of exactly the same process —and, what is more, both were taken to be absolutely identical with the attainment of Release.

Conclusion

The full range of Eastern thought concerning death has by no means been exhausted in this discussion of certain aspects of the Sinitic, Vedic–Hindu, and Buddhist perspectives. Important and quite distinct traditions that have been touched upon only briefly or not discussed at all include, among others, the Maoist in China, the Ajivaka and Jain in India, the Shinto in Japan, and the Bon Po in Tibet, as well as various forms of Islam and Christianity that are firmly established in several different Asian contexts. However, perhaps enough has been said to suggest something of the diversity, richness, and depth of the thought that has emerged as Eastern men have struggled with the enigmas and paradoxes of death.

Obviously there is no single "Eastern" way of formulating the problematics of death, or of resolving the ethical issues it poses. However, when the various Eastern conceptions are set over against the dominant attitudes that have developed in the modern West two points are worth emphasizing. First, the various Eastern views place a strong emphasis on the fact that meaningful efforts to extend human life expectancy must involve not only the utilization of medical procedures and techniques, but also the development of moral attitudes and styles of life that place men in harmony with the reality and rhythms of the universe in which they live. Second, the various Eastern views (with the exception of certain Taoist traditions which held out the hope that death could be permanently postponed) emphasize the importance of developing and cultivating disciplines, meditations, and insights which have the capacity to rob death of its destructive power and in some cases even to transform it into a positive opportunity for human fulfillment. Perhaps in our modern struggle against death we have now reached a point at which it would be both possible and advisable to take these traditional approaches and conceptions more seriously into account.

FRANK E. REYNOLDS

[Other relevant material may be found under PAIN AND SUFFERING, article on RELIGIOUS PERSPECTIVES; SUICIDE. For discussion of related ideas, see: BUDDHISM; CONFUCIANISM; HINDUISM; and TAOISM. See also: MEDICAL ETHICS, HISTORY OF, section on SOUTH AND EAST ASIA, articles on INDIA, PREREPUBLICAN CHINA, and CONTEMPORARY CHINA.]

BIBLIOGRAPHY

"Death and Disposal of the Dead." Encyclopaedia of Religion and Ethics. Edited by James Hastings. New York: Charles Scribner's Sons; Edinburgh: T. & T. Clark, 1912, vol. 4, pp. 411–511. Those who are interested in the conceptions reflected in the communal practices related to dying and death which have been largely bypassed in our own discussion should begin by consulting, for India and China, the relevant articles under the above general topic. For Buddhist communal practices in various areas, see pp. 485–497 on Japanese customs, and the works by Tambiah and Welch.

FREMANTLE, FRANCESCA, and TRUNGPA, CHÖGYAM, trans. The Tibetan Book of the Dead: The Liberation through Hearing in the Bardo. Clear Light Series. Berkeley: Shambhala Publications, 1975. A fascinating primary text which describes in detail the states through which, according to the Tibetan Buddhist conception, every individual passes in his journey from death to rebirth.

HOLCK, FREDERICK H., ed. Death and Eastern Thought: Understanding Death in Eastern Religions and Philosophies. Nashville, Tenn.: Abingdon Press, 1974. This collection of essays is very useful for gaining a further orientation to the topic. It contains five essays on various aspects of the Indian tradition (including one that focuses primarily on Buddhism), one dealing with China, and one on Japan in which specific attention is given to certain aspects of Japanese Buddhism. For the books that provide an overall orientation see Reynolds and Waugh, and Lemaître.

JAN YÜN-HUA. "Buddhist Self-Immolation in Medieval China." History of Religions 4 (1964): 243–268.

LAMOTTE, ÉTIENNE. "Le Suicide religieux dans le bouddhisme ancien." Academie royale des sciences, des lettres, et des beauxarts de Belgique: Bulletin de la classe des lettres et des sciences morales et politiques 5th ser., 51 (1965): 156–168.

LEE, JUNG YOUNG. Death and Beyond in the Eastern Perspective. New ed. New York: Gordon & Breach Science Publishers, 1974. An introductory book which should be consulted only with the greatest caution.

LEMAÎTRE, SOLANGE. Le Mystère de la mort dans les religions d'Asie. 2d ed. rev. & corr. Paris: Adren Maisonneuve, 1963. An introductory book which covers several major areas in very general terms.

NEEDHAM, JOSEPH. "The Drug of Deathlessness; Macrobiotics and Immortality-Theory in East and West." Science and Civilization in China. Vol. 5: Chemistry and Chemical Technology. Pt. 2: Spagyrical Discovery and Invention: Magisteries of Gold and Immortality. London: Cambridge University Press, 1974, pp. 71–127.

REYNOLDS, FRANK E., and WAUGH, EARLE H. Religious Encounters with Death: Insights from the History and Anthropology of Religion. University Park: Pennsylvania State University Press, 1977. This broadly cross-cultural collection contains fifteen essays, five of which concern "Eastern" traditions (three on Hinduism, one on Indian Zoroastrianism and one on Japanese Buddhist meditational techniques which emphasize the practice of dying).

SMITH, D. HOWARD. "Chinese Concepts of the Soul." Numen 5 (1958): 165–179.

TAMBIAH, S. J. "Death, Mortuary Rites and the Path to Rebirth." Buddhism and the Spirit Cults in North-East Thailand. Cambridge Studies in Social Anthropology, no. 2. London: Cambridge University Press, 1970, pp. 179–194.

WELCH, HOLMES. "Rites for the Dead." The Practice of Chinese Buddhism: 1900–1950. Harvard East Asian Studies, no. 26. Cambridge: Harvard University Press, 1967, pp. 179–205.

YÜ, YING-SHIH. "Life and Immortality in the Mind of Han China." Harvard Journal of Asiatic Studies 25 (1964–1965): 80–122.

III

WESTERN PHILOSOPHICAL THOUGHT

Philosophers, presumably like other humans, have always been aware of death, though the extent of their interest and concern has varied from individual to individual and from age to age. Special problems connected with death have arisen from time to time, though some—such as the question of survival and an afterlife—have persisted in various cultures. Not only individual differences but the emphases and assumptions of established traditions and the cultural atmosphere of which successive philosophical views have been a part have inevitably influenced thoughts about death. Changes in social, political, and economic conditions and in religious, artistic, and scientific outlook have thus affected attitudes toward death.

In Western philosophical thought six such cultural periods can usefully be distinguished: (1) ancient Greek philosophy, comprising (a) the pre-Socratics as background to (b) the classic philosophies of Socrates, Plato, and Aristotle; (2) Hellenistic, that is, Greco-Roman thought, especially the Epicurean, Stoic, and other schools of the post-Aristotelian ancient world and also contributions of Hebrew–Christian traditions that entered the stream of Western philosophy during this period; (3) medieval thought of both (a) the early Middle Ages and (b) from the eleventh to the fifteenth century, including the various Renaissance movements of the period; (4) early modern philosophy of the sixteenth and seventeenth centuries with their social, religious, and scientific revolutions and reformations; (5) philosophy in the eighteenth, nineteenth, and early twentieth centuries, the periods of "Enlightenment" and "Romanticism," of pre-Darwinian and evolutionary science; and (6) recent and contemporary philosophical thought in its positivistic and pragmatic critiques and in its existentialist emphasis on problems associated with death.

Ancient Greek philosophy

The pre-Socratics. In Jacques Choron's *Death and Western Thought*, which provides a partial basis for this article, the author writes in discussing the contemporary German philosopher Martin Heidegger (1899–1976): "Perhaps the new answer to death to which Heidegger is being led is the consoling certitude of the harmony between human existence and the ground of Being, which he believes Western man has not known or felt since the Pre-Socratics" (Choron, p. 240).

Harmony between man and nature (*physis*) was for the pre-Socratics an unquestioned assumption, not as for Heidegger and other moderns the outcome of subtle and sophisticated argument. Moreover the "harmony" assumed by the pre-Socratics was variously expressed in the references and quotations that survive in later writings and constitute the basis of knowledge of their views. Awareness of continuity and change pervades the thought of pre-Socratic scientist-philosophers. Their observation of the natural order, and of human life as part of it, sometimes leads to emphasis on elements that are permanent in the midst of change, sometimes to a sense of universal mutability. It is significant that those Greeks of the sixth and fifth centuries B.C. lived in outlying areas of the Greek world, in Asia Minor and in what today is Italy, though one can only speculate about the influence of that circumstance. What other factors led to various interpretations of continuity and change remain unknown: Parmenides stressed the fundamentally unchanging order of things; Heraclitus, the constant change in everything except the *Logos*, the unchanging law of change. The melancholy that seems to pervade Heraclitus's thought may well have been derived from his pervasive sense of mutability. Tradition contrasts Heraclitean pessimism with the view of Parmenides and also with a later figure, Democritus (born 460? B.C.), whose commitment to atomistic materialism was supposedly connected with a cheerful outlook.

In contrast to these and other observers of the natural order, including Empedocles, whose doctrine of the four elements—earth, air, fire, and water—left a lasting imprint on later theorists, the mathematician-musician Pythagoras (died 497? B.C.) alone presents a comprehensive doctrine with regard to death. Supposedly derived from traditional mystery cults, the Pythagorean view holds that after death souls transmigrate from one animate being to another.

The background of classic Greek philosophy, of which Socrates, Plato, and Aristotle are the principal spokesmen, includes in addition to Homer, Hesiod, and the pre-Socratics the dramatists Aeschylus, Sophocles, Euripides, and Aristophanes, and the historians Herodotus and Thucydides. Herodotus's *History of the Persian Wars* focuses on the glory of the Greek triumph over Persian power and surveys calmly the rise and fall, the life and death of whole civilizations. Herodotus offers a view of death as "no evil," perhaps better than life, indeed "the gods' best gift to man." Thucydides' tragic account of the history of *The Peloponnesian War* provides the immediate background for the drama of Socrates' life and death and the philosophy of Plato's dialogues. It should be noted that in contrast to the pre-Socratic philosophers the three spokesmen of classic Greek thought lived and taught in the center of Greek culture, Athens.

Socrates, Plato, and Aristotle.   Though countless scholars have labored to disentangle the specific strands of Socrates' thought from those of Plato, whose dialogues constitute the record of Socratic philosophy, this distinction is insignificant in regard to reflections on death since these are expressed most eloquently in the *Apology, Crito,* and *Phaedo,* which relate Plato's account of the trial, imprisonment, and execution of Socrates. Moreover, whether one accepts Plato's praise of Socrates for having brought philosophy down to earth to dwell among men, or agrees with Nietzsche's—and Heidegger's—view that Socrates' teaching disrupted the harmony between man and nature, it is Socrates—Plato's Socrates—who remains the primary philosophical fountainhead of Western ethical thought, including much subsequent thinking about death. This is true of later classical philosophy, of the traditions of Epicureanism as well as Stoicism and other Hellenistic philosophies, and of much of later Greco-Roman, medieval, Renaissance, and modern thinking.

The drama of Socrates' trial and execution is central to Plato's discussion of death though the *Apology, Crito,* and *Phaedo* can be supplemented by references in other dialogues, including the *Republic, Gorgias,* and *Symposium.* One need not take literally the passage in the *Phaedo,* the account of Socrates' last hours, likening death to the daily life of the philosopher: "Death, the separation of soul and body, is something which a philosopher who dies to the body every day he lives ought to welcome." And in the *Phaedo* he proclaims:

I desire to prove to you that the real philosopher has reason to be of good cheer when he is about to die, and that after death he may hope to obtain the greatest good in the other world. . . . Is death not the separation of soul and body? And to be dead is the completion of this; when the soul exists in herself, and is released from the body and the body is released from the soul what is this but death? [Plato, p. 447.]

It should be repeated that those words are spoken by Socrates as he faces immediate death and that there is no preoccupation with the theme of death in the Platonic dialogues. Moreover, though Plato's philosophy and particularly his theory of Ideas or Forms has been interpreted as separating the world of matter from the realm of spirit, the distinction by no means constitutes a sharp division in Plato's thought. For Plato, as George Santayana has expressed it in his *Life of Reason,* all things ideal have a natural basis and all things natural have ideal fulfillment or possibilities. Similarly, the radical separation of body and soul as presented in the *Phaedo* is by no means as sharp in other Socratic statements and may be read as the expression of Socrates' effort to comfort his friends rather than as a formal doctrine.

Though Aristotle did formulate and criticize the Platonic theory of forms or ideas, his own views of the relation of body and soul and of immortality in the life of reason are essentially Socratic and find many parallels in Plato's dialogues. In early writings attributed to Aristotle, the dialogue *Eudemos* and the *Protrepticos,* there are echoes of a Pythagorean transmigration theory and a view of the body as the soul's "prison." But the major works of Aristotle, notably the *De Anima,* treat the theory of transmigration as a myth. Here Aristotle regards the soul as the entelechy, the "form-giving cause," of the body just as seeing is the entelechy of the eye. For Aristotle, as for the pre-Socratics, the world of nature is of primary interest, and he views it, as they apparently did, as the setting of human life and continuous with human nature. But Aristotle follows the Platonic Socrates in the centrality of his interest in human beings in their social setting.

One notes that Aristotle's father was a physician and that Aristotle's absorption in biological studies may well be the most significant factor in his approach to ethical questions, including problems connected with death. By contrast, Plato's acceptance of mathematical models —not improbably a Pythagorean influence— surely affected his thinking, e.g., his theory of Forms or Ideas. Yet a common element, Socratic in its emphasis, is readily discernible.

Hellenistic thought

Aristotle's death in 322 B.C. has conventionally marked the end of classical Greek philosophy. Post-Aristotelian—Hellenistic as distinguished from Hellenic—thought continued many of the lines of classical philosophy. But even in the traditions of Platonism and Aristotelianism there were marked changes, and this is true of the several schools that claimed to derive from Socrates: Cyrenaics, Cynics, Skeptics and their successors the Epicureans, Stoics, and other Schools of the Greco-Roman world. Such interest as there had been in problems related to death among the pre-Socratics and in the philosophies of Socrates, Plato, and Aristotle had never been the central focus of their thought. But in the Hellenistic age, marked by what Gilbert Murray called a "failure of nerve," the questions of death and dying became a preoccupying and sometimes an obsessive concern.

A few external circumstances may be briefly summarized. The disastrous conclusion of the Peloponnesian War precipitated the decline and death of the Greek city-states. The tragic irony may be noted that it was Aristotle's most famous student, Alexander, who brought to an end the city-state, which made possible, according to Aristotle, a truly good life of free citizens. The transfer of imperial power to Rome brought with it the transfer of surviving elements of Hellenic culture: The Roman pantheon was expanded to accommodate the entire family of Olympian deities, and the closing of the schools of Athens led to their Roman substitutes. Roman power, far more expansive and efficient than the Greek, brought great military achievement; but the succession of wars and conquests—witness Tacitus (A.D. 55–117)—produced diminishing satisfaction. The wheels of fortune turned rapidly; great wealth and poverty coincided. Social and political problems abounded; the ancient gods, as Augustine (A.D. 354–430) later observed, proved unavailing. Ancient pieties sought to fortify themselves by turning to the East, to exotic faiths and mystery cults.

To such a world, Greek in its background, Roman in its laws and organization, the surviving philosophic schools of Epicureanism, Stoicism, and the rest brought their distinctive messages —not philosophy as continued Socratic inquiry, but rather prescriptions for a way of life and a way to face death.

Epicureanism. For Epicurus (341–270 B.C.) philosophy was not a love of wisdom as good in itself but rather as a "remedy for the soul." This distinction is indeed the watershed between Hellenic and Hellenistic philosophers, even though the latter claimed to look back for their inspiration to classical thinkers, notably to Socrates. Epicurus looked back to Democritus too, but knowledge of atomistic physics was no longer desired for itself but rather to give reas-

surance. Epicurus's remedies were designed to liberate men from fear of the gods, to assure them that death was a relief to be welcomed, that evil could be endured if it could not be avoided in cloistered gardens, and that a relatively good life could be attained in simplicity and seclusion. The bad reputation that Epicureans subsequently acquired is to be explained by their neglect of the duties of active public life and citizenship and their supposed "atheism." It should be noted, however that most Epicureans (e.g., the poet Lucretius, 96?–55 B.C.) retained the Olympiad as models of Epicurean *ataraxia*, life free from worry. Epicurean arguments against immortality were based on Democritean atomism; after death the soul, being material, made of the finest atoms, would quickly be dissipated. There is nothing to fear: No man will attend his own funeral. Life is a feast and we have banqueted; should not the worm as well?

Stoicism. Stoicism, though often contrasted with Epicureanism, shared its essential purposes: to provide a way of life designed to make existence bearable and a system of knowledge primarily valued as a foundation for ethics—in the case of Stoicism an ethics of rigorous duty and civic virtue. For the Greek Stoics (e.g., Zeno, 335–265 B.C.) physics had been basic; for the three great Roman Stoics, Seneca, Epictetus, and Marcus Aurelius, the ethics of *apatheia* (indifference) and *aequanimitas* (peace of mind) is all-important. Though they retain a traditional pantheism, sometimes suggesting an undogmatic monotheism in which Zeus is identified with the universe, these doctrines in Roman Stoicism are very tentative. So too, "living according to nature" is assumed to be equivalent with "living according to reason," which, in turn, interprets the "life of reason" as a life reasonably disposed to accept those evils that cannot be avoided or brought under control as necessary. Thus Epictetus declares in his *Discourses*:

When death appears an evil we must have ready to hand the argument that it is fitting to avoid evils, and death is a necessary thing. What am I to do? Where am I to escape it? . . . I cannot escape death: am I not to escape the fear of it? Am I to die in tears and trembling? For trouble of mind springs from this, from wishing for a thing which does not come to pass [Oates, p. 271].

For the Stoics death was an escape from otherwise unavoidable evil—the door was always open—and they held to the conviction (Seneca put it into practice) that suicide was a way out. It is curious how often it is forgotten that the Stoics gave suicide their approval, whereas Schopenhauer, who because of his avowed pessimism is widely though mistakenly believed to have supported suicide, in fact argues against it as an erroneous submission to "Will." It may be noted that the argument for the "open door" has been revived in recent times by Jean-Paul Sartre. For the French existentialist suicide represents a way for man to assert his freedom.

Seneca's prescription for escaping the fear of death by thinking of it constantly is characteristic of Stoic ethics, but Jacques Choron's assertion that Marcus Aurelius's *Meditations* are "meditations on death and almost nothing else" (Choron, p. 73) seems an exaggeration. Death and its inevitability are, indeed, of concern to the emperor-philosopher but there are numerous other interests.

Hebrew–Christian traditions.   There is a noble sobriety in the ethical doctrines of the Hellenistic schools, but, in contrast to the Socratic teaching from which they claimed to have been derived, their emphasis is negative—deliverance from evil, escape from an alien world, salvation from sin. Along with Epicureanism and Stoicism, other philosophical systems, some of them revivals of classic formulations such as neo-Pythagoreanism and neo-Platonism, offered themselves as cures for failure of nerve. And along with such philosophies men turned to exotic faiths to supplement or replace their traditional religion. Among these, in competition with Persian Mithraism and, later, Manicheanism, for example, came the promise of salvation through faith in Jesus of Nazareth as preached by Paul of Tarsus. The Old Testament, as well as the New, now entered the mainstream of Western culture, and the Hebrew–Christian ethic came to dominate Western thinking, including thought about death.

There is relatively little concern with death in the Hebrew scriptures. Though later ages stressed Adam's sin as having "brought death into the world and all our woes," the prevailing mood of Hebraism was expressed in the formulation of Koheleth that "there is a time to be born and a time to die" (Ecclesiastes 3:2). Between birth and death there should be a full life, and after death human souls (*rephaim*) may lead a shadowy existence in an afterworld (*Sheol*). Real immortality pertains to the race, rather than to individuals, and to vicarious immortality through one's descendants.

Christianity, though rooted in the Old Testament, reversed these emphases, and the Hebrew–Christian dispensation reflects the preoccupations of the Hellenistic age. Jesus of Nazareth and the Christian promise of divine love supplied a doctrine of salvation from evil— above all from the sins of concupiscence and sexual desire—a doctrine that offered the release of grace from the threat of everlasting hellfire and the hope of eternal blessedness. From the philosophical elements in Patristic theology, from Origen (185?–254?) to Augustine (354–430) to Thomas Aquinas (1225–1274), the natural world was viewed primarily as the scene of human salvation and humankind as essentially sinful, doomed to die and to suffer eternal damnation unless rescued by supernatural Grace.

Medieval thought

This was the framework within which medieval philosophers operated, using tools derived from ancient thinkers. They included Platonic traditions in a limited knowledge of the dialogues and, for scholastic philosophy, the available works of Aristotle, "master of all who know" in Dante's famous epithet. When more complete records came from the Arab world as a result of Muhammadan conquests and penetration of the Iberian peninsula, the teachings of Avicenna (980–1037) and Averroes (1126–1198) added to Western knowledge of ancient philosophy and scientific interests. To this increased understanding there were also contributions by medieval Jewish philosophers such as Abraham Ibn Ezra (1092–1167) and especially Moses Maimonides (1135–1204). These factors helped to modify medieval otherworldliness and twelfth- and thirteenth-century anticipation of the revival of naturalistic philosophy, literature, and art associated with the later Renaissance of the fifteenth century. Though the Renaissance and the sixteenth-century religious Reformation have often been viewed as terminating the Middle Ages, latter-day historians have recognized the earlier shift of emphasis and, on the other hand, the continuity of stress on sin and salvation in various aspects of Reformation thought, notably in the philosophy of Calvin (1509–1564).

Early modern philosophy (16th and 17th centuries)

The waning of the Middle Ages and the dawn of modernity was of course not a sudden shift. The transition was gradual, and elements that characterize modern culture can readily be discerned in late medievalism. The growth of capitalism and of national states, continuing Renaissance naturalism and new sciences took time to develop, and, correspondingly, aspects of a predominantly "medieval" religious culture persist into the seventeenth century and later. But from then on Western thought becomes predominantly secular and scientific.

Two thinkers express this outlook, and each has been called the father of modern philosophy: Francis Bacon (1561–1626) and René Descartes (1596–1650). The very titles of some of Bacon's books indicate his sense of the novelty of his outlook: *Novum Organum*, the *New Method* designed to replace the old methodology, the organon of scholastic Aristotelianism; and the *New Atlantis*, a forecast of cooperative, modern science, which anticipates developments in the investigation of nature until the eighteenth and nineteenth centuries' laboratory science, the practical applications of knowledge as power, the pragmatic mood in philosophy.

In his criticism of the Stoics Bacon echoes the view of his predecessor Montaigne, whose essay on death, "To Philosophize Is to Learn How to Die," concludes: "If we have learned how to live properly and calmly, we will know how to die in the same manner."

As for Bacon, so for Descartes "the sciences have a definitely practical aim, the harnessing of nature to the purposes of man. The will o' the wisp of his life was the conquest of death not only for the soul but also for the body" (Choron, p. 111). Like Bacon, too, Descartes's concern is to extirpate the fear of death, though unlike Bacon his chief argument is the traditional one of assurance of the survival of the soul. Cartesian dualism, the sharp dichotomy between body (*res extensa*) and mind (*res cogitans*) provides ground for Descartes's assurance but leaves the problem of their relationship, the "mind–body problem" of how two radically different kinds of thing can interact, as a continuing problem throughout modern philosophy.

In the context of the continuing preoccupation with the theme of death, a famous dictum of Spinoza (1632–1677) is to be read. He writes: "A free man, that is to say, a man who lives according to the dictates of reason alone, is not led by the fear of death. . . . He thinks, therefore, of nothing less than of death, and his wisdom is a meditation upon life" (Spinoza, bk. IV, prop. LXVII). There is no reason to accept critical interpretations of Spinoza that attempt to psychoanalyze him as himself harboring an extreme fear of death or suspect his argument "that death is by so much the less injurious to us as the clear and distinct knowledge of the mind is the greater" (bk. V, prop. XXVIII, note). This becomes especially cogent in the light of Spinoza's own criticism of simplistic rationalism (e.g., the Stoics) and his conviction that a lesser emotion can be displaced only by one that is more powerful, the most powerful being "the intellectual love of God or Nature" (*Amor intellectualis Dei—Deus sive Natura*).

Another mathematical genius, co-discoverer with Sir Isaac Newton of the calculus, was Gottfried Wilhelm von Leibniz (1646–1716). He reacted against what he took to be the excessive mechanism of dominant Cartesian views and sought to reconcile science and religion. In this context he distinguished mere unconsciousness from *absolute death* in which all perception would cease. This has confirmed the ill-founded opinion that some souls are destroyed, and the bad ideas of some who call themselves freethinkers and who have disputed the immortality of the soul" (Leibniz). Hence Leibniz argued that no animate being can "entirely perish in what we call death" and that "God will always conserve not only our substance, but also our person." Leibnizian optimism had wide influence in the eighteenth century as expressed in Alexander Pope's couplet seeing in "all discord, harmony not understood; all partial evil, universal good."

Philosophy in the 18th to 20th centuries

There were dissenting voices against the Leibnizian optimism. David Hume attacked the entire doctrine of immortality, and the French philosophes of the Enlightenment (D'Holbach, 1723–1789; Condorcet, 1743–1794; Diderot, 1713–1784) held it to be a "priestly lie." Consequently, "Fear of death is the only true enemy that has to be conquered, and that there is no afterlife makes us free from the power of the priests" (Choron, p. 135). Finally Voltaire in his *Candide* demolished Leibnizian optimism in his caricature of the philosopher "Dr. Pangloss."

In Immanuel Kant, Johann Gottfried Herder, Goethe, and the post-Kantian German philosophers there are fundamentally different views of the problems of death and immortality. Herder held that belief in a future life was universally natural to man. Goethe saw death as "Nature's stratagem to secure more abundant life," and his challenging phrase: *stirb und werde* (die and live anew) was echoed by post-Kantian philosophers of Romanticism. So was Kant's ethical argument for immortality: Though it cannot be established by "pure Reason," the requirements of moral necessity can be validated by "practical Reason" without which "the moral worth of actions, on which alone the worth of a person and even of the world depends in the eyes of supreme wisdom, would not exist at all" (Kant, p. 247). This conviction was followed by the philosophers of the Romantic period (Fichte, 1762–1814; Schelling, 1775–1854; Schleiermacher, 1768–1814) in the phrase of Arthur Schopenhauer (1788–1860): "Death is the true inspiring genius or the muse of philosophy" (Schopenhauer, vol. 3, p. 249).

For Georg Wilhelm Friedrich Hegel, Kant's moral argument had other implications. In Hegel's view "Death has the peculiar effect of uniting the individual with universal matter. The living individual is a particular person; once dead, however, he becomes, through bodily corruption indistinguishable from abstract being" (Hegel, p. 192). Hegel held immortality to be a quality of the living spirit, not an event in the future, and this view guided Hegel's follower, Ludwig Feuerbach. In his *Thoughts on Death*, Feuerbach argued that "Immortal life is the life which exists for its own sake and contains its own aim and purpose in itself—immortal life is the full life, rich in contents" (Choron, p. 191).

Søren Kierkegaard sets himself apart from all this. Attacking Hegel and traditional philosophy in general for concentrating on the "essence" of things as against the "existence" of the specific individual, Kierkegaard and the existentialists who follow his teachings emphasize the values of "immediate experience" in contrast to all metaphysical abstractions. In spite of Kierkegaard's attacks on traditional thought, existentialists have much in common with the attitude of Romanticist philosophers in their emphasis on the values of the individual, and like all exponents of "philosophies of life" they stress the significance of the crucial experiences of human lives, including the experience of death.

Friedrich Wilhelm Nietzsche, though influenced by Kierkegaard as well as by Schopenhauer, rejected the Romantic view of death as "the muse of philosophy" and argued that, though man's mortality is of the greatest impor-

tance for any philosophy of life, the act of dying is not. In his view the "will to die" can be countered by the affirmation of life in art and by the heroic acceptance of "eternal recurrence" in the experience of finitude.

Recent and contemporary thought

The individualism of Romanticists and of Kierkegaardian existentialists contrasts with an outlook that "developed during the 19th century and found its expression in Auguste Comte's positivism, an intellectualized form of nationalism." For Comte "society is composed of both the dead and the living. . . . For the dead have gone through the moment of change, and their monuments are the visible sign of the permanence of their city" (Ariès, p. 73).

Comtian sociological philosophy, though scientific and positivistic, was essentially pre-Darwinian in its perspective. Sharing a scientific outlook, the American pragmatists—Charles Sanders Peirce, William James, and John Dewey—were biologically oriented. Thus Peirce held that "death and corruption are mere accidents or secondary phenomena. Among some of the lower organisms, it is a moot point with biologists whether there be anything which ought to be called death" (Fisch, p. 109). With this naturalistic approach and, perhaps, as in the case of the "unalterable optimism of the dentists in an American small town . . . Relax, take it easy, it's nothing," as Jacques Maritain wrote in his *Reflections on America* (p. 91), pragmatists have focused attention on life, not death. However, there are significant reflections on death in William James's view that "life and its negation are beaten up inextricably together. But if life be good, the negation of it must be bad. Yet the two are equally essential facts of existence; and all natural happiness thus seems infected with a contradiction. The breath of the sepulchre surrounds it" (James, p. 139). Of course, James is writing about the attitude of "the sick soul" and from the viewpoint of a sympathetic psychologist.

Other philosophies indicating the importance of post-Darwinian biology include the vitalism of Hans Driesch (1867–1941) and the creative evolutionism of Henri Bergson (1859–1941). Bergson finds in his élan vital, the drive of life throughout reality, a ground for faith in life after death, and Alfred North Whitehead (1861–1947) finds comparable assurance by subsuming human immortality under the inclusive rubric of "the immortality of realized value."

More extensive treatments of the problems of death in late nineteenth- and twentieth-century philosophical thought are in works by Max Scheler and Georg Simmel. Contemporary existentialists devote great concern to the theme of death. Martin Heidegger places death in the very center of his consciousness as the way to "disarm" it and to offset "animal anxiety." Gabriel Marcel uses the despair evoked by the persistent consciousness of death to examine and deepen religious faith, and Jean-Paul Sartre finds in the experiencing of death ground for asserting human freedom.

Though contemporary philosophical analysts are disposed to reject "unanswerable questions" as meaningless, a respected spokesman for this point of view writes about death: "It is a meaningful question, because we can indicate ways in which it could be solved. One method of ascertaining one's own survival would simply consist in dying. It would also be possible to describe certain observations of scientific character that would lead us to accept a definite answer" (Schlick).

Though it is too soon to discern the philosophical implications of recent developments in the biological sciences and in medicine, a new concern for the dying and for human dignity in its final phases may be noted as characteristic of such movements as euthanasia and thanatology. In general it may be asserted that not since the later Middle Ages has there been as much consideration for problems associated with death as is evident at present. Although the anthropologist Geoffrey Gorer could assert in 1965 that there was a "conspiracy of silence" about death as though it were a "pornographic" subject, it is now clear that Philippe Ariès is accurate when he writes, in the early 1970s, that "death is once again becoming something one can talk about" (p. 103).

JAMES GUTMANN

[*Directly related are other articles in this entry:* WESTERN RELIGIOUS THOUGHT *and* DEATH IN THE WESTERN WORLD. *For a discussion of the meaning of death in other cultures, see the other articles in this entry:* ANTHROPOLOGICAL PERSPECTIVE *and* EASTERN THOUGHT. *For discussion of related ideas, see:* DEATH AND DYING: EUTHANASIA AND SUSTAINING LIFE, *article on* HISTORICAL PERSPECTIVES; MIND–BODY PROBLEM; *and* SUICIDE.]

BIBLIOGRAPHY

ARIÈS, PHILIPPE. *Western Attitudes Toward Death: From the Middle Ages to the Present.* Translated by Patricia M. Ranum. Johns Hopkins Symposia in Comparative History. Baltimore: Johns Hopkins University Press, 1974.

ARISTOTLE. *The Basic Works of Aristotle.* Edited by Richard McKeon. New York: Random House, 1941.

BROAD, CHARLIE DUNBAR. *Lectures of Psychical Research: Incorporating the Perrott Lectures Given in Cambridge University in 1959 and 1960.* International Library of Philosophy and Scientific Method. New York: Humanities Press; London: Routledge & Kegan Paul, 1962.

CHORON, JACQUES. *Death and Western Thought.* New York: Collier Books, 1963.

CORNFORD, FRANCIS MACDONALD. *From Religion to Philosophy: A Study in the Origins of Western Speculation.* The Library of Religion and Culture. Edited by A. J. Ayer. New York: Harper & Row, 1957.

DUCASSE, CURT JOHN. *Nature, Mind, and Death.* The Paul Carus Lectures, 8th ser. LaSalle, Ill.: Open Court Publishing Co., 1951.

FEIFEL, HERMAN, ed. *The Meaning of Death.* New York: McGraw-Hill, 1959.

FISCH, MAX HAROLD, ed. *Classic American Philosophers: Peirce, James, Royce, Santayana, Dewey, Whitehead: Selections from Their Writings.* New York: Appleton-Century-Crofts, 1951.

FLEW, ANTONY GARRARD NEWTON, ed. *Body, Mind, and Death: Readings.* New York: Macmillan Co., 1964.

GORER, GEOFFREY. *Death, Grief, and Mourning.* Problems of Philosophy Series. Garden City, N.Y.: Doubleday, 1965. First published in London as *Death, Grief, and Mourning in Contemporary Britain.*

HEGEL, GEORGE WILHELM FRIEDRICH. *Hegel: Selections.* Edited by Jacob Loewenberg. The Modern Student's Library, Philosophy Series. Edited by Ralph B. Perry. New York: Scribner, 1929.

JAMES, WILLIAM. *The Varieties of Religious Experience: A Study in Human Nature: Being the Gifford Lectures on Natural Religion Delivered at Edinburgh in 1901–1902.* New York: Longmans, Green & Co., 1928.

JOLIVET, RÉGIS. *Le Problème de la mort chez M. Heidegger et J.-P. Sartre.* Paris: Éditions de Fontenelle, 1950.

KANT, IMMANUEL. *Critique of Practical Reason: And Other Writings in Moral Philosophy.* Translated and edited by Lewis White Beck. Chicago: University of Chicago Press, 1949.

LAMONT, CORLISS. *The Illusion of Immortality* (1935). 4th ed. Introduction by John Dewey. New York: Frederick Ungar Publishing Co., 1965.

———. *Issues of Immortality: A Study in Implications.* New York: Henry Holt & Co., 1932. Ph.D. dissertation, Columbia University, 1932.

LEIBNIZ, GOTTFRIED WILHELM. *The Monadology and Other Philosophical Writings.* Translated by Robert Latta. London: Oxford University Press, 1898.

MARITAIN, JACQUES. *Reflections on America.* New York: Scribner, 1958.

OATES, WHITNEY JENNINGS, ed. *The Stoic and Epicurean Philosophers: The Complete Extant Writings of Epicurus, Epictetus, Lucretius, Marcus Aurelius.* New York: Random House, Modern Library, 1940.

PLATO. *The Dialogues of Plato.* Translated by Benjamin Jowett. New York: Random House, 1937.

SCHELER, MAX FERDINAND. "Tod und Fortleben." *Gesammelte Werke.* Vol. 10: *Schriften aus dem Nachlass* (1933). Edited by Maria Scheler. Bern: Francke, 1957, pp. 9–52.

SCHLICK, MORITZ. "Unanswerable Questions." *A Modern*

Introduction to Philosophy. The Free Press Textbooks in Philosophy. Edited by Paul Edwards and Arthur Pap. New York: Free Press, 1973, pp. 791–795.

SCHOPENHAUER, ARTHUR. *The World as Will and Idea.* Translated by Richard B. Haldane and John Kemp. 3 vols. New York: Scribner; London: Routledge & Kegan Paul, 1949.

SIMMEL, GEORG. "Zur Metaphysik des Todes." *Logos: Internationale Zeitschrift für Philosophie der Kultur* 1 (1910–1911): 57–70.

SPINOZA, BENEDICT DE. *Ethics: Preceded by On the Improvement of the Understanding.* Edited by James Gutmann. New York: Hafner, 1949. Based on the translation by William Hale White as revised by Amelia H. Stirling.

IV

WESTERN RELIGIOUS THOUGHT

1

DEATH IN BIBLICAL THOUGHT

The Old Testament

In Genesis 2–3, Israelite folk literature preserved and possibly combined two "explanations" (etiologies) of human mortality: (1) A protohuman couple, in primeval time, disobeyed their creator, and the two were placed under the sentence of death ("When you eat from [the tree of knowledge] you are doomed to die," 2:17). Presumably, they were created immortal and might have remained so. (2) The protohuman couple was created mortal. "The Man" (Hebrew: *ha-'adam,* later shortened to a proper name, Adam) was thought to have been fashioned from the soil (*ha-'adamah*) since humans are buried in the ground and their deteriorating bodies seem to blend into it. The image is that of the potter who fashions vessels from ceramic clay. Life results when the creator forces breath into the nostrils, resulting in a "living creature" (2:7). Presumably, mortality was intended, just as it was for all of the other "creatures" who are likewise fashioned from the soil (2:19). The couple is banished from the primeval garden lest they eat from the "tree of life."

The account can also be read as a continuous, integrated story: The couple forfeits access to the "tree of life" by their disobedience in eating from the "tree of knowledge." The result is that they must remain as they were created: mortal. However, later generations, particularly in the early Christian era, would read the unified story to mean that death was a tragic disruption of the Creator's plan. Thus, the second folk explanation will be indicative of Israelite and Jewish thought, while the first will predominate in Christian thought.

The term "death" is used in the Old Testa-

ment in at least three senses: (1) for biological cessation, the end of one's historical existence; (2) as a metaphor for those things which detract from life fully lived—illness, persecution, despair, etc.—e.g., God is described as one who "kills and brings to life" (1 Sam. 2:6), with no implication that biological death or resurrection is intended; (3) as an active power in opposition to the created order. This is usually only a literary vestige from the pre-Yahwistic period or from Israel's neighbors, e.g., when one of Job's friends describes deterioration of the body, he uses a formalized idiom: "the first-born of death consumes his limbs" (Job 18:13). He need not mean thereby what a non-Israelite likely would mean: that the god Mot (death), a demonic, autonomous power, had seized the person.

In Israelite anthropology there is nothing corresponding to the Greco-Christian concept of a "soul" (itself a very nebulous term). Humans are a totality, flesh animated by a life force (*nefesh* or *ruach*), which was thought to reside in the blood or in the breath. The departure of the life force results in death. The body, thus weakened, is placed in the tomb, where a subexistence was sometimes associated with it and especially with the bones. Hence, desecration of the remains was considered sacrilege (Amos 2:1). Sometimes a shadowy, weakened remnant of the person was thought to reside in the Underworld (Hebrew: *Sheol;* cf. the "shadows" of the Homeric Hades). For example, a medium claims to have made contact with the deceased prophet Samuel, still recognizable as an old man dressed in a robe (1 Sam. 28). However, such ideas and practices are largely vestiges of an older cult of the dead, which official Yahwism transforms, ignores, or forbids: The potent death-demons of neighboring cults are denied existence; mediums are to be executed (Exod. 22:18); priests are forbidden to participate in rituals for death and burial (Lev. 21); tomb gifts are vestigial (vessels are empty); the dead are reduced to a state approaching nonexistence and hence can scarcely influence the living (Eccles. 9:5–6); no judgment of the dead or expectation of resurrection is affirmed, save at the very end of the Old Testament period.

While there is a variety of responses to biological death (as one might expect from a collection ranging over at least a millennium), the predominant response in old age is one of calm acceptance. Considerable comfort seems to lie behind the oft-repeated refrain, "N died old and full of years" (Gen. 25:8). The fact of human mortality does not engender the belief that life is thereby meaningless. Laments do not focus upon biological death as a theological problem (2 Sam. 1:19–27). The question, "Why should I/we die?" is not asked except in situations where foolish action would lead to premature death (Gen. 47:15).

Occasionally the positive values of mortality are implied: the rebellious protohuman couple, Adam and Eve, barred from "the tree of life" (Gen. 3:22–24); the human life span is shortened in order to limit unacceptable behavior (Gen. 6:1–4); it was necessary for an entire generation to die before Israel could move on toward her ordained destiny (Num. 32:13); Job, overcome with pain and grief, observes that death would be a form of release (Job 3:1–19); the psalmist suggests that human finitude can be an incentive to seek the ultimate meaning of life (Ps. 90:12).

While the Wisdom literature most often is concerned with premature biological death (how to avoid it: "Fools die for lack of sense," Prov. 10:21), Ecclesiastes in particular focuses upon the fact of mortality. Wise or foolish, one fate comes to all, and thus all achievements are negated (Eccles. 2:15–22). Thus, one is forced to concentrate upon the present, which can be seen as a gift from God (Eccles. 3:1–15). Ultimate nihilism is overcome by keeping death within the domain of God's wisdom, even though it be incomprehensible to humans.

In sum, then, what happened after death was not a matter of religious importance, and mortality is calmly accepted as part of the definition of being human (a creature). Attention is focused almost entirely upon this world and its activities: responsible life in a covenant community called to serve God. Anything that interferes with life in this fashion is to be avoided and is metaphorically described as "death." Seemingly, anxiety about mortality has largely been transferred to anxiety about things that interfere with life at its fullest. Protest against biological death, apart from Ecclesiastes, is directed only toward: (1) premature death (Isa. 38:2–3, a response to a death-oracle at age 39); (2) an "evil" death, characterized by violence; and (3) severance of relationship with God ("For [those in] Sheol cannot thank thee, death cannot praise thee," Isa. 38:18). Some scholars think that the desire for unending relationship with God is the bridge that finally leads to assertion of life after death, e.g., in Psalm 73:23–26.

On occasion, attention is focused on, and

comfort derived from, those things which will survive the mortal human: one's reputation (Prov. 10:7; Sirach 44:8–9); male offspring to preserve one's memory and property (2 Sam. 18:18; Isa. 56:3–5; such desire may be a vestige of the ancestor cult, wherein the function of the eldest son was to bring offerings to the tomb); the elect, worshiping community Israel (Gen. 48:21); and God, who alone is immortal (Ps. 90; Hab. 1:12, Tiq. Soph.).

The intertestamental literature

In the Old Testament literature, the primary hindrance to Israel's corporate existence was a human tendency toward rebellion (Num. 11–16). The prophets proposed that the reverses of history might serve a didactic purpose, leading to an age of spontaneous obedience (Jer. 31:31–34), or that God would give the people a "new heart" (Ezek. 18:31; 36:26). Because of the failure of such reform to materialize, because of the disintegration of traditional social and economic structures after the fall of Jerusalem (587 B.C.), and because of the harshness of subsequent oppression by Babylonians, Persians, and Greeks, some persons found it impossible any longer to hope for the transformation of society through human initiative or response. Influenced by ancient conflict myths, the apocalyptic school of thought slowly developed, beginning toward the end of the Old Testament period. It proposed that a catastrophic divine intervention would be necessary in order to restore the world to the Creator's design. Death, increasingly viewed as an active power or agent (and later identified with the devil: Wisd. of Sol. 1:13; 2:23–24), would be eliminated from human experience (Isa. 25:8) and the deceased might even be resurrected to enjoy the new age (Dan. 12:1–3). The possibility of a semiconscious interim existence (usually in the Underworld) was then perceived, possibly influenced by contact with the anthropology of the Greek mystery religions: the life force and consciousness are fused into an entity able to survive cessation of bodily functions.

Intense and sustained persecution sometimes produced a positive evaluation of biological death. The paradigm of a martyred mother and seven sons is offered by 2 Macc. (second century B.C.): death, to be followed by resurrection, is much to be preferred to some forms of this-worldly existence. In the Wisdom of Solomon (first century B.C.), the traditional Old Testament stance is reversed: premature death of the righteous indicates that they are worthy of the divine presence (Wisd. of Sol. 3:4–5) and frees them from further suffering (Wisd. of Sol. 4:11). Thus, death need be a source of anxiety only to the wicked.

In the sectarian literature from the ascetic community at Qumran (the Dead Sea Scrolls, first century B.C.), biological death is scarcely an issue. Rather, attention is focused upon the possibility of transition from one this-worldly mode of existence to another—from what is metaphorically described as "death" to "life." Through membership in the Community, with its regimented life-style and esoteric scriptural lore, one can escape the human inclination toward evil, from the assaults of the "angel of darkness," and be in communion with the "heavenly hosts." This present possibility will be augmented by a final war, which will usher in an era of divine favor centered in the city of Jerusalem. (Whether and how the deceased will participate in this new age is still a matter of scholarly debate.)

By the second century B.C., the protohuman couple in the primeval garden was understood not only to have become mortal because of sin (a move in interpretation from etiology number two toward number one), but to have been the means whereby death grasped their descendants: "Woman is the origin of sin, and it is through her that we all die" (Sirach 25:24). This understanding will play a major role in the thought of some New Testament writers.

The New Testament

Although this literature comes from a narrow period of time (little more than a century), it contains a variety of perspectives, definitions, and emphases that cannot easily be harmonized. In general, it builds upon apocalyptic thought and develops death into a larger theological issue than has been the case previously.

The earliest spokesman, Paul (A.D. 50?), concentrates upon biological death as a consequence of sin (Rom. 6:23), unleashed by the disobedience of Adam and Eve (Rom. 5:19). He perceives sin as a power, related to the devil, that has infected the entire cosmos, setting it in opposition to the Creator's design (Rom. 8:22). Death is thus the enemy, the paradigm of all existence, the background of all patterns of possibility: demoralizing, challenging, and negating all human vitality and sense of purpose. It is not merely that the individual is mortal: It is that all existence must be perceived as futile, as

death-directed (Rom. 8:18–25). "Life" has been engulfed by "death." However, since death is a "historical" problem rather than a metaphysical one (i.e., "Adam" has been historicized), it is subject to a historical solution. Jesus, perceived as having risen from the dead, illustrates that the resurrection hope of apocalypticism is well founded and that the transition to the new age is imminent. The fact that death has been defeated, that God will shortly vindicate himself, makes it possible to perceive the cosmos in a new light, to see new possibility patterns, to "walk in newness of life" (Rom. 6:4). It is this new perception that now empowers the followers of Jesus to act. They believe that the power of death has been negated, although it temporarily continues to manifest itself biologically. That will cease at the transition to the new age, when all followers of Jesus, living or deceased, will be granted "immortality" (1 Cor. 15:53–54).

In the Synoptic Gospels, biological death is cited primarily as an incentive to prepare for the impending arrival of the new age; the insecurity and shortness of life serve as sanctions for obedience to the appeals of Jesus. Death, especially biological death, is not perceived as a serious theological problem. Little attention is given to the details of life after death.

In the latest Gospel, John, the apocalyptic theme of catastrophic transition to a new age (including the hope for resurrection of the dead), is pushed even farther to the margins of discussion. The quality of one's existence, here and now, becomes the issue. Biological death is not man's fundamental problem; it is how life is to be lived. Hence, when the author speaks of "eternal life," he is not thinking fundamentally of an apocalyptic transition to life without end still lying before the individual. Rather, "death" is a metaphor for a quality of existence that the followers of Jesus are able to transcend: They will "never die" (John 11:26), i.e., not be subject to a mode of existence, even though they will eventually biologically expire. The choice for humans is "eternal life" versus living "death."

Conclusions and implications

The Bible, like any other document, is heavily dependent upon the cultural milieu of which it is a part—a milieu radically different from that of the modern Western reader. This, plus the fact that biomedical technology has thrust upon us problems beyond the imagination of the biblical writers, makes it extremely hazardous to propose simplistic "contemporizations." Nonetheless, the following observations, restrictions, and implications are offered, tentatively, for those whose ultimate points of reference include the biblical tradition.

1. The Bible contains a variety of perspectives, which cannot be harmonized or easily systematized and need not be arranged in a hierarchy of values (such as, "the perspective[s] of Jesus are normative"). Such variety is a reflection of changing historical situations; it is an accurate perception of the ambiguity of reality. It may be a strength rather than a weakness, however frustrating this may be to the ethicist.

2. Death is more than biological cessation. The Bible's metaphorical use of the term corresponds, in part, to such modern perceptions as psychological death, social death, and spiritual death.

3. Life is more than biological functioning. Therefore, one's commitments should be directed to the conditions under which life in community is lived and to the values that make life meaningful (and the Bible has very definite ideas about what such conditions and values are, in social, economic, political, and religious terms). It is precarious to go beyond this and assert, as is sometimes done, that the lack of emphasis in biblical books upon biological life as intrinsically valuable (see, however, paragraph 4 below) would support an ethical stance in which extraordinary life-support systems should be withheld or withdrawn from some categories of dying patients.

4. The emphasis upon biological life as the result of the deity's creative act (Gen. 2:7, Ps. 104:30) and the insistence that even animal life cannot be taken without the enactment of a ritual which acknowledges God's sovereignty over it (Lev. 17:1–16; secular slaughter of an animal is regarded as murder, 17:4) serves as a caution against any simplistic human desire to terminate, directly or indirectly, the life of one who is suffering.

5. Physicians who tend to view death as an "enemy" to be overcome at all costs may feel more kinship with a New Testament stance (death as a "power," which God will soon eradicate) than with that of the Old Testament (death as a natural event).

6. Since the biblical thinkers could not conceive of existence in noncorporeal terms and thus forbade desecration of corpses or even bones, Orthodox Judaism quite logically has usually opposed autopsies and cremation as sacrilege.

7. The idea of life after death, being in some measure culturally and historically conditioned, may only with difficulty become a criterion in ethical decisions. In the biblical text itself, it is not used to devaluate this-worldly existence.

LLOYD BAILEY

[*Directly related are the entries* CADAVERS; EMBODIMENT; *and* JUDAISM.]

BIBLIOGRAPHY

BAILEY, LLOYD R. "Death as a Theological Problem in the Old Testament." *Pastoral Psychology* 22, no. 218 (1971), pp. 20–32.
BRUEGGEMANN, W. "Death, Theology of." *The Interpreter's Dictionary of the Bible: An Illustrated Encyclopedia.* 4 vols. and supp. *Supplementary Volume.* Edited by Keith Crim, Lloyd R. Bailey, Sr., Victor P. Furnish, and Emory S. Bucke. Nashville: Abingdon Press, 1976, pp. 219–222.
KECK, LEANDER E. "New Testament Views of Death." *Perspectives on Death.* Edited by Liston O. Mills. Nashville: Abingdon Press, 1969, chap. 2, pp. 33–98.
LAPP, PAUL W. "If a Man Die, Shall He Live Again?" *Perspective* 9 (1968): 139–156. *Perspective* is a journal of the Pittsburgh Theological Seminary.

2
POST-BIBLICAL JEWISH TRADITION

Rabbinic period

The rabbinic period (c. 200 B.C.E. to 500 C.E.) provided important ideas and practices, which had a crucial impact on the unfolding of the Judaic view of death.

Fate after death.   First, there was a definite expression of Jewish dogma concerning the fate of the person after death. The Pharisaic doctrine, which became normative both for Judaism and Christianity, was expressed in the phrase, *tehiat hametim,* the resurrection of the dead. This meant that death was not seen as the final end of existence. It was a prelude to the *olam haba,* the world to come. There is no doctrinal clarity as to the exact nature of the *olam haba.* Some believed that until the day of the resurrection (which would be ushered in by the Messiah) the soul slept waiting. The day of the resurrection would also be a day of judgment when the righteous would be ushered into the *olam haba.* Others believed that the soul enjoyed immortality in a disembodied state in the world to come. During this time there is a preliminary judgment; the wicked being purged in *Gehenna* (hell) and the righteous enjoying the delights of heaven. This would end when the time of *tehiat hametim* arrived, the souls rejoining the reborn bodies to live in eternal bliss. It is important to note that it was the resurrection of the body which was seen as the *final* consummation of salvation. It is also important to note that a religion which was, in general, loath to enunciate specific dogmas, insisted on the belief in the resurrection of the dead as one of the few specific doctrines considered to be indispensable for a believing Jew.

Customs and rituals surrounding death. The second important development during the rabbinic period was the formulation of specific customs and rituals surrounding death. The dying were to be treated with special consideration, even to the extent of withholding the entire truth about their condition so that they might not be thrown into despair. The obligation of *bikkur holim*, the visiting of the sick, especially the dying, was seen as very important. When death seemed to be drawing near, the person was advised to confess, "I acknowledge before Thee, O Lord my God and God of my fathers, that my life and my death are in Thy hands. May it be Thy will to heal me. But if death is my lot, then I accept it from Thy hand with love." Then came a simple confession of sin and a prayer: "May my death be an atonement for whatever sins and errors and wrongdoings I have committed before Thee. In Thy mercy grant me the goodness that is waiting for the righteous and bring me to eternal life." The confession ends with the historic affirmation of Jewish faith: "Hear, O Israel, the Lord our God, the Lord is One."

The dead are to be treated with dignity. Desecration of the body is forbidden, and burial must be immediate; it must be through interment in the soil; the dead are to be buried simply in white shrouds. The funeral is simple; the eulogy is for the honor of the deceased and the comfort of the bereaved. Close relatives observe a prescribed period of mourning, during which time they stay at home to receive friends and neighbors who come to console them, using the formula: "May the Lord comfort you amongst the mourners of Zion and Jerusalem." In later Judaism, these mourning customs were elaborated, the most important aspect being the obligation of the sons to recite the *kaddish*, a prayer in praise of God at every synagogue service for eleven months. This is seen as an expression of the commandment "Honor thy father and thy mother." In another later elaboration, the *kaddish* is recited also on the *yahrzeit*, the anniversary of the day of the death, and there are memorial prayers (the *yizkor*) during the important festivals of the liturgical year. The Judaic rites

of burial and mourning have been described as providing an "expression for grief, for strengthening family and community solidarity, honoring God and inculcating the acceptance of His will" (Eckhardt, p. 497).

Ethical rules in death and dying. A third element that was important during the rabbinic period was the formulation of rules of conduct in areas connected with death and dying. We find, for example, a formulation of the definition of death (the cessation of breathing and of the heartbeat); rules concerning the treatment of the fetus threatening the life of its mother (it should be destroyed); and the treatment of the terminally ill. The latter are in no manner to be *actively* deprived of even a moment of life. "The dying person is to be considered as living in all things" (Talmud, Shabbat, 151a). There is indication, however, that it is permissible to remove an "impediment which prevents the soul from leaving the body" (Code of Jewish Law, Yoreh Deah, 339). There is a condemnation of suicide, and persons who "destroy themselves willingly" are not entitled to the dignity of a funeral or mourning. Especially interesting is the stress on the dead as a source of ritual impurity, thus negating pagan notions of the apotheosis of the dead. This is, of course, biblical legislation spelled out in rabbinic codes.

Meaning of death. Fourth, the rabbis speculated as to the reasons why death came into the world. One school of thought held that death was the result of sin. Since there is no righteous man who does not sin, death is universal. Another school of thought believed that death was the natural course of events, reflecting the inevitable cycle of birth, maturity, and decay. The most striking statement expressing this attitude is the comment on Genesis I by the great rabbinic sage, Rabbi Meir, who was a second-century scholar. " 'Behold it was very good'—that refers to death" (Midrash, Bereshet Rabba 9:5). According to both schools, the fear of death is an element of human existence, and its contemplation should guard one from sin. Death for the Sanctification of the Name (martyrdom) was especially praiseworthy.

Post-talmudic period

In the post-talmudic period, two streams of thought expressed the principles of Jewish faith: the mystical school, whose classic work was the *Zohar*, The Book of Splendor, and scholastic philosophy, exemplified by the work of Moses Maimonides (1135–1204).

The mystical school. In the literature of the Jewish mystics there is, of course, an acceptance of the principles of normative Judaism. There is also an acceptance of the idea of the transmigration of soul (*gilgul*) as a form of completion of unfinished earthly tasks or as a form of punishment. In addition, there was the idea of *ibbur* (impregnation) which means the "entry of another soul into a man during his life" (Scholem, p. 348). *Ibbur* of a wicked man into the soul of another man is also called a *dibbuk* (something attached). These unwanted inhabitants could be exorcised only by special formulas. The mystical tendency within Judaism was sensitive to the demonic aspects of existence. This strengthened folk superstitions about the harm that the dead spirits might cause. Customs were added to standard Jewish practices such as covering mirrors in houses of mourning, avoiding cemeteries at special times, and guarding people in special circumstances against possible onslaughts by demons. It was also thought that the dead could intervene on behalf of their relatives and friends. These tendencies were strengthened in areas of Jewish settlement influenced by *hasidism*, a pietistic movement in Eastern Europe beginning in the eighteenth century that based many of its beliefs and customs on mystical teachings. The mystic-hasidic movement also developed extensive and imaginative descriptions of heaven and hell (Scholem).

Scholastic philosophy. The scholastic interpretation of Judaism, whose greatest figure was Moses Maimonides, identified intelligence as the most important part of the soul. It was this part of man which enjoyed eternal bliss, since it was concerned with eternal things, especially the nature of God. This meant that an individual's immortality and his real worth were gauged by the degree to which he had acquired knowledge of eternal truths. Immortality was seen as the soul's vision of God unencumbered by the body. According to Maimonides, the resurrected body would also die, the soul returning to paradise to enjoy the beatific vision of the godhead.

Late medieval times saw the creation of normative codes of Jewish law. The most important of these was that of Moses Maimonides called the *Yad Hachazak* (*Strong Hand*) and that of Rabbi Joseph Caro (1488–1575) entitled the *Shulhan Arukh* ("The Prepared Table"). It is to these works that Jews look for specific guidance as to how to treat the dying, how to relate to the corpse, how to mourn for the dead, obligations for self-sacrifice, etc. These codes together with their commentaries are the authoritative sources for Jewish practice until this day, especially for orthodox and conservative Jews.

Modern period

With the beginning of the modern period, reform movements affected Jewish law, tradition, and theology. There was in these movements little stress on the doctrine of the resurrection of the dead. In some liberal prayer books references to this dogma were removed. The idea of the immortality of the soul was preferred. This was evident in the work of Moses Mendelssohn (1729–1786), the first important Jewish thinker in modern times. The Pittsburgh Platform of the American Reform movement stated: "We reassert the doctrine of Judaism that the soul is immortal, grounding this belief on the divine nature of the human spirit, which forever finds bliss in righteousness and misery in wickedness. We reject as ideas not rooted in Judaism, the beliefs both in bodily resurrection and in *Gehenna* and Eden [hell and paradise] as abodes for everlasting punishment and reward" (Philipson, p. 357). Conservative and Orthodox Judaism retain references to the resurrection of the dead in the liturgy, reserving the right to interpret the doctrine as a symbol for the total salvation in God (both body and soul). The rise of reform Judaism also meant that some of the traditional practices were to be liberalized in the area of autopsies, burial, and mourning customs.

Some of the leading philosophers of contemporary Judaism have discussed the idea of death. Franz Rosensweig (1886–1929) opens his great work, the *Star of Redemption* (1921), with the words: "All cognition of the All originates in death; in the fear of death; and this mortal lives in this fear of death." Abraham Joshua Heschel (1907–1972) sees death as the "ultimate self-dedication to the divine. Death so understood will not be distorted by the craving for immortality, for this act of giving away is reciprocity on man's part for God's gift of life. For the pious man it is a privilege to die" (Riemer, p. 73). Writers such as Will Herberg have been influenced in their view of the doctrine of the resurrection of the dead by the writings of Reinhold Niebuhr. Herberg sees the doctrine as an expression of the basic theological assertion that fulfillment is "not a disembodied soul that has sloughed off the body, but the whole man—body, soul and spirit joined in an indissoluble unity" (Herberg, pp. 229–230).

In contemporary Judaism there is also some concern that Jewish funeral practices have become too elaborate and too expensive. There are calls for a return to the more simple rituals of ancient times.

Summary and conclusions

Several important conclusions emerge from the reflections on death in post-biblical Judaism:

1. There is an emphatic stress on the importance of human life. Therefore, to prolong a human life even for a short while is a good deed. Though death is inevitable, it is seen as an event to be opposed. Therefore, in general, traditional Judaism has been opposed to euthanasia, abortion, and suicide.
2. The dead are to be honored because they once had life. The human body, which houses the immortal soul of man, even when life has ceased, is entitled to be treated with dignity and respect. Therefore, in general, traditional Judaism has been opposed to autopsies for no real purpose, cremation, and displays of the dead.
3. There is emphasis on the reality of death. It is seen as a real event in which the real presence of the dead is removed. There is an emphasis on the communal loss as well as the communal responsibility to help mourners overcome the pain of their loss and to start life again. The dead are really dead. Therefore, they must be mourned and the survivors have to learn to live without them.
4. Yet, there is hope that death is not the end of the human drama. The doctrine of immortality and especially the resurrection of the dead means that humans are responsible for their deeds—a responsibility that will somehow be exacted even after death—but it also means that in God they will find their fulfillment and salvation. The purpose of these doctrines is not to make death easier but to enhance life.

Seymour Siegel

[*Directly related are the entries* Abortion, *article on* Jewish Perspectives; Cadavers, *article on* Jewish Perspectives; Death and Dying: Euthanasia and Sustaining Life, *article on* Ethical Views; Judaism; *and* Suicide. *See* Appendix, Section I, daily prayer of a physician ("prayer of moses maimonides").]

BIBLIOGRAPHY

GENERAL LITERATURE

"Death." *Encyclopaedia Judaica.* 16 vols. New York: Macmillan Co., 1972, vol. 5, pp. 1420–1427.
"Death, Views and Customs Concerning." *The Jewish Encyclopedia.* 12 vols. Edited by Cyrus Adler. New York: Funk & Wagnalls, 1901–1906. New ed. 1925, vol. 4, pp. 482–486.
Eckardt, A. Roy. "Death in the Judaic and Christian Traditions." *Social Research* 39 (1972): 489–514.
Heller, Zachary I. "The Jewish View of Death: Guidelines for Dying." *Death: The Final Stage of Growth.* Edited by Elisabeth [Elizabeth] Kübler-Ross. Englewood Cliffs, N.J.: Prentice-Hall, 1975, pp. 38–43.
Lamm, Maurice. *The Jewish Way in Death and Mourning.* New York: J. David, 1969.
Riemer, Jack, ed. *Jewish Reflections on Death.* Foreword by Elizabeth Kübler-Ross. New York: Schocken Books, 1974.

TALMUDIC PERIOD

Büchler, Adolf. *Studies in Sin and Atonement in the Rabbinic Literature of the First Century* (1928). Library of Biblical Studies. New York: Ktav Publishing House, 1967.
Finkelstein, Louis. *The Pharisees: The Sociological Background of Their Faith.* 3d ed. The Morris Loeb series. Philadelphia: Jewish Publication Society of America, 1962.
Schechter, Solomon. *Some Aspects of Rabbinic Theology.* New York: Macmillan, 1909.
———. *Studies in Judaism.* 3 vols. Philadelphia: Jewish Publication Society, 1896–1924, vol. 1.

MEDIEVAL PERIOD

Scholem, Gershom. *Kabbalah.* Library of Jewish Knowledge. New York: Quadrangle/ New York Times Book Co., 1974.
Trachtenberg, Joshua. *Jewish Magic and Superstition: A Study in Folk Religion.* Meridian Books and the Jewish Publication Society, no. 33. Cleveland: World Publishing Co., 1961.
Twersky, Isadore, ed. *A Maimonides Reader.* Library of Jewish Studies. New York: Behrman House, 1972.

MODERN PERIOD

Herberg, Will. *Judaism and Modern Man: An Interpretation of Jewish Religion.* Jewish Publication Society series, no. JP10. New York: Meridian Books, 1960.
Philipson, David. *The Reform Movement in Judaism.* Rev. ed. New York: Macmillan Co., 1931.

3

POST-BIBLICAL CHRISTIAN THOUGHT

Historians and theologians have sometimes called the twentieth century the "post-Christian" age, implying that Christian institutions and values have ceased to play a normative role in contemporary civilization. Arguable though this view may be, it is nevertheless true that positions popularly perceived to represent the tradition of Christian teaching have influenced debate in such areas of practical and theoretical bioethical concern as the definition of death, the propriety of life support for the terminally ill, and euthanasia. In fact, Christian theology has had little to say about death as a biological phenomenon. It has, however, been deeply concerned with the problem of the destiny of humanity, the fulfillment of the yearning for perfection of both the individual and the social order—and in this context the theological tradition has had much to say concerning the meaning of individual life and human history. This fulfillment has been discussed in terms transcending historical life. Thus, questions concerning the meaning of death in Christian thought have arisen largely in the context of discussions of (1) a postmortem destiny for the person and (2) the future of the Christian community.

The common modern assumption, both lay and clerical, has been that the immortality of the soul is a fundamental aspect of Christian doctrinal and credal development. Recent scholarship on biblical and post-biblical thought agrees, however, that the matter is very complex. The basic biblical concept is the resurrection of the body at the end of history (the "Last Times"), a doctrine that does not necessarily imply an active afterlife between death and the resurrection or inauguration of the Kingdom of God. Against this is set the doctrine of immortality, which presupposes an active afterlife for the disembodied soul. Some proponents of immortality have seen it as only filling the interim between death and resurrection; others have virtually assimilated resurrection within the concept of immortality. A sketch of the history of Christian eschatology must, therefore, be an account of the developments of these often polarized views. (By "eschatology," theologians mean both the vision of the consummation of history in the Last Times and the group of doctrines treating the destiny of the person from death through the Last Judgment.)

Early Christian thought

In the Judaic tradition, man was viewed as a unity whose death was regarded as a natural and, usually, final phenomenon. By New Testament times two developments had modified this ancient tradition. One was the indigenous development of apocalypticism and the related doctrine of the resurrection of the body, which formed an important element in the teaching of Jesus. This was basically a political—and certainly a corporate—doctrine arising from the yearnings of the people: In the fullness of his time God would gather his people—raising their dry bones—to participate in his fulfilled, perfect reign. The second development arose from contact with Hellenistic religious and philosophical notions of immortality. The Hellenistic notion

of immortality was that man's soul is released by death from the body, from entrapment in time and space. The most extreme version of the doctrine was the Neoplatonist teaching that the soul is an emanation of the One and thus is eternal in the senses of both preexistence and continuing existence.

So pervasive and common were the notions of the separability of soul and body and of the body's inferiority to the soul in the Hellenistic world to which the Gentile mission of the primitive Church was sent that it was inevitable some accommodation (linguistic, at least, if not conceptual) would have to be made to the doctrine of the soul and its immortality. Thus the basic traditional Christian definition of death as the separation of body and soul is as old as are investigations in the philosophical vein of the nature of the soul. The soul is often conceived as the divine element in the human and, hence, the object of salvation.

Yet the Church Fathers were reluctant in the extreme to speculate on the nature of the soul's existence following death or even to posit for it a conscious or active existence. For example, Irenaeus of Lyons in the second century speaks of the soul as waiting for the apocalypse of the Last Judgment in an "invisible place" and in an inactive state (*Against Heresies* V, 31). It was sometimes said the martyrs constituted an exceptional class whose souls might not have to await the resurrection to enjoy communion with the godhead. However, the generally conservative view of the postmortem destiny of the individual grounded in Hebrew apocalyptic literature continued to hold sway at the same time as room was made to accommodate the concept of a soul and the custom of prayers for the dead. Gregory of Nyssa, in *On the Soul and the Resurrection* (380?), may exemplify this continuity among the Greek fathers. The soul is the divine or immortal element in man; yet it "exists in the actual atoms" it animates. There is no cause to speculate on the locus of the soul after death, although (metaphorically) it can be said to tend to be drawn toward evil or good according to patterns set during life. Conscious of the writings of Plato and of the platonic tradition, Gregory nevertheless maintained that body and soul cannot fully exist in isolation from each other: The postmortem interim is primarily to be characterized as a period of waiting for their reunion at the resurrection.

The Latin or Western Fathers continue the same kinds of teaching. Augustine's early works (e.g., *Soliloquies*) are often regarded as Neoplatonic exercises on the nature of the soul and its knowledge of God. Yet Augustine broke off the *Soliloquies* before he got to the question of the nature of the soul's postmortem knowledge. His related and contemporary treatise, *On the Immortality of the Soul*, he himself later found uselessly obscure, and it is evasive on this issue. The letter (No. 147) on *The Vision of God* treats of the postresurrection knowledge of the godhead; and the great treatment of the subject is *The City of God*, in which Augustine is primarily concerned with the problem of history and its consummation.

Later theologians often pointed to the *Dialogues* of Gregory the Great (Pope, 590–604) as a locus classicus for the notion that the soul may undergo purgation after death, while it continues its active existence in the interim between the separation of body and soul and their reunion. Gregory deals in this work with the problem of miracles as signs of sanctity and with the nature of the contemplative (or monastic) life; and ultimately his concern is with miracles and visions of the afterlife as signs of sanctity. For Gregory, the souls of the perfect (as, for earlier writers, the souls of the martyrs) enjoy immediate beatification. There are no grounds to suppose, however, that the Pope does more than allow the possibility that divine judgment *may* be meted out in the period between death and the resurrection. Gregory is a great exponent of the biblical doctrine of eschatology; and in the sermons on the Gospels and other works, the emphasis is clearly on the consummation of all things and reunion of the soul and body.

Medieval developments

The same may be said of most theologians of the early Middle Ages (to approximately A.D. 1100). Nevertheless, the possibilities for an active postmortem existence inherent in the doctrine of the immortality of the soul did not go unnoticed. Many of the documents of the Apocryphal New Testament (i.e., writings with some claim to apostolic authority but rejected in the process of formation of the New Testament canon because they were of spurious authorship and questionable orthodoxy) pictured the soul (whether metaphorically or literally is often difficult to say) as having an active existence after death. The *Vision of Paul* is a particularly influential item in this group and is often regarded as an important source for Dante's *Divine Comedy*.

From it comes, for example, the tradition that the soul returns periodically to the body to castigate or to praise the body for the state the soul currently endures or enjoys; and from it descends likewise a tradition, in Latin and the Western vernacular languages, of the soul's didactic addresses to the body or of debates between the two.

The state of the question of the afterlife in the later Middle Ages is extremely complex. One possible generalization is that academic or scholastic theology absorbed the notion of an active afterlife for the soul into the doctrine of penance. At the same time, traditional eschatology and its literary topics continued to circulate widely, especially in popular and Benedictine monastic theology. Thus in the fourteenth and fifteenth centuries one continues to find corporate, communal, heroic Christology and eschatology in such more "popular" works as Langland's *Piers Ploughman* and the medieval drama, even while a more individualized eschatology and doctrine of the soul achieved dominance in works emanating from the universities and the mendicant orders. Meanwhile, however, didactic *exempla* (cautionary and exemplary narratives) of the soul's continued active existence had also permeated popular theology with what often seems to us a gruesome preoccupation with the morbid and with the corruptibility of the body. As Ariès has argued, this phenomenon probably reflects not so much a devaluation of life in the world or of the body as the realization that because life is short each moment of it is urgent in fixing one's eternal destiny and is to be highly valued.

For an appreciation of later developments in both Catholic and Protestant theology, it is necessary to dwell briefly on the development of the doctrine of purgatory within the framework of the teaching about penance and on the implications of this development for the notion of an active afterlife between death and the resurrection of the Last Day. In the social (feudal) metaphor for the work of Christ that became dominant with Anselm's *Cur Deus Homo?* (1097), mankind owed God so enormous a satisfaction or compensatory payment for unlawfulness or sinful breach of the covenantal relationship between creator and creature that only God himself in Christ could pay it. After Christ's atonement (or, for the individual, after baptism), the individual was responsible for new breaches. These penalties could be worked off on the basis of penances imposed by the Church in the penitential discipline. Should the penitent die before completing this task, or should the penance be imposed at confession at the point of death, it was conceived that postmortem purgation was allowed. Hence (in large part) the doctrine of purgatory and the notion of suffering were emphasized in discussion of the period following separation of body and soul; concomitantly, active bliss was posited for those who had no penance to complete or had already completed it; and it was argued the temporal church might grant postmortem mitigation of temporal penalties. These developments contributed materially to the shift in emphasis in Christian thought from the resurrection of the Last Times as inaugurating active future life to the fate of the soul between death and the resurrection. A judgment of the individual soul was said to take place at the instant of its separation from the body.

The great work of Thomas Aquinas illustrates this development. For Thomas, the resurrection and Last Judgment remain the necessary culmination of the history of the race and the individual; but primary interest is centered on the soul, the form of the body, which must, in the light of God's justice, receive merited reward as well as merited punishment. Thus the developments after the reunion of body and soul at the resurrection will confirm a judgment and state of being that essentially date from the moment of death—the only change being that some souls will have completed temporal purgation in this period.

Trends in modern Christian thought

One of the major theses of the Protestant reaction was against the excesses of the penitential doctrine of purgatory. Luther, Calvin, and other Reformers were still late medieval theologians, however; and although purgatory was anathema to them and their successors, increased emphasis on the afterlife of the soul before the resurrection remained characteristic of Protestant as well as of Catholic theology in the sixteenth century. For Calvin, for example, Christ's satisfaction for mankind's sins is absolutely sufficient; thus purgatory is unnecessary. But from the earliest versions of the *Institutes*, the immortality of the soul is "beyond controversy" for Calvin, and immortality seems to have greater force as the image of the postmortem destiny of humans than does resurrection. Thus both Catholic and Protestant theology entered the modern period with the idea of resurrection, the ancient corner-

stone of Christian eschatological teaching, retaining only a vestigial or metaphorical place in the theological system. The notion of an active postmortem existence enjoyed by far the greater prominence. (The sociological correlatives of these phenomena are well discussed by Ariès.)

The situation depicted above tended to persist in the modern period. Catholic theology from the Council of Trent (1545–1563) through the neo-Thomist period of the twentieth century followed approximately what was understood to be the position of Thomas Aquinas; and Protestant theology through neo-orthodoxy was based on the outlines laid down by the Reformers. Perhaps the greatest influence on both, but most especially the Protestants, was the rise of empiricism in the seventeenth century. For the empiricist, that which is true is that which is authenticated only by experience; and even revelation is an individual and subjective experience. The apocalyptic eschatology of early and medieval Christianity became an embarrassment, and more and more a spiritualized picture of the disembodied soul in the immediate afterlife took its place. Often the issue of divine judgment was evaded in "liberal" circles.

Not until the twentieth century has a sense of biblical eschatology been regained. At present, historical scholars generally agree that any Christian doctrine of immortality ought to be tempered in the light of the more community- and judgment-oriented eschatology of the earlier centuries, but there has been a general failure to communicate this consensus widely in the lay community. It might further be generalized that those who are more concerned with the state of the individual tend to emphasize immortality in their discussions of eschatology, and those more concerned with the social implications of Christianity tend to find the apocalyptic picture of the redeemed community gathered at the resurrection more meaningful.

Conclusions and observations

Recent studies in the history of Christian eschatology perhaps have not been adequately assimilated by students of Christian ethics, who have increasingly been drawn into debate on bioethical issues. This may be in part because discussion of the dogmatic problem of immortality and resurrection seemingly complicates the issues and in part because issues touching the problem of afterlife (even if viewed only metaphorically) are uncomfortable in the contemporary intellectual milieu. Yet eschatology, the doctrine of hope (together with the doctrine of Christ, which is the basic substance of Christian faith), is the basis and sanction for Christian ethics, the doctrine of love. The tenacity with which common opinion holds to what seems to many in academic theological circles a questionable view of the centrality of immortality and the active afterlife immediately following death is at the core of most difficulties concerning the Christian view of death. In order to address the bioethical implications of Christian ethics, it is necessary first to attempt to reconcile the apparent conflict between immortality, with its emphasis on the destiny of the individual, and resurrection, with its stress on the destiny of the community. The values of both views ought to be weighed carefully.

Regarding such matters as the definition of physical death, there seems little in theological reflection on the subject that helps or hinders in the determination of the moment at which what has been called the separation of body and soul occurs. In discussions of "death with dignity," Christian ethical thought should have suggestions to offer with an eye to reconciling the conflicts between the needs of the individual, the requirements of society, and the traditions of professional medical ethics. Death will always be a fearful event for the dying, their friends, and those who minister to them. There is now a widespread recognition that ethical concerns surrounding death should be faced and discussed rather than evaded, as they have tended to be since the rise of modern medicine and the transfer of care for the dying in urban society from home, church, and family to professional institutions and professional persons. Christian ethics needs to come to terms with Christian eschatology in order to help frame new and helpfully realistic approaches to care for the dying and to the new bioethical issues raised by modern research and applied medicine.

In the past, Christian thought has valued life in the world as the arena in which humanity's yearning and struggle for redemption are worked out. The moment of death thus has been one for assessment or judgment of the individual's contribution to that struggle. At best, Christian theology has reflected on death so as to emphasize the importance of life in the great drama of salvation. Some would say that, at its worst, Christian teaching has seemed to imply that worldly life—in contrast with the ultimate goal of beatific vision—is a status without value from which death is a release. Perhaps the most needed contribution of Christian ethics is to communicate more widely that Christian thought on death is neither so simple nor so "dogmatic" as it is sometimes perceived to be.

MILTON McC. GATCH

[*Directly related are the two preceding articles,* DEATH IN BIBLICAL THOUGHT *and* POST-BIBLICAL JEWISH TRADITION, *and the following article on* ARS MORIENDI. *For discussion of related ideas, see:* PAIN AND SUFFERING, *article on* RELIGIOUS PERSPECTIVES.]

BIBLIOGRAPHY

ARIÈS, PHILIPPE. *Western Attitudes toward Death: From the Middle Ages to the Present.* Translated by Patricia M. Ranum. Johns Hopkins Symposia in Comparative History. Baltimore: Johns Hopkins University Press, 1974.

BOASE, THOMAS SHERRER ROSS. *Death in the Middle Ages: Mortality, Judgement, and Remembrance.* Library of Medieval Civilization. New York: McGraw-Hill, 1972. Collects material from the iconography of medieval churches, manuscripts, and funerary monuments to illustrate both the learned and the popular theological traditions.

CHORON, JACQUES. *Death and Western Thought.* New York: Collier Books, 1963. More philosophical than theological in its focus, but a useful survey.

FROOM, LE ROY EDWIN. *The Prophetic Faith of Our Fathers: The Historical Development of Prophetic Interpretation.* 4 vols. Washington: Review & Herald, 1950–1954. Written from the point of view of the tradition that seeks clues in history and scripture to the approach of the Last Times, but a mine of information on the history of apocalyptic thought.

GATCH, MILTON McC. *Death: Meaning and Mortality in Christian Thought and Contemporary Culture.* New York: Seabury Press, 1969.

———. "Some Theological Reflections on Death from the Early Church through the Reformation." *Perspectives on Death.* Edited by Liston O. Mills. Nashville: Abingdon Press, 1969, chap. 3, pp. 99–136.

RAHNER, KARL. *On the Theology of Death.* Translated by Charles H. Henkey. Quaestiones disputatae, no. 2. New York: Herder & Herder, 1961. 2d ed. Freiburg: Herder; London: Burns & Oates, 1965. Very influential modern Catholic essay.

STENDAHL, KRISTER, ed. *Immortality and Resurrection: Four Essays.* Ingersoll Lectures, Harvard University, 1955–1959. New York: Macmillan, 1965.

4
ARS MORIENDI

Ars moriendi, or *The Art of Dying,* identifies an important subgenre of later medieval conduct literature. Like similar treatises on courtesy, courtship, education, recreation, and warfare, these little manuals on dying were meant to guide the reader's behavior on an occasion of some importance to him. Today, about three hundred manuscripts of the *Ars moriendi* survive along with a hundred or so incunabula, including both block-books and editions printed in movable type. The best evidence indicates that the first woodcut edition appeared by 1465, and the fact that some twenty percent of all surviving block-books are *Artes moriendi* is enough to show the extraordinary importance of these books for the history of early printing. Both Latin and vernacular texts (in seven modern languages, eventually) had appeared in both woodcut and printed form by 1475.

The *Ars moriendi* occurs in a longer and a shorter version. Almost all the manuscripts, the majority of the vernacular texts, and most of the typographic editions are of the longer version, which is divided into six sections: (1) a miscellany of quotations on death from Christian authorities; (2) advice to the dying man (*Moriens*) on overcoming temptations to faithlessness, despair, impatience, pride, and worldliness; (3) catechetical questions whose correct answers lead to salvation; (4) prayers and rules for imitating the dying Christ; (5) advice to persons attending the dying man; (6) prayers to be said by the attendants.

The shorter *Ars moriendi* seems to be an abridged derivative of the longer, which is about triple its size. The smaller work occurs in almost all the woodcut editions. A brief introduction and conclusion summarize the material contained in sections 1, 3, 4, and 5 of the longer version. The body of the shorter version corresponds to section 2 of the longer, but this material is transformed and dramatized as a *psychomachia*, a struggle between good and bad angels for the dying man's soul. *Moriens* must choose either the five vices mentioned in the longer text or their contrary virtues: faith, hope, love, humility, and detachment. In a shorter *Ars moriendi* eleven striking woodcuts in a fifteenth-century Flemish style illustrate the fight against temptation: five cuts for the virtues, five for the vices, and one for the eventual delivery of *Moriens*'s soul to the good angel.

The origins of the *Ars moriendi* are in the compendia of piety and doctrine that appeared when later medieval Church councils took steps to educate the laity in the fundamentals of Christianity. Jean Gerson's *Opus tripartitum* (before 1408) grew out of such concerns, and the third part of this work, titled *De arte moriendi*, is the source of much of the *Ars moriendi*. Other important sources are to be found in the Bible, the Fathers, medieval liturgies, papal and conciliar statements, medieval patristic collections, and later medieval devotional and doctrinal literature. The authorship of the *Ars moriendi* remains in doubt, but there is good reason to locate its composition in southern Germany, at the time of the Council of Constance (1414–1418), and with the Dominican Order.

Both the fifth section of the longer *Ars moriendi* and Gerson's *De arte moriendi* advise those who attend the dying man not to give him false hopes of regaining the health of his body. This is a commentary not only on the state of medicine in the later Middle Ages and on contemporary attitudes toward it but also on the Christian understanding of the death of the body. Since death was a beginning, not an end, there was no reason to take heroic measures to postpone it. Innocent III, whose decretals also found their way into the Ars moriendi, warned that none were to administer bodily medicine to *Moriens* until the ills of his soul had been cared for. The antecedents of this attitude are as old as Plato (*Charmides* 156–157) and the Gospels (Matt. 8:5–13; John 5:1–14).

The woodcut that depicts *Moriens*'s being tempted against faith also sets deathbed medicine in a problematic light. Three learned men, apparently physicians, stand in consultation at *Moriens*'s right while a demon points at them and whispers the words *"infernus factus est"* into the dying man's ear. Since the context of this illustration is the temptation against faith, and since other figures in it represent idolatry, suicide, and other errors, some authorities have concluded that the three figures in question are not physicians but heretics. If so, the demon who says "hell has been prepared" would be warning *Moriens* against the sin of heresy—hardly a typical concern for a dying Christian and, in any event, not the sort of advice a demon ought to be giving. In light of what the *Ars moriendi* says elsewhere about corporeal medicine, it is more likely that the demon is enticing *Moriens* into the error of caring for his physical health just at the moment when spiritual health ought to be his chief concern. The demon raises the prospect of damnation in order to frighten *Moriens* away from a good Christian death.

Johan Huizinga and other authorities have mentioned the *Ars moriendi* in the same breath with the *danse macabre*, plague books, grisly funerary art, and other manifestations of an obsession with death in the later Middle Ages, an obsession consequent, perhaps, upon the great plague, which arrived in Europe in 1348 and recurred for several centuries. While the great popularity of the *Ars moriendi* may support such a view, its contents generally do not. True, crowds of demons populate its woodcuts, and its *Moriens* looks like a dying man, but on the whole there is little of the macabre in the advice the *Ars moriendi* gives. Its purpose was not to terrorize but to point the way to a good death. It ended in the expectation of heaven, not with the horrors of hell.

For a society whose members viewed death as a passage to an afterlife, a manual on the art of dying had an eminently practical function. The recent tendency to see the *Ars moriendi* as a feature of a necrophile culture may tell us more about modern anxieties than about medieval attitudes.

BRIAN P. COPENHAVER

[*Other relevant material may be found under* DEATH, ATTITUDES TOWARD.]

BIBLIOGRAPHY

BOASE, THOMAS SHERRER ROSS. *Death in the Middle Ages: Mortality, Judgment, and Remembrance.* Library of Medieval Civilization. London: Thames & Hudson; New York: McGraw-Hill, 1972.

HUIZINGA, JOHAN. *The Waning of the Middle Ages: A Study of the Forms of Life, Thought and Art in France and the Netherlands in the XIVth and XVth Centuries.* Translated by F. Hopman. New York: Longmans, Green, 1949.

O'CONNOR, MARY CATHARINE. *The Art of Dying Well: The Development of the Ars moriendi.* Columbia University Studies in English and Comparative Literature, no. 156. New York: Columbia University Press, 1942. Still the fundamental work.

V

DEATH IN THE WESTERN WORLD

Death has been a "fact of life" for as long as humans can remember, but this in no way puts to rest their struggle to understand its meaning. Some conceptualization, beyond common sense, of a human individual or "person" is necessary in order to understand the problematic of death. Therefore, a few comments on this topic are in order before proceeding to a reflection on some of the more salient features of death as it has been understood in the Western world.

The person and the problematic of death

The human individual has often been viewed in the Western world as a synthesized combination of a living organism and a "personality system" (an older terminology made the person a combination of "body" and "mind" or "soul").

It is in fact no more mystical to conceive of a personality *analytically* distinct from an organism than it is to conceive of a "culture" distinct from the human populations of organisms who are its bearers. The primary criterion of personality, as distinct from organism, is an organization in terms of symbols and their meaningful relations to each other and to persons.

Human individuals, in their organic aspect, come into being through a process of bisexual reproduction. They then go through a more or less well-defined "life course" and eventually die. That human individuals die as organisms is indisputable. If any biological proposition can be regarded as firmly established, it is that the mortality of individual organisms of a sexually reproducing species is completely normal. The death of individuals has indeed a positive survival value for the species.

As Freud said, organic death, while a many-faceted thing, is in one principal aspect the "return to the inorganic state." At this level the human organism is "made up" of inorganic materials but is organized in quite special ways. When that organization breaks down—and there is evidence that this is inevitable by reason of the "aging process"—the constituent elements are no longer part of the living organism but come to be assimilated to the inorganic environment. Still, even within such a perspective on the human individual as an organism, life "goes on." The human individual does not stand alone but is part of an intergenerational chain of indefinite durability, the species. The individual organism dies, but if he or she reproduces the "line" continues into future generations.

But the problematic of human death arises from the fact that the human individual is not only an organism but also a user of symbols, who learns symbolic meanings, communicates with others and with himself through them as media, and regulates his behavior, thought, and feelings in symbolic terms. He is an "actor" or a "personality." The human "actor" clearly is not born in the same sense in which an organism is. The personality or actor comes into being through a gradual and complicated process sometimes termed "socialization."

Furthermore, there is a parallel—in my judgment, something more than a mere "analogy"—between the continuity of the "actor" and that of the organism. Just as there is an intergenerational continuity on the organic side, so is there an intergenerational continuity on the personality or action side of the human individual. An individual personality is "generated" in symbiosis with a growing individual organism and, for all we know, "dies" with that organism. But the individual personality is embedded in trans-individual action systems, both social and cultural. Thus the sociocultural "matrix" in which the individual personality is embedded is in an important sense the counterpart of the population–species matrix in which the individual organism is embedded. The individual personality "dies," but the society and cultural system, of which in life he or she was a part, goes on.

But what is it that happens when the personality "dies"? Is the death of a personality to be simply assimilated to the organic paradigm? It would seem that the answer is yes, for just as no personality in the human sense can be conceived as such to develop independently of a living organism, so no human personality can be conceived as such to survive the death of the same organism. Nevertheless, the personality or "actor" certainly influences what happens in the organism—as suicide and all sorts of "psychic" factors in illnesses and deaths bear witness. Thus, although most positivists and materialists would affirm that the death of the personality must be viewed strictly according to the organic paradigm, this answer to the problem of human death has not been accepted by the majority in most human societies and cultures. From such primitive peoples as the Australian aborigines to the most sophisticated of the world religions, beliefs in the existence of an individual "soul" have persisted, conceivably with a capacity both to antedate and to survive the individual organism or body. The persistence of that belief and the factors giving rise to it provide the framework for the problematic of death in the Western world.

Christian orientations toward death

Because the dominant religious influence in the history of the Western world has been that of Christianity, it is appropriate to outline the main Christian patterns of orientation toward death.

There is no doubt of the predominance of a duality of levels in the Christian paradigm of the human condition, the levels of the spiritual and the material, the eternal and the temporal. On the one hand, there is the material-temporal world, of which one religious symbol is the "dust" to which man is said to return at death. On the other hand, there is the spiritual world of "eternal life," which is the location of things divine, not human. The human person stands at the meeting of the two worlds, for he is, like the animals, made of "dust," but he is also, unlike the animals, made in the image of God. This biblical notion of man, when linked to Greek philosophical thought, gave rise to the idea in Catholic Christianity that the divine image was centered in the human "soul," which was conceived as in some sense an "emanation" from the spiritual world of eternal life. Thus arose the notion of the "immortal soul," which could survive the death of the organism, to be rejoined to a "resurrected" body. The hope of the resurrection, rooted in the Easter faith of the Christian community, was from the beginning a part of the Christian faith and provided another dimension behind the teaching on the immortality of the "soul."

The Christian understanding of death as an event in which "life is changed, not taken away" in the words of the traditional requiem hymn, *Dies Irae*, can be interpreted in terms of Marcel Mauss's paradigm of the gift and its reciprocation (Parsons, Fox, and Lidz). Seen in this way the life of the individual is a gift from God, and like other gifts it creates expectations of reciprocation. Living "in the faith" is part of the reciprocation, but, more important to us, dying in the faith completes the cycle. By the doctrine of reciprocation mankind assumes, it may be said, three principal obligations, namely, to "accept" the human condition as ordained by the Divine Will, to live in the faith, and to die in the faith—and to die in the faith means to die with the hope of resurrection. If these conditions are fulfilled, "salvation," life eternal with God, will come about.

This basically was the paradigm of death in Catholic Christianity. Although the Reformation did "collapse" some elements in the Catholic paradigm of dualism between the eternal and the temporal, it did not as such alter fundamentally the meaning of death in societies shaped by the Christian faith. Still, the collapse of the Catholic paradigm did put great pressures on the received doctrine of salvation. The promise of a *personal* "eternal life" became increasingly difficult to accept, and the doctrine of eternal punishment in "hell" proved even more difficult to uphold.

The conception of a "higher" level of reality, a "supernatural" world in which human persons survived after death, did not give way but became more and more difficult to "visualize" (along with the meaning of death as an event in which one gave life back to its Giver and in return was initiated into a new and eternal life) by simple extrapolation from this-worldly experience. In addition to the changes in conceptualization set in motion by the Reformation, the rise of modern science, which by the eighteenth century had produced a philosophy of scientific "materialism," posed an additional challenge to the Christian paradigm of death, manifesting itself primarily in a "monism" of the physical world. There was at that time little "scientific" analysis of the world of action, and there was accordingly a tendency to regard the physical universe as unchanging and hence eternal. Death then was simply the return to the inorganic state, which implied a complete negation of the conception of "eternal life," since the physical, inorganic world was by definition the antithesis of life in any sense.

Contemporary scientific orientations

The subsequent development of science has, however, modified or at least brought into question the monistic and materialistic paradigm generated by the early enthusiasm for a purely positivistic approach. For one thing, beginning in the nineteenth century and continuing into the twentieth the sciences of organic life have matured, thanks largely to placing the conception of evolutionary change at the very center of biological thought. This resulted in the view, which we have already noted, that death is biologically normal for individual members of evolving species.

A second and more recent development has been the maturing of the sciences of *action*. Although these have historical roots in the "humanistic" tradition, they have only recently been differentiated from the humanistic trunk to become generalizing *sciences*, integrating within themselves the same conception of evolutionary change that has become the hallmark of the sciences of life.

The development of the action sciences has given rise, as already noted, to a viable conception of the human person as *analytically* distinct from the organism. At the same time these sciences, by inserting the person into an evolutionary sociocultural matrix analogous to the physico-organic species matrix within which the individual organism is embedded, have been able to create an intellectual framework within which the death of the personality can be understood to be as normal as the death of the organism.

Finally, the concept of evolutionary change has been extended from the fields of the life sciences (concerned with the organism) and of the action sciences (concerned with the person-actor) to include the *whole* of empirical reality, and *at the same time* we have been made aware —principally by the ways in which Einstein's theory of relativity modified the previous assumptions of the absolute empirical "givenness" of physical nature in the Newtonian tradition— of the *relative* character of our human understanding of the human condition.

Thus there is now a serious questioning of absolutes, both in our search for absolutely universal laws of physical nature and in our quest for "metaphysical" absolutes in the philosophical wake of Christian theology.

The Kantian impact and the limits of understanding

The developments in a contemporary scientific understanding of the human condition are both congruent with and in part anticipated and influenced by Kant, whose work during the late eighteenth century was the decisive turning point away from both physical and "metaphysical" absolutism. Kant basically accepted the reality of the physical universe, as it is humanly known, but at the same time he "relativized" our knowledge of it to the categories of the understanding, which were not grounded in our direct "experience" of physical reality but in something "transcending" this. At the same time Kant equally relativized our conceptions of "transcendental" reality, whose existence he by no means denied, to something closer to the human condition. Indeed, it may be suggested that Kant substituted "procedural" conceptions of the "absolute," whether physical or "metaphysical," for "substantive" propositions.

While relativizing our knowledge both of the physical world, including the individual human organism, and of the "metaphysical" world, with its certitude about the immortality of the soul, Kant nonetheless insisted on a transcendental component in human understanding and explicitly included belief in personal immortality in the sense of eternal life.

With respect to the bearing of Kant's thought and its influence through subsequent culture on the problem of the meaning of death, I have already noted that he prepared the way, procedurally, for the development of the action sciences and their ability to account intellectually for the personality or "actor" experienced as one aspect of the human individual without the need to infer, of necessity, the existence of a spiritual soul existentially and not merely analytically distinct from the living organism. The action sciences, in a very real sense, attempt to provide a coherent account of human "subjectivity," much as Kant himself attempted to do in his *Critique of Judgment,* without "collapsing" the difference of levels between the physical and what may be called the "telic" realm.

The framework provided by Kant's thought is indeed congenial to the scientific perspective on the normality of the death of a person, conceived as an actor whose coming into existence is in symbiosis with a growing individual organism and whose individual personality, while continuing into a new generation in the same sociocultural system, can be understood to "die" in symbiosis with the same organism. Nonetheless, if Kant was right in refusing to collapse the boundaries of the human condition into the one vis-à-vis the physical world, the meaning of human individual death can no more be exhausted by that of the involvement of the human individual in a sociocultural system of more comprehensive temporal duration than can the meaning of our sensory experience of empirical reality be exhausted by the "impressions" emanating from that external world, or even the theoretical ordering of those impressions.

If Kant's fundamental position is accepted, then his skepticism about absolutes must apply to both sides of the fundamental dichotomy. Modern biology certainly must be classed as knowledege of the empirical world in his sense, and the same is true of our scientific knowledge of human action. In his famous terminology, there is no demonstrable knowledge of the thing in itself in *any* scientific field.

In empirical terms organic death is completely normal. We have, and acording to Kant we presumably can have, no knowledge of the survival of any organic entity after death except through the processes of organic reproduction, through which the genetic heritage does survive. Kant, however, would equally deny that such survival can be excluded on empirical grounds. This has an obvious bearing on the Christian doctrine of the resurrection of the body. If that is meant in a literal biological sense (though this is by no means universally the way in which Christians understand it), then the inference is clearly that it can never be proved, but it can still be "speculated" about and can be a matter of "faith," even though it cannot be the object of either philosophical or scientific demonstration.

The same seems to hold for the personality-action component of the human individual. Empirically, the action sciences can account for its coming-to-be and its demise without postulating its survival. But neither can they exclude the possibility of such survival. Thus the "eternal life" of the individual soul, although metaphysically unknowable, can, like resurrected bodies, be speculated about and believed in as a matter of "faith."

Thus, included in the victims of Kant's skepticism or relativization is belief in the cognitive *necessity* of belief in the survival of human individuality after death as well as belief in the cognitive *necessity* of belief in the nonsurvival of human individuality after death. Kant's relativization of our knowledge, both empirical and metaphysical, both closed and opened doors. It did, of course, undermine the traditional specificities of received beliefs; but at the same time and for the very same reason it opened the door, by contrast to scientific materialism, not merely to one alternative to received Christian belief but to a multiplicity of them.

This leaves us with the position that the problem of the meaning of death in the Western tradition has, from a position of relative closure defined by the Christian syndrome, been "opened up" in its recent phase. There is above all a new freedom for individuals and sociocultural movements to "try their hands" at innovative definitions and conceptions. At the same time, the "viability" of their innovations is subject to the constraints of the human condition, both empirical and transcendental, noted by Kant.

The problem of the meaning of death in the West is now in what must appear to many to be a strangely unsatisfactory state. It seems to come down to the proposition that the meaning of death is that, in the human condition, it cannot have any "apodictically certain" meaning without abridgement of the essential human freedom of thought, experience, and imagination. Within limits, its meaning, as it is thought about, experienced for the case of others, and anticipated for oneself, must be autonomously interpreted. But this is not pure negativism or nihilism, because such openness is not the same as declaring death, and of course with it individual life, to be "meaningless."

Conclusion

Insofar as it is accessible to cognitive understanding at all, the problem of the meaning of death for individual human beings must be approached in the framework of the human condition as a whole. It must include both the relevant scientific understanding and understanding at philosophical levels, and must attempt to synthesize them. Finally it must, as clearly as possible, recognize and take account of the limits of both our scientific and our philosophical understanding.

If the account provided in the preceding sections is a correct appraisal of the situation in the Western world today, it is not surprising that there is a great deal of bafflement, anxiety, and indeed downright confusion in contemporary attitudes and opinions in this area. Any consensus about the meaning of death in the Western world today seems far off, although the attitude reflected in this article would seem to be the one most firmly established at philosophical levels and the level of rather abstract scientific theory.

A very brief discussion of three empirical points may help, however, to mitigate the impression of extreme abstractness. First, though scientific evidence has established the fact of the inevitability of death with increasing clarity, this does not mean that the *experience* of death by human populations may not change with changing circumstances. Thus, we may distinguish between inevitable death and "adventitious" death, that is, deaths that are "premature" relative to the full life span, and in principle preventable by human action (Parsons and Lidz). Within the last century and a half or so, this latter category of deaths has decreased enormously. The proportion of persons in modern populations over sixty-five has thus increased greatly, as has the expectancy of life at birth. This clearly means that a greatly increased proportion of modern humans approximate to living out a full life course, rather than dying prematurely. Persons living to "a ripe old age" will have experienced an inevitably larger number of deaths of other persons who were important to them. These will be in decreasing number the deaths of persons younger than themselves, notably their own children, and increasingly deaths of their parents and whole ranges of persons of an older generation, such as teachers, senior occupational associates, and many public figures. Quite clearly these demographic changes will have a strong effect on the balance of experience and expectations, of the deaths of significant others, and of anticipation of one's own death.

Second, one of the centrally important aspects

of a process of change in orientation of the sort described should be the appearance of signs of the differentiation of attitudes and conceptions with regard to the meaning of the life cycle. There has indeed already been such a process of differentiation, apparently not yet completed, with respect to both ends of the life cycle (Parsons, Fox, and Lidz). With respect to the beginning, of course, this centers on the controversy over the legitimacy of abortion and the beginning of life. And concomitant with this controversy has been an attempt at redefinition of death. So far the most important movement has been to draw a line *within* the organic sector between what has been called "brain death," where irreversible changes have taken place, destroying the functioning of the central nervous system, and what has been called "metabolic death," where, above all, the functions of heartbeat and respiration have ceased. The problem has been highlighted by the capacity of artificial measures to keep a person "alive" for long periods after the irreversible cessation of brain function. The main point of interest here is the connection of brain function with the personality level of individuality. An organism that continues to "live" at only the metabolic level may be said to be dead as an actor or person.

Third, and finally, a few remarks about the significance for our problem of Freud's most mature theoretical statement need to be made. It was printed in the monograph published in English under the title the *Problem of Anxiety*. In this, his last major theoretical work, Freud rather drastically revised his previous views about the nature of anxiety. He focused on the expectation of the loss of an "object." For Freud the relevant meaning of the term "object" was a human individual standing in an emotionally significant relation to the person of reference. To the growing child, of course, his parents became "lost objects" in the nature of the process of growing up, in that their significance for the growing child was inevitably "lost" at later ages. The ultimate loss of a concrete human person as object—of cathexis, Freud said—is the death of that person. To have "grown away" from one's parents is one thing, but to experience their actual deaths is another. Freud's own account of the impact on him of the death of his father is a particularly relevant case in point.

Equally clearly an individual's own death, in anticipation, can be subsumed under the category of object loss, particularly in view of Freud's theory of narcissism, by which he meant the individual's cathexis of his own self as a love object. Anxiety, however, is not the actual experience of object loss, nor is it, according to Feud, the fear of it. It is an anticipatory orientation in which the actor's own emotional security is particularly involved. It is a field of rather free play of fantasy as to what "might" be the consequences of an anticipated or merely possible event.

Given the hypothesis that, in our scientifically oriented civilization, there is widespread acceptance of death—meant as the antithesis of its denial—there is no reason why this should lead to a cessation or even substantial diminution of *anxiety* about death, both that of others and one's own. Indeed, in certain circumstances the levels of anxiety may be expected to increase rather than the reverse. The frequent assertions that our society is characterized by pervasive denial of death may often be interpreted as calling attention to pervasive anxieties about death, which is *not* the same thing. There can be no doubt that in most cases death is, in experience and in anticipation, a traumatic event. Fantasies, in such circumstances, are often characterized by strains of unrealism, but the prevalence of such phenomena does not constitute a distortion of the basic cultural framework within which we moderns orient ourselves to the meaning of death.

Indeed, the preceding illustrations serve to enhance the importance of clarification, at the theoretical and philosophical levels, to which the bulk of this article has been devoted. This is essential if an intelligible approach is to be made to the understanding of such problems as shifts in attitudes toward various age groups in modern society, particularly the older groups, and the relatively sudden eruption of dissatisfaction with the traditional modes of conceptualizing the beginning and the termination of a human life and with allegations about the pervasive denial of death, which is often interpreted as a kind of failure of "intestinal fortitude." However important the recent movements for increasing expression of emotional interests and the like, ours remains a culture to which its cognitive framework is of paramount significance.

TALCOTT PARSONS

[*While all the articles in this entry are relevant, see especially the articles* WESTERN PHILOSOPHICAL THOUGHT *and* WESTERN RELIGIOUS THOUGHT. *Also directly related is* DEATH, ATTITUDES TOWARD. *For discussion of related ideas, see the entries:* EMBODIMENT; MIND–BODY PROBLEM; ABORTION; *and* DEATH, DEFINITION AND DETERMINATION OF.]

BIBLIOGRAPHY

BELLAH, ROBERT N. "Religious Evolution." *American Sociological Review* 29 (1964): 358–374.

BURKE, KENNETH. *The Rhetoric of Religion: Studies in Logology.* Boston: Beacon Press, 1961. Reprint. Berkeley: University of California Press, 1970.

CHOMSKY, NOAM. *Syntactic Structures.* Janua Linguarum, no. 4. 'S-Gravenhage: Mouton & Co., 1957.

DURKHEIM, ÉMILE. *The Division of Labor in Society* (1893). Translated by George Simpson. Free Press Paperbacks. Glencoe, Ill.: 1933, 1964.

——. *The Elementary Forms of the Religious Life* (1912). Translated by Joseph Ward Swain. London: Allen & Unwin, 1954. Reprint. Glencoe, Ill.: Free Press, 1976.

——. *Sociology and Philosophy* (1924). Enl. ed. Translated by D. F. Pocock. New York: Free Press, 1974.

FREUD, SIGMUND. *Beyond the Pleasure Principle* (1920). *Standard Edition*, vol. 18, pp. 7–64.

——. *The Ego and the Id* (1923). *Standard Edition*, vol. 19, pp. 12–66.

——. *The Future of an Illusion* (1927). *Standard Edition*, vol. 21, pp. 5–56.

——. *Inhibitions, Symptoms and Anxiety* (1926). *Standard Edition*, vol. 20, pp. 77–175.

——. *The Origins of Psycho-analysis: Letters to Wilhelm Fliess, Drafts and Notes, 1887–1902.* Edited by Marie Bonaparte, Anna Freud, and Ernst Kris. Translation by Eric Mosbacher and James Strachey. Introduction by Ernst Kris. New York: Basic Books, 1954.

——. *The Standard Edition of the Complete Psychological Works of Sigmund Freud.* 24 vols. Edited by James Strachey, Anna Freud, Alix Strachey, and Alan Tyson. London: Hogarth Press, 1955–1974.

HENDERSON, LAWRENCE JOSEPH. *The Fitness of the Environment: An Inquiry into the Biological Significance of the Properties of Matter.* In part delivered as lectures in the Lowell Institute, February, 1913. New York: Macmillan Co., 1913. Paperback ed. Boston: Beacon Press, 1958.

——. *The Order of Nature: An Essay.* Cambridge: Harvard University Press, 1917.

——. *Pareto's General Sociology: A Physiologist's Interpretation.* Cambridge: Harvard University Press, 1935.

KANT, IMMANUEL. *Critique of Judgment* (1790). Translated by James Creed Meredith. Oxford: Clarendon Press, 1964.

——. *Critique of Practical Reason and Other Writings in Moral Philosophy* (1788). Translated and edited by Lewis White Beck. Chicago: University of Chicago Press, 1949.

——. *Critique of Pure Reason* (1781). Translated by Norman Kemp Smith. London: Macmillan & Co., 1929.

LEACH, EDMUND R. *Genesis as Myth, and Other Essays.* Cape Editions, no. 39. London: Jonathan Cape, 1969.

LÉVI-STRAUSS, CLAUDE. *Structural Anthropology.* Translated by Claire Jacobson and Brooke Grundfest Schoepf. New York: Basic Books, 1963.

LOVEJOY, ARTHUR ONCKEN. *The Great Chain of Being: A Study of the History of an Idea.* The William James

Lectures delivered at Harvard University, 1933. Cambridge: Harvard University Press, 1936. Reprint. Harper Torchbooks, 1960.

MAUSS, MARCEL. *The Gift: Forms and Functions of Exchange in Archaic Societies* (1925). Translated by Ian Cunnison. Glencoe, Ill.: Free Press, 1954.

NOCK, ARTHUR D. *Conversion: The Old and the New in Religion from Alexander the Great to Augustine of Hippo.* London: Oxford University Press, 1933, 1961.

PARSONS, TALCOTT. *Social Systems and the Evolution of Action Theory.* New York: Free Press, 1977.

———; Fox, RENÉE C.; and LIDZ, VICTOR M. "The 'Gift of Life' and Its Reciprocation." *Social Research* 39 (1972): 367–415. Reprint. *Death in American Experience.* Edited by Arien Mack. New York: Schocken Books, 1973, pp. 1–49.

———, and LIDZ, VICTOR. "Death in American Society." *Essays in Self-Destruction.* Edited by Edwin S. Shneidman. New York: Science House, 1967, chap. 7, pp. 133–170.

WARNER, WILLIAM LLOYD. *The Living and the Dead: A Study of the Symbolic Life of Americans.* Yankee City Series, vol. 5. New Haven: Yale University Press, 1959. Reprint. Westport, Conn.: Greenwood Press, 1975.

WEBER, MAX. *The Protestant Ethic and the Spirit of Capitalism* (1904). Translated by Talcott Parsons. Foreword by R. H. Tawney. London: G. Allen & Unwin, 1930. Reprint. New York: Charles Scribner's Sons, 1958.

———. *The Sociology of Religion* (1922). Translated by Ephraim Fischoff. Boston: Beacon Press, 1963.

DEATH AND DYING: EUTHANASIA AND SUSTAINING LIFE

The article on HISTORICAL PERSPECTIVES *focuses on historical views of euthanasia and examines the origins of the ethical distinctions in contemporary thought. The second article,* ETHICAL VIEWS, *systematically examines the ethical issues involved in decisions affecting the termination of human life in a biomedical setting and discusses such questions as the right to die, and indirect and direct killing. The final article,* PROFESSIONAL AND PUBLIC POLICIES, *discusses the moral arguments for and against the different options in professional and public policy concerning euthanasia and the prolongation of life.*

I. HISTORICAL PERSPECTIVES   *Gerald J. Gruman*
II. ETHICAL VIEWS   *Sissela Bok*
III. PROFESSIONAL AND PUBLIC POLICIES
    Robert M. Veatch

I

HISTORICAL PERSPECTIVES

Introduction

This article will survey in historical context a number of key concepts of the modern era from the Renaissance on, concerning the ethics of sustaining and lengthening life or, contrariwise, hastening death. Such an outline is meant to help elucidate contemporary questions in biomedicine and to provide a useful perspective for the subsequent articles on ethics and on public policy.

The focus of this article on the modern era is not meant to imply that the questions treated here first appeared in the Renaissance but rather that it was then that they became readily relevant to the secular, scientific culture of the twentieth century. Already in prehistoric times, measures had been taken to hasten death, if we may judge from the observed practices of "primitive" cultures. In Graeco-Roman antiquity, there was a generally recognized "freedom to leave" that permitted the sick and despondent to terminate their lives, sometimes with outside help. The combination of tolerance and unconcern that allowed such practices was ended during the rule of Christianity in the medieval West. Although Christian charity brought a heightened responsibility to relieve suffering, the Sixth Commandment (Fifth Commandment in Roman Catholic and Lutheran traditions) seemed to prohibit absolutely the taking of the patient's life.

As to sustaining life, yearnings for extended longevity were characteristic in early folklore and found expression in the religion of ancient Egypt. With the Latin alchemy of the Middle Ages, an ambitious quest for the prolongation of life entered Western culture. On the one hand, man's dominion over nature inspired the thirteenth-century monk Roger Bacon to claim that Christian medicine would surpass pagan science by conquering senescence. On the other hand, medieval Christian thought was pervaded by a disdain for this-worldly considerations compared with the importance of supernatural salvation.

In contemporary discussions of biomedical ethics, euthanasia often is contrasted with the prolongation of life almost as if these aims inherently were opposed. This was not previously the case; the meanings of the terms have changed over the years. Until the seventeenth century, "euthanasia" generally referred to any means for an "easy" death; for example, by leading a temperate life or by cultivating an acceptance of mortality. However, upon entering the domain of medicine, with Francis Bacon's *Advancement of Learning* (1605), "euthanasia" increasingly came to connote specifically measures taken by the physician, including the possibility of hastening death. It is the latter meaning of a more rapid death that has been prevalent in the twentieth century, often in reference to the movement to reform legislation for that purpose.

With the onset of the idea of progress, the vision of the Christian alchemist Roger Bacon became secularized and adapted to the new sciences. The resulting belief I termed "prolongevity" (1956), i.e., the idea that it is possible and desirable to increase significantly the length of healthful, effective life by means of biomedical science. After the Enlightenment, biomedicine in general took on a sense of mission that may be called "meliorism," i.e., the belief that humanity can and should act to make this world better.

A different meaning of prolongation of life, more analogous to life sustaining, is "life support"—contingent measures to keep a patient alive who otherwise shortly would die. This aspect of modern biomedicine, growing out of heroic experiments in resuscitation, has evolved from temporary expediency to become long-term and routine, as in the various methods maintaining comatose patients and cases of renal failure. This development of life support has tended recently to pre-empt the meaning of "prolongation of life" thereby placing it in contradistinction to euthanasia. Moreover, it has tended to displace the popular import of "euthanasia" from active intervention to a passive withholding of "extraordinary" measures.

The evolution of these concepts and issues now will be examined more closely; the article proceeds in chronological order but will take the liberty in each era of drawing inferences directly to the present day (Kastenbaum and Aisenberg, chaps. 8, 9).

Renaissance humanism (1341–1626)

"Temperate" life and "natural" death are the concepts that connect euthanasia and the prolongation of life in Renaissance humanist thought. According to the prevalent physiological theory, each person is born with a certain amount of vital substance; if this is utilized with restraint in the course of a long life, death will be "natural" and benign. But if one's animating principle is consumed by unnatural, inordinate activity or disease, dying is agonized. This classical idea of easy dying was imbued by humanists with the values and rewards of Christian conduct: thus, "natural" connoted a better or higher kind of death. Luigi Cornaro's *Temperate Life* (1558 ff.), frequently consulted into the eighteenth century, featured both an easy ("holy")

terminus in advanced years and the prospect of longer life—up to 120 years.

In contrast to Cornaro, Francis Bacon was inspired by the promise of planned experimental research as the key to controlling bodily processes, either to lengthen life or, when indicated, to end it painlessly. He praised prolongevity as the "most noble" purpose of biomedicine, and he also considered "euthanasia," as he termed it, an essential area of medical skill. He inferred that relief of suffering is central in terminal care, and, accordingly, the physician sometimes may hasten death. Although their approaches differ, the intentions of Cornaro and Bacon are similarly in keeping with Christian humanist concepts of man's dignity and well-being: longevity liberated from the infirmities of senescence and dying freed from mortal pain.

The way of Cornaro, with its quietist reliance on nature, is an antecedent of passive euthanasia or "letting die." This standpoint persists in countries where the customs and judicial codes show traditional reverence for natural law. Omission of extraordinary measures continues to summon an imagery of natural death by "exhaustion" that seems preferable to the comparatively "unnatural" procedures of active euthanasia, connoting violent "extinction" and something of the illicit. Until recent decades, many patients did reach a condition of drastic debility where death appeared natural. However, there were many other instances in which nature seemed far from benevolent, and clinical mitigation was inadequate. Moreover, present-day care is inescapably a complex mixture of factors in which the natural, technical, and synthetic components cannot be separated. These considerations bring to mind Bacon's active interventionist aim of using nature's secrets to attain, for the moribund patient, a more *human* death. ("Exhaustion" and "extinction" are Aristotelian terms.)

Mercantilism and the social contract (1498–1714)

During two centuries of warfare, the Baroque ethos transformed Renaissance culture into an instrument of regimentation serving church, state, and the balance of trade. It should be noted that both Francis Bacon and Thomas More not only were humanists but also had official positions in mercantilist governments. The fierce competitiveness of mercantilism was defined by Bacon's maxim that what is gained in one place *must* be lost at another. And the same consciousness of limited resources appeared in More's *Utopia* (1516), which outlined the first organized *system* of euthanasia, in which patients with painful, hopeless diseases are advised by a panel of priests and magistrates to embrace a rapid death either by suicide or by the action of the authorities. Mercantilism favored energetic, mandatory direction of the individual; More's panel of advisers ruled as the "will of God." Humanist self-assertion was replaced by a calculating kind of heroic self-sacrifice that was concisely defined by the famous last words of Sir Philip Sydney (1586): "Thy need is greater than mine."

Amid the assumptions of scarcity economics, there arose a concept we may term "thrift euthanasia," which would permit the community to close off, by one means or another, lives requiring "undue" expenditure of inherently limited resources. The quantification of life-and-death questions was remarkably parallel to the managerial accounting in economic and political matters. The body thus has a fixed sum of vital force: enough, e.g., for "x" number of heart-beats or hours of work. Authorities, including the individual's own conscience, must vigilantly prevent any waste of vital powers (on loan from God and nature) in sexual indulgence, luxury, or even illness. In the contractual imagery of that era, death is a veritable *debt*, payable at three score years and ten, if not sooner. Suicide, however, was denounced as a personal indulgence violating the work ethic, according to which a lifetime of productive labor is equated with saintly suffering that may earn Christian redemption. There is room in heaven only for a "predestined" elite, and, likewise, the allotment of limited medical facilities favored a select few.

Mercantilist regimes would have furthered the prolongation of life only if it had been possible to increase the years of greatest productive vigor. They did not at all want larger numbers of aging persons. The scientific outlook, including statistics, was applied to the population rather to promote orderliness of flow from birth to death and an assured incremental by-product of net social profit. One may note analogous present-day interest in social strategies of selective implementation of birth control and suicide prevention while simultaneously withholding costly therapies, except in patients of unusual social "worth." Such trends are predictable in a century of war-time mobilizations, economic crises, and an apparent depletion of basic resources.

The thrift factor in euthanasia raises difficult problems concerning economics and the public policy aspects of biomedicine. On one hand, modernization creates the possibility of abundance in matters of human value (Fox); on the other, it is customary to submit to the presumed necessity for restrictive slice-of-pie allocations from a limited amount of social wealth. The latter assumption can be said to comport to an "ideology of death" (Marcuse), in that the point at which biomedicine ceases trying to prevent death and to restore health is decided not by inherently biological considerations but by social ones; and much of this bias toward economic scarcity stems from the power struggles of the seventeenth century.

Conflicts about euthanasia and the prolongation of life cannot be reduced to a quarrel between the religious and the laity or to a question of human rights per se. John Locke's *Treatise on Government* (1690), the landmark social-contract document of the liberal secular state, reasons that life not only is a right but also is an inalienable one: It can be neither taken nor given away. Markedly extended longevity did not seem to interest Locke; a physician as well as a philosopher, he always referred to life "preservation," a cautious word. Yet his idea of the natural persistence of the living organism (similar to Newton's concept of momentum) later stimulated Enlightenment theories of prolongevity.

Just as Locke was vigilant against tyrants' usurping of power, so also was he mistrustful that the people would willingly relinquish their God-given and natural prerogatives. Thus he did not condone a freedom to die. Patrick Henry's "liberty or death!" was more in keeping with Renaissance humanism than with Lockean liberalism. Thus, mercantilist tendencies toward euthanasia were blocked by Locke's philosophy in which life preservation, liberty, and the pursuit of property are inseparably interrelated. A possible exception would be a situation that violated integrity of person so grossly that basic contractual responsibilities ended. That would be comparable to a nation at the brink of justified revolution—a highly unusual occurrence.

Something that is "inalienably" invested cannot be disposed of at pleasure, just as the steward or servant of a merchant must guard and augment the wealth of his employer. This stewardship of life and property, to be accumulated rather than enjoyed, initiated hard-working industrial expansion but not greater personal freedom. Partly as a result of this, there is a bias in contemporary society (Arendt) against suicide and voluntary euthanasia, the means by which the individual could shorten his life in order to escape bad conditions; yet, where the individual might wish to lengthen his life, it becomes evident that precedence is given to the ongoing preservation of the governmental regime, the society, or the entire species.

The Enlightenment and the idea of progress (1687–1804)

Enlightenment thinkers, seeking to relax the rigidities of early liberalism, explored two major ethical pathways: hedonism and relativism. Jefferson, exemplifying the former trend, changed Locke's focus on the acquisition of property to a "pursuit of happiness." There were, however, definite limitations in Jefferson's approval of the pleasure principle: Although "cruel and unusual" reprisals against suicide were abolished, self-death nevertheless was to be "pitied" by public opinion. Jefferson thus continued the Lockean supposition that one who takes his own life must be "alienated," a word implying mental imbalance. This interpretation persists today in the assumption that one choosing suicide or euthanasia is temporarily "not himself" (Parsons and Lidz).

It was left to Bentham to affirm an unconditional hedonist rejection of suffering, rephrasing Hamlet: "To be *happy* or not to be at all." Also significant was Hume's philosophy recognizing that different persons and interest groups cannot be kept within Locke's severe formulation but should be permitted to express freely the *relative* truth which each discerns. This open-eyed acknowledgment by Hume of the variety of conditions led him to picture some cases in which the torments of illness justified "courageous escape." He also reasoned that, if mankind legitimately could seek to lengthen life, it follows that similarly life justifiably might also be shortened. Yet Hume and his associates were publicly conservative, and his own composure in terminal illness, in reality eased by potent drugs, was ascribed instead to his unique rationality and superior character. Such ambiguity severely restricted the impact of eighteenth-century libertarian thinkers. They were counterbalanced too by the growing influence of Rousseau's theory of the "general will," a more democratic and romantic version of the social contract. The general will became equated with rule by majority opinion, which frequently turned out to be con-

ventional and unenlightened about life-and-death issues.

Meanwhile, the Enlightenment faith in progress led to the elaboration of a number of ambitious, this-worldly alternatives to Christian salvation from death. There was, for example, intense interest in prolongevity. Benjamin Franklin boldly declared senescence to be not a natural process but a "disease" to be cured, and he predicted that longevity might reach a thousand years or more. The mathematician Condorcet speculated about virtually immortal life, an idea that has reappeared because of the present-day biomedical revolution (Harrington). The seeming lack of concern about euthanasia in Enlightenment biomedicine calls for further scholarly investigation. Present evidence indicates a heroic approach preoccupied with visions of large-scale research and public health programs, possibilities of much-increased life expectancy, and fascinating methods for restoration of persons "apparently" dead. Humane societies were devoted to resuscitation of the drowned and asphyxiated. Also characteristic of progressist medicine was curiosity about suspended animation by freezing or chemical means, a technique that might resolve the plight of the moribund in a completely new way. And there was much anxious apprehension regarding premature burial.

The invention of the now-maligned guillotine, to rid execution of the physical torture then customary, does indicate that research was done at least indirectly relevant to euthanasia. But during the Age of Reason, patients with unbearable pain or long-continued senility usually were considered mentally "alienated" by their extreme situation and not really responsible, thus causing a breakdown in doctor–patient communication. The paucity of eighteenth-century euthanasia debate reflects also the adoption of the reassuring natural-death model by the bourgeoisie. Their life-style aimed at the prudent accumulation of status and wealth during a life sufficiently long gradually to deplete vitality and thus conclude with a relatively easy demise at home; there at the death bed, blessings and property were transferred to the sons. Natural death thus acquired an aura of bourgeois comfort and the sentimental cult of the family. Life insurance was added, and there was a modicum of anticlerical thought to dispel "superstitious" fears. Money and connections made available the services of bedside physicians who applied measures, discreetly vague, for easier, and perhaps speedier, dying.

Positivist mortalism (1800–1906)

In order to see how Enlightenment heroic medicine became transformed en route to the present, it is necessary to examine the philosophy of positivism. The pattern for positivist thought actually was provided by medical practice, in particular the habitual strategem of using death as the pragmatic operative limit of clinical effort. Thus, Bichat in 1800 defined "life," in this common-sense way, as the ensemble of all the functions that *resist* dying. Medicine, he indicated, does not seek to conquer death or to preserve life interminably; the doctor strives only to slow down the tragically inevitable processes of decline. This medical "mortalism" (Foucault) removes death as a final catastrophe and instead spreads dying, as a series of little deaths, along the entire life span from birth on. Bichat, thus, subtly undermined progressist biomedicine.

Adopting Bichat's medical insight, Auguste Comte created a systematic *social* mortalism assuming that civilization inherently is beset by forces of decay and, upon reaching a mature stage, is fated to decline and fall. The worthwhile goal, he stated, is to avoid unprofitable "metaphysical" controversy and instead to utilize known, "positive" facts to stave off such social diseases as war and revolution, thereby preventing *premature* termination of Western civilization. To this purpose, he proposed that a corps of "sociologists" should employ an ensemble of ideas and beliefs, termed "ideology," to mold public opinion continuously to correlate with the everchanging requirements of modern society.

The positivist authorities were to control not only education but the entire process of human development. The life span was divided by Comte into functional age stages: childhood, youth, early adulthood, maturity, and retirement at sixty-three. Death usually would occur by age seventy, and seven years later a solemn judgment would select those whose "sanctified" remains merited interment in a monumental cemetery. Despite his pretentious thoroughness nearly all of Comte's notions were adopted, in one form or another, in Europe and the Americas during the latter nineteenth century. Indeed, the positivist model of expert intervention and guidance at each transitional life crisis still underlies current discussion of the moral role of biomedicine in death and dying.

Positivist-style medicine was effective in reducing the premature death rates of early life; but there is little sign that an aging population was desired or even responsibly foreseen. Comtean "Progress" carefully was balanced with "Order": In generational terms, youth represented innovation whereas the elders were an equally essential conservatism. Both birth control and death control were apprehended as potentially disruptive of smooth social functioning. In this calculated equilibrium, however, culture is not static, for industrial society requires incessant motion and change; but the positivist stream of novelty designedly lacked the profound ethical dimension of Enlightenment advance. Completely contrary to Condorcet's prolongevity, Comte held that death *contributes* to "Progress," a view continued today in the neopositivism of Parsons.

More studies are needed into positivist attitudes about euthanasia. Evidence now at hand indicates there was much less concern about the suffering and the ethical and legal prerogatives of patients than with their duty as citizens to set an inspiring example for the community. The sociologist Émile Durkheim, for example, was hostile to suicide and recommended that the individual's morale and "altruism" be strengthened by increased ties of "solidarity" with colleagues and family. George Eliot, the English writer, reflected positivist ideals in her philosophy of bearing life's pains "without opium." Later however, Eliot protested against the positivist doctrine that "pain is not an evil" (Guyau) and invented the word "meliorism" to emphasize the ethical imperative to better the world and, preeminently, to lessen human anguish. The introduction of anesthesia in the mid-nineteenth century also signified that professional and public attitudes could be favorable to pain prevention, as did William Munk's treatise on "euthanasia" as specialized care to ease the distress of the moribund. Yet positivist constraints are revealed in the unique honors paid to obstetric anesthesia (because it aided the function of motherhood) and in Munk's overly explicit disclaimers of hastening death. Similarly, Ilya Mechnikov's proposals to ameliorate senescence were restricted to so-called premature aging, and he invoked both natural death and an "instinct" of death to keep his project within positivist bounds.

A positivist kind of heroic medicine continues today in attempts to conduct an arduous, defensive "resistance" to death. This differs sharply from Enlightenment heroic medicine, with its aim of decisive life-affirming power over natural forces. The philosophes had been fascinated by prospects for the rapid restoration of effective health, either by resuscitation or by a reversal of senescence; in extremity, they considered suspended animation, with clear provisos for radical cure in the future. They had not wanted painfully to postpone dying, day by day, within a complex equilibrium between vectors of clinical endeavor and inevitable decline. In contrast to Enlightenment medicine, the tenacious positivist maintenance of life is in the social-contract tradition that there is a correct time of death which can be determined by a conflict of contending forces. Such a process has come to be criticized as a "prolongation of dying." Positivist medicine also demands extensive diagnostic and prognostic procedures, aside from curative purposes, in order to provide suitably exact or "positive" knowledge of the changing nature and timing of the fatality. Thus considerable efforts are taken to predict and record the fluctuating parameters of the case, while the medical team makes a suitable show of resistance to "premature" termination.

Revolt and neopositivism (1885 to the present)

In the latter nineteenth century, an intellectual and cultural rebellion began to gain ground against positivism. The most brilliant of the German antipositivists, Nietzsche, was intrigued by the idea that the "right" time for death could be decided not by calculation but by proud, "barbaric," egoistic choice. He scorned the "altruistic" self-denial of positivist ethics, and he praised suicide when "appropriate." However, Nietzsche himself, aware of a core of inner self-destructiveness, instead chose to endure and create despite his long years of painful illness. Confidence in freedom to choose death was undermined further by Freud's depth psychology of conflict and ambivalence. Like Nietzsche, Freud came to reject mortalism and affirmed the forces of life, Eros, against the "death drive," Thanatos.

An even more fundamental antipositivism came from the Russian philosopher Nicholas Fyodorov (1828–1903), who completely rejected the positivist ethos as a shattering betrayal of Christian charity and hope. Fyodorov was unique in his linking of an explicitly Christian vision of salvation with the promise of planned melioristic research. He demanded that science "begin to do" its immense task of actually saving humanity from mortality. The vaunted "progress" of the nineteenth century was derided by Fyodorov as, by and large, a parade of novel consumer products and deadly armaments. He also pointed out the ethical dilemma of generational displacement occurring in modern society in which youth

holds superiority merely by arriving at a later, "higher" stage of history. Such a sacrificial succession of generations was being justified by positivists and Darwinists, as in Winwood Reade's *Martyrdom of Man* (1872).

The triumph of Darwinism caused widespread withdrawal of sympathy from the ill and old, who were viewed as inferior and even parasitic beings. According to the important evolutionary theory set forth by August Weismann in 1882, nature programs higher organisms to die at the end of the years of reproduction; this was a severe blow to comforting notions about natural death. Even more ominous was the interpretation being given to Bichat's two-level hypothesis of mortality that contrasted brain death with that of the heart and lungs. It was implied that women, the aged, and the uneducated existed on a lower, less creative "vegetative" plane almost akin to the comatose; therefore, their dying was relatively uncomplicated and unimportant. In 1905 Osler, influenced by Weismann, set the cessation of creativity and the onset of "comparative uselessness" in men at age forty. At almost the same time, a leading German biologist, Ernst Haeckel, recommended that hundreds of thousands of "useless" persons be rapidly poisoned (Gasman).

Meanwhile, a new positivism, with a heroic, romantic bent and an emphasis on national-imperial mission, became the prevalent social ideology. ("Neopositivism" here refers to that ideology, not to logical-positivist philosophy.) Thus, on the eve of the First World War, Durkheim affirmed the primary role in ethics of personal sacrifice on behalf of the community. Another neopositivist theme was the "obligatory-gift" relationship, a modern industrial version of the social-contract theory, that holds each citizen morally accountable for putting his lifetime to socially productive and profitable use. This concept of life as an investment became the basis for the most cogent sociological study of American behavior regarding death and dying (Parsons and Lidz; Parsons, Fox, and Lidz).

Twentieth-century wars and revolutions brought the dire premonitions of Fyodorov to startling reality as entire generations were consigned to the "dustbin" of history. One's political or socioeconomic enemy was seen as a diseased, death-tainted force to be eradicated by the agencies of "real" or authentic life. During the First World War, each side claimed to be the champion of "life against death," and such ideological conflict persisted into the 1930s until it took a strangely twisted form in the Spanish fascist slogan, "Long live death!" With National Socialist racism, a "final solution" (1942 ff.) attempted to promote "racial health" by liquidating allegedly alien "races." This genocide program was titled "euthanasia," and techniques of efficient killing first were developed (1939–1942) in eliminating thousands of patients with chronic disease or mental illness. Such Nazi actions can be cited to exemplify an "opening wedge" argument against euthanasia. For that interpretation, it is necessary first to estimate the extent to which genocide actually represented the continuation of earlier eugenic and public health innovations. Secondly, one must consider the continued existence today of widespread cultural tendencies to evade social problems by victimizing a scapegoat category of people. The first, or social-medical, factor has been debated extensively, but it is the lethal expression of prejudice that is likely to prove the greater danger.

Conclusion

As we have seen, the terms "euthanasia" and "prolongation of life" are not necessarily antithetical. Both aims can be seen generally as expressions of the aspirations of modern culture to control the forces of nature. This article has indicated some of the viewpoints that have considered such newly acquired powers to be conducive to human freedom, dignity, and well-being. On the other hand, it has reviewed attitudes that would tend to bar or to delimit significantly such intervention. But it has not attempted to deal directly with the teachings of organized religions or with the more specialized literature of medicine and law. Instead, it has focused on those turning points in modern history that illuminate present-day secular cultural and intellectual currents as well as the influences of economics and social ideology.

It is questionable if today the young comatose patient is the prototype for the discussion of issues of death and dying. A more probable crucial issue is that of the elderly: a reservoir of relatively defenseless persons, perceived, through bigoted "ageism," as unproductive and pejoratively dependent. In them, modernization has created a population stratum that, in a state of nature or conditions of scarcity economics, "ought" to be dead. Here one confronts the recoil from the unfamiliarity of modernization, with its overturning of traditional age, sex, and generational patterns. To antimodern thinkers, an aging population seems a symptom of socio-

cultural decadence, and they typically have urged a revolt of the "young" against the "old"—sometimes arbitrarily defining a particular nation or race as young (Stern; Butler).

The perverse attraction to death that motivated genocide personnel (Alexander, 1949, "Destructive," "Molding") is not uncommon in contemporary society, in which the "necrophilous" personality aligns itself with technology's cold efficiency (Fromm). It may be that human history is veering toward the "death worship" foreseen by Orwell in *1984*—anonymous sacrifice of seemingly expendable individuals to the on-living social unit. When an unconditional mortalism prevails, human personality is stripped of significance and even reality (Borkenau). Thus, it is ethically necessary to challenge both mortalism and antimodernism (see also Veatch, chap. 8).

Genocide can be analyzed as part of a rebellion by desperately alienated masses of people against modernization—a regressive leap into an idealized past. To prevent that temptation, Ernst Nolte, in his profound study of the twentieth-century situation, suggests that human nature be considered something not yet fully formed, but rather engaged in a continuing process of unfolding realization through historical time. In this perspective, modernization is an alienating but necessary "transcending" of our familiar, incompletely moral world. In the open, adaptational dimension of human nature, there is an indispensable role for the therapeutic principle of biomedicine. For that task, mortalism can be replaced by an ethos in which life is the defining absolute and death the variable, "moving target." Discussion of euthanasia and prolongevity may once again come into affiliation with each other in the context of melioristic commitment. The great worth of individual human life is not yet a fact, but it is, for biomedical ethics, an essential goal.

GERALD J. GRUMAN

[*For further discussion of topics mentioned in this article, see the entries:* AGING AND THE AGED; DEATH, *articles on* WESTERN PHILOSOPHICAL THOUGHT *and* DEATH IN THE WESTERN WORLD; *and* SUICIDE. *Directly related are the other articles in this entry:* ETHICAL VIEWS *and* PROFESSIONAL AND PUBLIC POLICIES. *Also directly related are the entries* DEATH, ATTITUDES TOWARD; PAIN AND SUFFERING; *and* RIGHT TO REFUSE MEDICAL CARE. *For discussion of related ideas, see the entries:* CRYONICS; LIFE-SUPPORT SYSTEMS; LIFE; *and* MEDICAL ETHICS UNDER NATIONAL SOCIAL-

ISM. *Other relevant material may be found under* ETHICS, *articles on* TELEOLOGICAL THEORIES, UTILITARIANISM, *and* RULES AND PRINCIPLES; *and* MEDICAL ETHICS, HISTORY OF, *section on* EUROPE AND THE AMERICAS, *article on* MEDIEVAL EUROPE: FOURTH TO SIXTEENTH CENTURY.]

BIBLIOGRAPHY

[Documentation of primary sources, e.g., Bacon, Cornaro, Locke, Condorcet, Bichat, etc., is presented in the Gruman studies cited below.]

ALEXANDER, LEO. "Destructive and Self-Destructive Trends in Criminalized Society: A Study of Totalitarianism." *Journal of Criminal Law and Criminology* 39 (1949): 553–564.

———. "The Molding of Personality under Dictatorship." *Journal of Criminal Law and Criminology* 40 (1949): 3–27.

———. "War Crimes and Their Motivation: The Socio-Psychological Structure of the SS and the Criminalization of a Society." *Journal of Criminal Law and Criminology* 39 (1948): 298–326.

ARENDT, HANNAH. *The Human Condition.* Charles R. Walgreen Foundation Lectures. Chicago: University of Chicago Press, 1958.

BORKENAU, FRANZ. "The Concept of Death." *Death and Identity.* Edited by Robert Fulton. New York: John Wiley & Sons, 1965, pp. 42–56.

BUTLER, ROBERT N. *Why Survive?: Being Old in America.* New York: Harper & Row, 1975.

FOUCAULT, MICHEL. *The Birth of the Clinic: An Archaeology of Medical Perception.* Translated by A. M. Sheridan Smith. World of Man. New York: Pantheon Books, 1973. Reprint. New York: Vintage Books, 1975.

FOX, DANIEL M. *The Discovery of Abundance: Simon N. Patten and the Transformation of Social Theory.* Ithaca, N.Y.: Cornell University Press, 1967.

FROMM, ERICH. *The Anatomy of Human Destructiveness.* New York: Holt, Rinehart & Winston, 1973.

FYODOROV, NICHOLAS. "The Question of Brotherhood or Relatedness, and of the Reasons for the Unbrotherly, Dis-Related, or Unpeaceful State of the World, and of the Means for the Restoration of Relatedness." (1906). Translated by Ashleigh E. Moorhouse and George L. Kline. *Russian Philosophy.* 3 vols. Edited by James M. Edie, James P. Scanlan and Mary-Barbara Zeldin. Chicago: Quadrangle Books, 1969, vol. 3, pp. 16–54. Reprint. *Death As a Speculative Theme in Religious, Scientific, and Social Thought: An Original Anthology.* The Literature of Death and Dying. New York: Arno Press, 1977, pp. 16–54.

GASMAN, DANIEL. *The Scientific Origins of National Socialism: Social Darwinism in Ernst Haeckel and the German Monist League.* History of Science Library. New York: American Elsevier; London: Macdonald & Co., 1971.

GRUMAN, GERALD J. "An Historical Introduction to Ideas about Voluntary Euthanasia: With a Bibliographic Guide for Interdisciplinary Studies." *Omega: Journal of Death and Dying* 4 (1973): 87–138.

———. *A History of Ideas about the Prolongation of Life: The Evolution of Prolongevity Hypotheses to 1800.* Transactions of the American Philosophical Society, n.s. vol. 56, pt. 9. Philadelphia: 1966. Reprint. New York: Arno Press, 1977.

———. "Longevity." *Dictionary of the History of Ideas: Studies of Selected Pivotal Ideas.* 5 vols. Edited by Philip P. Wiener. New York: Charles Scribner's Sons, 1973–1974, vol. 3, pp. 89–93.

GUYAU, JEAN-MARIE. *The Non-Religion of the Future: A Sociological Study* (1887). New York: Schocken Books, 1962.

HARRINGTON, ALAN. *The Immortalist: An Approach to the Engineering of Man's Divinity.* New York: Random House, 1969.

KASTENBAUM, ROBERT, and AISENBERG, RUTH. *The Psychology of Death.* New York: Springer Publishing Co., 1972.

MARCUSE, HERBERT. "The Ideology of Death." *The Meaning of Death.* Edited by Herman Feifel. New York: McGraw-Hill, 1959. Paperback ed., 1965, chap. 5, pp. 64–76.

MUNK, WILLIAM. *Euthanasia; or, Medical Treatment in Aid of an Easy Death.* London: Longmans, Green & Co., 1887. Reprint. The Literature of Death and Dying. New York: Arno Press, 1977.

NOLTE, ERNST. *Three Faces of Fascism: Action Française, Italian Fascism, National Socialism.* Translated by Leila Vennewitz. New York: Holt, Rinehart & Winston, 1966.

PARSONS, TALCOTT, and LIDZ, VICTOR. "Death in American Society." *Essays in Self-Destruction.* Edited by Edwin S. Shneidman. New York: Science House, 1967, chap. 7, pp. 133–170.

———; Fox, RENÉE C.; and LIDZ, VICTOR M. "The 'Gift of Life' and Its Reciprocation." *Death in American Experience.* Edited by Arien Mack. New York: Schocken Books, 1973, pp. 1–49.

STERN, FRITZ. *The Politics of Cultural Despair: A Study in the Rise of the Germanic Ideology.* Berkeley: University of California Press, 1961. Reprint. Garden City, N.Y.: Doubleday/Anchor, 1965.

VEATCH, ROBERT M. *Death, Dying, and the Biological Revolution: Our Last Quest for Responsibility.* New Haven: Yale University Press, 1976.

II

ETHICAL VIEWS

Introduction

Every society has tried to stave off death and set limits to killing. But differences have arisen at times when living comes to be so painful or oppressive that some desire to die, perhaps even ask to be killed. In such cases of suicide and mercy killing, the prohibition on taking innocent life has collided with the demand for mercy in the face of intolerable suffering.

Arguments based on Judeo-Christian beliefs and/or natural law have traditionally formed the mainstay of the opposition to all such acts. To take an innocent life is, in these traditions, to usurp the right over life and death attributed to God. For some theorists of natural law, such acts violate the most fundamental human end of self-preservation. Others, both within and outside these traditions, have argued, on the contrary, that there are certain predicaments so agonizing that even the drive to self-preservation and the respect for all life are overpowered.

Throughout the discussions of these questions the issue is one of setting limits to what human beings can do to one another and to themselves when life is at stake. Should human beings ever have the right to seek their own death? If so, under what conditions? And should others be allowed to assist them in dying? Can innocent persons ever be rightfully put to death against their own will? What ethical lines against abuses and mistakes should be drawn by religion, by law, and in professional codes?

These problems have often been debated under the heading of "euthanasia," a word deriving from the Greek for "good death." Mercy for the suffering patient who desires to die has been the primary reason given by those who advocate legalizing voluntary euthanasia. But the word has been applied to such different acts, in such diverse circumstances, that much confusion has resulted. In spite of great differences among the views about rightful dying and allowable killing, the debates concerning the standards that ought to prevail have stressed time and again certain themes or aspects of the problems: (1) whether death is actively brought about or comes because support is withheld; (2) whether every conceivable effort should be made to ward off death; (3) what our responsibility is for death which has come through our action though we have not intended it; (4) whether death is voluntary or involuntary; (5) whether the agent brings death to himself as in suicide, or to another. In all these aspects efforts have been made to draw lines, to set procedures, and to make prohibitions that will protect the innocent and the unwilling.

This article attempts a systematic overview of these problems. It considers the different kinds of line-drawing and the protections that have been worked out in the face of human suffering, brutality, and coercion. And it examines the views concerning rights and powers to *decide* whether or not death should be sought by persons for themselves and for others.

Omission and commission

To omit is to leave undone, to fail or to forbear to perform an action that is within one's range of awareness and capability. To commit an act, on the other hand, is to perpetrate or perform it. Both "omission" and "commission" may be disapproved; one can be accused of omitting a lifesaving measure, or of committing a crime or a folly. They are narrower terms than "action" and "inaction," which generally signify the presence or absence of purposeful activity. In the context of what is done or not done to bring about *death,* they point to a basic distinction: that between death which is actively brought about and death which comes through the leaving out or neglecting of life-preserving measures. Thus to shoot someone is to commit an act; but to refuse help to the victim of the shooting is an omission. In discussions of euthanasia, the terms "active" and "passive" are often used to denote the same distinction. Jointly, active and passive euthanasia are then distinguished from a "natural" death.

The distinction between omission and commission is also a necessary one for setting limits to what must be done to preserve life. Legal, moral, and religious traditions have all regarded it as more crucial to specify the harm that people must not do to one another than the helpful acts they must not omit. Otherwise, everyone might be held responsible for all the accidents and deaths in the world from which they could conceivably have protected others. To sleep at night, for instance, rather than to patrol rivers and lakes looking for drowning victims would then be turned into a culpable omission. Clearly, this distinction between omission and commission corresponds to a fundamental limiting of human responsibility. And the failure to draw the distinction leads to fallacies such as that expressed in the loose phrase: "If you are not part of the solution, you are part of the problem."

While the distinction between omission and commission is necessary, however, it is obviously not sufficient. There are circumstances in which it is no defense at all to say that one did not do anything, and should therefore not be considered responsible for an accident or a death. A parent who does not feed an infant, or a doctor who fails to provide standard treatment to a patient in a case where he had a clear duty to act cannot merely argue that such inaction is justifiable *because* it is an omission.

There are circumstances, then, when such heavy responsibility can be assigned for *not* saving or prolonging a life, that the distinction between omission and commission evaporates. These are the circumstances where there is both a *relationship*—such as between parents and children, or in certain cases physicians and their patients—that entails duties to preserve life and to help, and also a chance that the help provided may succeed. In the law, similarly, inaction is held tantamount to action when there is a duty to act and failure to do so.

Intentional acts of killing are thus prohibited in almost all societies, the major exceptions being those of killing in war, in self-defense, and as lawful punishment. Omitting to save or prolong someone's life, on the other hand, has usually been viewed as only comparably wrong where there exists a *duty* to preserve that person's life and a chance of success. To omit help which it is a duty to provide constitutes abandonment.

But choices are not so simple, even in relationships where there are duties to patients and dependents. For it is increasingly possible to provide life support far beyond what many patients wish to receive. The very concept of "help" then comes into question, and a conflict arises as to whether to preserve the lives of such patients can realistically be thought of as "helping" them.

As a result, societies must now determine under what circumstances, even in relationships where there *is* a duty in some sense to take care of another and the ability to prolong life, omission is morally justified. The clearest case is one in which existing duty has ceased because the patient, while manifesting some physiological activities, is no longer alive. Another clear case is that in which the competent patient rejects the life-prolonging treatments available, thus releasing relatives and health personnel from any duty to prolong his or her life.

It is the effort to distinguish *further* criteria for justifying certain omissions that now preoccupies theologians, medical personnel, lawyers, and philosophers. At what cost to the patient in terms of suffering, effort, and exhaustion of resources can efforts to prolong life be carried on? And how are these efforts to be balanced against the neglect of others in need of assistance? Should the likelihood of success of such efforts be a factor in weighing the length to which they should be pushed?

In considering *omission* of action to prolong life under such complex circumstances, the debate has focused on the distinction between ordinary and extraordinary means. The debate concerning *commission*—concerning acts that can and cannot be performed so as to cause death—has centered on the distinction between direct and indirect action. In the next three sections,

these two kinds of distinctions will be taken up.

Ordinary and extraordinary means

Physicians have the moral and legal duty to continue appropriate care for patients once they have accepted such a responsibility in the first place. They may not abandon their patients. Yet it is possible for them to continue some kinds of support while not going to every length to prolong lives that are ebbing away, or when the support is useless, unavailable, or unwanted. They need not, for instance, provide resuscitation for a patient who is virtually certain not to survive the effort, even though resuscitation may be indicated for other patients with higher chances of survival.

How, then, can one know where and when it is permissible to omit certain life-supporting efforts, and which ones these should be? If a patient is in a permanent coma, should a respirator be employed? And should a patient near death from both painful cancer and debilitating heart disease be resuscitated? What if this patient develops pneumonia—should antibiotics be administered? Should surgery be undertaken on this patient to correct a condition unrelated to the cancer and the heart condition? And what measures can be omitted from the care of severely malformed newborns?

There is great need, then, for criteria permitting the omission of some life-preserving means at certain times. For this reason, health professionals have looked to the distinction stressed by Catholics, and adopted by many others, between ordinary and extraordinary means. Pope Pius XII said, in a widely cited address to an international congress of anesthesiologists, that "normally one is held to use only ordinary means [for the preservation of life and health]—according to circumstances of persons, places, times, and culture—that is to say, means that do not involve any grave burden for oneself and others" (Pius XII, p. 395).

Certainly, in clear cases, this distinction corresponds to a powerful intuition. We sense that there is a difference between resuscitating a dying man over and over again, on the one hand, and resuscitating someone who has a likelihood of continuing to live, on the other hand. We know that means exist in some hospitals not available in others. But in the many complex cases where one cannot be so certain, the frequent use of the term "ordinary means" has been ambiguous and self-serving. People have tended to say that what they wanted to omit was extraordinary; because of the vagueness of the term, it has been hard to pin down exactly what they meant, and thus to make a coherent argument in support or in contradiction. These terms have both normative and descriptive meanings; if they are not seen as separate, confusion results.

The basic use of the terminology is to signal a distinction between what is binding and what is not binding, between the mandatory and the merely allowable. When we ask "binding for what reason?" several different criteria emerge, often confusedly.

One distinction is between that which is helpful to prolonging life, and called ordinary, and that which merely prolongs the process of dying, and thus is extraordinary, useless, and at the very least not required. This is an important distinction, but it does not speak to all that concerns us about life support. For instance, say that a surgical procedure actually could prolong a life for a period of months, but at an extreme cost of pain for the patient and of resources for society, should it be considered ordinary? Most would follow Pope Pius in considering the gravity of the burden of life-support, thus rendering this first distinction insufficient.

A second distinction, frequently made by physicians, is that between standard treatment and unusual treatment, thought to be extraordinary. In this sense, food and shelter are basic and ordinary, whereas, at the other extreme, rare or experimental or expensive treatment is extraordinary. Again, this distinction speaks to only one factor, but it cannot cover all of what we mean by extraordinary. Take the case of the person dying of cancer in great pain, close to death, who develops pneumonia. Certainly, antibiotics are now part of the standard arsenal of medicine; yet many would consider it cruel and extraordinary to use them to prolong such a patient's care.

A third kind of distinction encompasses these two but stresses the *circumstantial* nature of what is considered ordinary and extraordinary. A procedure may be called extraordinary if there is *any* overwhelming reason why it ought not to be undertaken. Perhaps the procedure will leave the patient in intolerable pain or require resources not easily acquired; perhaps it is morally unacceptable, as when it requires taking an organ from an unwilling donor; or perhaps there is too small a chance of success or survival. According to such a distinction, antibiotics—by now standard or usual treatment in a number of

circumstances—might be extraordinary in the sense of not being morally necessary if they have to be flown in from far away in a snowstorm, or if the patient already suffers from a fatal illness and is in great pain.

A further question with respect to the use of the "ordinary–extraordinary" distinction is the following: To whose choices does it apply? Some hold that all that is ordinary is mandatory not only for health professionals but also for patients. Since life is not ours but God's, they argue, we cannot abandon it except in extraordinary circumstances, for ourselves or for others in our care.

A different view holds, on the other hand, that what the patient wants is part of what renders circumstances ordinary or extraordinary. For a Jehovah's Witness, for example, receiving a blood transfusion may be thought immoral, destructive of one's soul, and to be avoided at all costs, however common such a procedure has now become for many patients in our hospitals. For a patient who wishes to die at home, going to the hospital might prolong life considerably yet be considered morally extraordinary.

If the patient's own circumstances and desires are to be taken into account in this view of the two concepts, special difficulties will arise in the increasingly frequent circumstances where patients have lived past the point of being competent to express and enforce their desires. To some extent, this difficulty is being anticipated by the numerous "living wills" now being written in anticipation of just such circumstances. Another effort to cope with such a situation is represented by hospital policies concerning patient treatment in terminal stages of illnesses where continued life prolongation appears increasingly cruel or hopeless.

Stopping versus not starting a procedure

Many health professionals who recognize that a particular life-supporting treatment has become useless are reluctant to discontinue it, especially if the patient's life will ebb away as a result. Even if their patient is permanently unconscious, with no possibility of mental function left, they hesitate to turn off the respirator which keeps the body in partial "life." And they draw a distinction between *ceasing* such support and not starting it in the first place. For a patient similarly unable to regain consciousness, they might have no hesitation at all in deciding not to institute respirator support. But they do hesitate to cease existing support. In part, the hesitation flows from the fact that to stop the respirator or turn it down is itself an act—a commission—and thus surrounded by special precautions where life is at stake. But this need not be the case in all questions of stopping treatment. To cease giving medication, for example, is at times more clearly an omission than to cease respirator support.

Even when one has concluded, therefore, that a procedure may be omitted in a case where it is unquestionably extraordinary, one has to ask whether "omit" here means omit beginning a process, or whether it can also be extended to mean omit continuing it once started. Ramsey holds that there is no difference between the two; that the same moral warrant is required for deciding to stop "extraordinary" lifesaving treatments as for deciding not to begin to use them (Ramsey, p. 121). It is important to stress here the word "extraordinary." For there certainly *is* a great difference between the two types of decisions in most situations of life. Once we undertake some form of help, such as to house an orphan, for example, we have created an obligation not to cease it, greater than before we had stepped in.

But we need to specify what *kind* of cessation would be no different from not starting, even in the realm of extraordinary procedures. Ramsey's equation of the two may be correct only where extraordinary is taken to mean "death-prolonging." If a respirator merely prolongs the process of dying of an organism, with absolutely no hope of reversal, then the moral warrant for turning off the machine is the same as for not instituting such care in the first place. But other forms of extraordinary support *are* more difficult, morally speaking, to stop once they have been started. An extraordinarily expensive treatment, for example, such as the constructing of a special chamber where a single patient is kept free from infection, might not have been undertaken; if undertaken, it might not have been devoted to a particular patient. But to withdraw support from a patient in need once it has been undertaken and so devoted is of a very different moral order. A relationship has been created; expectations have been aroused. And while the withdrawal of support may be justified, such justifications must overcome the claims of the relationship and the expectations; this is not the case *before* the procedure has been undertaken.

Renée Fox and Judith Swazey describe similar difficulties for physicians in discontinuing treatment such as dialysis once they have begun, or deciding not to do successive renal implants on a patient who has rejected previous ones (Fox and Swazey, p. 323). Physicians then feel bound to their terminally ill patients in ways that make it nearly unbearable to cease treatment even where treatment is no longer indicated. There are psychological barriers in such cases which render stopping a procedure quite different from not starting it, quite apart from the moral reasons for and against such acts. From a moral point of view, the refusal of continued treatment by a competent patient may be seen as removing the duty to continue what has been started. What *makes* the treatment "extraordinary," then, is that the patient no longer wants it. Yet in practice it is much harder for a patient to secure the cooperation needed to cease dialysis or to leave the hospital than to refuse dialysis or hospitalization before beginning them. Stopping and not starting extraordinary forms of care, then, are felt differently, and have different moral and psychological warrants in a number of situations. But where a procedure is merely death-prolonging, stopping and not starting are much more alike.

Direct and indirect

Indirect acts are defined as those not directly aimed at or attained. Direct acts, on the contrary, are those with results that are either intended or take effect without intermediate instrumentality. Aiming and attaining—these concern the two separate domains of intention and causality. One or the other, or both together, may be at issue in writings on "indirect killing." Thus Joseph Fletcher (p. 147) calls euthanasia "direct" if life is ended actively, as by swallowing something or pulling out a tube, while "indirect" euthanasia is allowing death to come (ibid.). And Pope Pius XII describes the omission of resuscitation efforts for a dying patient as "never more than an indirect cause of the cessation of life" (Pius XII, p. 397).

A second meaning of "indirect" is one in which death *is* actively caused, but only indirectly. There may be human or mechanical intermediaries to trigger off the actual killing. This can happen at great distance in space and time, as where villages are bombed from planes by military personnel knowing that people will be killed, yet never confronting the victims face to face. Those who kill indirectly in this sense often feel that the indirectness reduces or even removes their moral responsibility for the consequences of their actions. Indirectness, here, serves as a *psychological* buffer; whether or not their *moral* responsibility is in reality reduced, indirect killers sometimes believe that it is.

It is when "direct" and "indirect" are used in a third sense to describe the intention guiding the act which results in death, however, that an especially important moral distinction is illuminated. For while the taking of life is clearly ruled out in most instances, there are certain cases in which action *leads* to death while it is not primarily *intended* to do so. (The same is true of omissions where there is a duty to act.) And in these cases the actions are sometimes seen as more readily justifiable.

Thomas Aquinas made this distinction very clear with respect to self-defense. If a man is attacked and kills his attacker, his intention is to defend himself, even though the effect of his action is also to take a life. This kind of action is characterized by the fact that there are at least two consequences of the action, one good, the other bad, and that the good consequence is the one primarily intended (Thomas Aquinas II-II, 64, 7).

An act of killing, according to this third distinction, is characterized as "direct" or "indirect" according to its goal or purpose. "Indirect euthanasia" would then refer to killing by an action that is primarily intended to relieve suffering (or promote some other good) but is also known to be potentially lethal. By contrast, the term "direct euthanasia" would describe any situation in which the death of the patient is the primary goal. The textbook case of indirect killing is the "merciful overdose"—where fatal doses of narcotics are administered to a terminal patient in unbearable pain. Here the action is characterized as indirect because the real purpose in giving the drugs is held to be to relieve the patient's pain rather than to cause his death. The motive is in fact often a mixed one where a "merciful overdose" is administered. The act is therefore one, often, of both direct and indirect killing; it differs from the clear indirectness described by Aquinas in acts of killing in self-defense.

Clearly, not all actions that do severe damage in the pursuit of some good consequence can be thus defended. To give an overdose of narcotics to save a child from the pain of a curable illness is not excused by the self-professed good intention of the agent. Here we have a case of morally unjustifiable indirect killing. Yet it is equally clear that there are times when we require a moral distinction between two situations in which identical results, equally foreseen, have been achieved with very different intentions. This question has long been debated (in Catholic moral philosophy) in terms of the principle of double effect, which presents four criteria guiding conduct in a dilemma arising from an action with several effects, one bad and at least one good (McCormick, 1973, pp. 1–112). The four criteria are the following: (1) The act itself must be good or morally indifferent; it cannot be morally evil. (2) The evil effect must not be intended, merely allowed. (3) The good effect must flow from the action and not from the bad effect; that is, the bad effect must not be the means to the good. (4) There must be a proportionately good effect, sometimes called a "commensurate reason," to overcome the evil effect—some proportionate reason for allowing the evil to occur.

It is often possible to make a clear distinction between intended wrongs and wrongs foreseen but not intended, using these four criteria (Fried, p. 186). But in difficult or borderline situations, all four become hard to evaluate. The second, which asks that the agent's intention not be aimed at producing the evil effect, then becomes especially elusive. A mere personal claim of innocence of intention on the part of the agent is obviously not sufficient. Yet the knowledge others can have of his intentions is of necessity limited.

At times when people disagree as to whether an act results in any evil effects in the first place, moreover, the distinction is persuasive only for those who on separate grounds believe there is an evil effect, or believe that such evil effects must not be intended for whatever reason. Thus for a woman to take drugs that are needed for a uterine disease but have the foreseeable yet unintended side effect of making her sterile would be permissible in Catholic moral philosophy. It would represent an indirect sterilization (McCormick, 1973, p. 3). But to take the same drug in order to achieve sterility would be a direct sterilization, and as such forbidden. For many others, on the other hand, neither direct nor indirect sterilization requires such special efforts at justification, since they see no "evil effect" in either.

Richard McCormick has suggested that intention be judged in terms of "proportionate reason" (ibid., p. 69). Such proportionate reason is held to exist when (1) the value at stake is at least equal to that sacrificed; (2) there is no other way of salvaging it here and now; and (3) its protection here and now will not undermine it in the long run. Using such a distinction, one can justify certain crisis choices such as that of the truck driver confronted with running into either two men or a busload of children, or that of giving narcotics to still the intolerable pains of a dying person at the risk of speeding the moment of death. But if alternatives do exist, such as narcotics that do not threaten life or a different path for the truck driver, the indirectness of the intention is called into question. Particular care must therefore be taken to assess the attitudes of those potentially involved in an act of euthanasia. Clearly a doctor or nurse could not legitimately be said to have the relief of pain as a primary intention in a case where narcotics are administered in doses known to exceed the quantity required to achieve analgesia, or where the patients show no signs of suffering in the first place (e.g., the comatose patient).

But while the direct–indirect distinction reflects our instinctive sense of the moral significance of right intention, it does not show us how to transcribe this moral sentiment into firm rules of decision making. While there are clear cases of direct and indirect killing, there is a "gray area" between them. Even as we gain insight into current problems, moreover, the issue of indirectness will develop new facets. The justification for the "merciful overdose" depends on the contingency that the most adequate analgesics for many terminal patients happen to have debilitating side effects. If this connection is broken by pharmacological advance or increased sophistication in the use of existing drugs, medicine will have lost this means of coping with the question of how long to try to prolong the lives of terminal patients in great pain. Even without these specific developments, life-support systems are bound to improve in general, so that it will be increasingly relevant to ask whether the length of a patient's life should be compromised for the sake of some other good. Thus the issues surrounding the distinction between direct and indirect euthanasia, particularly the question of the moral significance of right intention, are likely to assume even greater importance with the advance of biomedical technology.

Voluntary and involuntary dying

Every society, then, has set limits to killing. But the more that can be done to *prolong* a life that is ebbing away, the more necessary it becomes also to set limits to avoid assault and battery upon helpless, at times unwilling, victims in the name of prolonging their lives. All the distinctions mentioned up to now represent efforts made through the centuries to separate the permissible from the impermissible in these regards.

There is another indispensable distinction, however; that between voluntary and involuntary dying. It concerns the *attitude* of the person whose life or death is at stake.

Voluntary dying represents a vast spectrum of attitudes, from the peaceful acceptance with which death can be greeted to acts of suicide and euthanasia. It can encompass many choices, such as asking to be kept home from the hospital, ceasing to struggle against disease, or asking medical personnel to assist in suicide or even to perform acts of killing. A voluntary death can be achieved through suicide, through martyrdom or sacrifice for the welfare of others; it can also take place through voluntary euthanasia or mercy killing where what is at issue is the welfare of the victims themselves.

Nonvoluntary dying occurs in all acts of killing of unwilling or nonconsenting victims— either those who expressly oppose dying or those who are unable to express any opinion at all. Infanticide and the killing of unconscious patients, even when undertaken for merciful purposes, differ from voluntary dying since the persons killed have expressed no desire to die. And "involuntary euthanasia" refers to such programs of exterminating the sick and the disabled as were undertaken by the Nazis and others.

Some hold that the distinction between voluntary and involuntary dying is so important that it obviates all the previous ones mentioned. So long as a person *wants* to die, they say, and has a powerful reason for such a desire, it ought not to matter whether death comes by omission or commission, or what means are used, or whether there is direct or indirect intention to take life. Thus, advocates of the legalization of voluntary euthanasia hold that it ought to be possible actively to bring death by poison or other means to a suffering and dying individual requesting such assistance (Williams, 1957).

Religious arguments. Others have maintained their opposition to all kinds of suicide and mercy killing. Chief among them are Christian writers closely connected with the tradition of natural law. Other religions may outlaw these acts summarily or permit them under certain circumstances. But without strong prohibitions, Christianity, with its explicit outlining of the nature of life after death, would run the risk of tempting believers to speed death in order to achieve such a new life. Thus St. Augustine pointed out that if suicide were permissible in order to avoid sin, then it would be the logical course to choose for all those who were fresh from baptism. The "epidemics" of suicides among early Christians show that there have been times when those temptations were very great and help to explain the strong condemnation of suicide by Christian writers such as Augustine and Thomas Aquinas.

The great majority of the religious arguments supporting the condemnations of suicide hold that the individual has no right to desire to end his life (nor therefore to ask another to end it) since the right over life and death belongs exclusively to God, who is held to have given human beings the prescription not to kill. This prescription, however, has never been interpreted as being without exceptions. Even within the religious traditions, some have asked why suicide and voluntary euthanasia could not be exceptions, just as are killing in self-defense and killing in just wars for Christian theologians. Such an exceptional status is nevertheless denied to voluntary dying by most writers in the Christian tradition. To want to end one's life is thought to go against God's right; the right of God over life and death corresponds, they have held, with a duty on the part of men to protect their lives even from themselves. For most religious theorists of natural law, suicide and mercy killing would violate the natural end of self-preservation.

Proposals to legalize voluntary euthanasia. Proposals to legalize euthanasia would permit acts of both omission and commission resulting in death, given certain safeguards (Kamisar; Williams). The requirement that the patient should have *requested or consented expressly* to the act of euthanasia is clearly the most important of these safeguards, a requirement thought by sponsors of such proposals to provide a simple and clearcut distinction between voluntary and nonvoluntary dying. However, such a requirement raises new, and perhaps even more difficult, problems of how to draw a clear line. These problems are always present when consent is involved and are especially grave when a person's life is at issue. Opponents ask, Is there not an important distinction between request and consent in the first place? Might there be a danger of slipping from request to resigned acquiescence? Might there be a risk of someone's asking to die out of a concern for the burden he places

on his family? How does one determine whether the request or the consent is not the result of a temporary aberration or of medication-induced confusion or depression? Or what if the desire to die is based upon an unrealistic view of the present situation, or of the prognosis for the future, based on false or insufficient information? And how is the situation altered if the patient requesting to die has dependents? (Cantor.)

In order to meet some of these concerns, a number of additional requirements, beyond mere consent or request, are suggested by those in favor of allowing voluntary euthanasia: The patient must be over the age of twenty-one; the agent must be a physician who should have consulted with another physician or with some specified authority; sometimes a period of time is required between the request for euthanasia and the act itself during which the patient's possible change of mind must be heeded.

Given such safeguards, these advocates argue that it is cruel to prolong intense suffering on the part of someone who is mortally ill and desires to die. Mercy dictates intervention. A secondary argument holds that a person has the *right* to decide whether he should continue to live or not, and that such a decision can be reached after rationally weighing the benefits of continued living against the suffering involved. If a person has such a right, it is held, then it cannot be wrong for him to ask another to help him carry out his desire, nor can it be wrong for another to do so.

Opponents argue first that acts of killing would not, in fact, always truly be merciful for the patients requesting them. There are risks that some patients might die as a result of an error in the prognosis of their disease. Others might die who could have recovered as a result of a new approach to their illness such as that provided when penicillin came into use. Still others might die who did not really wish to die, given the difficulties already mentioned of knowing whether the request for euthanasia is genuine and, even if genuine, is truly in the best interest of the patient. They point to the familiar cases where patients have pleaded to be allowed to die, only to recover with gratitude that the physician did not respond to their plea.

Secondly, these critics argue, even where dying would be more merciful, and even if patients have the right to determine whether they want to continue to live or not, such a right provides the justification for *suicide* and for the *refusal of life-prolonging treatment*, but not for another to engage in an act of killing. "Helping" a person to end his life is seen as fundamentally different from helping him to build a house or to find his way; and the question of whether the killing is helpful or harmful, lawful or prohibited, cannot, therefore, be decided merely by establishing that the victim asked for help.

The third argument stresses the small number of those who would actually be helped by new legislation. There is general agreement that very few of the cases publicly debated under the rubric of euthanasia would fit the requirements suggested in the different proposals. True, many persons suffer, and many are near death, but those who suffer *and* are near death and who are willing and able to ask, in a manner acceptable to courts and to physicians, to be killed, constitute a much smaller group. All acts of euthanasia contemplated by relatives or friends would be ruled out. And the familiar cases of infanticide sometimes referred to as euthanasia would also be ruled out, both because of the absence of consent by the victim and because the victim is under the age of twenty-one.

Most important, those *not competent* to give consent, even if they are over the age of twenty-one, would not fit the requirements. Those who are legally incompetent—such as great numbers of the retarded—have not been held capable of initiating procedures to resist medical treatment. Much less, then, would they be able to request euthanasia. Those who are physically unable to communicate, such as patients in coma, would likewise be excluded from consideration by euthanasia legislation requiring consent, in spite of the fact that much public concern with euthanasia stems from an awareness of the conditions under which their lives are prolonged.

Nevertheless, if these were the only objections to euthanasia, they might well be overcome through careful safeguards. Even if euthanasia does not always represent the most beneficial act for patients, and even if there are possibilities of cures, those few patients who would request euthanasia, it could be argued, ought to have the right to decide whether or not they wish to take such odds and continue to suffer, or choose to die. Even if helping someone to die differs from other forms of help in that it involves destruction, and even if administered euthanasia differs from suicide, given that the act is lawful and the agent willing, those who *want* to perform such acts could be empowered to do so. And even if very few would actually request euthanasia, their small number does not in itself bar provid-

ing them with relief. Finally, problems of competence and incompetence could be carefully worked out here, as elsewhere, in medicine and law. All of these factors, then, so long as they are considered purely on an individual basis, fail to make a sufficient case against voluntary euthanasia.

These factors take on new significance in the light of the most serious risks which the acceptance of voluntary euthanasia opens up—risks to social structures, and thus to individuals who have *not* requested euthanasia. These are risks of abuses and errors that might result from a relaxation in the present strong prohibitions against killing. Rules may be misapplied. Practices may be extended to groups of patients beyond the original few who fit the strict requirements. Distinctions may be blurred, so that patients may come to die without having requested euthanasia, perhaps quite against their wishes. The fears of such risks are supported by a concern for the defenselessness on the part of groups such as the newborn or the senile, and by a lack of confidence in the social resistance to harming them.

Suicide. Suicide has often been held to be an exception to the prohibitions universally placed upon taking innocent life. It does not pose the same threats to the social fabric as legalized voluntary euthanasia. There is much less to be feared from a spread of abuses and mistakes. And since suicide is the killing of self, there can be no concern, as in situations where others are the agents, about the brutalization of those professionals asked to participate in taking lives.

In the long debates concerning suicide, it has always been assumed that most suicides should be prevented; the disputed cases have been those where a person seems to be laboring under the compulsion of some painful and inevitable misfortune (Plato IX, 8). Such debates have then focused on the question of the duties owed by persons in respect to their own life. Some have held that, in killing oneself, one need only consider one's own life. Others have held, on the contrary, that duties concerning one's life are owed to God, to the state, to nature, and to one's family, or to some combination of these. Hume argued that, when a man is miserable enough to contemplate suicide, he is not obligated to give society the questionable benefit of living on at the expense of great suffering for himself. Nor could suicide be a transgression of the duty to God since God has already given men the power to alter the course of survival in building dwellings or inoculating children for smallpox (Hume). As for the duty to oneself, Hume argued that no one would kill himself if it were best for him to remain alive, and stated that he intended his arguments for suicide to restore men to their native liberty.

Kant, on the contrary, held that suicide violates man's duty to himself in the most fundamental way and thus is opposed to the supreme principle of all duty. He held that to destroy the subject of morality in one's own person is to root out the existence of morality itself from the world so far as this is in one's own power (Kant).

The growth of the discussion of rights in the last two centuries has brought to the fore the question of whether or not there is a right, more basic than all others, over one's own life. The act of suicide is no longer held to be a crime in many societies. While great efforts are still made to prevent most suicides, some categories of justifiable suicide may come to be set apart, where prevention of the suicidal action may not be undertaken. In such cases, the role of the physician in providing the means for suicide is once again in question, as it was in antiquity.

Conclusion

The distinctions surveyed above represent deeply felt differences. They often succeed in marking off regions of abuse or injustice and in exploring complex dilemmas. But these distinctions are at times very hard to draw. There are borderline regions between omission and commission, between extraordinary and ordinary means, between indirect and direct killing, and between voluntary and involuntary dying. We do not always possess clear natural lines.

Such a realization is sometimes thought to imply that all distinctions are useless, so long as they are not mirrored in nature. But it is crucial to see that, even though a line is not drawn in nature, it may well be needed in practice. Most norms are of this nature. Sometimes the precise location of the line drawn is somewhat arbitrary, as with age limits for driving, yet some line is clearly needed.

All social policy requires the drawing of lines, and those drawn to protect against killing are among the most universal. Prohibitions have to be established and distinctions made even where human affairs are uncertain and hard to classify. Such lines are troubling because they can seem arbitrary or harsh. Yet they are necessary in order to avoid considering afresh each new choice that arises. The most important question

remains: Who is to draw the different lines, within what bounds, and with what degree of accountability?

SISSELA BOK

[*For further discussion of topics mentioned in this article, see the entries:* DOUBLE EFFECT; *and* SUICIDE. *Also directly related are the entries* DEATH; DEATH, ATTITUDES TOWARD; *and* DEATH, DEFINITION AND DETERMINATION OF. *For discussion of related ideas, see the entries:* ACTING AND REFRAINING; CARE; HEALTH AS AN OBLIGATION; INFANTS; LIFE-SUPPORT SYSTEMS; *and* RIGHT TO REFUSE MEDICAL CARE.]

BIBLIOGRAPHY

AUGUSTINE. *The City of God* 1.17,19,20,21. Translated by Demetrius B. Zema and Gerald G. Walsh as *Saint Augustine.* Vol. 6: *The City of God, Books I–VII.* Introduction by Étienne Gilson. The Father of the Church: A New Translation, vol. 8. Edited by Roy Joseph Deferrari. New York: 1950, bk. 1, chaps. 17, 19, 20, 21; pp. 46–47, 49–54.

BEHNKE, JOHN, and BOK, SISSELA, eds. *The Dilemmas of Euthanasia.* Garden City, N.Y.: Anchor Press/Doubleday, 1975.

BRIM, ORVILLE G., JR.; FREEMAN, HOWARD E.; LEVINE, SOL, and SCOTCH, NORMAN A., eds. *The Dying Patient.* New York: Russell Sage Foundation, 1970.

CANTOR, NORMAN L. "A Patient's Decision to Decline Life-Saving Medical Treatment: Bodily Integrity versus the Preservation of Life." *Rutgers Law Review* 26 (1973): 228–264.

CRANE, DIANA. *The Sanctity of Social Life: Physicians' Treatment of Critically Ill Patients.* New York: Russell Sage Foundation, 1975.

FLETCHER, JOHN. "Abortion, Euthanasia, and Care of Defective Newborns." *New England Journal of Medicine* 292 (1975): 75–78.

FLETCHER, JOSEPH. "Elective Death." *Ethical Issues in Medicine: The Role of the Physician in Today's Society.* Edited by E. Fuller Torrey. Boston: Little, Brown & Co., 1968, chap. 7, pp. 139–157.

FOOT, PHILIPPA. "The Problem of Abortion and the Doctrine of the Double Effect." *Oxford Review,* no. 5 (1967), pp. 5–15. Reprint. *Moral Problems: A Collection of Philosophical Essays.* 2d ed. Edited by James Rachels. New York: Harper & Row, 1975, pp. 59–70.

FOX, RENÉE C., and SWAZEY, JUDITH P. *The Courage to Fail: A Social View of Organ Transplants and Dialysis.* Chicago: University of Chicago Press, 1974.

FRIED, CHARLES. "Right and Wrong—Preliminary Considerations." *Journal of Legal Studies* 5 (1976): 165–200.

GOUREVITCH, DANIELLE. "Suicide among the Sick in Classical Antiquity." *Bulletin of the History of Medicine* 43 (1969): 501–518.

GRUMAN, GERALD J. "An Historical Introduction to Ideas about Voluntary Euthanasia, with a Bibliographic Survey and Guide for Interdisciplinary Studies." *Omega* 4 (1973): 87–138.

HUME, DAVID. "Of Suicide." *Essays Moral, Political, and Literary.* 2 vols. Edited by T. H. Green and T. H. Grose. The Philosophical Works of David Hume, vols. 3–4. London: Longmans, Green, & Co., 1875, vol. 2, pp. 406–414.

KAMISAR, YALE. "Some Non-religious Views against Proposed 'Mercy-Killing' Legislation." *Minnesota Law Review* 42 (1958): 969–1042.

KANT, IMMANUEL. *Grundlegung zur Metaphysik der Sitten* (1785). Translated and edited by H. J. Paton as *The Moral Law: Kant's Groundwork of the Metaphysic of Morals.* New York: Barnes & Noble, 1967.

KOHL, MARVIN, ed. *Beneficent Euthanasia.* Buffalo, N.Y.: Prometheus Books, 1975.

KÜBLER-ROSS, ELISABETH. *On Death and Dying.* New York: Macmillan Co., 1969.

McCORMICK, RICHARD A. *Ambiguity in Moral Choice.* The 1973 Père Marquette Theology Lecture. Milwaukee: Marquette University Press, Theology Department, 1973.

————. "To Save or Let Die." *Journal of the American Medical Association* 229 (1974): 172–176.

MAGUIRE, DANIEL C. *Death By Choice.* Garden City, N.Y.: Doubleday, 1974.

PIUS XII. "The Prolongation of Life." *The Pope Speaks* 4 (1958): 393–398.

RACHELS, JAMES. "Active and Passive Euthanasia." *New England Journal of Medicine* 292 (1975): 78–80.

RAMSEY, PAUL. *The Patient as Person: Explorations in Medical Ethics.* The Lyman Beecher Lectures at Yale University, 1969. New Haven: Yale University Press, 1970.

THOMAS AQUINAS. *Summa Theologiae* II-II 64,7; Response. Translated by the Fathers of the English Dominican Province as "Whether It Is Lawful to Kill a Man in Self-defense?" *Summa Theologica: First Complete American Edition.* 3 vols. Vol. 2: *Second Part of the Second Part, QQ. 1–189 and Third Part, QQ. 1–90, with Synoptical Charts.* New York: Benziger Brothers, 1947, question 64, article 7, pp. 1471–1472; especially p. 1471.

VEATCH, ROBERT M. *Death, Dying and the Biological Revolution: Our Last Quest for Responsibility.* New Haven: Yale University Press, 1976.

WILLIAMS, GLANVILLE L. *The Sanctity of Life and the Criminal Law.* James S. Carpentier Series, 1956. New York: Alfred A. Knopf, 1957.

III
PROFESSIONAL AND PUBLIC POLICIES

Ethical issues and ethical positions are reflected in explicit philosophical arguments about caring for dying patients, the right to refuse life-saving medical treatment, and the active termination of human life. They are also reflected, at least implicitly, in professional and public policies related to death and dying. Some of these policies deal with the definition of death, the use of cadaver organs for transplantation and other purposes, suicide, and what dying patients should be told. These policies are discussed in the relevant entries elsewhere in this Encyclopedia and are not examined here. Many of the most important and controversial policies deal, however, with the decision to let a dying patient die or to intervene actively to cause death for reasons of mercy. It is such policies that will be examined in this article.

It might be argued on moral grounds that in principle there ought to be no policies regarding letting dying patients die or active intervention to cause death; that such matters should be left in the hands of God or fate. It could be a matter of hospital, professional, or public policy that in all cases everything possible must be done to preserve the life of every dying patient. That policy itself, however, reflects a particular ethical commitment—the commitment to the preservation of life at all costs. While individuals may have held (or thought they have held) such a moral policy position, no society, government, professional, or religious group has even taken such a position. Generally it is recognized that as a matter of policy some things that can be done to preserve life ought not to be done or at least ought not to be required. Different societies and different professional groups have, however, from time to time held different policy positions apparently reflecting different moral positions regarding such decisions.

What follows is a systematic review of policy options focusing first on policies related to professional groups and organizations—that is, policies appropriate for physicians, hospitals, and other professionally organized bodies. Then this article will turn to more public policies: informal policy mechanisms for individual patients as well as laws establishing policies regulating death and dying decision making.

Policies favoring professional decisions

One broad group of policies relating to the care of the dying focuses on the responsibility of the individual professional or group of professionals to use discretion in deciding when it is appropriate to stop care of a dying patient. This discretion is normally exercised in a context of legal limits established by the society. Even contemporary society considers active killing of a terminally ill patient even on grounds of mercy to be an offense (Baughman, Bruha, and Gould, pp. 1203–1204; St. John-Stevas, p. 264). The details of these laws will be discussed later in this article. Such law, moreover, is generally reflected in professional codes and policies.

Policies favoring decision making by physicians. Policies permitting or supporting individual professional decision making focus on the use of professional judgment whether to stop or refuse to initiate treatment of a dying person. Traditionally in Western society this has been seen as part of the physician's prerogative, indeed responsibility. Although occasionally it is suggested that a decision by a physician (at least without court authorization) to let a patient die should and would be treated as a homicide, there has never been a prosecution in the United States for such a decision, and there are no reports available of conviction in other jurisdictions. In fact courts have consistently supported the rights of patients to refuse treatment for any reason whatsoever provided the patient is competent and the treatment is being offered for the patient's own good rather than the good of another (as in public health cases). There have even been decisions supporting such treatment-stopping decisions when they were made by others on behalf of an incompetent patient. Thus, even though the law does not permit a physician to decide to kill for mercy actively, it has generally tolerated reasonable decisions by physicians that treatment should not go on.

This procedure is being endorsed more explicitly in some countries as the debate about the care of the dying becomes more public. For example, the Swiss have had significant public debate about the policy of physician discretion. In 1975 a Swiss physician, Urs Peter Haemmerli, was arrested and accused of murdering by starvation elderly patients at Triemli City Hospital where he was chief of medicine. The patients were described as paralyzed, unconscious persons for whom there was no chance of successful treatment. He was cleared of the charges, the court finding that in nine cases specifically under review "the withholding of nourishment was justified by the fact that it appeared useless to continue feeding a patient whose brain had ceased to function" (Culliton). Although the case could be and has been interpreted as a justification of the policy of permitting physicians to use discretion, there was much confusion over the issues. At some points, arguments were presented that the patients were dead according to brain criteria. At most the Haemmerli decision can be interpreted as justifying the physician's decision in cases where the patient's condition resembled the ones in this case.

In the aftermath of this case the Swiss Academy of Medical Sciences in 1977 issued guidelines for physicians claiming for the physician wide discretion. The Academy favored permitting doctors to discontinue medication as well as technical measures such as respirators, blood transfusions, hemodialysis, and intravenous nourishment when use of these measures "would mean for the dying an unreasonable prolongation of sufferings and if the [patient's]

basic condition has taken an irreversible course."

Many physicians in other countries share the view that they should be permitted to use their judgment in such cases. In France, fifty-three percent of physicians surveyed by the French edition of *Medical Tribune* in 1976 said they would consider "omission of an action which hastens the end" when faced with a terminal patient whose suffering seems unbearable (Joly and Neron). Yet it is still an open question whether professional discretion is the most appropriate policy and, indeed, whether it is legal. It could still be illegal to exercise such discretion even if professional medical groups within a country favored such a policy.

The moral objections to this policy of "individual physician" decision making are of two kinds. One group of opponents objects substantively to the position that physicians should ever be placed in a position of deciding not to do something that they could do to save a life. Another argument focuses more on procedure than on substance. A policy of full professional autonomy in deciding when treatment should be stopped could force treatment on patients who do not want it. It could also lead to stopping treatment on a patient who wants the treatment to continue. It is argued that at least for competent patients this professional decision making is an unacceptable policy. The Swiss directive is qualified to the extent that it insists that doctors must "respect the will of the patient" when such wishes can be expressed even if it does not correspond with what is called the medical indications. The House of Delegates of the Medical Society of the State of New York in 1973 approved a statement that appeared to reject the role of the professional as decision maker, yet holds on to the notion insofar as the physician must approve the decision made by the patient and/or his family. This contrasts with the more patient-centered policy adopted by the American Medical Association's House of Delegates later that same year. The AMA made clear that it rejected active killing, but recognized the right of the patient or his family to make treatment-stopping decisions at least in cases where death is imminent.

The arguments against a policy of granting the individual physician or the medical profession as a whole the authority to make such decisions is grounded variously in the fear that the physician may not adequately know the values of the patient, that the physician may hold special professional values (such as the duty to preserve life) that should not be inflicted on the patient, or that patient and familial freedom and integrity require a policy of removing such authority from the professional realm.

Policies using hospital committees.   All of these difficulties with the policy of permitting the individual physician to decide when and if treatment should be stopped have led to proposals that a committee of professionals be used to make such decisions (Veatch, 1977). In the United States such a policy received great impetus from the case of Karen Ann Quinlan, where a "hospital ethics committee" was required by the judgment of the Supreme Court of the State of New Jersey to review the case (*In the Matter of Karen Quinlan*).

Several proposals for transferring decision-making authority to committees have been put forward (Teel; Rabkin, Gillerman, and Rice). Some committees actually have begun the process although often in more of an advisory than a final decision-making capacity (Critical Care Committee of Massachusetts General Hospital). The policy of having a committee rather than an individual physician make the decision to stop treatment is put forward for several reasons. It is seen as a way of neutralizing the individual biases that a single physician might possess. It is also thought to be a way of diffusing authority for such decisions.

Yet there are objections to the committee approach as well. Although a committee might in principle eliminate the idiosyncratic biases of the individual physician, if it were made up of physicians, it would in no way eliminate any systematic biases that physicians as a group might have. Furthermore, it would not give authority to individual values, rights, and responsibilities of the patient or his family. It is also argued that, although diffusion of personal responsibility for the decision may be psychologically satisfying for the physician, it is a morally risky procedure. Rather, it is argued by opponents of the committee mechanism, someone should have clear responsibility for such a crucial decision. They also argue that, while the individual physician may have personal knowledge of the patient's beliefs and values about treatment stopping, the more impersonal committee can never have this crucial knowledge except indirectly.

There is debate over the various functions that such a committee might perform. In the *Quinlan* court opinion a "hospital ethics committee" was to determine whether "there is no reasonable possibility of Karen's ever emerging from her present comatose condition to a cognitive, sapient state"; that is, they are to confirm prognosis. They are not given the task of reviewing, approving, or disapproving the decision to stop treatment. One task for such committees, then, is to review prognosis, while leaving to others the decision about what to do about stopping treatment. Other committees such as the Critical Care Committee of the Massachusetts General Hospital see themselves much more as advisers to the individual physician. Still other committees deal with problems of allocating scarce resources (such as deciding who receives a single hemodialysis machine when more than one patient needs it) or of general hospital policy. These functions should be kept quite separate from the use of a committee to decide when and if to stop treatment.

Policies favoring patients, other lay persons, and public bodies

The problems with policies focusing on the decision making of individual medical professionals and professional committees have led to consideration of other types of policies with more direct involvement of patients, other lay people, and the public as a whole. Some policies emphasize the role of personal communication by individuals in anticipation of a day when they may not be able to take an active part in deciding whether treatment should continue. Another type of public policy involves legislation to clarify the rights and responsibilities of various actors in decisions about stopping treatment and about active killing for merciful reasons.

Personal communication policies

Living wills and their rationale.   There are a number of responses to the awareness that increasingly decisions must be made about the stopping of medical treatment that prolongs the dying process. One has been the advocacy of informal communication undertaken while a person is of sound mind. Such communication has the objective of indicating the person's wishes regarding terminal care. The most important development has been the preparation of a model document called a "living will." The document, prepared and distributed by the Euthanasia Educational Council, the successor organization to the Euthanasia Society of America, is in the form of an informal letter addressed to "my family, my physician, my lawyer, my clergyman; to any medical facility in whose care

I happen to be; to any individual who may become responsible for my health, welfare, or affairs."

The movement to informal and formal personal expressions of wishes in "living wills" and similar documents has been taken up in many countries in addition to the United States. In Sweden a group called "The Right to Our Death" has promoted such communication as well as legislation. Reportedly thousands of Swedes have signed such documents. In Denmark a group called "My Life Testament" reports similar activity. Similar groups exist in Switzerland and Britain. There is less formal activity in Catholic Europe, such as Italy and France, although groups there are also advocating the "right to die."

The model living will of the Euthanasia Council in the United States includes this request: "If the situation should arise in which there is no reasonable expectation of my recovery from physical or mental disability, I request that I be allowed to die and not be kept alive by artificial or 'heroic' measures." The letter, by itself, is a "request." It probably has no legally binding effect. An earlier version of the document explicity said it was not legally binding.

Other individuals and groups have prepared other versions of such informal communications. The "Christian Affirmation of Life" has since 1974 been distributed by the U.S. Catholic Hospital Association. It includes a more theological introduction, but its operative language is remarkably similar to the Euthanasia Council's document, saying, "I request that, if possible, I be consulted concerning the medical procedures which might be used to prolong my life as death approaches. If I can no longer take part in decisions concerning my own future and there is no reasonable expectation of my recovery from physical or mental disability, I request that no extraordinary means be used to prolong my life."

Objections to these policies. There have been several criticisms of the informal letter devices. They are not, by themselves, legally binding documents, so that if one is worried that he will be treated in a situation where he would not want to be (or would not be treated in a situation where he would want to be) the documents will, at most, provide some guidance; they cannot give a legal guarantee that one's wishes will be followed.

Another criticism is that such documents may be written while one is healthy—perhaps many years before one is critically ill when the document would have to be used. It has been argued that one might change one's mind in the interim. This is said to decrease the reliability of such documents. On the other hand defenders have countered that, while it is true that the writer may have changed his mind, it is more reasonable to presume that the views explicitly set forth in such documents rather than some other views are his current convictions.

Another problem with the letters is that, in part because they are written while one is healthy, they are necessarily very vague. One cannot describe all of the possible conditions under which one may be critically ill. Some physicians have attempted to write much more explicit and specific instructions regarding their own treatment, including such items as the number of minutes without breathing after which resuscitation should not be attempted. It is doubtful than even a well-trained physician could envision all of the specific events that might occur many years in the future. Furthermore one's desire for treatment may depend not only on the medical facts but also on one's life situation. In any case the medical lay person is not able to write instructions with such specificity.

Alternative communications. One alternative that is still in the category of personal communications by individuals prior to the time they are terminally ill is the preparation of a "power of attorney" document that would have as its objective not the specification of conditions under which treatment should or should not be given, but the designation of someone—a spouse, relative, lawyer, clergyman, or friend—as one's agent for the purpose of refusing treatment should the writer become incapable of exercising his own judgment. Some such power of attorney forms include general guidelines to instruct the agent and to make clear to others evaluating the agent's actions what the writer's wishes are. The device leads to decisions made at the critical time by an agent rather than in advance by the writer. It is meant to be legally binding. It provides another alternative for personal expression of wishes about terminal care.

Legislative options. A more formal public policy is also evolving rapidly for the regulation and structuring of decisions concerning death and dying in both case law and legislative proposals. The case law has grown out of court decisions evaluating the right of individual patients or their agents to refuse medical treatment. Several hundred cases in the United States have given substantial clarity to the policy growing on the common law foundation. [This case law is examined in the article RIGHT TO REFUSE MEDICAL CARE.] The legislative options have been receiving increasing attention since about 1970.

Common law countries have traditionally been governed by prohibitions against homicide and suicide, but the precise application to decisions pertaining to the terminally ill has never been clear. The movement to statutory law began in Great Britain in the 1930s with the establishment of the Voluntary Euthanasia Legislation Society. A bill was introduced into the House of Lords in 1936 sponsored by the British society. The bill required that a person sign an application asking to be put to death before the euthanasia could be carried out. The person had to be over twenty-one and suffering from an incurable and fatal disease accompanied by severe pain. Apparently active killing of the one signing such a document was envisioned. The application signed in the presence of two witnesses was to be submitted to a "Euthanasia Referee" appointed by the Minister of Health who was to review the case.

In 1937 a euthanasia bill had been introduced into the Nebraska legislature. About the same time the Euthanasia Society of America was founded by the Reverend Charles Potter. It had first intended to include nonvoluntary euthanasia for eugenic purposes. The legislation proposed for Nebraska had similarly made provision for nonvoluntary killing. A survey of physicians in 1941 indicating resistance to this led the society to limit its activities to voluntary euthanasia. In 1946 a committee including 1,776 physicians worked for legalizing euthanasia in New York State. A bill was introduced into the state legislature in 1947. Reaction to the Nazi experience with compulsory euthanasia for medical as well as genetic reasons combined with the failure of the American movement to distinguish between active killing and omission of treatment led to a diminishing of interest until the late 1960s. At that point increasing use of only partially successful life-extending technologies maintaining individuals in a prolonged debilitated state together with the evolution of an American egalitarian and individual civil rights movement led to a new round of legislative activity. The American legislative proposals rapidly increased in number and variety. Three basic types of legislation appeared. (1) The first type, following the earlier pattern,

would make active killing legal—normally upon request. (2) The second is limited to omission of treatment, but would attempt to clarify the policy regarding decision making in the case of incompetent patients. (3) The third type simply clarifies the rights of the individual to refuse medical treatment and to write a document to take effect should the person become incompetent.

Legislation proposing active killing. The legislative activity in the late 1960s began with the introduction of a bill into the British Parliament that would have made it lawful "for a physician to administer euthanasia to a qualified patient who had made a declaration that is for the time being in force" (Downing, pp. 201–206). Even though the law regarding certain stopping and omission of treatment is unclear, in every country in all legal systems active killing even for mercy and at the request of the one killed is an offense (Silving, p. 378). In modern continental European codes of criminal law motive can be a mitigating factor. The Prussian Landrecht in 1794 imposed a penalty, similar to negligent killing, for "killing with intention believed to be good" of a deadly wounded or otherwise dying person (ibid., p. 368). The codes of Wuerttemberg of 1839 and of Thuringia of 1850 and of other German states also imposed reduced penalty when killing took place at the request of a fatally ill person (ibid.). The Norwegian Penal Code of 1902, which is still in effect, has a similar provision, as do the Russian Penal Code of 1903, the Polish Code of 1932, similar codes in the Baltic countries, the Netherlands, Italy, Norway, Germany, Switzerland, Austria, and Spain (ibid.; Meyers). The 1933 Penal Code of Uruguay provides, "The judges are authorized to forgo punishment of a person whose previous life has been honorable where he commits a homicide motivated by compassion, induced by repeated requests of the victim."

In Germany as well as Switzerland mercy killing is classified not as murder but as manslaughter. German policy is unique in being influenced by the experience of the Nazi period. The eugenic idea of the "life not worthy to be lived" and the life that was a useless burden on the community was crystallized in Karl Binding's publication *Die Freigabe der Vernichtung Lebensunwerten Lebens* (permitting the extermination of life not worth living), but the idea is traced to Luther. One interpretation has it that the German mass extermination program can be traced to the attitude toward the nonrehabilitable sick

(Alexander), but others argue that the racist ideology of a pure *Volk* was the critical element behind both the euthanasia program and the "Final Solution" (Dawidowicz, p. 131). It is true that in late 1938 or early 1939 Hitler received a request from the father of a deformed child asking that the child be killed. He turned the request over to Brandt to investigate with authorization to inform the physicians, in Hitler's name, to carry out the euthanasia. In the spring of 1939 the killing of the mentally deficient and physically deformed children was regularized. In July he turned to the murder of the adult insane and rapidly to the "non-Aryans" and racially unfit. The historical debate, however, centers on whether these beginnings actually led to the development of a new moral policy—the first step on a "slippery slope"—or simply served as a convenient starting point for the execution of a policy already implied in Nazi notions of racial health, without which the whole development would not have occurred.

In contrast under Roman, canon, and common law and under English and American statutory penal law consent or request of the victim is irrelevant and the mercy motive is not a guilt-mitigating factor (Meyers, p. 155; Silving, p. 380). In England the Royal Commission on Capital Punishment in 1953 concluded "reluctantly" that voluntary euthanasia could not be taken out of the category of murder (Meyers, p. 146). Thus if there was to be a change it would have to be by statute. "Euthanasia" was defined in the British bill proposed in 1969 as "the painless inducement of death." A qualified patient was "a patient over the age of majority in respect of whom two physicians (one being of consultant status) have certified in writing that the patient appears to them to be suffering from an irremediable condition." An "irremediable condition" was "a serious physical illness or impairment reasonably thought in the patient's case to be incurable and expected to cause him severe distress or render him incapable of rational existence." The declaration made by the patient was one requesting "the administration of euthanasia at a time or in circumstances to be indicated or specified by me or, if it is apparent that I have become incapable of giving directions, at the discretion of the physician in charge of my case."

Similar bills following the British model were introduced into the legislatures of the state of Idaho in 1969 and Oregon in 1973. All of these bills would have permitted active killing. Further

they would have required the request of the patient executed in writing. The criticism of the bills has been strong on several grounds. The most direct opposition comes from those who object to active killing on moral grounds. The distinction between active killing and omission of treatment is deeply rooted in the moral conscience. Consistently in opinion polls only a small portion favor legalization of active killing while omission of treatment under specific conditions receives substantially more support. Active killing other than on the request of the patient has been found particularly morally objectionable whether the killing is proposed on humanitarian or eugenic grounds. On the other hand, active killing upon the request of the competent patient, as is proposed in the above draft bills, meets the needs of relatively few patients, because those who are sufficiently competent to execute the document are usually not in a condition in which they would request the action. Especially when omission of treatment in order to let the dying process continue (with pain controlled by adequate medication) is an available alternative in all or virtually all cases, the proposals for a policy of legalization of active killing upon request have received little public support.

Laws clarifying decision-making authority. A second type of legislative proposal was introduced into the Florida state legislature by physician-legislator Walter Sackett in 1970. It would have provided that "any person, with the same formalities as required by law for the execution of a last will and testament, may execute a document directing that he shall have the right to death with dignity and that his life shall not be prolonged beyond the point of meaningful existence." The bill went on, however, to clarify who should make such a decision in the case of a patient incompetent by reason of mental or physical incapacity. The first authority was a spouse or person or persons of first degree of kinship. If there were no relatives, it provided that "death with dignity shall be granted any person if in the opinion of three physicians the prolongation of life is meaningless." The bill, which never passed either house in Florida, was the first model focusing on the decision-making authority of guardians or agents for the incompetent patient. A somewhat similar bill was introduced in the legislature of West Virginia in 1972. There are other variants proposed on this model (Veatch, 1976, pp. 164–203). Some would give the first authority to someone designated by the individual while competent, by making use of a power-of-attorney type of instrument. This would avoid difficulties when an individual does not want the next of kin to make the decision, when he does not want to burden the next of kin, or when there is more than one person of equal degree of kinship. Some variants propose that, in cases where there are no relatives, a court-appointed guardian be used rather than a group of physicians. All of these models presume the existing legal remedy of judicial review whenever there is reason to suspect that the designated guardian is acting foolishly or maliciously.

These proposals avoid the moral objections to active killing. The main opposition has come from those who believe that no one other than the patient should be given the responsibility for making such treatment-stopping decisions or believe that relatives cannot be trusted to make them in the interest of the individual who is not competent. It is also argued that it places an undue burden on the family. The rebuttal emphasizes the presumed authority given parents to make decisions about accepting or rejecting treatment on behalf of their children. It is also argued that there has been little difficulty with such a policy when backed by the right of the court to intervene if necessary. Critical to the defense of the policy is a theory of the rights and responsibilities of the family. Defenders claim that the family is not only in the best position to speak for the interests of the patient, but has a moral obligation to do so. It is part of the nature of being a good family member even if at times the task is burdensome. The importance of the family in protecting the rights and interests of an incompetent member was central to the most important court case in this area, the case of Karen Ann Quinlan. Defenders of this type of legislation argue that someone must make decisions about what constitutes appropriate care of the incompetent dying patient. Those decisions should be based on the religious and ethical values of the patient if the patient had been competent. Or if the patient has never been competent, then the family, functioning within the limits of the law, may speak through the next of kin as the proper presumed guardian for purposes of initiating decisions to refuse treatment.

Legislation clarifying the right to refuse treatment. A third type of bill is much more modest in its intent. It would not make active killing legal even upon request. It would not even clarify the decision-making process for the incompetent

patient. It simply affirms the right of the competent patient to refuse medical treatment—a right already existing in U.S. law—and makes legal certain written instructions should the patient become incompetent. One of the legal problems in American jurisdictions has been that, even though it is clear that the competent patient could refuse any treatment whatsoever, it has not been clear that the refusal would remain valid if a patient lapsed into incompetency.

Walter Sackett, having experienced defeat of his previous proposals, introduced such a bill into the Florida legislature in 1973. It provided that any person may at any time execute a document directing that medical treatment designed solely to sustain the life processes be discontinued. Resistance to this bill (defeated by a close vote) came from some who opposed any legislation in this area and others who felt the bill did not go far enough. A similar bill was introduced into the Massachusetts legislature that year and in the next few years similar bills were proposed in at least thirty-nine states.

On 30 September 1976, the governor of the state of California signed the first law providing for what was called a "natural death" (California Health and Safety Code). The law specifies that "any adult person may execute a directive directing the withholding or withdrawal of life-sustaining procedures in a terminal condition." The directive is a statement of a desire that "my life shall not be artificially prolonged." It is limited to very narrow conditions when "I should have an incurable injury, disease, or illness certified to be a terminal condition by two physicians, and where the application of life-sustaining procedures would serve only to artificially prolong the moment of my death and where my physician determines that my death is imminent whether or not life-sustaining procedures are utilized."

One line of objection has come from those who argue that this is an opening wedge for more offensive euthanasia proposals or is, in itself, morally offensive in surrendering the obligation to prolong life as long as possible. Stronger objection has come, however, from those who argue that the bill is either not needed or does not go far enough. Some have argued that in the light of the already existing right to refuse medical treatment the statute adds nothing and in fact, by being limited to certifiably terminal illness, may give the impression that those who are not certifiably terminally ill do not have the right to refuse lifesaving medical treatment. The statute at least makes clear that, if you execute such a document at least fourteen days after becoming certifiably terminally ill, the directive must be followed by the physician, unless revoked, or the physician will be guilty of professional misconduct. This legal authorization of the written document was never clear before the passage of the California bill.

The bill, however, does not remove the fear of those who execute a document or a "living will" before they are certifiably terminally ill. In such a case "the attending physician may give weight to the directive as evidence of the patient's directions regarding the withholding or withdrawal of life-sustaining procedures and may consider other factors. In this case the patient's written instructions are still not binding. In fact, the physician is authorized as never before to make his own decision over and against the expressed wishes of the patient and cannot be criminally or civilly liable for failing to follow the document. Furthermore the family is given only a marginal role of presenting information rather than the key responsibility as advocated by those supporting the type of policy discussed above.

Not only does the document allow substantial physician discretion; it defines terminal illness very narrowly. A terminal condition is defined as one that is incurable "regardless of the application of life-sustaining procedures" and "would, within reasonable medical judgment, produce death, and where the application of life-sustaining procedures serve only to postpone the moment of death of the patient." Thus a patient with severe physical or psychological suffering from hemodialysis is not terminally ill, because if treated he can live indefinitely. Those supporting the moral traditions that recognize this kind of grave burden to justify refusal of treatment (e.g., in the "extraordinary means" ethic) would find this unacceptable. Similar bills have been considered in many states and passed in several. Policy regarding the never competent patient and the patient who lapses into incompetency without executing a document or executes one before being certifiably terminally ill remains vague in all American jurisdictions as does policy on these matters in other countries.

Conclusion

Policy choices must be made by individual patients, their families, physicians, hospitals, and governments. The policies, both professional and public, relating to the decisions about the care of the dying patient have incorporated and must incorporate basic positions on the key ethical issues. The policy choices reflect stances on the value of life, the meaning and importance of freedom, and duties to society and individuals.

ROBERT M. VEATCH

[*Directly related are the entries* ACTING AND REFRAINING; INFANTS, *article on* PUBLIC POLICY AND PROCEDURAL QUESTIONS; *and* RIGHT TO REFUSE MEDICAL CARE. *For discussion of related ideas, see the entries:* CHILDREN AND BIOMEDICINE; DEATH, ATTITUDES TOWARD; INFORMED CONSENT IN THE THERAPEUTIC RELATIONSHIP, *article on* LEGAL AND ETHICAL ASPECTS; LIFE; MEDICAL ETHICS UNDER NATIONAL SOCIALISM; *and* PAIN AND SUFFERING. *See also:* DEATH, *articles on* WESTERN PHILOSOPHICAL THOUGHT *and* DEATH IN THE WESTERN WORLD; DEATH, DEFINITION AND DETERMINATION OF; *and* SUICIDE. *See* APPENDIX, SECTION I, PRINCIPLES OF MEDICAL ETHICS, WITH REPORTS AND STATEMENTS (AMERICAN MEDICAL ASSOCIATION).]

BIBLIOGRAPHY

ALEXANDER, LEO. "Medical Science under Dictatorship." *New England Journal of Medicine* 241 (1949): 39–47.

ARISTOTLE. *Politics.* 7.16 1334B-1336A.

BAUGHMAN, WILLIAM H.; BRUHA, JOHN C.; and GOULD, FRANCIS J. "Euthanasia: Criminal, Tort, Constitutional, and Legislative Questions." *Notre Dame Lawyer* 48 (1973): 1203–1260.

California Health and Safety Code. Sec. 7185. Div. 7, pt. 1, chap 3.9, The Natural Death Act.

Critical Care Committee of the Massachusetts General Hospital. "Optimum Care for Hopelessly Ill Patients." *New England Journal of Medicine* 295 (1976): 362–364.

CULLITON, BARBARA J. "The Haemmerli Affair: Is Passive Euthanasia Murder?" *Science* 190 (1975): 1271–1275.

DAWIDOWICZ, LUCY S. *The War against the Jews: 1933–1945.* New York: Holt, Rinehart & Winston, 1975.

DOWNING, A. B., ed. *Euthanasia and the Right to Death: The Case for Voluntary Euthanasia.* Contemporary Issues series, no. 2. London: Peter Owen, 1974.

In the Matter of Karen Quinlan. 2 vols. Vol. 2: *The Complete Briefs, Oral Arguments, and Opinion in the New Jersey Supreme Court.* Introduction by Daniel N. Robinson. Arlington, Va.: University Publications of America, 1976.

JOLY, JEAN-MICHEL, and NERON, MICHEL. "Fifty-three Percent of French GPs Would Consider Passive Euthanasia." *Medical Tribune,* 19 May 1976, pp. 1, 12.

MEYERS, DAVID W. *The Human Body and the Law: A Medico-Legal Study.* Chicago: Aldine Publishing Co., 1970.

PLATO. *Republic.* 5.6 460A.

RABKIN, MITCHELL T.; GILLERMAN, GERALD; and RICE, NANCY R. "Orders Not to Resuscitate." *New England Journal of Medicine* 295 (1976): 364–366.

ST. JOHN-STEVAS, NORMAN. *Life, Death, and the Law:*

Law and Christian Morals in England and the United States. Bloomington: Indiana University Press, 1961.

SILVING, HELEN. "Euthanasia: A Study in Comparative Criminal Law." *University of Pennsylvania Law Review* 103 (1954): 350–389.

TEEL, KAREN. "The Physician's Dilemma. A Doctor's View: What the Law Should Be." *Baylor Law Review* 27 (1975): 5–9.

VEATCH, ROBERT M. *Death, Dying, and the Biological Revolution: Our Last Quest for Responsibility.* New Haven: Yale University Press, 1976.

———. "Hospital Ethics Committees: Is There a Role? Some Possible Functions . . . and Problems." *Hastings Center Report* 7, no. 3 (1977), pp. 22–25.

WILLIAMS, GLANVILLE. *The Sanctity of Life and the Criminal Law.* James S. Carpentier series, 1956. New York: Knopf, 1957; London: Faber & Faber, 1958.

DEATH, ATTITUDES TOWARD

The simple expression "attitudes toward death" encompasses a complex of interrelated but far from identical concepts. The first term, *attitudes*, is recognized as having cognitive, affective, and behavioral components, so we must consider how people think about death, how people feel about death, and how people behave in regard to death.

Nor is the term *death* a unitary concept. When used in this context, it normally includes the dying process, the moment of death, and the state of being dead. Each of these may be perceived as something imminent or something indefinitely far off in time, as something that will happen to oneself or that will happen to others, as something attended to as an abstract concept or as something personal and real. "Attitudes toward death," then, includes, for example, how I feel about my being dead, what I think about your being in the process of dying, and how I behave in response to a funeral procession.

Attitudes, by definition, are relatively enduring, but they also occur within a context. Thus global statements about either an individual or a culture as being death-denying or fearful of death require careful delineation. An individual might properly be described as death-denying, yet he or she might discuss the latest grotesque homicide with glee. Western culture is generally described as death-denying, yet newspapers are filled with accounts of death; cemeteries and mortuaries are visible to the casual passerby; and an immense number of expressions using the word *death* and its derivatives have crept into Western languages. In order to understand death-related behavior at any given moment, it is necessary to understand the broad social con-

text, the immediate situation, and the life history and present circumstances of the individual affected.

Another concern in understanding the death attitudes of an individual or of a community is the process through which such attitudes are communicated. The attitudes of individuals can be ascertained by asking them how they think or feel, by observing their behavior (how they adopt health practices, drive automobiles, observe religious rituals, participate in life-threatening activities), by asking others who know them, by evaluating their creative output (literature, painting, music), or by some of the more subtle kinds of measures developed by behavioral scientists over the years.

A similar tactic can be used to understand the death attitudes of a community (e.g., society, culture, subculture, people, group). In both instances, we must attend to both the most frequent responses/occurrences and the variation of responses/occurrences. However, whether our focus is the individual or the community, we need to remain alert to the potential for error in the information. Broadly speaking, such error can arise from three sources: distortions and misrepresentations in what various individuals or other sources communicate; ambiguities and incompleteness in the message; and biases and inaccuracies in the interpretation.

Because the likelihood of error arising from these sources is substantial, caution is required in translating the results of any attitude studies into policy, programs, or practice. Feifel and Branscomb have pointed out that responses to death-related stimuli are very different when elicited at the level of conscious awareness from those elicited at levels of less conscious awareness. This makes the research base for policy decisions more problematic, since the decisions are so significant and the research is still so new. A particularly relevant instance is the attitude toward permitting people to die if they want to. Results of one study indicated that about half the respondents agreed that people should be given this prerogative, especially if they are in pain or dying anyway. Of those who did not approve, explanations primarily revolved around the belief that only God has the right to take a life (forty-nine percent) or that there is always hope (thirty-two percent) (Kalish and Reynolds). The ethical issue is not only whether or not to allow a person to die, or even whether or not to accelerate the dying process, but the prior issue of how to evaluate survey data when the implications are literally matters of life and death.

Attitudes of persons facing their own imminent death: stage approaches

The work of Elisabeth Kübler-Ross has undoubtedly had greater influence on both theory and clinical practice than any previous writing. Based on many discussions with terminally ill persons, plus other sources of information, Kübler-Ross described five stages through which dying persons were seen to move: (1) *denial* and isolation, (2) *anger* and resentment, (3) *bargaining* and an attempt to postpone, (4) *depression* and sense of loss, and (5) *acceptance*. Kübler-Ross views this progression as both normal and adaptive, especially when the final stage of acceptance is reached and maintained. Medical caretakers are encouraged to enable their dying patients to advance through the stages, albeit at their own rate, hoping for minimal regression—that is, without returning to denial or anger after a subsequent stage has been attained. Inadequate medical or psychosocial care is often held responsible when a patient who has come to accept his or her coming death returns to a less adaptive stage.

Both the value of the stage approach and its validity have been questioned by others. Concern has been expressed that the stages have become so familiar to many health and social practitioners, as well as to the patients themselves and their families, at least in North America, that there is danger of the stages becoming a self-fulfilling prophecy. It is difficult to ascertain whether the stages are universal, modal, culture-bound, or even adaptive, since no consistent research findings have been reported, and medical clinicians themselves are in disagreement. One summary of the existing literature (Schulz and Alderman) reports little published support for the stages as occurring in the indicated sequence, but the stages appear to provide a useful framework for those who work with terminal patients. Kübler-Ross cautions that the sequence is not immutable, that many patients move back and forth or even maintain two or more stages virtually simultaneously. Kastenbaum reflects the concerns of many workers in the field when he states that "the rapid acceptance of the stage theory of dying has quite outdistanced any attempt to examine the theory empirically or logically . . . and no

effort has been made to test out the theory as it continues to become more widely disseminated and applied" (p. 42).

There is little doubt that Kübler-Ross's name is better known than that of anyone else working on the concerns of death and dying or that her stages are the single best-known piece of information extant. Given the lack of empirical validation of her work and the extent to which her stages have been questioned by other knowledgeable persons, an ethical question arises as to the degree to which her writing should function as a basis for policy or practice. The emerging ethical issue is whether her five stages are not merely descriptive but also optimally adaptive and, if the latter, whether policy should encourage practice to intervene with dying persons to increase the probability that they will pass successfully through all five stages in time to die having reached the stage of acceptance. That this kind of intervention is already being practiced is common knowledge; the degree to which it is good or poor practice has not yet been determined.

Attitudes of persons facing their own imminent death: other approaches

Other investigators, using quite different methodologies and asking different questions, have emerged with other kinds of insights. One question that has been studied on several occasions is the desire of dying persons to know of their terminal condition. Through interviews with the dying, evidence has accumulated that not only do they wish to have a reasonable understanding of their prognosis but, given the opportunity, most will spontaneously mention awareness of their own condition, even though relatively few had received official medical diagnosis (Hinton, 1966). Those with dependent children and those in greater physical distress were more likely to indicate awareness.

Weisman adds another dimension to understanding the awareness the dying person has of his or her own condition. "Somewhere between open acknowledgement of death and its utter repudiation is an area of uncertain certainty called *middle knowledge*" (Weisman, p. 65). He continues his warning to avoid attempts to establish firm categories: "Patients seem to know and want to know, yet they often talk as if they did not want to be reminded of what they have been told" (ibid., p. 66).

The ability of dying patients to cope psychologically with their impending death has also been investigated. Although previous neurotic symptoms are apparently not related to effective coping, such factors as being physically comfortable, having good marital relationships, having good interpersonal relationships in general, expressing greater life satisfaction, and maintaining open communication about dying all appear prognostic of more positive attitudes in the face of death (Carey, pp. 435–438; Hinton, 1975, pp. 99–110; Kalish).

Certain qualities appear to enable dying persons to survive longer than statistically predicted by their illness. Those patients who outlive anticipated life expectancy are more likely to have good relationships with others and to maintain a higher level of intimacy with family members and friends, even to the time of death. They were also capable of requesting and receiving considerable support, in terms of both medical care and emotional relationships. These individuals were able to accept the reality of having a serious illness, although they often rejected the idea that death was inevitable (perhaps another self-fulfilling prophecy). Similarly, they were seldom deeply depressed, but they were quite likely to express resentment about various aspects of their treatment and illness (Weisman and Worden, p. 70). Such qualities obviously resemble those described in the previous paragraph.

Given these initial findings, including the suggestion that outliving the life tables may be in part a function of being able to express resentment about both health condition and health care, should health caretakers encourage the development of such characteristics among the dying? Since these qualities would be difficult to develop at the time of dying and would, in most instances, need to have occurred previously, are health caretakers ignoring their responsibilities by not participating in health education and mental health programs that would improve family relationships and the ability of patients to request support? Further, since accepting the reality of the prognosis also appears to be life-extending, what responsibilities do physicians and others have to encourage that kind of understanding? All of this appears to lead us back to a familiar dilemma: When it is learned that nonmedical factors contribute to good or poor health, are physicians who are trained to deal with medical factors also responsible to their patients for improving other aspects of their

lives? This dilemma is no less acute for the terminally ill patient than for any other person.

It readily becomes obvious that the dying process and, therefore, attitudes toward it and toward one's own imminent death vary greatly as a function of numerous factors. Glaser and Strauss describe one such factor, the death trajectory, in considerable detail. The cause of death, the pace of decline, and perceptions the patient has of his or her condition all affect death attitudes. A patient dying from lung cancer faces a much different situation from that of a patient who is being rushed to the hospital with a second major coronary; each will undoubtedly differ in attitudes from the patient whose self-inflicted gunshot wounds did not lead to immediate death or the patient whose first stroke has left much of his or her body paralyzed.

Other relevant situational factors include the kind and extent of pain and discomfort and the effectiveness in controlling discomfort; the kind and extent of familial support, which reflects past family relationships; the expectations the patient has of dying, which may be influenced by both cultural and personality factors; the age, and sex, familial roles, extent of unfinished projects, and unresolved tensions in significant human relationships; and location (home, hospital, nursing home, hospice) in which the dying process is occurring.

Attitudes of persons not facing their own imminent death

Innumerable studies have been conducted to determine how various segments of the public feel about death or how they respond to situations in which death is a factor. These have been carried out with psychiatric patients, the elderly, children, adolescents, parents of dying children, physicians, nurses, nursing home personnel, various religious and ethnic groups, the ubiquitous university student, hospital patients, and general respondent populations (Hinton, 1972; Kastenbaum and Aisenberg, pp. 40–246).

Probably the most comprehensive study, based on a quota sampling design, was directed by Kalish and Reynolds. More than four hundred adults in the Los Angeles area were interviewed for one hour each; respondents were about evenly divided among blacks, Japanese Americans, Mexican Americans, and Anglo-Americans; among young, middle-aged, and old; and among men and women. Results showed many significant differences between groups and emphasized the importance of social role as a factor in death attitudes.

A relevant and particularly significant treatise by Becker not only placed fear and denial of death as *the* major determinant of human motivation, but also reinterpreted many Freudian concepts as based on decay, deterioration, and awareness of finitude rather than on Freud's original sex-related considerations (pp. 11–46). Becker posits a "healthy-minded" argument versus a "morbid-minded" argument regarding the fear and denial of death. The former assumes that fear of death is learned and, therefore, can be unlearned or, even better, never learned at all as the result of "healthy" early learning. The latter assumes that the fear of death is natural and is present in everyone, that it is "the basic fear that influences all others, a fear from which no one is immune, no matter how disguised it may be" (p. 15). Optimum learning and social environment can reduce the fear, or terror, but cannot eliminate it; indeed, Becker contends that much of our behavior arises from just such attempts to reduce the fear of death, not the least of which are our attempts to be in control, to attain power, and to relate to transcendent phenomena.

The position one takes regarding the nature and origin of the fear of death thus obviously relates to one's perceptions as to how to reduce this fear or whether to try. For those whom Becker terms "healthy-minded," the attempt to reduce the death fears of others through educational and therapeutic programs might be perceived as virtually a responsibility; for the "morbid-minded," the task called for would have more modest results. Further, if one continues to follow Becker, he would have to deal with the use of rituals and adherence to concepts of transcendence to reduce death fears, while others might espouse more familiar kinds of learning. Thus pedagogy, therapy, and ethics intertwine in the wake of religion and values.

Attitude surveys are not consistent with Becker's assumptions. One review of the literature has shown that, when asked directly, only a small proportion of individuals will admit fear of death (Kalish). Although this could be considered an indication of extensive denial rather than low fear of death, it is more likely that death fear is so complex that direct attitude questions do not effectively probe its meaning for most individuals.

Attitudinal studies of correlates of death fear have also been reviewed, and it was found that high fear is related to high scores on measures of depression, impulsivity, hysteria, manifest anxiety, need for heterosexual activity, need to be succorant, and low need for change. Conflicting results have emanated from studies of religiousness and death fear, with the less religious stating the higher fear of death. However, when curvilinear rather than linear functions were tested, it appeared that the highest death fear was found among persons who were intermediate in religiousness and who were irregular churchgoers, while both the non-religious and the devoutly religious displayed considerably less fear (ibid.).

Differences in responses from the ethnic communities did not follow any particular patterns, but could be interpreted primarily in terms of the ethnology of the community. Thus, of four ethnic groups, Japanese Americans were more likely than others to say they would try very hard to control the way they showed their emotions in public following the death of a loved one; Mexican Americans and black Americans were most likely to say that the death of an infant is less tragic than the death of persons of other ages; white Americans were most likely to have made out a will and least likely to agree that "accidental deaths show the hand of God working among men." When asked directly how they felt about death, Japanese and Mexican Americans were more likely than the others to say they were afraid.

It is important to keep in mind that attitude surveys measure what people say they feel or believe, which presumably correlates with what they actually feel or believe. The common assumption made concerning people's fear of death is that appropriate interventions will help reduce the fear. That this is true is most probable, but the nature of the optimum kinds of interventions is less certain. On the one hand, death educators believe that proper early learning experiences will keep fear of death to a minimum; on the other hand, other experienced persons believe that death fears are maximally reduced through reducing fears of abandonment and loss of control. These are not mutually exclusive, but they most certainly point to differing ameliorative approaches.

Attitudes of professionals

Work-related involvements with the dying and the dead are found in many vocational fields: medicine, nursing, social work, ministry and chaplaincy, cemetery and funeral work, florist industry, police, military, and a variety of others. Much related literature has been critical of the professionals for focusing too much on their specific task and not relating to the feelings of dying persons and their families. This criticism has frequently been directed toward physicians. Thus one study describes its findings as showing "a number of deficiencies and discrepancies in our approach to the terminally ill patient." Such studies emphasize "the patient's desire for complete openness and honesty in discussions regarding diagnosis and prognosis, the physician's reluctance to be that candid, the resident's relative lack of concern for the patient's emotional needs, and the social worker's tendency to minimize the problem" (Mount, Jones, and Patterson, p. 741). Feifel and his colleagues provide additional supportive data showing that a sample of eighty-one physicians exhibited more fear of death than either a group of physically ill persons or a group of healthy normal individuals.

The issue of communication between the dying patient and the health caretakers has been extensively discussed, and the overwhelming weight of opinion seems to support the view that open awareness is, for most dying persons, an optimum setting. Nonetheless, large numbers of physicians have indicated in surveys that they seldom or never inform their patients about their own death (Fitts and Ravdin). With amazing consistency, however, individuals indicate themselves as capable of and desiring the necessary information to understand their prognosis, while being less certain that others are similarly deserving (Kalish and Reynolds). This has been shown equally true for physicians themselves.

A question that is frequently posed is whether individuals who have not fully handled their own feelings about their own death are capable of working effectively with others who are dying. Although no empirical evidence is available, the weight of professional opinion is that people who have great difficulty with their own feelings concerning death will definitely have trouble relating to others who are dying. This does not mean, however, that all vestiges of death fear must be eliminated prior to working with the dying, or that physicians who have not worked through their feelings about death are ineffective in working medically with the dying. Rather, it suggests two possibilities. First, those physicians who prefer avoiding the psychosocial relationship with their dying patients should consider

requesting the help of another relevant person to supplement their own functioning; second, physicians and others who have extensive contact with dying persons should develop their own support system, if they lack support through family members, since the professional person's confrontation with death and loss may prove destructive of both his work-related and his personal involvements.

Conclusion

Many issues, not all of which have been touched upon here, arise in any discussion of attitudes toward death. Substantive issues include the effects of religious belief systems on the ability to deal with death and dying, the implications of changing funerary and burial practices, the possible emergence of a new group of professionals trained particularly to work with the dying, the reasons why death has become a significant concern among sociomedical and behavioral scientists and practitioners at this time, and many more. Although a modest body of research and commentary now exists, the data and the insights are just beginning to accumulate.

At the same time, ethical issues are seen as increasingly important. Among the more important ethical issues, aside from those mentioned previously in this article, are the implications of brain death; the right of an individual to opt for euthanasia or suicide; the issue of who should participate in the decision for an abortion; the potential for psychological damage to research participants in death attitude studies; the validity of what people state on a questionnaire about their attitudes toward death and whether this should be perceived as a base for policy; the need to change the health-care financing system to permit new kinds of care for the dying; the development of standards for persons working in one-to-one relationships with the dying; the need for standards for death educators, especially those serving in the public school system; and the impact of these new death education programs on their students.

There appears little reason to doubt that the current interest in death and dying is not merely a fad but has become a fashion. The degree to which the fashion will embed itself into the social fabric of Western and other nations is still unknown.

RICHARD A. KALISH

[*Directly related are the entries* RIGHT TO REFUSE MEDICAL CARE; *and* TRUTH-TELLING. *Other relevant material may be found under* DEATH; DEATH AND DYING: EUTHANASIA AND SUSTAINING LIFE, *articles on* ETHICAL VIEWS *and* PROFESSIONAL AND PUBLIC POLICIES; DEATH, DEFINITION AND DETERMINATION OF; *and* SUICIDE. *See also:* CARE; *and* THERAPEUTIC RELATIONSHIP.]

BIBLIOGRAPHY

BECKER, ERNEST. *The Denial of Death.* New York: Macmillan Publishing Co., Free Press, 1973. An analysis of the pervasive meaning of death for all human activity; written by a social anthropologist, but based more on writing and thinking associated with psychology and philosophy.

CAREY, RAYMOND G. "Emotional Adjustment in Terminal Patients: A Quantitative Approach." *Journal of Counseling Psychology* 21 (1974): 433–439. A study, based on ratings of chaplains, of factors related to emotional adjustment in dying patients.

FEIFEL, HERMAN, and BRANSCOMB, ALLEN B. "Who's Afraid of Death?" *Journal of Abnormal Psychology* 81 (1973): 282–288. Measures death fear in several populations at three awareness levels: conscious, fantasy, and below the level of awareness.

————; HANSON, SUSAN; JONES, ROBERT; and EDWARDS, LAURI. "Physicians Consider Death." *Proceedings of the 75th Annual Convention of the American Psychological Association.* Washington: 1967, vol. 2, pp. 201–202. Reports a segment of a larger study on attitudes of physicians, nurses, critically and terminally ill persons, and healthy persons regarding death and dying.

FITTS, WILLIAM T., and RAVDIN, I. S. "What Philadelphia Physicians Tell Patients with Cancer." *Journal of the American Medical Association* 153 (1953): 901–904. A mail survey of physicians in Philadelphia disclosed that only a minority regularly informed their patients concerning their terminal prognosis.

GLASER, BARNEY G., and STRAUSS, ANSELM L. *Awareness of Dying.* Chicago: Aldine Publishing Co., 1965. A comparison of various awareness contexts, for example, open awareness, mutual pretense, suspicion awareness. In each context, the extent to which the dying person is aware of his prognosis and the significance of his awareness for communication with others is discussed.

————, and STRAUSS, ANSELM L. *Time for Dying.* Chicago: Aldine Publishing Co., 1968. Describes the results of a grounded theory study of dying trajectories, based on extensive observations and interviews.

HINTON, JOHN M. *Dying.* 2d ed. Studies in Social Pathology. Edited by C. M. Carstairs. Baltimore: Penguin Books, 1972. A review of death and dying, with particular attention to the dying patient and the role of the caretaker.

————. "Facing Death." *Journal of Psychosomatic Research* 10 (1966): 22–28. A study based on interviews with terminally ill patients; includes discussion of related studies.

————. "The Influence of Previous Personality on Reactions to Having Terminal Cancer." *Omega* 6 (1975): 95–111. An investigation of mood, satisfaction with care, and life satisfaction of patients with terminal cancer; numerous correlates are statistically evaluated.

KALISH, RICHARD A. "Death and Dying in a Social Context." *Handbook of Aging and the Social Sciences.* Edited by Robert H. Binstock and Ethel Shanas. Handbooks of Aging Series. Edited by James E. Birren. New York: Van Nostrand Reinhold, 1976, pp. 483–503. An overview of death and dying in the later years.

————, and REYNOLDS, DAVID K. *Death and Ethnicity: A Psychocultural Study.* Los Angeles: University of Southern California Press, 1976. A research monograph based on the findings of a three-year study; data are reported across ethnic groups and within ethnic groups.

KASTENBAUM, ROBERT. "Is Death a Life Crisis?: On the Confrontation with Death in Theory and Practice." *Life-Span Developmental Psychology: Normative Life Crises.* Edited by Nancy Datan and Leon H. Ginsberg. The Fourth West Virginia University Conference on Life-Span Developmental Psychology, 1974. New York: Academic Press, 1975, pp. 19–50. An examination of how death is seen as a variable, event, state, analogy, and mystery.

————, and AISENBERG, RUTH. *The Psychology of Death.* New York: Springer Publishing Co., 1972. A comprehensive book discussing the entire range of thought, research, and theory concerning death and dying, with particular emphasis on psychological factors.

KÜBLER-ROSS, ELISABETH. *On Death and Dying.* New York: Macmillan Co., 1969. The now classical description of five stages in the dying process, accompanied by extensive case materials.

MOUNT, BALFOUR M.; JONES, ALLEN; and PATTERSON, ANDREW. "Death and Dying: Attitudes in a Teaching Hospital." *Urology* 4 (1974): 741–748. A survey of staff and patients regarding specific issues concerning the role of health caretakers for the terminally ill. Results showed that members of different health professions perceived their roles and their own effectiveness much differently from members of other health professions or the patients themselves.

SCHULZ, RICHARD, and ALDERMAN, DAVID. "Clinical Research and the Stages of Dying." *Omega* 5 (1974): 137–143. A critical evaluation of both research and commentary concerning various stage theories of dying.

WEISMAN, AVERY D. *On Dying and Denying.* Foreword by Herman Feifel. New York: Behavioral Publications, 1972. A thorough discussion of what dying means and how it takes place, written by a highly experienced psychiatrist.

————, and WORDEN, J. WILLIAM. "Psychosocial Analysis of Cancer Deaths." *Omega* 6 (1975): 61–75. A determination of which psychosocial factors are related to living beyond the statistical prognosis for specific cancer conditions.

DEATH, DEFINITION AND DETERMINATION OF

I. CRITERIA FOR DEATH   *Gaetano F. Molinari*
II. LEGAL ASPECTS OF PRONOUNCING DEATH
                    Alexander Morgan Capron
III. PHILOSOPHICAL AND THEOLOGICAL
     FOUNDATIONS   *Dallas M. High*

I
CRITERIA FOR DEATH

Introduction

Technical advances in medicine now permit maintenance and support of cardiac and respiratory function in man long after massive or even total destruction of the brain. Conversely, in specially equipped operating rooms the biological integrity of the human brain can be protected and maintained for extended, though finite, periods of time, while the function of the heart and lungs is deliberately but reversibly suspended in order to permit successful open-heart surgery. Whereas previously cerebral function and cardiorespiratory function were intimately mutually dependent, modern medical technology permits dissociations among individual vital functions. These dissociations have outstripped the usefulness of a monolithic set of criteria for the pronouncement of death based upon the vitality of a single organ system.

Terminology

Borderline states between life and death have been recognized for many years (Mollaret and Goulon; Bertrand et al.) and a series of often lyrical, sometimes practical neologisms has evolved very rapidly to identify varying degrees of biological integration and survival short of complete cognitive, sentient life. Such terms include coma depassé, coma-vigil, artificial survival, and more recently irreversible coma and persistent vegetative state. Many of these terms have been defined only descriptively; some have been used quite precisely and have been correlated pathologically with massive brain destruction; others correlate with smaller lesions in specific but critical brain centers.

In dealing with current medical developments, the terms cerebral death and brain death have crept into common usage among physicians. While the cerebrum is a part of the brain with distinctive ontogenetic and phylogenetic characteristics, the adjective "cerebral" is often used imprecisely. Terms such as cerebral circulation and cerebral vasculature refer to the blood supply to the entire brain rather than to the cerebrum specifically. Many physicians use the terms "brain death" and "cerebral death" interchangeably, while a few insist on precise distinctions, adding "cortical death" as yet another entity (Korein).

The former group uses the term brain death or cerebral death in contradistinction to cardiac death. The others equate the irreparable destruction of a part of the organ with the "death" of that part. Still others equate certain microscopic characteristics of individual nerve cells with cellular "death." These terms are still more confusing to those outside of medicine, because they imply that there are different kinds of death.

Better terms for the more generic application of "brain death" and "cardiac death" are death as determined by neurological criteria and death as determined by cardiological criteria.

To distinguish among cortical death, cerebral death, and brain death implies that there are degrees of death stratified in accordance with the hierarchical organization of the nervous system. Throughout this treatise, the use of ambiguous, controversial, or confusing terms will be avoided. However, that will not always be possible when referring to the work of some authors.

Classical criteria

The signs of life used in day-to-day medical care, routinely observed, measured, and recorded on hospitalized patients' daily records, are body temperature, pulse, respiratory rate, and blood pressure. While determination of these vital signs is generally left to the nursing staff, their absence may be used as criteria for death only by a physician. Therefore, the pragmatic but traditional criteria for death have been the cessation of heartbeat or cardiac pulse, respiration, blood pressure, followed by a fall in body temperature as determined or confirmed by a physician. The first three are eminently more practical than the last; in fact, the pronouncement or declaration of death is rarely delayed until the body temperature falls.

Despite the ready availability of physiological monitoring of cardiovascular functions, such as electrocardiography, no moral, medical, or legal principles mandate the use of the most sensitive technical device available to determine death under ordinary circumstances. Nonetheless, when such equipment is already in use in operating rooms and in coronary care units, the increased sensitivity afforded the physician is exploited. Death has not usually been declared in the presence of electrical evidence of cardiac function, even though blood pressure, pulse, and respiration have disappeared. It should also be noted that no medical policy or legal precedent specifies a duration of time over which the classical criteria must persist.

Irreversible coma

Coma is defined as a pathological state of depressed consciousness from which the patient cannot be aroused even by painful stimulation. Coma may be caused by a wide variety of disease states that affect the entire brain or merely a strategic part of the brain. When the cause of the coma is known, and that cause is a disease known to be irreparable, a state of irreversible coma exists, a coma from which there is no hope of recovery.

Irreversible coma merely predicts death without return of consciousness; it neither implies that death has occurred nor does it predict precisely when death will occur. Patients in irreversible coma may have portions of the nervous system intact, which permit blood pressure, pulse, respiration, and normal body temperature to persist indefinitely without artificial or mechanical support.

Irreversible destruction of the entire brain

Respiratory movement is initiated by centers within the primitive brain or brain stem; but cardiac muscle has the intrinsic properties of excitability and contractility independent of nervous system control. Hence, the complete destruction of the brain, including loss of spontaneous respiration, may occur while the cardiovascular system continues to function autonomously. Apnea (the absence of spontaneous respiration) has been considered by most medical authors to be a cardinal sign of total brain destruction. Other practical and reliable indices of brain-stem function are the cephalic reflexes, or those reflexes the presence of which require anatomical, physiological, and biochemical integrity of specific brain-stem centers.

Pupil size, pupillary reactions to light, eye movement in response to passive head movement (oculocephalic), eye movement in response to caloric stimulation of the inner ear (vestibulo-ocular), pharyngeal, swallowing, and cough reflexes, in addition to respiration, all are determined by the activity of specific brain-stem centers.

Therefore, the basic criteria for the suspicion

of a totally destroyed brain are unresponsive coma, apnea, and absent cephalic reflexes. When these criteria are judged to be permanent, the brain may be considered irreversibly destroyed. However, two reversible causes of coma are also known to produce this constellation of clinical signs, namely, drug intoxication and low body temperature. Allen and his associates have recently analyzed and reported the predictive and discriminative value of the clinical findings in individuals suspected to have irreversibly destroyed brains. In addition to clinical signs, most authors have recommended either objective confirmatory tests, prescribed durations for persistence of the clinical signs, or both, in order to determine if a brain is irreversibly destroyed and to pronounce death on that basis in jurisdictions authorizing such pronouncement (Allen et al.).

Prolonged nonfunctional state

In its 1968 report, the Harvard Committee on Irreversible Coma described the clinical and electroencephalographic characteristics of the nonfunctioning brain. A prerequisite the Committee required was the exclusion of patients with drug intoxication and hypothermia, the reversible conditions known to depress cerebral function, reflex activity, and electrical activity measured by the electroencephalogram (EEG).

In the absence of hypothermia and drug intoxication, the Committee suggested that concomitant unresponsive coma, apnea, absence of cephalic reflexes, absence of spinal reflexes, and an isoelectric electroencephalogram were characteristic of patients with a nonfunctioning brain. Persistence of all these features for twenty-four hours was thought adequate grounds to consider the nonfunctioning state permanent. Although the Committee expressed some doubt about the necessity for the absence of spinal reflexes, that group, in fact, equated brain death with the "permanently nonfunctioning brain."

Clinical experience

Mohandas and Chou recommended far less stringent criteria. Their data suggested that, in patients who have known brain damage of a type known to be irreparable, no spontaneous movement, apnea, and absent brain-stem reflexes persistent for twelve hours, predict an invariably fatal outcome (Mohandas and Chou). While these criteria may predict eventual death with certainty, they rely totally on the responsible physician's diagnostic skills, his knowledge of the natural history of the specific disease diagnosed, and his confidence in the universal applicability of statistical outcome data. Not only do these criteria admit to the possibility of human error at multiple levels, they fail to distinguish the dead from the dying brain. Moreover, in an analysis of 503 prospectively studied brain-death suspects, seventeen patients would have met these criteria even while they had evidence of cerebral activity electroencephalographically (Walker and Molinari).

Cardiovascular collapse

A study undertaken in 1973 in Japan concluded that a diagnosed gross primary brain lesion, deep coma, bilateral dilated pupils with absent pupillary and corneal reflexes (a selection of specific brain-stem reflexes), and an isoelectric EEG characterize moribund patients. Furthermore, the Japanese group observed that a fall in the blood pressure of 40 mm of mercury and persistent low blood pressure for six hours signal the imminence of death (Ueki, Takeuchi, and Katsurada).

These criteria redirect the major focus for the difference between irreversible coma and imminent death from the neurological characteristics of the patients back to classical circulatory system criteria. The progressive and irreversible failure of another of the "vital signs," namely blood pressure, is used as the decisive factor, adequate for termination of artificial support mechanisms.

Scandinavian criteria

At a symposium on this subject, reported in 1972 (Ingvar and Widén), criteria were recommended for use in Scandinavia incorporating the combination of clinical features, cerebral electrical activity, and arrest of the circulation to the brain (regional or local circulatory arrest).

The symposium participants suggested that patients could be dead who had known primary or secondary brain lesions, unresponsive coma, apnea, and absence of all cerebral functions including brain-stem reflexes; a single electroencephalogram showing no biological activity, and radiological evidence of shutdown of the cerebral blood vessels were considered confirmatory objective evidence of a nonviable brain. Furthermore, they postulated that failure to demonstrate perfusion of cerebral arteries, using standard X-ray methods, on two trials twenty-five minutes apart, indicates impairment of circulation to the point of total destruction of the brain.

These criteria are very attractive, because (1) they utilize multiple parameters independently measured and thereby are cross-confirmatory; (2) they eliminate the need to exclude drug intoxication and other metabolic disturbances by biochemical methods, since these etiologies do not grossly affect the cerebral vasculature, and therefore brain circulatory patterns are normal; and (3) they reduce the requirement for persistence of the criteria to the absolute minimum (twenty-five minutes). These criteria therefore equate death by neurological criteria with total brain infarction.

The collaborative study of brain death

A prospective collaborative study of deeply comatose, apneic patients was undertaken in the United States and published in 1975 (Walker). Five hundred and three patients were followed by clinical and electroencephalographic examinations at regular intervals until outcome. Pathological confirmation of the clinical diagnosis of brain death was sought in all fatal cases coming to autopsy.

The findings of that study were somewhat unsettling. First, opinions regarding the histological characteristics of the brains from respirator-dependent patients varied among pathologists, even those specializing in nervous system diseases (Moseley, Molinari, and Walker). Second, in some patients the pathology failed to confirm the clinical diagnosis of total brain destruction (Walker, Diamond, and Moseley). A few patients who were pronounced dead after prolonged periods of coma, apnea, absence of cephalic reflex activity, and electrocerebral silence showed few changes at autopsy of the types reputed to indicate nerve-cell death. Conversely, a few who continued to record biological activity in the EEG until the moment of final cardiac arrest showed postmortem changes consistent with long-standing, advanced, and widespread cellular death in the brain. While reasons for these variations exist, it seems clear that the morphological changes of neuronal death lag behind the physiological and biochemical end points of irreversibility. Therefore, one cannot expect objective confirmation of the clinical diagnosis of death by neurological criteria by the postmortem changes perceptible by light microscopy.

Third, in objective screening of blood samples from deeply comatose patients more instances of drug ingestion (or administration) were uncovered than had been suspected clinically. Even in clear cases of attempted suicide by massive drug overdose, quantitative measurements of the offending drug in the blood were disproportionately low compared to the severity of the clinical syndromes produced. Qualitative identification of drugs alone and in combination was limited by the adequacy of local screening techniques and procedures. The absence of a history of drug ingestion in comatose patients does not exclude the possibility of their presence in the blood. Drugs taken by the patient before a severe accident involving brain injury or, indeed, drugs given therapeutically for convulsions caused by the cerebral disease, may contribute to the overall depression of clinical and electrical indices of nervous system function; consequently the presence of any amount of drugs in the blood introduces doubt as to the irreversibility of the clinical syndrome.

Therefore, it seemed highly desirable to resort to criteria for irreversible destruction of the brain that would be independent of the nature of the disease or cause of the coma (Walker). The criteria recommended for use in Scandinavia seemed to meet this requirement, but in the 503 cases studied in the United States only seventeen X-ray studies of the circulation were performed (Walker and Molinari). The latter fact probably represents the reluctance of American physicians to subject their moribund or desperately ill patients to even slight additional risk. Moreover, neither the equipment required nor respirator-dependent patients themselves are portable, so obtaining X-ray confirmation is a major operational problem. Therefore, these criteria seem impractical.

Indirect assessment of the cerebral circulation is possible, however, by any of a number of parameters. Several ophthalmological methods for indirect assessment of the cerebral circulation have been reported over the years (Pines; Kevorkian; Lobstein, Tempe, and Payeur). Echoencephalography permits ultrasonic detection of brain pulsations at the bedside (Uematsu and Walker). The perfusion of the cerebrovascular bed may be detected using tracer amounts of innocuous radioisotopes and portable equipment (Braunstein et al.). Although none of these techniques has been studied in a large sample of patients, preliminary tests of validity and reliability of the radioisotope technique compared to contrast (X-ray) angiography have been promising (Korein et al.).

Conclusion

This article has traced a spectrum of descriptive criteria for death based upon a variety of clinical observations, often confirmed by one or more of the currently available diagnostic techniques.

It is evident from the criteria described that concepts of death vary among medical authors, ranging from inevitable mortality to documentary evidence of total destruction of the brain.

The determination that death will occur in critically ill or brain-injured patients has never been a diagnostic problem. The prediction of the moment at which death may be pronounced using classical cardiorespiratory criteria is more difficult but becomes simpler as cardiovascular and respiratory system physiology deteriorates. The concept that death may occur while the cardiorespiratory physiology is being artificially sustained is a by-product of modern medical technology. While pronouncement of death based on neurological criteria seems reasonable and practical, proof of the accuracy of that pronouncement is not always possible.

The criteria used in pronouncing death while certain organs continue to show signs of function continue to be enigmatic to physicians and scholars alike. May the destruction of the most complex portion of the organ, the brain, alter the nature of the organism, man? May the total destruction of the organ be equated with the death of the organism? Does the proximity or imminence of death permit a declaration of death? The criteria discussed above presume that one or more of these issues may be decided in the affirmative.

GAETANO F. MOLINARI

[Directly related are the other articles in this entry: LEGAL ASPECTS OF PRONOUNCING DEATH and PHILOSOPHICAL AND THEOLOGICAL FOUNDATIONS. See also: DEATH AND DYING: EUTHANASIA AND SUSTAINING LIFE; DECISION MAKING, MEDICAL; and LIFE-SUPPORT SYSTEMS.]

BIBLIOGRAPHY

Ad Hoc Committee of the Harvard Medical School to Examine the Definition of Brain Death. "A Definition of Irreversible Coma." *Journal of the American Medical Association* 205 (1968): 337–340.

ALLEN, NORMAN; BURKHOLDER, JAMES D.; COMISCIONI, JOHN; and MOLINARI, GAETANO F. "Predictive Value of Clinical Criteria in Cerebral Death." *Neurology* 26 (1976): 356–357. Abstract.

BERTRAND, IVAN; LHERMITTE, FRANÇOIS; ANTOINE, BERNARD; and CUCROT, HENRI. "Nécroses massives du système nerveux central dans une survie artificielle." *Revue Neurologique* 101 (1959): 101–115.

BRAUNSTEIN, P.; KOREIN, J.; KRICHEFF, I.; COREY, K.; and Chase, N. "A Simple Bedside Evaluation for Cerebral Blood Flow in the Study of Cerebral Death: A Prospective Study on 34 Deeply Comatose Patients."

American Journal of Roentgenology, Radium Therapy and Nuclear Medicine 18 (1973): 757–767.

INGVAR, DAVID H., and WIDÉN, LENNART. "Hjärndöd: Sammanfattning av ett symposium." [Brain death: abstract of a symposium]. *Läkartidningen* 69 (1972): 3804–3814.

KEVORKIAN, JACK. "Rapid and Accurate Ophthalmoscopic Determination of Circulatory Arrest." *Journal of the American Medical Association* 164 (1957): 1660–1664.

KOREIN, JULIUS. "Neurology and Cerebral Death—Definitions and Differential Diagnosis." *Transactions of the American Neurological Association* 100 (1975): 210–212.

———; BRAUNSTEIN, PHILLIP; KRICHEFF, IRVIN; LIEBERMAN, ABRAHAM; and CHASE, NORMAN. "Radioisotopic Bolus Technique as a Test to Detect Circulatory Deficit Associated with Cerebral Death." *Circulation* 51 (1975): 924–939.

LOBSTEIN, ANDRÉ; TEMPLE, JEAN-DANIEL; and PAYEUR, GEORGES. "La Fluoroscopie rétinienne dans le diagnostic de la mort cérébrale." *Documenta Ophthalmologica* 26 (1969): 349–358.

MOHANDAS, A., and CHOU, SHELLEY N. "Brain Death: A Clinical and Pathological Study." *Journal of Neurosurgery* 35 (1971): 211–218.

MOLLARET, P., and GOULON, M. "Le Coma dépassé." *Revue Neurologique* 101 (1959): 5–15.

MOSELEY, JOHN I.; MOLINARI, GAETANO F.; and WALKER, A. EARL. "Respirator Brain: Report of a Survey and Review of Current Concepts." *Archives of Pathology & Laboratory Medicine* 100 (1976): 61–64.

PINES, N. "The Ophthalmoscopic Evidence of Death." *British Journal of Ophthalmology* 15 (1931): 512–513.

UEKI, K.; TAKEUCHI, K,; and KATSURADA, K. "Clinical Study of Brain Death." Fifth International Congress of Neurological Surgery, Tokyo, 7–13 October 1973. Presentation no. 286.

UEMATSU, S., and WALKER, A. E. "A Method for Recording the Pulsation of the Midline Echo in Clinical Brain Death." *Johns Hopkins Medical Journal* 135 (1974): 383–390.

WALKER, A. EARL. "Cerebral Death." *The Nervous System*. 3 vols. Edited by Donald B. Tower. Vol. 2: *The Clinical Neurosciences*. Edited by Thomas N. Chase. New York: Raven Press, 1975, pp. 75–87.

———; DIAMOND, EARL L.; and MOSELEY, JOHN. "The Neuropathological Findings in Irreversible Coma: A Critique of the 'Respirator Brain'." *Journal of Neuropathology and Experimental Neurology* 34 (1975): 295–323.

———, and MOLINARI, GAETANO F. "Criteria of Cerebral Death." *Transactions of the American Neurological Association* 100 (1975): 29–35.

II
LEGAL ASPECTS OF PRONOUNCING DEATH

The recently developed capability of biomedicine to sustain vital human functions artificially has presented new problems for the public and its legal institutions as well as for medical practitioners. Determining that a person has died is no longer the relatively simple matter of ascertaining that his heart and lungs have stopped functioning. Mechanical respirators, electronic pacemakers, and analeptic and tensive drugs give the appearance of circulation and respiration in what is otherwise a corpse. As lay people became aware of those medical developments in the 1960s, an undeniable need arose for change in the public policy on when and how death could be declared. The great drama of heart transplantation, beginning with the operation performed in Cape Town, South Africa, on 3 December 1967 by Dr. Christiaan Barnard, was all the more astonishing because a heart taken from a woman who had been declared "dead" beat in a living man's chest in place of his own.

Although cardiac transplantation provides the boldest illustration of medicine's new powers, the need for a new way of determining whether death has occurred extends to the far more numerous cases of lengthy, intensive maintenance of moribund patients long after they would have formerly ceased living. In some of those patients, medical intervention can end because it has been successful in permitting recovery to occur, and in others it terminates because the patient's bodily systems have so totally collapsed that circulation and respiration cannot be maintained. But in a significant number, deep in coma from trauma or deterioration, artificial support is successful enough to be continued indefinitely, with no prospect that the patient will ever recover but also no point in sight at which bodily functioning will cease so long as medical care continues.

The response of the medical profession in the 1960s was to develop new criteria, which rely on irreversible changes in the central nervous system, to guide physicians in determining that death had occurred in artificially maintained patients. According to the criteria suggested by an ad hoc committee of the Harvard Medical School and generally followed by American and British physicians, death may be declared when the clinical signs of brain activity—such as response to external stimuli, spontaneous respiration, movements, and reflexes—are absent for twenty-four hours; an isoelectric electroencephalogram confirms the diagnosis (Ad Hoc Committee, pp. 337–338). The Mollaret criteria used in France, like the Harvard criteria, measure indicators of continued brain function, while the methods employed in Austria and Germany search for the preconditions for brain function, such as intracranial blood circulation (Van Till, pp. 139–144). Despite this divergence in reasoning and method, the underlying consensus that emerged in the medical profession was that the total and irreversible absence of brain function is equivalent to the traditional indicators of death. The new medical criteria were not in accord with the common understanding of the lay public nor with the rules embodied in custom and law. Anglo-American common law, for example, requires the total cessation of *all* vital functions ("Death"). Two issues are thus presented: an issue of process—how ought lawmaking bodies to respond to the changes in medical practice and doctrine?—and one that concerns product—what changes should be made in the law?

Process: the authority to frame definitions

Let the physicians decide. A number of routes have been advanced for arriving at a new "definition of death" that would encompass a neurological understanding of the phenomenon. (The commonly employed phrase, "definition of death," is useful shorthand but should not be taken to mean the *explanation* of a fact but rather the *choice* about the significance of certain facts in the task of determining whether, and when, a person has died.) Some commentators have proposed that the task should be left to physicians, because the subject is technical and because the law might freeze the definition prematurely, leading to conflicts with the developments that will inevitably occur in medical techniques (Kennedy, pp. 946–947). Yet the belief that defining death is wholly a medical matter misapprehends the undertaking. At issue is not a biological understanding of the inherent nature of cells or organ systems but a social formulation of humanhood. It is largely through its declaration of the points at which life begins and ends that a society determines who is a full human being, with the resulting rights and responsibilities. So long as the standards being employed by physicians to pronounce death in individual cases are stable and congruent with community opinion, most people are content to leave the entire matter in medical hands. But the underlying extramedical aspects of the definition become visible, as they have recently, when medicine either departs or appears to depart from the common understanding of the concept of death.

Since physicians have no special competence on the philosophical issue of the nature of human beings and no special authority to arrogate the choice among definitions to themselves, their role is properly one of elucidating the significance of various vital signs. Nevertheless, medical statements on death help to frame the relevant issues, and the attention devoted to the subject by the biomedical professions has been a major stimulus to the process of redefinition. The public might decide to reject the medical view if, for example, it concluded that a prognosis based on the new brain-oriented criteria cannot be sufficiently accurate. A new definition will be forthcoming not simply to accommodate biomedical practitioners' wishes, but as a result of perceived social need and of evidence that brain tests for death are as reliable as the traditional heart–lung tests. The public might also reject the medical view that brain-oriented criteria ought to be used even if it were convinced of their reliability in measuring brain function if that public did not share the medical profession's concept of personhood.

Let the courts decide. The medical definitions may take on legal status were the courts to defer to them as the issue arose in litigation. In the United States and other common law countries, law is to be found not only on the statute books but in the rules enunciated by judges as they resolve disputes in individual civil and criminal cases. Faced with a factual situation that does not fit comfortably within the existing legal rules, a court may choose to formulate a new rule in order to reflect current scientific understanding and social viewpoints more accurately.

Nonetheless, there are problems of principle and practicality in placing primary reliance on the courts for a redefinition of death. Like the medical profession, the judiciary may be too narrowly based for the task. While the judiciary, unlike the medical profession, is an organ of the state with recognized authority in public matters, it still has no means for actively involving the public in its decision-making processes. Judge-made law has been most successful in factual settings embedded in well-defined social and economic practices, with the guidance of past decisions and commentary. Courts operate within a limited compass—the facts and contentions of a particular case—and with limited expertise; they have neither the staff nor the authority to investigate or to conduct hearings in order to explore such issues as public opinion or the scientific merits of competing "definitions." Consequently, a judge's decision may be merely a rubberstamping of the opinions expressed by the medical experts who appeared before him. Moreover, testimony in an adversary proceeding is usually restricted to the "two sides" of an issue and may not fairly represent the spectrum of opinion held by authorities in the field.

In the cases in which parties first argued for a redefinition, the courts were unwilling to disturb the existing legal definition. Such deference to precedent is understandable, because everyone needs to be able to rely on predictable legal rules in managing one's affairs and cannot always be overcome by arguments on the merits of a new rule. As recently as 1968 a California appellate tribunal, in a case involving an inheritorship issue, declined to redefine death in terms of brain functioning despite the admittedly anachronistic nature of an exclusively heart–lung definition.

In light of possible judicial adherence to existing but outmoded rules, reliance on the judicial route to a new definition of death is likely to create a considerable period of uncertainty, which is especially unfortunate in an area where private decision makers must act quickly and irrevocably. An ambiguous legal standard endangers the rights, and in some cases the lives, of the participants and fosters public confusion. A physician's choice of one course over another may depend less on his or her view of their relative merits than on his or her willingness to face a court challenge on the issue.

The unfortunate consequences for physicians and patients of the unsettled state of the common law definition of death is illustrated by three American cases. In the first, *Tucker* v. *Lower*, which came to trial in Virginia in 1972, the brother of the man whose heart was taken in an early transplant operation sued the doctors, alleging that the operation was begun before the donor had died. The evidence showed that the donor's pulse, blood pressure, respiration, and other vital signs were normal but that he had been declared dead when the physicians decided these signs resulted solely from medical efforts and not from his own functioning, since his brain had ceased working. The trial judge initially indicated that he would adhere to the traditional definition of death, but he later permitted the jurors to find that death had occurred when the brain ceased functioning irreversibly, and a verdict was returned for the defendants. Since the court did not explain its action, the law was not clarified, and future parties face continued uncertainty.

The other two cases arose in 1974 in California when two transplant operations were performed using hearts removed from the victims of alleged crimes. The defendant in each case attempted to interpose the action of the surgeons in removing the still-beating heart of the victim as a complete defense to the charge of homicide. One trial judge accepted this argument as being compelled by the existing definition of death, but his ruling was reversed on appeal, and both defendants were eventually convicted. This graphic illustration of legal confusion and uncertainty led California to follow a third route to redefining death, the adoption of a statutory definition.

Let the legislatures decide. The legislative process permits the public to play an active role in decision making and allows a wider range of information to enter into the framing of standards for determining death. That is important because basic and perhaps controversial choices among alternative definitions must be made. For example, some commentators have argued for a new concept of death as solely the cessation of the higher faculties of the brain upon which cognition and personality depend (Veatch). Faced with this option, all legislatures have thus far concluded that it is preferable instead simply to restate the existing understanding of death, based on the recognition that, if cardiac and pulmonary functions have ceased, brain functions cannot continue, and if there is no brain activity and respiration has to be maintained artificially, the same state (i.e., death) exists. Because they provide prospective guidance, statutory standards have the additional advantage of dispelling public and professional doubt, thereby reducing both the fear and the likelihood of cases for malpractice or homicide against physicians. The greatest danger of legislation is poor draftsmanship, which can best be addressed in the context of particular examples.

Product: the contours of a definition

The general principles for drafting a statute on death grow out of the objectives that the statute ought reasonably to serve. First, the phenomenon of interest to physicians, legislators, and the public alike is a human being's death, not the "death" of his cells, tissues, or organs. This step will resolve the problem of whether to continue artificial support in only some of the cases of comatose patients. Additional statutory guidance may also be desired by society concerning the cessation of treatment in patients who are alive by brain or heart–lung criteria but for whom further treatment is considered (by the patients or by others) to be pointless or degrading. This question of "when to allow to die" is distinct from "when to declare death."

Second, the merits of a legislative "definition" are judged by whether its purposes are properly defined and how well the legislation meets those purposes. In addition to its cultural and religious importance, society needs a definition of death for a number of decisions having legal consequences; besides terminal medical care or transplantation, those include homicide, damages for the wrongful death of a person, property and wealth transmission, and determination of insurance, taxes, and marital status. From this it can be argued that a single definition is inappropriate because different policy objectives may exist in those different contexts (Dworkin, p. 631). No special purposes requiring separate definitions have been suggested, however, and a single definition of death seems capable of being applied in a wide variety of contexts, as indeed the traditional definition has been.

A different rationale for multiple definitions of death may be drawn from the philosophical debate over the nature of death. Death may be viewed as a process since not all parts of the body cease functioning equally and synchronously (Morison, pp. 695–696). But society, through generally accepted medical and social practices and in its laws, recognizes that a line can and must be drawn between those who are alive and those who are dead (Kass, p. 701). The ability of modern bioscience to extend the functioning of various organ systems may have made knowing which side of the line a patient is on more problematic, but it has not erased the line. The line drawn by society is an arbitrary one in the sense that it results from human choice among a number of possibilities, but it need not be arbitrary in the sense of having no acceptable, articulated rationale.

Having a single definition to be used for many purposes does not, needless to say, preclude reliance on other events besides death as the trigger for some decisions. Most jurisdictions, for instance, make provision for the distribution of property and the termination of marriage after a person has been absent without explanation for a period of years, and some term this a "presumption of death," although a person covered by such a determination could not be treated as a corpse were he actually still alive (Capron, pp. 642–643). Similarly, a status such as "total, irreversible loss of cognitive abilities" might be established as the predicate for distributing the bulk of a terminally ill person's estate; it would not, however, be an alternative definition of

death and would need to be surrounded by procedural safeguards not necessary for such a definition.

Another principle of legislative drafting is that the standards must be uniform for all persons. It is, to say the least, unseemly for a person's wealth or potential social utility as an organ donor to affect the way in which the moment of his death is determined.

It is often beneficial for the law to move incrementally, particularly when matters of basic cultural and ethical values are implicated. Thus, what is needed is a modern restatement of the traditional understanding of death that will tie together the accepted cardiopulmonary standard with a new brain-based standard that measures the same phenomenon: the irreversible cessation of the integrated functioning of the three vital systems together.

Finally, in making law in a highly technological area, care is needed that the definition be at once sufficiently precise to determine behavior in the manner desired by the public and yet not so specific that it is tied to the details of contemporary technology. Such flexible precision can be achieved if the definition is confined to the general *standards* by which death is to be determined, for example, the irreversible cessation of spontaneous respiration or the irreversible loss of the ability to respond or communicate. The law can then leave to the continually developing judgment of biomedical practitioners the establishment and application of appropriate *criteria* and specific *tests* for determining that the standards have been met. To illustrate, deep coma, the absence of reflexes, and the lack of spontaneous muscular movements and respiration are among the criteria that have been proposed for determining that one standard—irreversible cessation of spontaneous brain functions—has been met (Ad Hoc Committee, pp. 337–338). Those criteria are implemented in turn by certain tests, such as applying painful stimuli, observing respiration and reaction to light, and performing electroencephalography at specified intervals. As medical understanding and technique develop, new tests and criteria may be established that will provide simpler, less expensive, and even more accurate means of fulfilling the standards set by the law.

Movement toward legal definitions

As one would expect, adoption of a modern definition of death has come about mostly through legislation; the court cases involving the issue have seldom eventuated in appellate opinions providing a new standard of general applicability, and medical practices, although better understood and more widely accepted by the public, still lack explicit legal sanction in most places.

The first statutes on the definition of death, which were addressed primarily to organ transplantation, erred on the side of generality. The British Human Tissue Act 1961, the Danish Act of 1967, and the Uniform Anatomical Gift Act, which was proposed in 1968 and adopted in all American jurisdictions by 1971, leave the standards for death too undefined to be any guide for the decisions of physicians called upon to declare death (Meyers, p. 113). The legislation enacted in France in April 1968, which was also intended to facilitate transplantation, went to the opposite extreme and defined death in clinical terms as occurring when an artificially maintained patient has lesions incompatible with life and has a flat electroencephalographic tracing for at least ten minutes.

Although not free from problems, the legislation adopted in a number of American states since 1970 has steered a middle course between excess generality and undue specificity. Nonetheless, the first American legislation, enacted by the State of Kansas in 1970, suffered in other respects. First, it set forth cardiopulmonary and brain definitions separately and without explaining their relationship. The practitioner is given no guidance on when one or the other is to be applied, and the public is left with the impression that they are two separate phenomena rather than two ways of measuring the same thing. This is especially unfortunate since the legislation was adopted to assist heart transplantation, and a lay person could interpret it as permitting doctors to use a new definition—"brain death"—to declare a person dead earlier than would be possible under existing law. The second problem with the Kansas statute is that it speaks in terms of pronouncing death when further efforts are "hopeless" or appear not to be successful. Such language wrongly implies that legislation defining death extends to passive euthanasia, that is, ceasing treatment on a dying patient in order to permit death to occur when no hope of recovery remains.

A model statute suggested in 1972 provides two interconnected general physiological standards for identifying the two primary manifestations of the phenomenon of death:

A person will be considered dead if in the announced opinion of a physician, based on ordinary standards of medical practice, he has experienced an irreversible cessation of spontaneous respiratory and circulatory functions. In the event that artificial means of support preclude a determination that these functions have ceased, a person will be considered dead if in the announced opinion of a physician, based on ordinary medical practice, he has experienced an irreversible cessation of spontaneous brain functions. Death will have occurred at the time when the relevant functions ceased [Capron and Kass, p. 111].

This proposal, which has since been adopted in several states, applies equally to all persons and not merely to those who are potential organ donors or even those who are hospitalized at the time of death. The legislation gives legal sanction to declaring a person dead based on an absence of all neocortical and lower brain activity without being tied to any particular medical procedures. Thus it would permit use of either the so-called Harvard criteria, which are generally accepted in the United States, or other accepted methods, such as those followed in Europe, which measure blood flow in the brain (Van Till, pp. 143–144). The specific practices prevailing in an area would be a matter of fact in each case, recognizing that more than one set of procedures may reach the necessary degree of certainty to be adopted by physicians.

In 1975 the American Bar Association endorsed similar legislation but defined death solely in neurological terms: "For all legal purposes, a human body with irreversible cessation of total brain function according to usual and customary standards of medical practice, shall be considered dead" (American Bar Association). This proposal has the advantage of removing the last trace of the "two deaths" misconception; yet it ignores the fact that physicians will continue in most cases to employ cardiopulmonary tests, which are easier to perform, more accessible and acceptable to the lay public, and perfectly adequate for determining death in most instances. In recognition of that fact, the California legislature in adopting an ABA-type bill added a clause permitting physicians to continue to employ "usual and customary" standards. Such legislation thereby resurrects the "two deaths" concept while failing to explain the connection between the new and the traditional measures.

Unfulfilled obligation: education for change

As can thus be seen, the movement toward a modern formulation of the bases for pronouncing death has not been completed. In some societies that task may be left to the medical profession, since the problems faced in medical practice have provided the impetus for change. Tradition as well as sound policy suggests, however, that the ground rules for decisions about individual patients should be established by public authorities. Whether the new legal definition emerges from the resolution of court cases or from the legislative process, it will be greatly influenced by opinion from the medical community. Recognition that the standards for determining death are matters of social and not merely professional concern only serves to underline the education of the public on this subject as an important ethical obligation of the profession.

ALEXANDER MORGAN CAPRON

[*Directly related is* DEATH AND DYING: EUTHANASIA AND SUSTAINING LIFE, *article on* PROFESSIONAL AND PUBLIC POLICY. *See also the other article in this entry,* CRITERIA FOR DEATH; *and the entry* ORGAN DONATION.]

BIBLIOGRAPHY

Ad Hoc Committee of the Harvard Medical School to Examine the Definition of Brain Death. "A Definition of Irreversible Coma." *Journal of the American Medical Association* 205 (1968): 337–340. The highly influential statement by Harvard physicians and others on the means for determining an irreversible loss of total brain functioning.

American Bar Association. "Section of Insurance, Negligence and Compensation Law (Report No. 102)." *Summary of Action Taken by the House of Delegates of the American Bar Association, 1975, Midyear Meeting.* Chicago: 1975, p. 19. Reprint. *American Bar Association Journal* 61 (1975): 463–466. Recommends a definition of death as an irreversible cessation of total brain function.

CAPRON, ALEXANDER MORGAN. "The Purpose of Death: A Reply to Professor Dworkin." *Indiana Law Journal* 48 (1973): 640–646. Argues in favor of developing a definition that comports with social reality and can be employed in as many legal settings as it suits.

———, and KASS, LEON R. "A Statutory Definition of the Standards for Determining Human Death: An Appraisal and a Proposal." *University of Pennsylvania Law Review* 121 (1972): 87–118. General discussion of the procedures and objectives for lawmaking on this subject.

"Death." *Black's Law Dictionary.* 4th rev. ed. St. Paul, Minn.: West Publishing Co., 1968, p. 488. Common-law definition of death.

DWORKIN, ROGER B. "Death in Context." *Indiana Law Journal* 48 (1973): 623–639. Contends that the law should be framed in terms of the consequences of cessation of human functioning and not in terms of a single definition of death.

KASS, LEON R. "Death as an Event: A Commentary on Robert Morison." *Science* 173 (1971): 698–702. Refutes Morison's thesis that death does not occur at an identifiable time and explores the social rules that follow from this view.

KENNEDY, IAN MCCOLL. "The Kansas Statute on Death: An Appraisal." *New England Journal of Medicine* 285 (1971): 946–949. Criticizes the Kansas legislation in detail; urges that the defining of death be left in medical hands.

MEYERS, DAVID W. *The Human Body and the Law: A Medico-Legal Study.* Edinburgh: Edinburgh University Press; Chicago: Aldine Publishing Co., 1970. Useful survey of American, British, Scottish, and Continental law on euthanasia, sterilization, etc.

MORISON, ROBERT S. "Death: Process or Event?" *Science* 173 (1971): 694–698. Contends that death is a process, not a single event; examines the ethical implications for physicians.

VAN TILL-D'AULNIS DE BOUROUILL, ADRIENNE. "How Dead Can You Be?" *Medicine, Science and the Law* 15, no. 2 (1975), pp. 133–147. Compares American diagnositic criteria with those used in France, Austria and Germany; also differentiates ceasing artificial maintenance from murder or active euthanasia.

VEATCH, ROBERT M. "The Whole-Brain–Oriented Concept of Death: An Outmoded Philosophical Formulation." *Journal of Thanatology* 3, no. 1 (1975), pp. 13–30. Examines the current concept of brain death from philosophical and medical viewpoints.

III
PHILOSOPHICAL AND THEOLOGICAL FOUNDATIONS

Every definition of death presupposes some form of philosophical and/or theological reflection. It may be explicit by way of careful reasoning and presentation of beliefs about the meaning of life and death (or in conceptual analysis, about the terms "life" and "death"), or it may all be implicit as is a cultural sensibility. Even if a person believes that the definition of death is a purely medical issue, the justification of such a claim must proceed on philosophical or theological grounds. On the other hand, if it is recognized that definitions and meanings of death are valuational, then philosophical or theological considerations, whether lay or professional, are primary. The strong version of this claim argues that a concept of death is never medically, empirically verifiable. Weaker versions of the claim regularly argue that any concept of death involves consideration of a family of ideas, such as, "human," "life," "birth," "soul," and "consciousness," which appeal, in part, to philosophical and theological notions. In bioethics, the philosophical–theological question regarding death is often posed in the following way: What is essential to the nature of man the loss of which would warrant calling an individual dead?

Although some philosophers would claim that attempts to determine the essence of anything are misleading, there is a long tradition in philosophical inquiry and theological doctrine to determine what is significant about man in just that way. Moreover, many contemporary bioethicists believe that, if a sufficiently simple, clear, and satisfactory answer can be given, its relevancy to criteria in determining an individual's death is immediate. For example, the widely known "Report of the Ad Hoc Committee of the Harvard Medical School to Examine the Definition of Brain Death" offers criteria for irreversible coma and tells us nothing of what is essentially significant about the nature of man. Although bioethicists do not argue that the Harvard committee should have specified the latter, many do argue that, unless the essential nature of man is somewhere satisfactorily formulated, no one can fully decide whether a set of criteria is appropriate.

Belief in the human soul

According to one widely popular view in Western religious tradition, man is distinctive by possession of a soul. In its simplest form such a view defines death (and the moment of death) as the departure of the soul from the earthly body. This view usually presupposes that a union of body and soul is essential to the spatiotemporal existence of man. The destruction of this union, whether the soul is affected or not, constitutes death and is very often interpreted as "death of the body." As to what a "soul" is, there is no general agreement. Apart from the popular view, some theologians have put forward rather sophisticated understandings of "soul." For example, Ladislaus Boros in *The Mystery of Death* argues for an interpretation of Thomistic metaphysics which denies that man is a composition of two things. The essence of man is a single whole in which the body is the whole work of the soul, and the body is included in the actuality of soul. The essence of man is a unity, not a duality. Consequently, the separation of the soul and body is not a simple separation of two existent things. Death affects both corporeality (body) and the form (soul), yet the soul as "subsistent form" remains indestructible. Consequently, on this Thomistic interpretation, death is defined as destruction not only of the body and the soul–body unity, but destruction of the soul insofar as it appears in material concretion. The clinical implications of this belief are far from clear. Some believers might be willing to assert that it means nothing more than a definitional specification of the "moment of death," irrespective of the practical problems of determining that moment. Alternatively, the belief

may be taken as an argument that opposes efforts to define death in any empirical and quantifiable manner. Other theologians have argued that the word "soul" is best used as an indicator of value and in no way names a spiritual substance or entity (Hick, pp. 1–29). In this case talk of a soul is seen as mythology, which reveals a people's belief in the intrinsic value and worth of a human individual.

Contemporary philosophers generally have not placed much credence in talk of a soul and have, instead, chosen to expose the mistakes of conceiving of the soul (or mind) as a substance. However, Ludwig Wittgenstein (1889–1951) did suggest that talk of a soul is an appropriate way of thinking of a human being. It is to admit of higher life; not to believe that a human being possesses a soul, but to have "an attitude towards a soul" (Wittgenstein, 1953, p. 178e). As such, human life cannot be exhaustively explained as a phenomenon of natural objects.

Process or event?

Some philosophers and physicians argue that the traditional or literary concept of death as a definite event which occurs at a specific moment is mistaken. It is argued that death should be conceived as a gradual process. This view finds support in the empirical knowledge that some parts of the body may disintegrate while others continue indefinitely. More important, it follows directly from a philosophical claim that no system fails all at once or, for that matter, no system can cease altogether and, hence, become nothing. Charles Hartshorne, in following the work of Alfred N. Whitehead, offers just that argument (Hartshorne). According to Hartshorne, death can never mean sheer destruction, including references to individual persons, since the "ego" is not identical with any single configuration of atoms or particles. There are no essential features necessary to the individual. Yet an individual does not "de-become." Death is merely the affixing of a particular quantum of reality. Death is the "last page" of the book, affixed, perhaps, retrospectively and somewhat arbitrarily. The answer to the basic question of death, as Hartshorne sees it—How rich and how complete is the book?—spells the tragedy or lack of tragedy of the quantum.

As an extension of the process view to bioethical questions, Robert Morison argues that the practical judgments concerning death can be solved by use of a cost-benefit analysis concerning the worth or worthlessness of life prolongation, an analysis that is remarkably close to what Hartshorne defines as the basic question of death. Morison holds that the usual bioethical question of "when an individual is dead" is not distinct from but is an instance of the question, "When is a person's life no longer worth prolonging?" Hence, the practical matter of death certification is seen as a value judgment, not a question of fact. According to Morison we need to abandon both efforts to define a moment of death and attempts to establish precise empirical criteria for death determination, since no real border between life and death exists (Morison).

There are, however, several objections to the process view. One objection consists in defending conceptual distinctions either overlooked or discounted by the process proponents. Dying should be distinguished from death, and both of these from aging. The question of when a life is no longer worth prolonging should be distinguished from the question of when in fact a person is dead (Kass, pp. 698–700). Another objection charges that the process view denies the reality of death by making it an empty concept or by using the term as a highly qualified metaphor. Finally, many persons argue that if one can legitimately claim an enduring self-identity (not necessarily substance) from birth till death or an identity of the organism as a whole, then the processive understanding of both the individual and death must be challenged for confusing character, biography, personality, and bodily function with the organism as a whole or the self as an agent.

Brain and consciousness

Focus of attention on a neurological locus of the essential nature of the human being is widespread. It has arisen not only through increased empirical knowledge of the neurological system, especially the brain, but through the continued interest of philosophers in the philosophic-scientific aspects of the mind–body problem, including efforts to understand such concepts as consciousness, remembering, and reasoning. The extension of such interests to a brain-oriented concept of death has arisen chiefly out of increased medical ability to transplant organs, together with increased ability to sustain heart and lung functions artificially. A brain-oriented concept of death might use the following kind of argument: If consciousness, remembering, reasoning, etc., are essential to the nature of man, and if these features are identical with processes of the brain, then the loss of brain processes (brain death) is sufficient warrant to call a person dead, i.e., the essential features of a person are absent.

One widely debated form of philosophical persuasion that would attempt to give some credence, at least by implication, to the above form of argument is "the identity thesis," a hypothesis of the identity of consciousness and brain processes (Rosenthal). Because the thesis generally claims that the confirmation must be the result of scientific-neurophysiological investigation, it can claim no higher status than a hypothesis. Basically, the arguments for the thesis take the form of answering objections and attempting to show that the thesis is neither self-contradictory nor self-evidently false. The thesis proposes that consciousness (a) is identical with brain processes (b) in the sense that what is true of (a) is true of (b) without the identity's becoming trivially true as in the case of "bachelors are identical with unmarried males." Statements about (a) and (b), so it is claimed, can have different meanings but identical references. It is not a thesis that consciousness and other mental states are merely associated with or dependent upon brain processes, which everyone would grant, but rather that consciousness and other mental states are factually discernible as brain processes. For the concept of death, this implies that, although the statements "Jones is dead" and "Jones's brain is dead" may have different meanings, they have identical factual references. That is, if brain processes are absent, there can be no other factual reality to death. Loss of consciousness, reason, etc., is nothing more than the diminution of brain processes.

It should be noted that "the identity thesis" has not to date received decisive empirical verification or general acceptance, even though as a hypothesis it has received two decades or more of discussion. However, many neurologists do generally *assume* in their model of explanation that conscious mental processes can be interpreted, without remainder, as material processes. But the neurological model is the philosophical basis of the empirical investigation and as such cannot confirm the identity thesis without circularity. Additionally, it runs the risk of being logically untenable, on the ground that totally different propositions cannot have an identical reference. On the other hand, John C. Eccles, a noted neurophysiologist, claims refutation of the strong version of the identity thesis and has gone so far as to suggest that the neurological model of the brain be amended. Similarly, Sir

Francis Walshe, a neurophysiologist who from time to time has reflected on the philosophical implications of his own enterprise, has argued that neurobiology, dominated by mechanistic and reductionistic ideas, has not provided an adequate account of consciousness and that "identification" efforts have produced a cluster of paradoxes (Walshe).

Efforts to define the death of a person as "death of the brain" encounter other philosophical difficulties as well. It is regularly pointed out that the argument for the identification either begs the question or makes an equivocal claim that conscious life, capacity for reasoning, acting, etc., "reside" in the brain. If the term "reside" is taken to mean "associated with" or "necessarily conditioned," then the argument will not yield the conclusion of identification of so-called brain death with "death of a person" since necessary conditions always leave open the possibility of a reality more comprehensive than the conditions themselves. On the other hand, if "reside" is taken to mean "consciousness is the same as brain processes," then a reckless extension of predicates of the human being to nonhuman beings or objects may be the result. For example, while it is appropriate to say "Jones knows that it is raining" it is a logically dubious personification to say "Jones's brain knows that it is raining" when knowing is accurately taken as a predication of a person (Kenny, pp. 65–74). Likewise, it may well be inadequate to argue from "Jones's brain is dead" to "Jones is dead." By analogy, clearly one would want to avoid argument from "Jones's brain has an undersupply of blood" to "Jones has an undersupply of blood." The difficulty over the "brain death" designation consists of both a reckless extension of predicates and a lack of precision regarding the meaning of brain dysfunction, for surely at death the brain does not cease to exist even though the human being, Jones, does. Just as the human being as a whole thinks, knows, and is conscious, not the brain *in vacuo* as it were, so, too, the human being as a whole dies, and not simply that certain functions cease in a brain. The recent impulse to discover a neurological locus of death coupled with a latent sense for whole entities may well account for the crude and paradoxical nature of the "whole-brain-oriented concept of death." That is to say, a "whole-brain-oriented concept of death" attempts to be more precise about the essential features of man than the heart-lung oriented concept of death, yet by focusing on the destruc-

tion of the whole brain it runs the risk of "false positive tests for life"—the same criticism to which the heart-lung oriented concept has been subjected. This has led some bioethicists to argue that the essential nature of man must be specified in terms of more precisely limited anatomical characteristics (Veatch). Nevertheless, caution is still needed. Even if one does distinguish between the whole-brain-oriented concept and the narrower higher-brain-oriented concept, any brain definition of death may well be subject to the philosophical criticism that it is "a curious revenant of the old soul–body dualism" (Jonas, p. 139), an exaggeration of the brain, forming a new dualism of brain and body, just as once the soul was exaggerated in attempting to understand the nature of personal identity.

The logic and ontology of death

Among twentieth-century philosophers, Martin Heidegger and Ludwig Wittgenstein have contributed most notably to discussions of death. Heidegger has made his impact by developing a voluminous existential phenomenology keyed to the subject, especially in *Being and Time,* while Wittgenstein has made impact by a few aphoristic comments about death, especially in *Tractatus Logico-Philosophicus.*

Heidegger's focus on the subject of death is ontological in character; that is to say, he claims that one's awareness of death raises the fundamental questions of what it means for anything to be. The chief feature of Heidegger's work is a theory of the meaning of death which shows that facing one's own personal death concretely offers life a purposefulness and urgency that otherwise would be lacking. The problem of death for Heidegger is not the death of others but clearly "my own death," i.e., death in the first person. Death is unique in the sense that no one else can die my death although it is still the case that not everyone lives his own life. Death is the termination of me and is not just one event among other events or possibilities on the horizon. This means that any phenomenological explanation of death must include more than an investigation of the disintegration of animal structure. Not only does awareness of death provide a frame of reference for one's own authentic existence, but an accurate account of human existence is not "full" or "complete" without proper attention to death. In this sense, death, too, is essential to human nature since it provides the proper perspective for viewing the totality of human existence even if it cannot be something one can experience. Death is the inevitable end of all experience, the end of existence, and the annihilation of one's being.

At the very least, Heidegger's analysis, as applied to bioethical questions, underscores the point that the meaning and definition of death are not essentially experiential issues. Anyone who might claim that he does not yet know what death is because he has not experienced it has only revealed conceptual confusion. More important, perhaps, Heidegger's account provides a forceful account of man's finitude by focusing on meaning as possibility, not actuality, since the question of the ontological actuality of my death cast in any experiential sense is a meaningless question. The parallel questions of what it means to be and what it means not to be are answerable by Heidegger's account not by inquiring into what man's essential nature is but by looking to possible existence, as awareness of death incites authentic existence, and possible nonexistence.

Wittgenstein, on the other hand, has provided some illumination of the logical peculiarities of the concept of death in a few brief remarks. He says, "As in death, too, this world does not change, but ceases. Death is not an event in life. Death is not lived through. . . . Our life has no end in just the way in which our visual field has no limits" (1933, 6.431, 6.4311). Wittgenstein's remarks exhibit quite precisely that death is not a concept characterized as an experience. In this way Wittgenstein's analysis shows the radical force of the concept of death. Although the death of another person may entail certain empirical propositions predicated by observers, there cannot be any empirical predication by the person who is dead. That is, one cannot seriously conjugate the verb "to die" in the past tense, first person singular (Poteat). So far, such a view of death raises serious questions about the appropriate use of such locutions as "Death is a part of life."

What is often overlooked is the peculiar logic of using the term "death" with reference to the world—"as in death . . . the world ceases." At first sight Wittgenstein's claim may appear contrary to all evidence or simply an illicit transition from "my world" to "the world." Not surprisingly, he shares company here with Heidegger and some other existentialists in showing that, in a significant sense, our death cannot be imagined if it is merely a cessation of experience (Van Evra, p. 176), and, as a corollary, he is affirming that in a significant sense only subjects die. The "world" and the use of the expression "the world of objects" is not only parasitic upon subject terms, but also "the world" or "the world of objects" becomes a logical impossibility without subjects. Strictly speaking a world only of objects or a world with only demonstrative references (the, this, that), if imaginable, would be a world in which there is no death. As a result, it makes sense to say that in death the world ceases. To assert that this is an illicit transition from "my world" to "the world" is in fact to entertain an equivocal concept of "world" as well as to assert the impossible priority of a world of objects. Wittgenstein also claims that life has no end in the way that our visual field has no limit. There is no limit to our visual field in the sense that the limit cannot be seen. Death is an analogous limit and is just as inexperienceable and literally inconceivable. To do otherwise is to be within the boundary. But this further means that death is best understood as an "ordering device" analogous to the notion "absolute zero" in thermodynamics and cannot be characterized as an extensional state (Van Evra, pp. 173–175). Such an analysis is opposed to the view that there can be an "awareness" of death as if it were a living recognition (a seeing) of the limit.

Irreducible structure of life

Alongside the strong philosophical warnings about the confusions arising from imagining death to be a thing or an existing entity, there is a strong contemporary, antireductionistic persuasion that the structure of human life itself is not explicable in "thing" language. Rather, an existent being must be seen to have an operating principle as a comprehensive entity that is not simply the sum total of operational principles of parts of the whole. If the "self," "person," or "human being" is not a fully reductive concept, then "grocery lists" of the characteristics of human nature or what is essential to man are at the very least inadequate. These lists have ordinarily included such functions as capacity for experience, rationality, remembering, social interaction, integration of bodily functions, consciousness, and others. Among the most notable alternatives to reductionism is the contribution of Michael Polanyi, a physician, physical chemist, and philosopher. His later work has prompted several advances in philosophical biology.

In several places Polanyi offers arguments and analogies exhibiting the irreducible structure of life (1958, pp. 327–405; 1969). His arguments conclude that an "operational principle" of a comprehensive entity has a reality of its own that is not reducible to lower-level principles. While the constituent particulars (and their laws) set conditions for the successful operation of a comprehensive entity, the conditions can apply to a variety of circumstances. The operational principle of the comprehensive entity provides what Polanyi calls the "boundary control" which forms the frame of relevancy, i.e., enables us to say which of many laws (conditions) are relevant. Thus, a comprehensive entity functions as a system of higher and lower orders, but the relationship of the levels of orders is asymmetrical. For example, certain physiochemical laws continue operation even when a comprehensive entity is smashed, as in the case of a clock. As a result, a comprehensive entity should not only be acknowledged as different from the aggregate of its parts, but the meaning of any part of a fully functioning comprehensive entity must be attended to from the higher operational principle of the entity. That is why it is tempting, but fallacious, to transfer the operation of the comprehensive entity to one or several constituent particulars.

On this view one must give attention to the successively higher levels of operational principles in order to understand and ascribe meaning to life. One set of operational principles always leaves open the possibility of yet another, higher operational principle. Consequently, a description of life and normal functioning requires an antecedent knowledge of the operational features of the comprehensive entity. As a counterpart, recognition of malfunction requires use of the higher order operational principle in order to determine the relevancy of many laws which may apply at a lower level.

Although Polanyi has not applied his findings to the issue of death, there are implications that directly follow (High). Not only is it impossible to give a complete physiochemical topography of a living organism, but acknowledgment of the higher operational principles of a comprehensive entity is paramount. The latter provide the basis for death recognition by way of determining the relevancy of ascertaining that certain functions have failed. It is never a simple matter of saying "This organ has failed; therefore, this person is dead." Indeed, that is why some physicians and bioethicists insist that in death the human being as a whole (as distinguished from whole human being) dies or that it is the individual who dies and not just an organ. In this sense

it is quite correct to say that organs do not die, persons do. This means not only that the concept of death must be kept distinct from medical criteria of death, but such criteria must be accorded no higher status than contingent clues, evidence, and justification for acknowledging that an individual, a person, has ceased to exist. Attempts to "locate death" in less than a comprehensive way are at best misleading, and the clues, evidence, and justifications must always be seen as open-ended and incomplete. On such a view, death is the termination of existence of an individual comprehensive being, a person, and not simply a dysfunction of one or more constituent particulars of that individual being, however much the latter may be used as evidence of individual demise or cited as causes of death. Even though certain dysfunctions or changed functions of constituent particulars, e.g., the brain, may be entailed by saying "I will die," the answer to the question of what is essentially lost or absent in death is on this view surprisingly simple and clear: myself.

Conclusion

The alternative candidates for specifying the essence of man and the philosophical/theological debates about conceptual foundations of death are complex and varied. The issues remain open-ended and invite increased attention from bioethicists and the public. However, it is not a logical necessity that the conceptual foundations must have universal agreement before criteria can have validity, even though the degree of confidence that can be placed in criteria will depend on the acceptability of those conceptual foundations.

Two salient features seem to have emerged from the current debates and are likely to have an influence on the continued discussions. First, the primacy of the person or person as a whole has gained a renewed status in understanding death. Whatever else may be said of characteristics or losses of particular functions, the debates constantly remind us that it is the person who dies. Second, a fairly clear distinction has emerged between a definition (or concept) of death and criteria for certifying death. As a result the debates may have inadvertently shown that the so-called traditional definition of death (cessation of circulation and respiration) was not a definition at all, popular assumptions to the contrary. Rather it was and is a set of criteria for determining that an individual has died, however much the criteria may need revising.

Twentieth-century man has not encountered a new death or a need to update death, popular language to the contrary, but has gained, perhaps, a renewed sensitivity to mortality.

DALLAS M. HIGH

[*Directly related is* DEATH, *articles on* EASTERN THOUGHT, WESTERN PHILOSOPHICAL THOUGHT, *and* WESTERN RELIGIOUS THOUGHT. *Other relevant material may be found under* EMBODIMENT; LIFE; MIND–BODY PROBLEM; *and* PERSON. *See also:* BIOLOGY, PHILOSOPHY OF.]

BIBLIOGRAPHY

BOROS, LADISLAUS. *Mysterium mortis: Der Mensch in der letzten Entscheidung.* Otlen und Freiburg im Breigau: Walter-Verlag, 1965. Translated by Gregory Bainbridge as *The Moment of Truth: Mysterium mortis.* London: Burns & Oates, 1965. And as *The Mystery of Death.* New York: Herder & Herder, 1965. Reprint. New York: Seabury Press, 1973.

Death Inside Out: The Hastings Center Report. Edited by Peter Steinfels and Robert M. Veatch. Preface by Daniel Callahan. A Harper Forum Book. New York: Harper & Row, 1975.

ECCLES, JOHN CAREW. *The Understanding of the Brain.* New York: McGraw-Hill Book Co., 1973.

HARTSHORNE, CHARLES. "Time, Death, and Everlasting Life." *The Logic of Perfection, and Other Essays in Neoclassical Metaphysics.* LaSalle, Ill.: Open Court Publishing Co., 1962, pp. 245–262.

HEIDEGGER, MARTIN. *Being and Time* (1927). Translated by John Macquarrie and Edward Robinson. The Library of Philosophy and Theology. London: SCM Press, 1962.

HICK, JOHN. *Biology and the Soul.* Arthur Stanley Eddington Memorial Lectures, no. 25. London: Cambridge University Press, 1972.

HIGH, DALLAS M. "Death: Its Conceptual Elusiveness." *Soundings* 55 (1972): 438–458.

JONAS, HANS. "Against the Stream: Comments on the Definition and Redefinition of Death." *Philosophical Essays: From Ancient Creed to Technological Man.* Englewood Cliffs, N.J.: Prentice-Hall, 1974, pp. 132–140.

KASS, LEON R. "Death as an Event: A Commentary on Robert Morison." *Science* 173 (1971): 698–702. Reprint. *Death Inside Out*, pp. 71–78.

KENNY, ANTHONY J. P. "The Homunculus Fallacy." *Interpretations of Life and Mind: Essays around the Problem of Reduction.* Edited by Marjorie Grene. London: Routledge & Kegan Paul; New York: Humanities Press, 1971, pp. 65–74.

MORISON, ROBERT S. "Death: Process or Event?" *Science* 173 (1971): 694–698. Reprint. *Death Inside Out*, pp. 63–70.

POLANYI, MICHAEL. *Personal Knowledge: Towards a Post-Critical Philosophy.* Chicago: University of Chicago Press, 1958.

———. "The Structure of Consciousness" and "Life's Irreducible Structure." *Knowing and Being: Essays.* Edited by Marjorie Grene. Chicago: University of Chicago Press; London: Routledge & Kegan Paul, 1969, pp. 211–224, 225–239.

POTEAT, WILLIAM H. "'I will die': An Analysis." *Philosophical Quarterly* 9 (1959): 46–58.

ROSENTHAL, DAVID M., ed. *Materialism and the Mind–Body Problem.* Englewood Cliffs, N.J.: Prentice-Hall, 1971.

VAN EVRA, JAMES. "On Death as a Limit." *Analysis* 31 (1971): 170–176.

VEATCH, ROBERT M. "The Whole-Brain-Oriented Concept of Death: An Outmoded Philosophical Formulation." *Journal of Thanatology* 3 (1975): 13–30.

WALSHE, FRANCIS. "Personal Knowledge and Concepts in the Biological Sciences." *Intellect and Hope: Essays in the Thought of Michael Polanyi.* Edited by Thomas A. Langford and William H. Poteat. Durham: Duke University Press, Lilly Endowment Research Program in Christianity and Politics, 1968, pp. 275–314.

WITTGENSTEIN, LUDWIG. *Philosophical Investigations.* Translated by G. E. M. Anscombe. Oxford: Basil Blackwell, 1953.

———. *Tractatus Logico-Philosophicus.* Translated by C. K. Ogden and F. P. Ramsey. Introduction by Bertrand Russell. International Library of Psychology, Philosophy and Scientific Method. London: Kegan Paul, Trench, Trubner & Co., 1933.

DECISION MAKING, MEDICAL

To make medical decisions in an ethical fashion, neither good intentions nor sound knowledge of fact is sufficient. There is no substitute for a careful analysis of the issues. A rational theory has been elaborated for optimizing decisions. In practice it falls short at two points. For most diseases many of the empirical facts are missing—frequencies of diseases and distributions of diagnostic findings in them, for instance. This defect is readily remediable in principle. A more elusive problem is the development of an appropriate theory of values.

This article shall first explain the general characteristics of decisions, paying some attention to those peculiar to medical practice. The formal principles for the well-characterized problem will then be briefly discussed.

General characteristics of medical decisions

Explicitness. An appropriate course of action in medicine is to be chosen by reflection on sound fact and with as clear a discernment as possible of the immediate and long-term consequences. Analysis cannot be subordinated to custom, nor should data be limited to the purported truths of textbooks, however well respected. Embarking on a sequential course of action—i.e., one modified conditionally on the intermediate outcomes—requires some provision for unfavorable outcomes.

Revocability. Some procedures are irrevocable (gastrectomy); some are doubtfully revocable (vasectomy); some are revocable (simple colostomy); and some involve recurrent acts (a regimen of insulin). The onus of decision is evidently greatest where the process in irrevocable.

The critical and the decisive. While the basis for a decision is not necessarily critical, the execution often is. There may be unresolvable doubt as to whether a patient has a perforated peptic ulcer; but the decisive policies—to operate or not—admit of no compromise. Some actions may be graduated—for instance, the amount of insulin given to a patient with a doubtful diabetic coma; others (e.g., tying the femoral artery) do not allow gradations.

Uncertainty. Decisions must commonly be made in the face of uncertainties of various types.

1. Personal ignorance on the part of the physician due to inexperience (in which case consultation is advisable). It may reflect culpable incompetence.

2. Illusory knowledge, based on what "everyone knows," quoted, but without good evidence, in influential textbooks. Policing this area is a corporate responsibility of the medical profession and especially of the academic leaders. Close reading of the literature suggests that the responsibility is not taken so seriously as it should be.

3. A limited corpus of knowledge about diseases only recently recognized or rarely encountered.

4. Incompleteness of data concerning the individual patient due to serious risks involved (e.g., myelography, though highly informative, is not lightly undertaken); or legal constraint (where permission is denied for a test by parents); or a test, though harmless and scientifically sound, that is morally offensive to the patient or doctor (e.g., reading the patient's private diary for evidence of mental disease).

5. An emergency decision that may have to be made without information that would take perilously long to obtain. Also, there may be insufficient time for reflection.

Conflicts. There are two broad kinds of conflicts. Intrapersonal conflicts are those in which the beneficiary is one person. For instance, amputation of a leg for osteogenic sarcoma mutilates the patient but offers him relief of pain and a chance of cure. The principle of doing what is best for the patient may not dispose of the problem because of the incommensurability between length of life, disability, pain, and so

forth. But at least the patient can be a party to all aspects of the decision.

Interpersonal conflicts are a different matter. They may call for altruism (e.g., donation of a kidney), where there are dangerous opportunities for insidious moral pressures. Free consent of the patient may not be possible (e.g., commitment of a psychotic patient for the public safety). They may offer nothing at all to the deprived party (e.g., a test may be denied because the laboratories are overloaded). Insufficient thought has been given to relative and absolute absence of constraints. The right to reproduce, which, even among the mentally retarded, is widely respected, cannot be absolute; however, when the density of population is low it may be mistaken for an absolute principle.

Pragmatism. Decisions, by nature pragmatic acts of the will, are not necessarily capricious but can be arrived at by conscientious, rational arbitration of the facts and arguments. Such an imperfect formulation can be ethically acceptable for reasons of urgency when even vacillation and postponement themselves may constitute implicit decisions. There is a real peril of mistaking for an essential principle such imperfect grounds for arbitrary decision. For instance, to prevent exploitation, the law protects the mentally retarded, e.g., in making contracts. To make such laws feasible legislators must arbitrarily define the mentally competent. Such an arbitrary pragmatic decision should not be endowed with an essential character from which a body of ethical theory should be deduced. If we believed in hard and fast categories—e.g., "the normal" and "the abnormal"—criteria for *one* decision would suffice for *many* decisions. A sound test of the validity of such a classification is how far we would be prepared to define it when the area of its application is *indefinite*.

Judgment. The professional person, unlike the scholar, may be forced to make decisions even in the face of insufficient knowledge. The gaps in knowledge are filled in by an indefinable quality, "professional judgment," the need for which is not in dispute. But such judgment— as Alvan Feinstein has so aptly pointed out—is not a substitute for knowledge, for the responsibility to amass knowledge, or for conscientious pursuit of whatever method or process of reasoning the problem may demand (Feinstein). It is not a substitution of sentiment for rationality, nor should it be an ornate rationalization for personal prejudices or a defense for neurotic guilt.

Professional judgment is appropriate in the more elusive evaluations—for reconciling conflicting but not clearly commensurable factors, or in marshaling common sense when all else fails.

Simplicity and practicality. Especially in emergencies, practical considerations may require simplifications. There may be logistical problems: A neurosurgeon may not be available quickly enough to deal with head injuries, or there may be insufficient staff to cope with a massive disaster. Alternatively the defect may lie in the lack of a formed attitude for dealing with foreseeable contingencies. The former class of problems reflects what society can afford. The second class of problems is less easily evaded. While a physician cannot be expected to solve any ethical problem instantaneously and infallibly, he could be prepared for many of them with formal training in the theory of making decisions and with sound prescriptions for the major types of cases he will encounter. That he is not usually so prepared is a lamentable comment on medical curricula. Simplicity and practicality are commonly used as evasions of responsibility to the point of slovenliness. Indeed, the foregoing example illustrates the difference between responsibility as a virtue and as a sentiment. Industrial poisoning with anthracite (which is slow) is not necessarily less important than rapid industrial poisoning with carbon monoxide; but *sentiments* of responsibility are much more easily evoked in the latter case.

Formal theory of decision making

In the past, medical ethics has commonly been cast in syllogistic terms. For practical phenomena, at least, deductive and inductive logic may be recast as special cases of a more general probabilistic decision theory, which should now replace the older methods. George Polya expounds the broad principles of such a theory in logical terms; there are several statistical (Lindley; Ferguson) and even clinical (Murphy) counterparts. A fundamental assumption of the formal theories of medical decision making that presents the most formidable difficulties is that all the penalties—loss of life, pain, disability, embarrassment, shame, loss of money, moral affront, etc., whatever cannot be immediately deduced from brute fact—can be condensed accurately into one mathematical function of the variables on which the decision is to be based. In the same accurate way, the benefits

(relief of a disability, beauty, fertility, improved sense of well-being) can also be expressed as a mathematical function of those variables. Benefit may be viewed as negative cost, and a single mathematical formula may be produced, to which we give the technical name *cost function.* It may be positive, in which case treatment does not seem warranted (the cost exceeding the benefit), or negative. If there are several strategies, that which gives the highest negative cost would be the appropriate one.

Much of the attempt to adapt general ethics to medicine has been based on the assumptions of unambiguous diagnoses and fixed costs. Mature consideration suggests the need for a more elaborate structure. There are at least three major components in such a structure.

1. *Probability.* A patient may have six fingers, easily established by examination. Most diagnoses are not of this kind. A common principle is to make the most likely diagnosis and act accordingly. But, as we shall see, this is not the most reasonable strategy.

2. *Nosological characteristics.* Some few conditions are clearly categorical (a traumatic Colles fracture of the wrist, for example). Then treatment and prognosis will be the same almost regardless of the findings, which are important only for diagnosis. The degree, as well as the presence, of the disease may bear on decisions (for instance, coronary disease). In some instances (e.g., "essential hypertension") the findings alone matter: The "diagnosis" does not in itself make any difference to either treatment or prognosis.

3. *Fixity of cost.* In some diseases, such as metastatic (disseminated) cancer, the cost functions are but slightly influenced by the stage of the disease. In certain infectious diseases, the cost of not treating varies according to the current threat to life (e.g., pneumonia), the prospects for preventing irreparable damage (e.g., tuberculosis), and the risks of spread (e.g., smallpox).

Ethical theorists have formulated their ideas on what medical theorists have supposed (often unrealistically) that sound practitioners do. They have thus tended to separate artificially these three major components. For example, arteriosclerosis is a disease; it has a serious prognosis, and therefore treatment is justified. It is not at all clear what it means to say that arteriosclerosis is a disease, because it is difficult to give a watertight definition of a disease. But there is no need to invoke the category "disease" to make rational decisions. The responsible physician has tended to argue broadly that what benefits a patient is warranted, and what does not is unwarranted. The fiction that an ethical decision proceeds in three mutually isolated steps has led to inconsistencies in diagnostic practices. For instance, in the course of one weekend a hospital changed the diagnosis of "sociopathic personality" from a nondisease to a disease because of the changing judicial principles about insanity as a legal defense (*Rosenfield* v. *United States*).

But decision theory would sustain the de facto practice of accepting a "rate of exchange" between uncertainty of diagnosis and cost. For instance, in a disorder of the spinal cord a test for vitamin B_{12} deficiency would be warranted on bare suspicion, because the cost of not treating (in what is a curable disorder) is disastrous. Surgeons demand a less certain diagnosis of appendicitis in a child than in an adult, because peritonitis is so much more devastating a complication in a child.

The treatment of secondary syphilis, once the diagnosis is made, on whatever grounds and with however much uncertainty, will be the same. However, the treatment of high blood pressure varies from inactive vigilance to elaborate and urgent medication: It is not the diagnosis but the floridness of the manifestations that dictates the course of action. Indeed, it matters little what the physician calls the condition or even how he classifies it. Pickering and Platt (to revive a famous controversy) have held diametrically opposite views about the nature of "essential hypertension" but manage cases in much the same way (Murphy).

Ideally we proceed as follows: Where diagnosis is uncertain we define probability distributions of the findings conditional on certain diseases. Particular signs or certain ranges of values may be exceptional in one state, common in another. But all competing diagnoses must be conscientiously considered. An atypical form of a common disease may be a more likely diagnosis than a typical form of a rare disease. The differential diagnoses of a large spleen would differ in emphasis in West Africa and St. Louis, or even from clinic to clinic in the same hospital. Again, diagnosis will be colored by family history. What might be called "tics" in a patient taken at random would be viewed as highly significant early signs if the patient's father had Huntington's chorea. The probabilistic assess-

ment, then, depends on at least three major components: (1) the prior probability of the disorder; (2) the impact of ascertainment (the means by which the patient comes to the attention of the clinician); and (3) the conditional probability of the findings if the patient has the conjectured disease.

These three separate quantities multiplied give the joint probability. If the finding is clearly categorical—for instance the Babinski sign—the result will be a joint probability of two events: first that the sign is present; and second that the patient has, say, multiple sclerosis. If the finding is a measurement on a continuous scale (e.g., a blood sugar level), the result will be a probability density, that is, roughly an index of the relative probability of the result in some defined small neighborhood of the actual observation. (Most of the measurements will be subject to error.)

With this broad background, I shall try to *illustrate* principles. We are torn between realistic examples and uncomplicated explanations. The clinician will object with some truth that "nobody makes decisions on a single datum"; but while an analysis based on many tests would be more plausible, the mathematical manipulation would be correspondingly more complicated.

Intrapersonal and interpersonal decisions

Intrapersonal decisions. The objective is to make the cost as negative as possible. There are two major types of problems.

First, consider cases in which the category to which the patient belongs is known or (what is equivalent) there is only one category. Examples might be arteriosclerotic gangrene of a toe, where the basis for decision is to be the blood flow; and blood pressure level in the absence of diseases—e.g., chronic nephritis or Addison's disease—that perturb it. In both cases the prognoses are related to the measurement. Then the basis for decision is to compare the whole future cost function with treatment (since treatment itself carries some side effects, danger, expense, temporary disability, etc.) with that without treatment. If the former is the greater, there seems to be no place for treatment. Note that in this instance diagnosis does not matter. It is immaterial whether we identify some class of blood pressure levels as "hypertensive."

A special modification may be mentioned. The measurable characteristic may show catastrophic changes in prognosis. In cancer cases the prognosis is markedly different in patients with and those without distant spread, but it scarcely matters how many metastatic lesions are recognized. The cost function with treatment would thus show a sudden leap up as the number of secondaries increases from 0 to 1, since the benefits are drastically curtailed and perhaps completely abolished. A similar case would be the degree of distention of the aorta in the Marfan syndrome, since at some critical point it will rupture, and the surgical mortality abruptly increases when it does.

Second, it may not be known with certainty to which of two or more categories a patient belongs. We must be content with a probabilistic assignment, which will depend on the joint probability functions discussed previously: The problem is one of discrimination. The cost function may itself be a function of the discriminating variable. For instance, red cell sedimentation rate aids in the diagnosis of rheumatism; it is also a prognostic index, and a guide to the efficacy of treatment. In general, then, we have at least four sets of cost functions to deal with: with and without the disease and with and without treatment. If the presence of the disease is in some doubt, the appropriate cost function would be a mixture of the two cost functions according to their relative plausibilities, and likewise for the benefit functions. A rational criterion of action is to minimize the (average) cost function. (This principle would also determine which of several regimens of treatment, all beneficial, should be picked.) The cost functions might also incorporate other factors (e.g., age, sex) that in the particular case bear on prognosis and side effects but not treatment or categorization. In view of the composite origin of the cost function, in making decisions one cannot rationally separate the probabilities and the costs; and an infallible categorization is neither necessary nor, in some cases, even intelligible.

Interpersonal decisions. In some degree the clinician has always been aware of the conflicting demands of more than one person: between the mother and the child at birth, or in distributing his attentions during a physical disaster. But for the most part his main responsibility has been to the individual patient, and the conflicts are intrapersonal. Certain modern procedures—mass screening, routine physical examination, annual examinations, and multiple channel analyzers—have shifted emphasis from the care of the sick to the anticipation of sickness in the symptomless. The profound change in prior probabilities (most of the characteristics in

these newer procedures being a priori unperturbed by illness) means that specificity and sensitivity must receive more attention. Screening tests (e.g., listening to the heart) are generally simple, harmless, and cheap, whereas confirmatory tests, such as cardiac catheterization, are often complex, dangerous, and expensive.

So some principles of selection, inevitably fallible, must be used. The patient, and even the personal physician, may find it hard to accept the idea that the patient's interests are being sacrificed to a more deserving case and that what is being optimized is not the patient's interests but the public good. Where the limiting factor is not cost but what is available (professional skill, supplies of a drug, etc.), more or less serious ethical problems arise in subordinating the good of society as a whole to the partisan demands of the patient or vice versa. The only defense for this policy choice would be a political one, which is outside the scope of this discussion.

EDMOND A. MURPHY

[*Directly related is* THERAPEUTIC RELATIONSHIP, *article on* CONTEMPORARY MEDICAL PERSPECTIVE. *For further discussion of topics mentioned in this article, see the entries:* ACTING AND REFRAINING; PRAGMATISM; *and* RISK.]

BIBLIOGRAPHY

FEINSTEIN, ALVAN R. *Clinical Judgment.* Baltimore: Williams & Wilkins, 1967.
FERGUSON, THOMAS SHELBURNE. *Mathematical Statistics: A Decision Theoretic Approach.* Probability and Mathematical Statistics, A Series of Monographs and Textbooks, no. 1. New York: Academic Press, 1967.
In re Rosenfield. 157 F. Supp. 18 (D. D. C. 1957).
LINDLEY, DENNIS VICTOR. *Making Decisions.* New York: Wiley-Interscience, 1971.
MURPHY, EDMOND A. *The Logic of Medicine.* Baltimore: Johns Hopkins University Press, 1976.
POLYA, GEORGE. *Mathematics and Plausible Reasoning.* 2 vols. London: Oxford University Press; Princeton: Princeton University Press, 1954.

DECLARATION OF GENEVA
See APPENDIX, SECTION I, DECLARATION OF GENEVA.

DECLARATION OF HELSINKI
See APPENDIX, SECTION II, DECLARATION OF HELSINKI.

DEFINITION OF DEATH
See DEATH, DEFINITION AND DETERMINATION OF.

DEMOGRAPHY

See POPULATION ETHICS: ELEMENTS OF THE FIELD, *article on* THE POPULATION PROBLEM IN DEMOGRAPHIC PERSPECTIVE.

DENTISTRY

I. ETHICAL ISSUES IN DENTISTRY
        Clifton O. Dummett
II. PROFESSIONAL CODES IN AMERICAN DENTISTRY
        Chester R. Burns

I
ETHICAL ISSUES IN DENTISTRY

The pursuit of modern dentistry is beset with a number of moral and social issues, which have inundated the profession and affected its daily practice to a considerable degree. Additionally, dramatic changes in the medical profession are having a profound influence on dentistry and have served to alert dentists to the possibilities of similar modifications.

Ethical issues

Among the contemporary ethical and social issues confronting the dental profession are those relating to accountability of dental health professional personnel; high-risk procedures; informed consent for dental and oral health services; peer review and quality of services; dental malpractice; expenditures for comprehensive dental care; dental professional advertising; denturism (unqualified, illegal practice of dentistry in any form on the public); dental auxiliary utilization and interprofessional relations; dental care of the aged and critically ill patients; community dentistry's responsibilities; dental experimentation in human subjects; and ethical emphases in undergraduate, postgraduate, graduate, and continuing dental education.

Oral disease prevention and oral health care for all people, advantaged and disadvantaged, are important responsibilities of community dentistry. Ethical issues are involved when it is recognized that implementation of these objectives requires interprofessional cooperation by all providers of health care. Some subjects have stimulated more attention than others. Extensive publicity has attached to propaganda stressing the need for dentures without emphasis on the equal need for the scientific knowledge that should undergird the technical expertise. This trend in consumerism places dentists in an adversary role in relation to the laboratory technicians whose outspoken proponents advocate direct denture fabrication, bypassing the dentist.

Dentists in general and oral surgeons in particular are sensitive about the question of informed consent—especially as regards the after-effects of anesthesia and X-ray, and clear statements of costs prior to initiating treatment procedure. Interest in the issue of informed consent is due largely to the growth in numbers of patients who have instigated legal action and the sympathetic juries who have made awards on the basis of the absence of informed consent. While the public has an increasing concern about patients' rights, burgeoning costs of malpractice insurance pose similar concerns among physicians and dentists. Peer review—the review of a clinician's services by his professional equals—is becoming an essential component of those dental care delivery systems which are sincerely interested in their accountability to the public for high-quality services. Increasing expenditures for health care have continued to occupy a large share of the public's attention. Consumers of hospital, medical, and dental services complain that health-care costs are rising at twice the rate of the cost of living; thus dentistry is caught up in the problem of justice in health-care delivery. With the professed aim of reducing health-care costs through competition, some states have introduced legislation that would allow various health professionals to advertise. Dental professional advertising has remained a perennial example of unethical practices. Its reevaluation may be one of the outcomes of court declarations with regard to legal and medicopharmaceutical advertising. The oft-stated shortage of health manpower as a primary factor in the health-care "crisis" has revived wide interest in dental auxiliary utilization and has fostered innovations in duty assignments and personnel relations. Even though dental care of the aged and the critically ill has not as yet occupied center stage in the attentions of professional planners, there have been stirrings from senior citizens whose numbers as well as oral health needs have steadily increased. The rights and responsibilities of these persons as well as those of all other consumers of health care have given impetus to renewed demands for a stricter accountability of dental clinicians.

Because the emphases in dental education usually have been oriented toward the acquisition of technical skills, there probably has not been the highest appreciation of the differences that distinguish dentistry as a health profession from the general series of profit-motivated occupations. There is growing recognition among many of today's professional leaders that schools of dentistry in the United States need to review and expand their curricula in the teaching of dental ethics and related health professional topics.

Dentist–patient relationship

The highly specialized knowledge relating to comprehensive treatment of oral diseases has been one reason for patient dependence upon the dental practitioner for the protection of the patient's interests. The quality of protection is directly related to the dentist's maintenance of high professional standards, altruistic ideals, and dedicated service.

The possibilities of patient exploitation have always been plentiful, and there are numerous examples in which improprieties have occurred. Publicity accorded several indiscretions and numerous individual unethical practices have alarmed a trusting public. Public opinion polls have demonstrated increasing lapses in the public's confidence in the occupational and personal integrity of all professionals—physicians and dentists included. As a result, many Americans are accepting greater responsibility for their own oral health and are attempting to maintain individual control over their medical, dental, and hospital care. Such developments have affected traditional dentist–patient relationships in which dental clinicians consistently made the choices of therapy for their patients. There is some evidence that dentists are gradually agreeing to study and accept the viewpoints of patients much more than they did in earlier times.

Dental education

The dental schools' responsibilities for student indoctrination in ethical considerations have remained as clearcut as ever; yet there are indications of a less than desirable effectiveness. In a longitudinal study of professional socialization in which 270 dental students from three dental schools in California participated, Morris and Sherlock reported that professional ethics declined steadily, while cynicism increased, especially in the clinic years.

There is consensus among significant numbers of dental students that their attitudes toward the profession underwent some objectional transformations during their clinical apprenticeships. This is the way it has been for generations of dental students—which suggests that the clinical faculty may also be in need of sensitization to human values in dental care.

In dental schools generally, there are few if any teachers appointed with sole or primary commitments in dental ethics instruction. Most teachers are either dentists who have developed an interest in ethics as it would apply to dentistry, or dentists who have no interest in the subject but nevertheless have been arbitrarily assigned to teach it. It would be unusual to find an ethicist teaching in a dental school.

Prompted by some of the changes in medical education, which include the expansion of the teaching of medical ethics, a few dental educators have been pressing for similar expansion in the teaching of dental ethics. The problems are common to medical and dental schools: The demands of currently established technical courses hinder the recognition, economic support, and ideological consideration of new courses.

Social issues in dental ethics

The American Dental Association's Code of Ethics and the various state dental codes have established laudable guidelines and ethical norms for dentists in their interpersonal relationships, but the dental profession has been reluctant to admit that it had an ethical responsibility in reference to the larger social issues. The quest for human and civil rights in the 1950s and 1960s in the United States compelled all health professions to weigh a professed adherence to ethical principles against widespread practices of discrimination on the basis of race, religion, and national origin. Following the U.S. Supreme Court rulings against segregated education in 1954, dental schools were obliged to reassess their admissions policies, which had denied minorities unhampered access to a dental education. Additionally, the country's social upheaval had an impact on the individual practitioners who were called upon to put dental ethical behavior above regional customs and personal prejudices. Many white practitioners of medicine and dentistry in the United States were guilty of unethical behavior in that they withheld or diluted their services in the delivery of health care to minorities. Moreover, many white dentists resisted admitting minority dentists into local and national dental societies.

In 1958 increased pressures to remove discriminatory barriers prompted the American Dental Association's Board of Trustees to request ADA constituent societies to make a study of the Association's bylaws to see that licensure and adherence to the principles of ethics were the sole essential qualifications for membership in the Association.

Conclusion

Past experiences underscore the unnecessary tensions and confusion created by an unwillingness to face forthrightly the ethical dilemmas in many sensitive areas of dental practice. No less urgent, complex, or far-reaching are contemporary issues that have been opened to public scrutiny. Dentists will have to make some difficult decisions based upon ethical considerations.

Thus academicians, general practitioners, and their representative organizations must make a joint effort to formulate an attainable, ethical base supportive of the delivery of high-quality oral health services. Objective appraisal and careful reorganization of the tenets of various codes must be accomplished within the framework of a morality that recognizes the vagaries of human behavior.

CLIFTON O. DUMMETT

[*Other relevant material may be found under* AD-VERTISING BY MEDICAL PROFESSIONALS; AGING AND THE AGED, *article on* HEALTH CARE AND RE-SEARCH IN THE AGED; INFORMED CONSENT IN THE THERAPEUTIC RELATIONSHIP; JUSTICE; MEDICAL ETHICS EDUCATION; *and* PATIENTS' RIGHTS MOVE-MENT. *See* APPENDIX, SECTION IV, AMERICAN DENTAL ASSOCIATION.]

BIBLIOGRAPHY

"An Act to Amend Section 1680 of and to Repeal Section 651, 651.2, 651.3, 651.4, 2556 and 3129 of the Business and Professions Code Relating to Advertising by Professionals." SB 1974, 1976 sess., State of California. Introduced 23 March 1976 by Senator John F. Dunlap (D.-Napa). Sent to Committee on Business and Professions. Short title: "Price Advertising."

DUMMETT, CLIFTON O. "A Chronology Updated—Recent Events in the Negro's Advancements in Dentistry in the U.S." *Quarterly of the National Dental Association* 21 (1963): 145–201.

———. "Year 2000: Community Dentistry." *Journal of the American Dental Association* 82 (1971): 280–285.

GOLDBERG, ARTHUR J. "Ethics in the Professions." *Journal of the American College of Dentists* 42 (1975): 218–223.

GOLDIAMOND, ISRAEL. "Protection of Human Subjects and Patients: A Social Contingency Analysis of Distinctions Between Research and Practice, and Its Implications." *Behaviorism* 4 (1976): 1–41.

Great Britain, Radioactive Substances Advisory Committee. *Code of Practice for the Protection of Persons Against Ionizing Radiations Arising from Medical and Dental Use.* 3d ed. London: Her Majesty's Stationery Office, 1972.

JONSEN, ALBERT R., and HELLEGERS, ANDRÉ E. "Conceptual Foundations for an Ethics of Medical Care." *Ethics of Health Care: Papers of the Conference on Health Care and Changing Values, November 27–29, 1973.* Edited by Laurence R. Tancredi. Washington: Institute of Medicine, National Academy of Sciences, 1974, pp. 3–20. Reprint. *Ethics and Health Policy.* Edited by Robert M. Veatch and Roy Branson. Cambridge, Mass.: Ballinger Publishing Co., 1976, pp. 17–34.

LAWS, PRISCILLA W. *Medical and Dental X-Rays: A Consumer's Guide to Avoiding Unnecessary Radiation Exposure.* Washington: Public Citizen Health Research Group, 1974.

MORRIS, R. T., and SHERLOCK, B. J. "Decline of Ethics and the Rise of Cynicism in Dental School." *Journal of Health and Social Behavior* 12 (1971): 290–299.

PARISH, JACK R. "Professional Conduct in Dental School and After." *Journal of Dental Education* 32 (1968): 326–329.

VEATCH, ROBERT M. and SOLLITTO, SHARMON. "Medical Ethics Teaching: Report of a National Medical School Survey." *Journal of the American Medical Association* 235 (1976): 1030–1033.

II
PROFESSIONAL CODES IN AMERICAN DENTISTRY

The quest for ethical ideals in American dentistry has been intimately associated with the evolution of professional organizations. By 1859, the year of the founding of the American Dental Association, there were ten local dental societies, two state societies, and four dental colleges. Nineteen years after the American Medical Association adopted a code of ethics, and in spite of opposition expressed by numerous dentists, the American Dental Association adopted a code at its sixth annual meeting in 1866 (American Dental Association, 1866; Burns).

There were many similarities between the code for physicians and the one for dentists. Dentists should exhibit firmness, kindness, and sympathy toward their patients. They should be temperate, make no false promises, and explain their professional procedures. A dentist should be a gentleman in all relationships and never speak disparagingly of a colleague's practices. Physicians and dentists should avoid interprofessional conflicts by recognizing distinctions between their specialized interests. Dentists, like physicians, were expected to honor the public's trust by exposing all quacks.

In 1880 the American Dental Association made adoption of its code a mandatory requirement for membership, as had physicians some twenty-five years previously (American Dental

Association, 1881). As with the physicians' code, the code of dental ethics had no provision for enforcement. By the turn of the twentieth century, only one dentist had lost his membership in the American Dental Association for unprofessional conduct.

In 1897 the Southern and American associations merged to form the National Dental Association, and two years later a revised code was adopted (National Dental Association). The revision contained two significant changes: encouragement of consultations and permission to use cards and newspaper announcements for advertising names and office addresses.

In 1922 the national organization of dentists assumed its original name, the American Dental Association, and adopted a new, substantially different code of ethics. Previous claims about mutual duties of the profession and the public and about interprofessional duties of dentists and physicians were omitted. Statements about the obligations of dentists to patients were summarized in a single exhortation: The dentist should conduct himself "in accordance with the Golden Rule." The remaining sections of the code dealt exclusively with transactions among dentists. A new section in the revised code of 1928 required dentists to report "illegal, corrupt, or dishonest conduct on the part of any member of the dental profession" to the proper authorities. A mechanism for judging and punishing unethical dentists was described in a note appended to the code. The code of 1928 also urged dentists to be good citizens and to conduct themselves as members of a profession "whose prime purpose is service to humanity" (American Dental Association, 1947).

A revision for 1936 included sections about patents, contracts, and group practices (ibid.). The duty to report illegal and unethical conduct was omitted in the revision of 1944, as were the imperatives to be good citizens and serve humanity. The codes of 1928, 1936, and 1944 had an important disclaimer: The ideals of these codes would not "cover the whole field of ethics for the members of the profession." Two very significant sentences were added in the code of 1944: "There are many obligations assumed by those who choose dentistry as their life's work, in addition to those included in the foregoing statements. To know the answers to most questions not presented in this code, we need but to be guided by the Christian rule to do unto others as we would have others do unto us" (ibid.). This conclusion allowed for ethical pluralism

and liberal interpretations; but it was also an invitation to oversimplify the ethical conflicts generated by the emerging social and technical complexities of twentieth-century dental practice.

A rewritten code, principles unchanged, was adopted in 1950 (American Dental Association, 1950, 1954). The Judicial Council of the American Dental Association subsequently converted the sections of this code into a set of "principles of ethics," which was approved in October 1955 and revised slightly in November 1958 (American Dental Association, 1958). Traditional ideals of professional loyalty and honor were substained, but important changes reflected new demands of educators, and allied professionals and paraprofessionals, as well as increasing pressures from both community and governmental groups for more attention to dental health broadly conceived, including fluoridation and preventive practices. A revision of the *Principles* occurred in 1960 and again in 1974 (Conway and Rutledge; American Dental Association, 1975). The Judicial Council of the American Dental Association continues to offer advisory opinions based on their interpretations of these *Principles*.

Repeatedly revising and reassessing their codes, American dentists have discovered norms that would uphold rights for professional self-regulation and provide means for intraprofessional policing. For individual dentists, a set of principles is an elaborate loyalty oath, with disobedience leading to dishonor and disfranchisement. These principles also constitute a bill of professional rights for dental practitioners. American communities may honor these rights and acknowledge the distinctiveness of their associated values if dentists, as groups and individuals, fulfill the obligations associated with the rights.

CHESTER R. BURNS

[See APPENDIX, INTRODUCTION, *article on* CODES OF THE HEALTH-CARE PROFESSIONS; *and* SECTION IV, AMERICAN DENTAL ASSOCIATION. *Directly related is the other article in this entry:* ETHICAL ISSUES IN DENTISTRY.]

BIBLIOGRAPHY

American Dental Association. "Code of Dental Ethics." *Transactions of the American Dental Association* 6 (1866): 401–405. Legislative history appears on pp. 228, 234, and 238 of the same volume.
———. "Code of Ethics." *Digest of Official Actions, 1922–1946.* Chicago: 1947, pp. 199–211. Digest containing official actions: Constitution and Administra-

tive By-Laws; Code of Ethics, each with all changes, 1922–1946.

————. "Ethics." *Digest of Official Actions, 1946–1953.* Chicago: 1954, pp. 118–120.

————. *Principles of Ethics,* Chicago: 1958. Pamphlet.

————. "Principles of Ethics." *Journal of the American Dental Association* 90 (1975): 184–191.

————. "Revised Code of Ethics to Be Considered at Atlantic City Meeting." *Journal of the American Dental Association* 40 (1950): 612–615.

————. "Standing Resolutions." *Transactions of the American Dental Association* 21 (1881): 36.

BURNS, CHESTER R. "The Evolution of Professional Ethics in American Dentistry." *Bulletin of the History of Dentistry* 22 (1974): 59–70.

CONWAY, BERNARD J., and RUTLEDGE, C. E. "The Ethics of Our Profession." *Journal of the American Dental Association* 62 (1961): 333–342.

National Dental Association. "Code of Ethics: Report of Committee." *Transactions of the National Dental Association* 3 (1899): 481–483. Legislative history appears on p. 17 of the same volume.

NOYES, EDMUND. *Ethics and Jurisprudence for Dentists.* Chicago: W. B. Conkey Co., 1923.

DEONTOLOGICAL ETHICS

See ETHICS, *article on* DEONTOLOGICAL THEORIES.

DESCRIPTIVIST ETHICS

See ETHICS, *article on* NON-DESCRIPTIVISM.

DETERMINISM

See FREE WILL AND DETERMINISM.

DIALYSIS

See KIDNEY DIALYSIS AND TRANSPLANTATION.

DISCLOSURE

See TRUTH-TELLING; INFORMED CONSENT IN THE THERAPEUTIC RELATIONSHIP; INFORMED CONSENT IN HUMAN RESEARCH; INFORMED CONSENT IN MENTAL HEALTH; PRIVACY; CONFIDENTIALITY.

DISEASE

See HEALTH AND DISEASE; MENTAL ILLNESS.

DOUBLE EFFECT

In an effort to stipulate the conditions under which one may rightfully cause evil, e.g., the death of another person and in particular an innocent person or of oneself, Roman Catholic moral theologians developed what has come to be called "the principle of double effect." Though this principle has been of major concern princi-pally to writers within the Roman Catholic tradition, the moral questions that it raises have been and are of interest to writers in other traditions. They have special relevance to many important problems in bioethics, e.g., abortion, euthanasia, and medical experimentation. This article will (1) provide a preliminary description of the principle, its underlying presuppositions, and its purpose; (2) offer a brief sketch of its historical development and the typical cases to which it has been applied; and (3) discuss some of the major contemporary debates centering on an understanding of the principle.

Description of the principle

As commonly formulated, the principle stipulates that one may rightfully cause evil through an act of choice if four conditions are verified: (1) the act itself, prescinding from the evil caused, is good or at least indifferent; (2) the good effect of the act is what the agent intends directly, only permitting the evil effect; (3) the good effect must not come about by means of the evil effect; and (4) there must be some proportionately grave reason for permitting the evil effect to occur (Mangan, p. 43; Conway, p. 137; Grisez, *Abortion*, p. 329; McCormick, p. 1; Curran, pp. 173–174).

Two of the major presuppositions of the principle around which contemporary discussion centers are that there is a morally significant difference between intending evil and permitting evil (condition 2) and that it is wrong to use an evil means to obtain a good end (condition 3). Condition 3, in short, rejects the view that a good end can justify an evil means, and some of the Roman Catholic defenders of the principle hold that this rejection is grounded in revelation, specifically in Romans 3:8 (Farraher, p. 71; Conway; Kelly, pp. 59–60).

The purpose of the principle is not, as some have recently suggested (Callahan, pp. 428–429), to allay subjective scruples about a "dirty" conscience, but rather, as others (Ramsey, pp. 207–211) have observed, to limit the area of moral ambiguity in "hard" cases by specifying the objective criteria for determining to what extent we can cause evil in the pursuit of good. Whether the principle is in fact capable of achieving this purpose is another question and is related to the debates to be considered later.

Historical development

Scholars agree that the principle was not fully formulated until the middle of the seventeenth century, but there is lively debate over its precise historical development. Some, for example Mangan, argue that the principle was basically, although by no means clearly, expressed in the thirteenth century by Thomas Aquinas in his discussion of killing in self-defense (in the *Summa Theologiae* II–II, 64, 7), and that it was in reference to this teaching that such sixteenth- and seventeenth-century authors as Thomas de Vio Cajetan (1468–1534), Louis Molina (1536–1600), Thomas Sanchez (1550–1610), and, in particular, the Salmanticenses (the Discalced Carmelites of Salamanca), preeminently Domingo de Santa Teresa (1600–1654), made the principle more and more explicit.

Others, inclining to the position of J. Ghoos, maintain that the principle is in no way entailed in Aquinas's teaching on killing in self-defense and that its development was stimulated by an endeavor to bring together two notions that were distinguished by Aquinas, namely, the "indirect voluntary" and the "voluntary in its cause." For Aquinas these were distinct concepts, with the first (*Summa Theologiae* I–II, 6, 3) referring to an effect that came about by the failure to act, and the second (ibid., I–II, 77, 7) referring to an effect that was willed not in itself but in its cause. For Aquinas, in other words, the "indirectly voluntary" was conceptually akin to the modern notion of refraining from acting, and Aquinas clearly held that a person is morally responsible for evils that result from such omissions if that person can and ought to take the action necessary to prevent the evil from occurring. During the sixteenth and seventeenth centuries these two terms gradually became synonymous, having the meaning that "voluntary in its cause" had in Aquinas, and these terms figured prominently in the evolution of the principle of double effect. Its precise formulation, according to this interpretation, was the work of John of St. Thomas (1589–1644) in his *De bonitate et malitia actuum humanorum*.

No matter which historical interpretation is correct, there is an undeniable close conceptual affinity, manifest in contemporary discussions of the principle (Grisez, *Abortion*, pp. 326–329, "Toward a Consistent," pp. 73–79; Ramsey, p. 220; Curran, pp. 174–182), between the reasoning at work in Aquinas's teaching on killing in self-defense and that entailed in the principle of double effect. Aquinas clearly held that a person may rightfully choose to defend himself from attack even if his act of self-defense will result in the death of the assailant, provided that (1) the agent intends only to preserve his own life (a good) and does not intend to kill the assailant (an evil) in order to protect himself, and (2) the force used to repel the attack is proportionate. This measured act of self-defense is justified because the good of life merits protection and one can rightfully protect this good by appropriate acts so long as choosing to do them does not of necessity require setting one's will on the foreseen evil. The reasoning involved in this argument closely parallels that expressed in the first, second, and fourth conditions of the principle of double effect. The difficulty is in reconciling the argument given by Aquinas with the third condition, a subject to which we shall return.

It is noteworthy that in the subsequent historical development of the principle of double effect the majority of Roman Catholic moral theologians did *not* use it to justify killing in self-defense. Although Cajetan did so (Mangan, p. 52), most writers in subsequent centuries, beginning with Molina in the sixteenth and continuing until very recent times, argued that one could rightfully intend to kill an aggressor, even one materially and not formally unjust, in self-defense (ibid., p. 54, n. 25).

During the sixteenth and seventeenth centuries the principle was applied typically to cases involving the loss of semen brought on by sexual desires that unavoidably arose while a person was engaging in otherwise unobjectionable pursuits and to cases involving the causing of scandal. The theologians of the era used the principle to justify, for example, a medical student's research even if it should cause him to ejaculate and to condone a young maiden's stroll through the village even if, modestly attired as she might be according to the customs of the day, she foresaw that her promenade would provoke lustful desires on the part of village rubes (Ghoos, pp. 40–47). It was also applied to cases involving the killing of the innocent, particularly in war, and to exposing oneself to mortal danger for a good cause (Mangan, pp. 54–55).

Eventually the principle was given wider application, particularly during the nineteenth century by Jean Pierre Gury in his often reedited and influential *Compendium Theologiae Moralis* (ibid., pp. 59–60; Connell, p. 1021), until it came to embrace almost the entire field of moral theology. It is invoked today to cope with many problems of crucial importance in bioethics, for instance, abortion, euthanasia, suicide, the hazards of medical experimentation, and the ethics of procreation (contraception and sterilization). The way the principle is commonly understood and applied can be well illustrated by taking the example of abortion. Until the relatively recent past Roman Catholic writers used the principle to justify abortions in ectopic pregnancies and in hysterectomies to remove a cancerous womb. In such instances the intention and the immediate effect of the act is the removal of a pathological organ (the fallopian tubes or uterus) that happens to contain a fetus. The removal of the fetus and its subsequent death are neither directly willed nor directly done (Bouscaren, pp. 147–155). As commonly understood, however, the principle cannot justify procedures involving "direct" abortions, even if such procedures are necessary in order to save the mother from imminent death, not even if it is morally certain that both mother and fetus will die if nothing is done (ibid., pp. 3–16; Grisez, *Abortion*, p. 179). In the latter type of case, it is commonly held, the principle is inapplicable inasmuch as the third condition is not capable of being fulfilled.

Contemporary debates on the principle

There seem to be inconsistencies in the application of the principle, e.g., allowing abortifacient procedures when organs are pathological while refusing them if no pathology exists although death of both mother and fetus is imminent. Partly for this reason but more basically because of serious difficulties in understanding the significance of its requirements, in particular conditions 2 and 3, there has recently been a lively discussion of the principle by many authors interested in bioethical problems.

One group of writers focuses on the second condition: that the evil be permitted and only indirectly intended whereas the good alone is to be directly intended. Williams (pp. 280–291) and Fletcher (1973) argue that this distinction is dishonest at worst and meaningless at best, although central to the reasoning of those who see a vast moral difference between killing a person for merciful reasons and allowing a dying person to die by refusing to continue the use of life-prolonging but extraordinary and morally optional techniques. For Williams and Fletcher the distinction is simply specious and an instance of moral quibbling inasmuch as the result is the same: A person dies. Defenders of this distinction, crucial to condition 2, have responded by pointing out that this criticism is predicated upon a consequentialist or utilitarian understanding of human action and that a significant difference is at stake inasmuch as the result is obtained in radically different ways: In the one instance the person dies from some

underlying disease or injury that it is no longer reasonable to combat, whereas in the other instance the person dies from an act truthfully describable as killing (Dyck, pp. 100–105).

Possibly Williams and Fletcher have confused the distinction between directly intending evil and only indirectly intending or permitting evil with the distinction between acting and refraining. The distinctions are not the same. If a person refrains from acting to save another's life when he can and ought to do so (e.g., if he fails to throw a drowning person a life preserver when he can easily do so), he is morally responsible for that person's death. His act of refraining from doing what he can and ought to do is the equivalent of doing the evil deed with direct intent.

With Williams and Fletcher, Aune claims that the distinction between intending and foreseeing, also central to condition 2, is indefensible (Aune). This claim seems unfounded. For instance, a dentist clearly foresees that in extracting an impacted wisdom tooth he will inflict pain on his patient. Yet he is surely not intending the pain that he will inflict. Were he properly intending the infliction of pain, his act could hardly be said to be one of proper dentistry (Grisez, *Abortion*, pp. 327–329). In fact, if a dentist does properly intend pain, his patients would be well advised to go elsewhere.

Somewhat similarly to Aune, Foot, while admitting the validity in theory between intending and permitting/foreseeing, contends that it is quite subsidiary to the distinction between positive and negative duties and argues that it is not reasonable to claim that a person can be held to be not morally responsible for the unintended yet foreseeable effects of his actions (Foot). Thus, should a shopkeeper knowingly sell poisons to someone who he knows will use them to kill others, he cannot avoid responsibility for the subsequent deaths. Although Foot's comments have some validity, they do not substantively affect the principle. The act, unwarrantable in the example given, would not be justifiable on grounds of the principle of double effect insofar as its fourth requirement would not be capable of fulfillment.

Another group of critics (Knauer; Van der Marck; Van der Poel; Janssens) take as their point of departure the third condition of the principle. They argue that in its traditional understanding this third condition has been interpreted too materialistically. They maintain that in instances such as killing in self-defense the evil effect (the death of the assailant) is physically direct and is the means to the good effect; and in making this argument some, for instance Knauer (pp. 138–141) and Janssens (pp. 116–133), explicitly appeal to the teaching of Aquinas on killing in self-defense. Although these authors differ markedly among themselves, they agree in making a crucial distinction between physical (ontic, premoral, or nonmoral) evil and moral evil. They then concur in holding that one can rightfully intend the physical (ontic, premoral, or nonmoral) evil, e.g., death, sterilization, mutilation, so long as a proportionate good or commensurate good will be served.

On this interpretation of condition 3, condition 2 becomes almost superfluous. In fact, some of these authors, e.g., Van der Marck (pp. 56–58) and Van der Poel (pp. 207–210) see no real meaning in the distinction between the directly and indirectly intended. Knauer retains the terminology of direct–indirect, but he so modifies its meaning that, as critics note, the distinction becomes inoperative and its function is supplanted by the notion of the commensurate good (Grisez, *Abortion,* p. 331; McCormick, pp. 11–12).

The general thrust of this critique has been accepted by others (Curran; McCormick) although each objects to specific features in the arguments advanced by Knauer, Van der Poel, and Van der Marck. McCormick believes that their arguments converge with others recently advanced and that they can be summarized by saying that it is morally permissible to intend directly an evil, in its physical (ontic, premoral, or nonmoral) sense, in itself but not for itself. This is true as long as there is a proportionate reason. If there is no proportionate reason, then the evil is intended not only in itself but for itself and thus becomes morally, and not merely physically, evil. McCormick himself admits the validity of the direct–indirect distinction but holds that it is of limited value and simply means that a greater proportionate reason is necessary if one is directly to intend the evil and not merely to permit it or intend it only indirectly (McCormick, pp. 68–106).

A third group of authors, preeminently Grisez and Ramsey, basically accept the principle of double effect. They reject the interpretation given above inasmuch as they believe that it is not only in effect a repudiation of the principle but an acceptance of a consequentialism (cf. also May). With the above group, however, Grisez and Ramsey agree that the third condition of the principle was too restrictively understood in the past. They grant that the evil effected may be direct physically but argue that it is permissible only if it is an unavoidable concomitant or aspect of an act that in itself is immediately targeted on the good (Grisez, *Abortion,* pp. 333–346; "Toward a Consistent," pp. 87–91; Ramsey, pp. 211–222). Although these authors also disagree among themselves, they agree that any evil effected through human acts can be morally justifiable only if it is "indirect," that is, a partial concomitant of an act that is directly intended and targeted on the achievement of the good. In their judgment, a human person makes himself to be morally evil if he chooses to do deeds in which he of necessity makes evil to be the precise end of his will, that is, of his person.

The argument over the meaning of the principle, and in particular of conditions 2 and 3, continues. It centers on some of the most critical issues in ethics and moral theory. Those who accept the principle, even as reinterpreted by the third group of authors discussed, hold that we are very limited in the evil that we may rightfully cause in our pursuit of the good and consequently are inclined to be very much opposed to abortion, artificial insemination, in vitro fertilization, nontherapeutic experimentation on children, etc. On the other hand, those who reject the principle or reinterpret it along the lines of the second group of authors discussed are more ready to accept procedures that give promise of securing proportionately good results despite the harm entailed.

WILLIAM E. MAY

[*Directly related is* ACTING AND REFRAINING. *This article will find application in the entries* ABORTION, *articles on* ROMAN CATHOLIC PERSPECTIVES *and* CONTEMPORARY DEBATE IN PHILOSOPHICAL AND RELIGIOUS ETHICS; CONTRACEPTION; DEATH AND DYING: EUTHANASIA AND SUSTAINING LIFE; HUMAN EXPERIMENTATION; INFANTS, *articles on* ETHICAL PERSPECTIVES ON THE CARE OF INFANTS, *and* INFANTICIDE: A PHILOSOPHICAL PERSPECTIVE; STERILIZATION, *article on* ETHICAL ASPECTS; *and* SUICIDE. *Other relevant material may be found under* ETHICS, *articles on* TELEOLOGICAL THEORIES *and* UTILITARIANISM; RELIGIOUS DIRECTIVES IN MEDICAL ETHICS, *article on* ROMAN CATHOLIC DIRECTIVES; *and* ROMAN CATHOLICISM.]

BIBLIOGRAPHY

AUNE, BRUCE. "Intention and Foresight." *Journal of Philosophy* 63 (1966): 652–654. Abstract of a symposium paper.
BOUSCAREN, TIMOTHY LINCOLN. *The Ethics of Ectopic*

Operations. 2d ed., rev. Milwaukee: Bruce Publishing Co., 1944.

CALLAHAN, DANIEL J. *Abortion: Law, Choice, and Morality.* New York: Macmillan Co., 1970.

CONNELL, F. J. "Double Effect, Principle of." *New Catholic Encyclopedia.* New York: McGraw-Hill Book Co., 1967, vol. 4, pp. 1020–1022.

CONWAY, WILLIAM. "The Act of Two Effects." *Irish Theological Quarterly* 18 (1951): 125–137.

CURRAN, CHARLES E. "The Principle of Double Effect." *On-going Revision: Studies in Moral Theology.* Notre Dame, Ind.: Fides Publishers, 1975, pp. 173–209.

DYCK, ARTHUR J. "An Alternative to the Ethics of Euthanasia." *To Live and to Die: When, Why, and How.* Edited by Robert H. Williams. New York: Springer-Verlag, 1973, pp. 98–112.

FARRAHER, JOSEPH J. "Current Theology: Notes on Moral Theology: Suicide and Moral Principles." *Theological Studies* 24 (1963): 69–79.

FLETCHER, JOSEPH FRANCIS. "Ethics and Euthanasia." *To Live and to Die: When, Why, and How.* Edited by Robert H. Williams. New York: Springer-Verlag, 1973, pp. 113–122.

———. *Morals and Medicine: The Moral Problems of the Patient's Right to Know the Truth, Contraception, Artificial Insemination, Sterilization, Euthanasia.* Foreword by Karl Menninger. Princeton: Princeton University Press, 1954.

FOOT, PHILIPPA. "The Problem of Abortion and the Doctrine of the Double Effect." *Moral Problems: A Collection of Philosophical Essays.* Edited by James Rachels. New York: Harper & Row, 1971, pp. 29–41. 2d ed. 1975, pp. 59–70. Also *Oxford Review* 5 (1967): 5–15.

GHOOS, J. "L'acte à double effet: Étude de théologie positive." *Ephemerides Theologicae Lovaniensis* 27 (1951): 30–52.

GRISEZ, GERMAIN GABRIEL. *Abortion: The Myths, the Realities, and the Arguments.* New York: Corpus Books, 1970, pp. 179, 321–346.

———. "Toward a Consistent Natural-Law Ethics of Killing." *American Journal of Jurisprudence* 15 (1970): 64–96.

KELLY, GERALD. "Current Theology: Notes on Moral Theology, 1951: General and Pastoral." *Theological Studies* 13 (1952): 59–63, especially pp. 59–61.

KNAUER, PETER. "The Hermeneutic Function of the Principle of Double Effect." *Natural Law Forum* 12 (1967): 132–162.

JANSSENS, LOUIS. "Ontic Evil and Moral Evil." *Louvain Studies* 4 (1972): 115–156.

MCCORMICK, RICHARD A. *Ambiguity in Moral Choice.* The 1973 Père Marquette Theology Lecture. Milwaukee: Marquette University Press, 1973.

MANGAN, JOSEPH T. "An Historical Analysis of the Principle of Double Effect." *Theological Studies* 10 (1949): 41–61.

MAY, WILLIAM E. "Becoming Human in and through Our Deeds." *Becoming Human: An Invitation to Christian Ethics.* Dayton, Ohio: Pflaum Publishing, 1975, chap. 4, pp. 79–112.

RAMSEY, PAUL. "Abortion: A Review Article." *Thomist* 37 (1973): 174–226.

VAN DER MARCK, WILLIAM H. M. *Toward a Christian Ethics: A Renewal in Moral Theology.* Translated by Denis J. Barrett. Westminster, Md.: Newman Press, 1967.

VAN DER POEL, CORNELIUS J. "The Principle of Double Effect." *Absolutes in Moral Theology?* Edited by Charles E. Curran. Washington: Corpus Books, 1968, pp. 186–210.

WILLIAMS, GRANVILLE LLEWELYN. *The Sanctity of Life and the Criminal Law.* New York: Alfred A. Knopf, 1957.

DRUG INDUSTRY AND MEDICINE

Medical practice in the industrially advanced countries is heavily oriented toward drug treatment, necessitating a more or less intimate tie between physician and drug manufacturer. Despite the potential conflict between the manufacturer's pursuit of profit and the physician's duty to his patient, until the early 1960s the interests of the three parties were considered to be in harmony—industry's desire for new products coinciding with that of the physician and patient for more effective therapy. However, the revelations of the U.S. Senate and House committees chaired by Estes Kefauver, Gaylord Nelson, Edward Kennedy, and others have cast doubt upon this harmony.

Development and use of drugs

Does industry's economic need for new and patentable drugs really promote the health of the public? If not, what can be done about it? The 1969 *Final Report* of the DHEW (U.S. Department of Health, Education, and Welfare) Task Force on Prescription Drugs defined "rational prescribing" as "the appropriate selection of a drug—the right drug for the right person, in the right amounts at the right time" (U.S. DHEW, p. 21). The relations between the drug industry and the medical profession can best be analyzed in terms of whether industry's demand for new products distorts this ideal of "rational prescribing."

Pharmacological education. After acknowledging that the American physician, who prescribes $25,000 worth of drugs every year, often does so in an irrational way, the *Final Report* states that "lack of knowledge and sophistication in the proper use of drugs is perhaps the greatest deficiency of the average physician today" (ibid., p. 23; Council on Economic Priorities, p. 27). Paradoxically, the physician who spends his professional life prescribing drugs knows relatively little about them.

Many authorities have ascribed this deficiency to the limited and inadequate pharmacological education of physicians. The medical school graduate lacks the background to examine critically the claims of industry for its products—contrary to the true aim of medical education and to medical tradition. This happens because initiative in drug development has passed from the medical profession and the medical schools to the pharmaceutical industry, distinguishing modern medicine from all previous eras when the pharmacist was subordinate to the physician. The change began in the 1880s with the introduction of "proprietary remedies"—medicines and medicinal mixtures promoted to the public and the profession for use in specific diseases or conditions (Coulter, pp. 417 ff.). The advertising of "proprietaries" in medical journals was initially considered unethical, undermining the physician's traditional responsibility for knowledge of his instruments of cure, but the profession used "proprietaries" more and more, and the de facto situation was legitimized in 1903 by an appropriate change in the Code of Ethics of the American Medical Association (AMA).

A medical journal in 1905 contrasted the resulting situation with "forty years ago [when] the physician who prescribed a medicine without some knowledge of its composition and effects was considered to have violated the Code of Ethics and regarded by his professional brethren with suspicion. There has been a great change" ("Action of Gases on Bacteria").

The change has meant that today medical schools and physicians simply perform the pharmacological tasks assigned them by the drug industry. Since drug research is often essential to professorial advancement, the drug industry underwriting such research has a measure of control over the pharmacological thinking of physicians and professors who might otherwise offer a counterweight to industry views. The company providing the drug for investigation and the financing often influences the design of the study—which may be used more to advertise the given product than to yield scientific data (Goddard). Some pharmacological research in medical schools is government funded, but its role is often merely one of disproving (at public expense) the claims of some company for a drug upon which it has already earned a profit (University Group Diabetes Program, *Diabetes* XIX [1970], p. 467). The involvement of industry in pharmacological education is hence a source of serious ethical conflict between the profit motive and the health needs of the public.

Informed consent. The competition among drug companies leads to pressure on physicians conducting clinical trials. Henry K. Beecher was one of the first, in 1966, to call attention to the consequence—failure, in many cases, to obtain patient consent to excessively dangerous experiments (Beecher). Some of the more striking examples cited by him were: the withholding of appropriate treatment from 109 servicemen with streptococcal respiratory infections, giving rise to two cases of acute rheumatic fever and one of acute nephritis; the administration of a drug to fifty healthy mentally retarded children and juvenile delinquents to ascertain if the drug caused liver damage, leading to a high incidence of hepatic dysfunction in the group after four weeks of the trial; and the administration, to forty-one randomly selected patients, of a drug known to cause aplastic anemia, so that many developed toxic bone-marrow depression. Beecher gave fifteen other instances and stated that examination of 100 consecutive human studies published in a leading journal indicated that twelve appeared to have been conducted without obtaining patient consent.

The problem of informed consent becomes acute in the case of children, mental defectives, and prisoners (U.S. Congress, Senate, Select Committee on Small Business, pt. 14, pp. 5689–5702). Prisoners are employed extensively by the so-called proof mills often used by drug companies to generate evidence favorable to their product (ibid., pp. 5702 ff.).

Duration of drug trials. The appropriate duration of a drug trial is another ethical issue related to industry's desire to market its products rapidly. Adverse reactions and lack of efficacy may take years to become manifest. The antidiabetic drug Orinase (tolbutamide) had been available since 1956 and was grossing the manufacturer more than $50 million a year when a 1970 study by a group of medical schools demonstrated it to be a cause of cardiovascular disease (University Group Diabetes Program, 1970, 1971). But this became evident only after a patient had taken the drug for three years. The first oral contraceptive was approved for sale in 1957, but only in the late 1960s did physicians become convinced that substances in them caused blood clotting.

Drug companies and their clinical investigators have refused to do follow-up studies of subjects of drug trials when subsequent research has shown such drugs to pose a previously unsuspected threat to health (U.S. General Accounting Office, pp. 37–49).

Reporting and labeling. Another series of ethical issues arises at the reporting stage of the clinical trial. It has been stated that one pharmaceutical company suppressed the report of one of its investigators showing its antidiabetic drug, Diabinese, to cause "side effects" (central nervous system damage, jaundice) in twenty-seven percent of the test subjects (Mintz, 1967, pp. 17–18). The U.S. General Accounting Office (GAO) reported in 1973 that internal controls in drug trials were often inadequate, with physicians involved in the human phase not being alerted in time to unfavorable results of animal studies (U.S. GAO, 1973, pp. 33–36). The U.S. Food and Drug Administration (FDA) has charged a number of drug companies and their officers with concealment and even falsification of experimental data (Silverman and Lee, pp. 64–67).

The same issues arise in connection with the label and package insert for a new medicine. Former FDA Commissioner James Goddard wrote, "This is extremely important to the pharmaceutical companies because this is where the money is. They have to convince the physician that this is the best possible product in its field. FDA, on the other hand, must make sure that the advertising claims remain within the bounds of scientific evidence" (Goddard). One company's package insert for Diabinese began: "Side effects are generally of a transient and non-serious character" (Mintz, 1967, p. 18). In 1971 the U.S. Department of Justice charged a drug company and two of its officers with mislabeling a product used to diagnose for hepatitis—failing to report that it was only thirty-five percent effective ("Abbott Firm Charged"). Still another drug firm, with $70 million in annual sales of its estrogen compound Premarin, used to treat menopause, failed to note on its package insert that the substance had been implicated as a cause of uterine cancer; a company vice-president, moreover, distributed to physicians a letter deriding the possibility of such a relationship ("FDA Criticizes Firm's Letter"; Mintz, " 'Misleading' Drug Promotion Letter?"; Mintz, "Reversing a Stand.")

Advertising and marketing of drugs

Drug industry pressure on physicians and the ethical conflicts associated with this become most acute in the advertising and marketing phase. With 7,000 single entities and 3,000 compounds available on prescription, not to mention an estimated 100,000 additional "over-the-counter" (nonprescription) preparations, a heavy investment in promotion is needed to bring any one of them to the physician's attention. The prescription drug industry spends more than $1 billion a year for promotion—about $5,000 for each of the 200,000 prescribing physicians in the United States (a sum larger than the 1970–1971 teaching budgets of all U.S. medical schools).

Companies manufacturing "over-the-counter" drugs spend another $1 billion or more in advertising. In 1972 $24 million was spent merely to promote Bayer Aspirin, and $11 million to promote Bufferin (Silverman and Lee, pp. 214–215). Since the consumer is rarely able to judge the truth of these claims, he can be easily misled.

About 25,000 "detail men" visit physicians to dispense information on their company's latest product. Two billion free samples are distributed annually to physicians, pharmacists, and medical students. Free color television sets, freezers, and other objects of value are presented to physicians as inducements to prescribe "correctly." All-expense-paid seminars are organized in Bermuda and other exotic locations to inform physicians of the latest drug-industry wonders (ibid., pp. 55–57).

All evidence indicates that these stimuli affect prescribing patterns. It is humanly impossible for the physician to keep abreast of this torrent of products. A professor of pharmacology testified at the Nelson hearings that he could barely keep up with the new offerings in his subspecialty, let alone the whole field (U.S. Congress, Senate, Select Committee on Small Business, pt. 2, p. 461).

The problem of obtaining reliable information on drugs is compounded by the existence of about 5,000 medical journals in the world, publishing upwards of 100,000 articles a year (May). This huge volume of information serves the interests primarily of advertisers and publishers. Companies use them as advertising vehicles, overwhelming the physician not only with the advertisements themselves but also with article after article on the product that is being heavily promoted at the time. Or they confuse legitimate scientific inquiry by placing articles designed to reflect industry views.

In 1970 four of the five trade journals with the largest advertising volume were medical—with *Medical Economics* ($11 million gross) in the lead (Silverman and Lee, p. 56). An authoritative observer estimated that a medical journal such as this earns for its owners a profit of forty percent of the income from advertisements and subscriptions, since no payment is made for contributions (U.S. Congress, Senate, Select Committee on Small Business, pt. 10, p. 3948).

Since profitability depends directly on the volume of advertisements, the commercial pressure on editorial boards is immense. A former editor of the *Journal of the American Medical Association* testified in 1969 that the "lack of ethical standards" within the AMA was a major cause of the misleading and tendentious advertising of drugs (ibid., pt. 14, p. 5723). In 1972 the AMA abolished its Council on Drugs, which had apparently exerted a modest restraining influence (Silverman and Lee, p. 292). A critic reported: "The AMA could no longer keep both an effective Council on Drugs and the support of drug advertisers. One of them had to go" (ibid.).

Overprescribing of drugs

Promotional pressure leads to overprescribing by physicians. A. Dale Console, former medical director of E. R. Squibb and Sons, estimated that only half the U.S. consumer's drug bill is medically justified (U.S. Congress, Senate, Select Committee on Small Business, pt. 11, p. 4491). Louis Lasagna wrote that physicians prescribe antibiotics for sixty percent of their patients with colds, even though these medicines are ineffective against the common cold (Silverman and Lee, p. 290). Harry Dowling, a specialist in infectious diseases and former chairman of the AMA Council on Drugs, has stated that the average patient needs an antibiotic once every five or ten years, while enough is manufactured every year to treat two illnesses of average duration for every man, woman, and child in the United States (Kunin, Tupasi, and Craig, p. 556). Between 1960 and 1970 the production of antibiotics increased by 320 percent. The average hospital patient receives from six to ten different medicines during his stay (Gardner and Cluff, p. 83).

Overprescribing has caused an epidemic of "adverse reactions" and doctor-induced (iatrogenic) disease. From ten to eighteen percent of hospital patients manifest an "adverse reaction," with a five percent case fatality (ibid., pp. 77–78). The cost of treating such iatrogenic illness is estimated at $4.5 billion a year in the United States; and while there is still a need for adequate data, the death rate from such disease is estimated at between 30,000 and 130,000 per year (the death rate of U.S. servicemen during the Second World War was 80,000 per year) (Silverman and Lee, p. 265; U.S. Congress, Senate, Committee on Labor and Public Welfare, pt. 5, pp. 1545–1546).

Significant morbidity and mortality have been associated with the use of tolbutamide in diabetes, chloramphenicol in infectious diseases, isoproternol as an inhalant in asthma (in the United Kingdom), isoniazid in tuberculosis, and potassium-thiazide diuretics (still commonly prescribed in pregnancy) (Davidson, p. 853; Silverman and Lee, pp. 59–61, 249–250). Chloroquine sulphate taken for rheumatoid arthritis has caused blindness, neomycin used for diaper rash and dihydrostreptomycin have been associated with deafness (a recent survey of Americans found a higher than expected incidence of deafness in those born since the onset of the antibiotic age) (Kagan, p. 306). The immunosuppressive drugs used to overcome "rejection" during organ transplants can cause cancer; a number of drugs, including thalidomide, oral contraceptives, and tranquilizers have been linked with stillbirths and fetal deformation (Janerich, Piper and Glebatis; Yalom, Green and Fisk; Silverman and Lee, p. 65). New drug-resistant bacterial strains, especially the "gram-negative" variety, have emerged and are estimated to cause an additional unnecessary 100,000 deaths a year, particularly in hospitals (Kagan, p. 306; Kunin, Tupasi, and Craig, p. 556).

One particularly tragic example concerns the development of cervical cancer in the daughters of women who had received diethylstilbestrol during their pregnancies twenty years earlier (Herbst, Ulfelder, and Poskanzer).

This leads to the question of the long-term impact of overprescribing and incorrect prescribing. Pierce Gardner and Leighton Cluff have noted that little attention is being paid to the "delayed untoward effects of drugs," in particular their role in the later development of cancer and degenerative diseases (Gardner and Cluff, p. 85). Since "adverse reactions" to drugs often take the form of heart and circulatory difficulties, arthritis, or cancer, it seems reasonable to associate the ever increasing incidence of these three chronic diseases with the observed overprescribing of today's medicine. The conversion of iatrogenic disease into chronic disease deserves greater attention than it has received.

The increasing drug dependency of American culture and, especially, the involvement in illicit forms of drug use are in part generated and maintained by the enthusiastic prescribing of the medical profession.

The physician himself is likely to be affected adversely, since these powerful substances with a general and diffuse impact on the organism lead him to neglect diagnosis (Lasagna). A. Dale Console testified, "Advertising and promotion efforts encourage the doctor to believe there is an easy way to practice medicine. They offer larger and larger shotguns which make pinpoint diagnosis, or for that matter any diagnosis at all, a pedantic exercise and a troublesome inconvenience that only the less well-informed academic bothers with" (U.S. Congress, Senate, Select Committee on Small Business, pt. 11, p. 4486). The "fixed-combination" antibiotics, which held forty percent of the drug market until banned by the FDA in 1968, were prime culprits in leading physicians to bypass diagnosis, but all the "broad spectrum" drugs available for use today have the same effect (ibid., pp. 4482–4483; Silverman and Lee, pp. 109–110).

U.S. Food and Drug Administration

Prior to the adoption of the Kefauver–Harris Drug Amendments of 1962 the U.S. Food and Drug Administration bore responsibility only for drug safety. The manufacturer reported the results of his tests, and the FDA reached a decision.

As a result of the thalidomide disaster (introduction into general use of a sedative and hypnotic drug that was found to cause malformation of infants born to mothers using it during pregnancy) and the Kefauver hearings, the Food, Drug, and Cosmetic Act was strengthened by three new provisions in 1962: (1) The FDA must be kept informed of the progress of tests of investigational drugs (i.e., drugs not yet approved by the FDA); clinical investigations must be preceded by sufficient preclinical studies to ensure reasonable safety; clinical investigations must be planned and executed by qualified investigators, and their names must be provided to the FDA. (2) On the basis of material submitted by the manufacturer the FDA decides whether or not the drug is effective in the way represented. (3) The FDA bears responsibility for ensuring that prescription drug advertising contains adequate information on effectiveness, side effects, and counterindications for the use of the drug advertised.

While observers credit this agency with improved regulatory performance since 1962, the ethical problems outlined above—relating to the pharmacological competence and human weakness of the prescribing physician, on one hand, and the commercial power of the drug industry on the other—are probably not amenable to substantial improvement as a result of any action that could be taken by the FDA.

Conclusion

The relationship between the medical profession and the drug industry is "unhealthy, and in many ways corrupt," as A. Dale Console expressed it, but at the same time economically beneficial to both parties (U.S. Congress, Senate, Select Committee on Small Business, pt. 11, pp. 4480–4481). The physician acts de facto as promoter and distributor of the products of industry, while these substances, in turn, enable him to process a large number of patients during the working day (the average length of an office visit in American practice is ten to twelve minutes).

To the extent that he acquiesces in this relationship the physician abandons his traditional role of master of his instruments of cure—and even, to some extent, that of diagnostician. Since his professional status is derived from the presumed possession of this knowledge, this status has been impaired by the medical profession's over-close relationship with the drug industry (Talalay, pp. 245–246).

The consequence for the American public is apparently about 200,000 avoidable deaths every year (the total number of deaths in the United States was 1.9 million in 1972), together with the observed increase in chronic disease. Some might ask if these factors do not actually outweigh the profession's contribution to the public health (Illich).

Two questions still await a satisfactory answer. Is a continuing stream of new pharmaceutical products beneficial to the public health, given the medical profession's demonstrated inability to understand and use them properly? Does the existing system of informing physicians about drugs promote adoption of the most scientific modes of treatment, or are the interests of a scientific medicine overwhelmed by those of the drug industry?

Undoubtedly public health would improve and many ethical problems would disappear if the volume of drugs available for use were vastly reduced, following the prescription given more than a century ago by Dr. Oliver Wendell Holmes. But the likelihood of this is minimal, as is that of a more effective governmental or social control over the manufacture and use of medicinal drugs. On the other hand, it is difficult to see why the public must remain passive while the medical profession and the drug industry work out their relationship at society's expense.

HARRIS L. COULTER

[*For further discussion of topics mentioned in this article, see the entries:* HUMAN EXPERIMENTATION; *and* PHARMACY. *Also directly related are the entries* PRISONERS, *article on* PRISONER EXPERIMENTATION; RESEARCH POLICY, BIOMEDICAL; *and* THERAPEUTIC RELATIONSHIP. *See also:* ADVERTISING BY MEDICAL PROFESSIONALS; *and* RISK. *See* APPENDIX, SECTION I, MEDICAL ETHICS: STATEMENTS OF POLICY DEFINITIONS AND RULES (BRITISH MEDICAL ASSOCIATION); *and* SECTION IV, AMERICAN PHARMACEUTICAL ASSOCIATION.]

BIBLIOGRAPHY

"Abbott Firm Charged in Drug Labeling Case." *Washington Post*, 8 May 1971, p. A3.

"Action of Gases on Bacteria." *Ohio State Medical Journal* 1 (1905): 82.

BEECHER, HENRY K. "Ethics and Clinical Research." *New England Journal of Medicine* 274 (1966): 1354–1360. The first critique by a physician of unethical practices in drug trials.

COULTER, HARRIS LIVERMORE. *Divided Legacy: A History of the Schism in Medical Thought.* Vol. 3: *Science and Ethics in American Medicine: 1800–1914.* Washington: Wehawken Book Co., 1973. A history of medical ethics and of the nineteenth-century relations between the medical profession and the drug industry.

Council on Economic Priorities. *In Whose Hands? Safety, Efficacy, and Research Productivity in the Pharmaceutical Industry. Economic Priorities Report* 4, no. 4–5 (1973). Critical examination of drug-industry claims by a consumer organization.

DAVIDSON, JOHN K. "The FDA and Hypoglycemic Drugs." *Journal of the American Medical Association* 232 (1976): 853–855. Criticizes the profession's use of tolbutamide in diabetes.

DOWLING, HENRY FILLMORE. *Medicines for Man: The Development, Regulation, and Use of Prescription Drugs.* New York: Knopf, 1970. A general discussion of the relations between the medical profession and the drug industry; less critical and insightful than the similar book by Silverman and Lee.

"FDA Criticizes Firm's Letter on Estrogen Drugs." *Washington Post*, 14 January 1976, p. A3.

GARDNER, PIERCE, and CLUFF, LEIGHTON E. "The Epidemiology of Adverse Drug Reactions: A Review and Perspective." *Johns Hopkins Medical Journal* 126 (1970): 77–87. One of the early warnings about the iatrogenic disease epidemic.

GODDARD, JAMES A. "The Drug Establishment." *Esquire*, March 1969, pp. 117–121, 152, 154. A former FDA Commissioner takes a skeptical look at the drug industry.

HARRIS, RICHARD. *The Real Voice.* New York: Macmillan Co., 1964. A scholarly account of the Kefauver hearings, but short, unannotated, and unindexed.

HERBST, ARTHUR L.; ULFELDER, HOWARD; and POSKANZER, DAVID C. "Adenocarcinoma of the Vagina: Association of Maternal Stilbestrol Therapy with Tumor Appearance in Young Women." *New England Journal of Medicine* 284 (1971): 878–881.

ILLICH, IVAN. *Medical Nemesis: The Expropriation of Health.* New York: Pantheon, 1976. A highly articulate and heavily documented polemic against the medical profession: "The medical establishment has become a major threat to health."

JANERICH, DWIGHT; PIPER, JOYCE M.; and GLEBATIS, DONNA M. "Oral Contraceptives and Congenital Limb-Reduction Defects." *New England Journal of Medicine* 291 (1974): 697–700.

KAGAN, BENJAMIN M.; FANNIN, SHIRLEY L.; and BARDIE, FELIX. "Spotlight on Antimicrobial Agents—1973." *Journal of the American Medical Association* 226 (1973): 306–310. A critique of the prescribing of antibiotics.

KUNIN, CALVIN M.; TUPASI, THELMA; and CRAIG, WILLIAM A. "Use of Antibiotics: A Brief Exposition of the Problem and Some Tentative Solutions." *Annals of Internal Medicine* 79 (1973): 555–560. Another critique of the prescribing of antibiotics.

LASAGNA, LOUIS. "The Pharmaceutical Revolution: Its Impact on Science and Society." *Science* 166 (1969): 1227–1233. Points out that medical care has suffered in consequence of the availability of too many new medicines.

LOWBURY, EDWARD JOSEPH LISTER, and AYLIFFE, G. A. J. *Drug Resistance in Antimicrobial Therapy.* Springfield, Ill.: Thomas, 1974. On the prescribing of antibiotics and the consequent emergence of new and resistant disease strains.

MAY, CHARLES D. "Selling Drugs by 'Educating' Physicians." *Journal of Medical Education* 36 (1961): 1–23. Also in United States, Congress, Senate, Select Committee, *Competitive Problems*, pt. 10, pp. 3938–3957. Calls attention to the misleading claims made by drug manufacturers.

MINTZ, MORTON. *By Prescription Only.* 2d ed. rev. Boston: Beacon Press, 1967. Issued originally in 1965 as *The Therapeutic Nightmare.* A classic study of the Kefauver hearings and the drug industry.

———. "'Misleading' Drug Promotion Letter?" *Washington Post*, 9 January 1976, p. B1.

———. "Reversing a Stand on the 'Pill'." *Washington Post*, 12 January 1976, p. B2.

Pharmaceutical Manufacturers Association. *Annual Survey Report, 1973–1974.* Washington: 1975. Gives sales and research statistics of PMA members.

SILVERMAN, MILTON, and LEE, PHILIP R. *Pills, Profits, and Politics.* Berkeley: University of California Press, 1974. A comprehensive account of the drug industry and medicine—scholarly, readable, and objective.

"Status of Problem of Usage of Tolbutamide—Preliminary Statements: FDA Statement, Friday, May 22, 1970." *Diabetes* 19 (1970): 467.

TALALAY, PAUL, ed. *Drugs in Our Society.* Baltimore: Johns Hopkins Press, 1964. One of the earlier examinations of the drug industry and medicine. Some of the contributions are very original, objective, and enlightening.

United States, Congress, Senate, Committee on Labor and Public Welfare, Subcommittee on Health. *Examination of the Pharmaceutical Industry, 1973–1974.* 93d Cong., 1st & 2d sess. Hearings on S. 3441 and S. 966. 6 pts. Washington: Government Printing Office, 1973–1974. The Kennedy hearings.

——, Congress, Senate, Committee on the Judiciary, Subcommittee on Antitrust and Monopoly. *Administered Prices in the Drug Industry.* 86th Cong., 2d sess. Pursuant to S. Res. 238. Washington: Government Printing Office, 1960–1961, pts. 14–26. *Drug Industry Antitrust Act.* 87th Cong., 1st & 2d sess. Pursuant to S. Res. 52 on S. 1552. 7 pts. Washington: Government Printing Office, 1961–1962. The Kefauver hearings, which first brought these issues to public attention and led to adoption of the Kefauver-Harris Amendments to the U.S. Food, Drug and Cosmetic Act.

——, Congress, Senate, Select Committee on Small Business, Subcommittee on Monopoly. *Competitive Problems in the Drug Industry.* 93d Cong., 2d sess. 28 pts. Washington: Government Printing Office, 1967–1975. The Nelson hearings.

——, Department of Health, Education, and Welfare, Task Force on Prescription Drugs. *Final Report: February 7, 1969.* Washington: Government Printing Office, 1969. A highly critical account of the prescribing practices of U.S. physicians and of drug-industry influence on the medical profession, compiled by a group of experts.

——, General Accounting Office; and United States, Department of Health, Education, and Welfare, Food and Drug Administration. *Supervision over Investigational Use of Selected Drugs.* Report to the Subcommittee on Reorganization, Research, and International Organizations, Committee on Government Operations, United States Senate. Washington: Comptroller General of the United States, 1973.

University Group Diabetes Program. "A Study of the Effects of Hypoglycemic Agents on Vascular Complications in Patients with Adult-onset Diabetes: I. Design, Methods, and Baseline Results." *Diabetes* 19 (1970): 747–783. "II. Mortality Results." *Diabetes* 19 (1970): 789–830. "IV. A Preliminary Report on Phenformin Results." *Journal of the American Medical Association* 217 (1971): 777–784. A ten-year, government-financed study conducted in 12 university medical schools and covering over 800 patients, most of whom were followed for eight years, this showed that tolbutamide—used in the treatment of about 1.5 million diabetics in the U.S. alone—is attended with a higher incidence of cardiovascular complications and mortality than when patients are treated with insulin or by dietary adjustment.

Yalom, Irvin D.; Green, Richard; and Fisk, Norman. "Prenatal Exposure to Female Hormones: Effects on Psychosexual Development in Boys." *Archives of General Psychiatry* 28 (1973): 554–561. Examination of the children of diabetic mothers who received estrogen and progesterone to prevent pregnancy complications suggests that prenatal sex hormone levels may influence some aspects of postnatal psychosexual adjustment in boys.

DRUG TRIALS

See Human Experimentation, *article on* basic issues; Drug Industry and Medicine.

DRUG USE

I. DRUG USE, ABUSE, AND DEPENDENCE
Robert Neville
II. DRUG USE FOR PLEASURE AND TRANSCENDENT
EXPERIENCE
Sidney Cohen

I
DRUG USE, ABUSE, AND DEPENDENCE

Drugs that affect thought, mood, or behavior have been used for a great many purposes. L. J. West lists ten: (1) to restore normal function, under conditions of disease, disorder, or discomfort, in either medical or nonmedical contexts; (2) to improve performance under various conditions; (3) to alter learning; (4) to reinforce behavior either positively or negatively; (5) for recreation; (6) to explore the inner self either of others or of oneself; (7) for the symbolic purposes of showing willingness to take risks, of demonstrating maturity, of defying prohibitions and controls, of belonging to peer groups, and of marking the transition from one culture to another; (8) to achieve mystical experience or partake of religious rites; (9) to manipulate others; and (10) to foster social or political policies by weakening the enemy or manipulating those dependent on drugs (West).

A wide range of drugs is available for one or several of these purposes, including sedatives and hypnotics, stimulants, psychedelics and hallucinogens, opiate narcotics, volatile solvents, nonnarcotic analgesics, clinical antidepressants, and the major tranquilizers. In light of West's list of purposes for drug use, alcohol, nicotine, and caffeine should be added, along with drugs used as "truth serum," those used for crowd control or to disorient individuals, and those drugs being developed to enhance or suppress sensory experience, including aphrodisiacs (Evans and Kline).

This article will deal with fundamental value questions associated with individual drug taking for whatever purpose, under four headings: (1) moral attitudes; (2) abuse and dependence; (3) criminality; and (4) drug abuse rehabilitation programs.

Moral attitudes

The range of attitudes toward drug taking extends from positive encouragement for easy access and use of drugs, whenever they do something someone wants and the costs to the user and others are acceptable, to the feeling that drugs should be used, if at all, only in desperate situations, because they involve an unnatural manipulation of one's mind and body and because they serve as unnecessary crutches. Whether one views drugs as problematic depends on the position occupied in the spectrum between those two extreme attitudes.

Indeed, those at the permissive end may look to drugs not only as remedies for abnormal functioning but as producing states that are better than normal. Let us put aside the instrumental use of drugs in religious or "self-revelation" contexts, a use that Robert Veatch in 1974 called "neo-Protestant"; an interpretation of drug use reflecting this perspective was given by Weil in 1972. People indulge in some drugs, for instance alcohol and marijuana, because of the pleasant consciousness they bring and because they facilitate enjoyable social times. The permissive attitude sees drugs as avenues to enjoyable experiences and evaluates the costs of drug taking quite differently from the attitude that approves drugs, if at all, only in therapeutic contexts where the cost–benefit question would include the risks of using drugs to get well.

Permissive attitudes toward drugs are often tied to larger views of life. Life is difficult even without crises for most people, and drugs can be seen as helping them through life's difficulties. Many people take caffeine and nicotine for a lift and alcohol to blur sharp edges, and in recent years millions of people in America have come to count on mild tranquilizers. Yet, if there were no drugs, many conditions that the drugs are used to alleviate might be considered entirely normal—just the frustrations and pains of daily living.

Those with a restrictive attitude toward drugs, on the other hand, might say the problems should be faced directly for what they are, not with a drugged response. Those whom Klerman called "pharmacological Calvinists" emphasize the seriousness of life. Life is not something to be "gotten through" but rather a task in which to achieve. The truths of life are to be faced directly, even when they are unpleasant and when nothing can be done about them. The honesty, sincerity, and directness of one's own response is a great value, according to this perspective; indeed, it is an important goal to be able to respond to life with singleness of heart (Klerman). Psychoactive drugs interpose an externally conditioned level of response between the work and one's perceiving and willing heart so that true integrity is difficult if not impossible.

Drugs, according to the restrictive attitude, should be used, if at all, only instrumentally, where a necessary condition of defining their benefit is their enabling one to live with honesty and seriousness. Robert Veatch, Associate for Medical Ethics, Institute of Society, Ethics, and the Life Sciences at Hastings-on-Hudson, has argued that the "Protestant drug ethic" disapproves of drugs that give pleasure but approves those that increase achievement, e.g. caffeine.

But why, ask more permissive people, should life be taken so seriously? Does not life itself mock our efforts? Why not take harmless pleasures where we can?

The value sets of those along the permissive–restrictive spectrum probably reflect personality types and social orientations that are systematically reinforced by more pervasive elements than the results of drug attitudes alone. The philosophic merits of the positions do not segregate neatly. The restrictive position is probably correct in holding that an honest and serious approach to life is a great value. The permissive position is equally correct in pointing out that pleasures and crutches are also great values. The restrictive position that taking drugs just to get through life is likely to lead to a falsification of experience and perhaps even a lessened ability to cope is probably right, although surely some situations are handled better, both experientially and in terms of objective outcome, with the aid of drugs. Those on the permissive end of the spectrum may point out rightly that drugs can enrich experience, which is both pleasant and beneficial.

Some issues dividing the permissive and restrictive approaches really have nothing to do with drugs. Is there an obligation to experience things directly and from the heart? Always? Under what conditions? Is there a moral or social right of private choice regarding what to experience and what pleasures to seek? (Veatch has a fine discussion of the problem of a choice.) Why do some people with crutches learn how to walk and others to love crutches?

Conflicts between attitudes, of course, are not the only moral issues involved in drug use, social commentators remind us. There are objective social situations that may be said to "drive" some susceptible people to drugs. Deprived of the pleasures of love, friendship, and self-satisfaction, a person looks more favorably on the pleasures of drug experiences. Should this be taken as warranting drug pleasures for the unfortunate, or rather as a call to action in remedying the lack of love, friendship, and self-satisfaction? Economic hardship and frustration, boredom, anomie, and countless other aspects of industrial society encourage people to take a mechanical approach to control of their responses to life. But perhaps those objective situations need amendment as much as the victims need balm.

It should be noted that, in discussing the morality of resorting to drugs in some situations, seemingly minor drugs such as caffeine and nicotine have been grouped with major ones such as alcohol and tranquilizers. This should not be taken to imply that there are no differences of seriousness among drugs. But regarding attitudes, there seems to be a carryover from one drug to another; if drugs are perceived to be valid ways out of troubles and into happiness, then which drug is used is a matter of context, expectations, availability, and costs.

Abuse and dependence

The language of drug use and abuse reflects the values and interests of the speakers. For instance, the World Health Organization Expert Committee on Drug Dependence defines drug abuse as "persistent or sporadic excessive drug use inconsistent with or unrelated to acceptable medical practice." Of course, one must determine what constitutes "excessive" use. But does the definition mean to suggest that some excessive drug use might be consistent with, or part of, acceptable medical practice? Does it suggest that using drugs for purposes or in dosages inconsistent with or unrelated to acceptable medical practice is what constitutes excessive use? At the very least, that definition supposes that medical goals such as treatment of mental illness or alleviation of physical pain determine legitimacy in drug use, and that using psychoactive drugs at dosage levels causing significant effects for nonmedical purposes—such as pleasure, consciousness alteration, or narcosis—is in fact drug abuse, or close to it. Questions are frequently raised about the standing the medical profession has to define use and abuse.

Sometimes drug abuse is loosely identified with drug "addiction." The tendency of medical professionals now, however, is to drop reference to addiction and speak of drug "dependency" instead. The World Health Organization distinguishes psychic from physical dependence and defines them in the following ways: *Psychic* dependence is

A compulsion that requires periodic or continuous administration of a drug to produce pleasure or avoid discomfort. This compulsion is the most powerful factor in chronic intoxication with psychotropic drugs, and with certain types of drugs may be the only factor involved in the perpetuation of abuse even in the case of the most intense craving. Psychic dependence, therefore, is the most universal characteristic of drug dependence. Operationally, it is recognized by the fact that the dependent continues to take the drug in spite of conscious admission that it is causing harm to his health and to his social and familial adjustment, and that he takes great risks to obtain and maintain his supply of the drug [Isbell and Cruściel].

Physical dependence is defined as:

A pathological state brought about by repeated administration of a drug and that leads to the appearance of a characteristic and specific group of symptoms, termed an abstinence syndrome, when the administration of the drug is discontinued or—in the case of certain drugs—significantly reduced. In order to prevent the appearance of an abstinence syndrome the continuous taking of the drug is required. Physical dependence is a powerful factor in reinforcing psychic dependence upon continuing drug use or in relapse to drug use after withdrawal [ibid.].

It is not at all necessary that people who are drug dependent thereby are drug abusers. Where the need for the drug is easily satisfied and where the effects of being on the drug do not impair activity, dependence may not dominate life. Many people dependent on barbiturates or opiates (morphine or heroin when easily obtained) can lead otherwise apparently successful lives; alcoholics, on the other hand, usually find it difficult under the influence of excessive drink to function normally even though the drug is easily available. If drug abuse is "bad use," drug dependency itself may not involve bad use. dependency itself may not involve bad use.

Some aspects of drug abuse have less to do with the effects of the drugs themselves than with the social factors necessary for their use. Illegal drugs are obtained in criminal ways, communities may be disrupted, economic productivity of the users and those who must care for them may be adversely affected, and the life of drug pursuit sometimes crowds out other important aspects of living.

The borderline between drug use and drug abuse often varies with diverse cultures. Acceptable alcohol consumption is a case in point. Diverse attitudes are held toward illegal activity, the importance of being "responsible" at all times, and many other factors. Many people would say that use is abuse when the user or others are definitely harmed by the use, although there is wide variability in considering what harm is in contrast to "acceptable cost."

To determine whether a certain drug use is abuse, and if so how bad, is a very difficult undertaking. Because drugs affect subjective experience, and people are different, even the same drugs in the same contexts have different meanings and effects. And then contexts differ too, as well as the histories of the individuals and groups involved. Moral judgments about drug use and abuse then must involve a complex weighing of a variety of factors, some of which will be discussed next.

Self. Drugs affect the person taking them. They have direct perceptible qualities, and except in the case of mild stimulants the usual case is that people take drugs to feel good. But the direct experience of drugs is also the culmination of previous strands of experience; drugs have a meaning depending on how ready the user is for them. "Trips" are good or bad; expectations and habits are reinforced or disoriented, depending on the drug, setting, and physical state. Taking drugs also has future consequences for the person's self, affecting his body, his future habits and expectations, his commitments and preparedness for life. It can be fairly said that no responsible and thorough judgment about a person's drug use can justifiably be given without a systematic interpretation of what that use means in the individual's direct experience, as a culmination of what he brings to the experience, and as a cause of its future effects. A moral evaluation of all of this entails direct reference to philosophical values concerning personal life-style of enjoying, achieving, and being free.

Interpersonal relationships. Drugs affect not only the user but also those with whom he is associated; his personal relationships mediate the effects of the drugs on himself. Psychoactive drugs are significant in interpersonal relations in many ways. They color the user's interpretation of those relationships, encouraging perhaps "good feeling," perhaps feelings of paranoia. They may affect the functions of relationships in personal growth; for instance, a classic psychoanalytic interpretation of heroin addiction views it as a way of fixing on passive oral dependence on one's mother (Radó). Drugs also affect the way others perceive the user. And, most of all, the activity of drug procurement and taking affect a person's health and also his ability to friends of drug users must accommodate themselves to the life of drug use, whether this means tolerating tobacco smoke, covering up for an alcoholic, or coping with a criminal junkie. For people whose lives are dominated by drug taking, this activity can be the most important determinant of personal relations, cutting them off from some people and putting them in touch with others. Drug use may require a superficiality in personal relationships that prevents serious ongoing emotional encounter.

Social career. Over and above one's personal experiences and relationships, a person generally has a career. This involves him in educational, familial, and economic institutions; in the long run a person's career is the shape of his life, his trajectory from birth to death. Drugs affect a person's health and also his ability to participate effectively in the institutions important for his career. Drugs can speed or impede education and productivity. They can make for tenser or more relaxed family structures. The wide differences in social, economic, and cultural classes affect participation in the institutions important for social development, and the moral meaning of drugs varies accordingly; for instance, amphetamines approved as helping middle-class hyperkinetic children to learn in school are sometimes viewed by lower classes as threats of social control.

Economic effects. Over and above the direct economic impact of drug use on the user's life, drug use affects the overall economy. Users are more or less productive, depending on the drugs, the circumstances of use, and the measure of productivity. Furthermore, the use of many psychoactive drugs is illegal, and this has enormous impact on the overall economy of societies. Users frequently must steal in order to pay for their drugs, and law enforcement agencies must be sustained to deal with this. In impoverished neighborhoods the social organization of drug use may be such as to prevent effective social and political organization; as in most things, the poorest people suffer most from the unfortunate consequences of drug use. This is true for legal drugs, such as alcohol, as well as for illegal ones, such as heroin and cocaine. It should be noted that economic effects are values for a larger society than that of the user and his personal contacts; therefore, the larger society has an interest in his drug taking that may be quite alien to his own real interests, and an issue of social versus individual good may be involved. Who should decide when a user's use is abuse so detrimental that something should be done about it?

Cultural implications. Any activity of sufficient magnitude to make an economic difference in society also makes a cultural difference. At the very least drug taking and the attitudes of various groups toward it partly define the values of a culture. A high frequency of alcohol use, for instance, or use of opiates may signify that people feel impotent to improve a condition from which they suffer. The tolerance of generally disapproved drug use is a measure of the permissiveness of a society. The acceptability of drug use of various sorts indicates where a society draws some significant lines distinguishing public from private spheres. Some people see drug abuse as a call for the treatment of a larger social pathology. Others see it as a justification for the regulation of drug use even when the users do not feel victimized by their use; this paternalism has been a dominant American attitude toward narcotic drug use.

Criminality

Drugs of various sorts are indeed abused by some, and frequently by those least able to help themselves—those suffering most from social inequalities and from psychological unreadiness to face the pressure of their social situation. For these reasons, as well as on moralistic grounds, societies have attempted to control drug use through taxation and prohibition. Actually, not all social policies regarding drugs have aimed at reducing drug use; the Opium Wars of the nineteenth century offer a counterexample. But most legislation has been against drugs; witness, in the United States, the experiments with prohibition of alcohol in the early part of this century and the attempt to control narcotics through the Harrison Act. Alfred R. Lindesmith has detailed the history of governmental policies in the United States to stop or contain the use of various drugs (1965).

One line of objection to the legal regulation of drug use is from a very individualistic libertarian, such as Thomas Szasz. What a person does in private is his own business, and the society has a right to intervene only when the private practice clearly has social harm. Now most of the social harm of drug use, the libertarian argument goes, derives from the fact that certain drugs are illegal. Whatever reasons a person might have for initiating the use of illegal drugs, the continued use involves him in a drug culture, associating with those who make their living dealing in illegal substances, and frequently paying for the drugs through illegal activity. As mentioned above, when an illegal drug culture becomes dominant in a particular segment of society, that segment finds it very difficult to organize itself or make use of the legitimate social institutions. Many people besides libertarians would agree with the following view: "It is clear that the *social and legal policies*, if ostensibly developed to control or prevent the use of some mind-altering drugs, are the cause of the main social problems that we find with those drugs" (Fort, p. 223).

But what about those who abuse legal drugs, for instance, alcohol? The libertarian position answers this, first by pointing out that Prohibition caused more problems than it solved and second by arguing that alcoholism is a private matter. Of course, some people will be hurt by alcoholism; certainly drunks should be prohibited from driving or otherwise endangering people's lives. But if a person chooses to ruin himself with drugs, that is his right (but it should be understood that society has no obligation to take care of him afterward).

The libertarian position usually is argued from two premises, one theoretical, one empirical. The theoretical premise is that individuals should be allowed to do what they want unless their exercise of liberty seriously endangers others. The empirical premise is that governmental attempts to regulate private affairs generally make matters worse; such policies are difficult to enforce and frequently create an opposition with greater powers of evil than the private matter under regulation.

There are several liberal (not libertarian) arguments against these premises. First, it is very hard to draw the line between private effects of drug use and those that might be harmful to others. Even when a drinker drinks alone and only alone, his drinking deprives others of his company and perhaps of his efforts on which they may have a claim. Tobacco smoke affects those nearby who are not smoking. At the very least, drug use affects the economy, and may do so harmfully.

Second, for a person to confine the effects of his drug use to a private sphere, he must have considerable resources to provide that cushion. For instance, he must relieve his family of the responsibility for caring for him when he suffers drug-induced sickness. Whereas this might be possible for rich people, it often is not for poor people. In conditions of poverty there is little privacy, and everyone suffers the burdens of all. So the conservative theoretical argument is class-biased.

Third, part of the impetus behind drug control legislation derives from the same motive as the control of food quality and of drugs for medical use. Basically the argument is that the public by and large is not in a position to protect itself from being abused by drugs. Just as consumers generally cannot judge the purity of the foods offered for sale and are at the mercy of physicians regarding the medicines offered to them, so people need protection against psychoactive drugs. People, particularly if they are young, do not know what they are getting into when they begin to smoke, drink, or use illegal drugs. And by the time they find out, the dependence on the drug and the involvement in the drug life-style may be so powerful that only heroes can get out.

Fourth, control of drugs is not as unsuccessful as critics complain. On the one hand, people are affected by what society legitimates and what it prohibits. Even if the laws are unenforceable, there are some who will not partake solely because of legal prohibitions, and there are some who will lose their resistance to harmful peer pressure if the legal sanctions are removed. On the other hand, *direct* prohibition may not be as effective as other forms of control. Legalizing drugs but making them available through specially controlled channels, as Great Britain currently does for narcotics, may be an effective way of reducing drug use.

Yet another perspective, neither conservative nor liberal, sees the whole focus on governmental regulation of drugs to be a mistake. The problem is not the chemicals people use and abuse, but the people who use them and the society in which they must live.

To consider the social critique first, it will be recalled that Marx called religion the "opiate of the masses." The interesting point is the supposition about opiates. Why do people need opiates? Because their lives are dehumanized and alienated from the activities providing real value and pleasure. The real problem is not the chemicals, which might well be used harmlessly if there were no pressures for abuse; the problem is the society. Consequently, the effort to prohibit

or control psychoactive drugs both detracts attention from the real problem and serves to support the social status quo. If the means by which people suffer can be curtailed through repressive controls, then the roots of the suffering can be left as they are, to the benefit of those in power who profit by the social arrangements. According to this radical view, even the best-intentioned of liberals merely reinforce the interests of those in power to keep basic conditions as they are while dealing with only the more blatant symptoms of human suffering.

From this perspective both the conservative and liberal views are mistaken also on the nature of personal responsibility. The conservatives are mistaken in believing that moral norms apply only to relations among people; the liberals are wrong in saying merely that the public has an interest in those interpersonal relations. Rather, persons and societies are bound by obligations regarding the quality of life, whether or not they happen to accept the obligations and regardless of their utility or disutility. For instance, a person makes promises that bind his future self, and ought therefore to make himself able to fulfill those promises. Drug use should be thought of in the light of obligations to personal and social value. The fundamental problem for this radical position is: Who decides what the obligations are? A secondary problem is determining when people should be forced to fulfill their obligations.

In all of these arguments it is apparent that the social response to drug use and abuse raises basic issues of freedom, social control, and social and personal values. These are well focused in the problem of drug rehabilitation programs.

Rehabilitation

If a person perceives his drug use as abuse and seeks professional help, the ethical problems surrounding rehabilitation are those of behavior control therapies employed as extensions of self-control. But in most cases drug abuse is also perceived by society as a problem *for* society. Societies, then, intervene in their own interest, providing rehabilitation opportunities or rehabilitation programs, sometimes as legal alternatives to incarceration for criminal offenders. Most rehabilitation programs, besides aiming to be therapeutic for the abuser, are exercises in social control for the intended benefit of the society. Rehabilitation programs in the United States are aimed mainly at narcotic and alcohol abusers, who may use other drugs incidentally. Users of other illegal drugs such as marijuana and LSD are treated simply as criminal offenders if they do not also use narcotics. The following brief discussion considers treatment programs moving from "least change" in the abuser to "most change."

Heroin maintenance. Heroin maintenance policies allow heroin addicts to receive their drugs in prescribed dosages from licensed agents of the state, usually family physicians. In an account of British and American experiences with heroin maintenance, we find that American clinics flourished from 1912 to 1924; since 1924 British physicians have legally maintained addicted patients on opiates, although since 1966 the dispensing of heroin has been permitted only through special clinics; family physicians continued to supply other opiates and synthetic narcotics (Brecher, chap. 13). Heroin maintenance has the advantage of assuring chemically controlled preparations, greatly reducing the dangers of toxicity and overdosage. It also reduces or eliminates the criminal aspects of the addict's life having to do with procuring and paying for his drugs and removes the black market underground from the heroin business. Addicted individuals are then enabled to lead more stable and productive lives, other things being equal.

But on this policy individuals are not rehabilitated regarding their addiction itself, and probably not regarding the causes of their addiction. And so, critics point out, even though a legally approved and orderly life is possible, the very causes that led to addiction in the first place remain and are likely to continue to upset the addicts' lives. Furthermore, even though heroin may be a benign drug in controlled dosages, it still dulls the user's perception of life, according to the critics. Heroin maintenance is principally a policy of social control to solve a social problem. Although the user's drugs become safe and legal, making his life better in important ways, heroin maintenance is not therapeutic for the individual in the sense of improving his life in those areas that led to drug abuse.

Methadone maintenance. Methadone is a drug chemically similar to heroin, although different from heroin in that it does not, when taken orally in the usual prescribed dosages, produce the feelings of euphoria typical of initial heroin experiences. Addicts are maintained on methadone with the same motives as in heroin maintenance: providing a safe and legal drug, and

allowing addicted persons to live a more stable and productive life. Similar objections regarding nonrehabilitation apply. Methadone is preferred to heroin mainly because it is not illegal.

In the United States, however, methadone maintenance programs typically are administered as programs for drug addicts, frequently related to courts, not as medicinal treatments provided by family physicians. This means that the "social organization" of the methadone programs is quite different from the heroin maintenance policy in Great Britain. Persons in the program are gathered and typed for their drug problems (whereas patients of a given physician have a common need of medical treatment, but not the same disease or need). Many methadone program centers have indeed become headquarters for the sale of illegal drugs, since they are common meeting grounds for interested personnel. Furthermore, methadone maintenance programs are blatant forms of social control, creating a physically dependent population subject to the policies of the social agencies.

Mixed treatments. Other rehabilitation programs aim to make users drug-free and to improve their psychological and economic capabilities. These involve either immediate detoxification or the use of methadone in progressively smaller doses until the user is no longer physically dependent. Alcohol and barbiturate detoxification are also handled in medically supervised ways. After detoxification various regimens of personal and group therapy are undertaken, and efforts may be made to secure the addicts some employment and to stabilize their home lives. How the approaches are mixed depends on the specific services and talents in each program, and also on what seems best for each drug user. Mixed treatment programs are highly variable in their effectiveness (*American Journal of Drug and Alcohol Abuse;* Mandell and Goldschmidt).

The degree to which mixed treatment programs are "rehabilitatively ambitious" depends upon both the program ideology and the kind of population served. Some programs count themselves successful if their clients, for a specified period of time, remain drug-free, commit no crimes, hold steady jobs, and maintain intact homes or living situations. "Drug-free" varies in meaning from merely not using the illegal or addictive drugs from which the person was detoxified all the way to avoiding all psychoactive drugs, including nicotine and alcohol. Programs that have comprehensive lists of drugs from which one should be free tend also to have high standards of psychological rehabilitation. Their treatments aim to penetrate to the reasons why people use drugs in the first place, and often focus on the concept of the "addictive personality." The degree to which a person's drug problem is a matter of personality or social condition probably depends on many independent factors.

Therapeutic communities. Therapeutic communities, deriving from the initial experiments with Alcoholics Anonymous and Synanon, are founded on the belief that rehabilitation requires the total immersion of the drug abuser in a treatment program (Yablonsky). Frequently staffed by former addicts or graduates of the program, therapeutic communities aim to break down psychological defenses and personality structures of their members on the grounds that those personalities are in need of thorough revision; the means for this are often group criticism sessions that appear brutal and sadistic to observers. Positive aspects of people's personalities are supposed to be reinforced, and the addicts' lives are reorganized in positive personal and social ways. Frequently therapeutic communities run businesses employing their own members, or place their members in local businesses. Some communities believe that members must remain in the community for life, having substituted dependence on the community for dependence on drugs. Other communities attempt to graduate their members to independent lives. Critics of therapeutic communities point out that they reinforce dependence so that a person becomes dependent or "psychologically addicted" to the community in nearly all aspects of his life, particularly regarding his feelings of self-worth. A person dependent on drugs alone at least has the possibility of compartmentalizing his dependence and perhaps treating that alone. Defenders of the communities answer that dependence on a community is still better than the life of crime and addiction, and that most drug-dependent people do not have strong enough personalities to live independently while compartmentalizing drug dependence.

Rehabilitation programs: conclusion. In the United States the development of drug rehabilitation programs has been affected by feelings in some quarters that drug abusers should be punished as well as rehabilitated, and also by ideological quarrels about goals and about who should be served. It is very difficult to determine scientifically the success rates of various treatment modalities, partly because most programs have not been set up so that accurate record keeping has a high priority and partly because reports by addicts about their drug use, criminal records, and social status cannot be trusted.

One of the greatest moral problems is that rehabilitation programs often promise what they are unlikely to fulfill, with two results. First, drug rehabilitation programs gain social and legal power over people that is often not justified by the programs' intent, i.e., mere rehabilitation; this also displaces responsibility from the user to the programs. Second, drug abusers frequently are not helped, and both they and society still have drug problems that need resolution. For these reasons, some critics of restrictive policies believe the illegal drugs should be decriminalized, that heroin and methadone maintenance programs should be instituted through regular channels of medical care, not special drug agencies, and that minimal goals of rehabilitation should be adopted. Then drug abusers can seek more ambitious kinds of rehabilitation on their own, encouraging better means of therapy and minimizing dependence on rehabilitation programs of controversial effectiveness.

ROBERT NEVILLE

[*Directly related are the entries* BEHAVIOR CONTROL; *and* PSYCHOPHARMACOLOGY. *For further discussion of topics mentioned in this article, see the entries:* ALCOHOL, USE OF; *and* PATERNALISM.]

BIBLIOGRAPHY

American Journal of Drug and Alcohol Abuse 2 (1975): 1–138. An issue devoted to the Drug Abuse Reporting Program (DARP).

BAZELON, DAVID L. "Drugs That Turn on the Law." *Journal of Social Issues* 27, no. 3 (1971), pp. 47–52.

BRECHER, EDWARD M., ed. *Licit and Illicit Drugs: The Consumers Union Report on Narcotics, Stimulants, Depressants, Inhalants, Hallucinogens, and Marijuana—Including Caffeine, Nicotine, and Alcohol.* Boston: Little, Brown & Co., 1972.

Drug Abuse Survey Project. *Dealing with Drug Abuse: A Report to the Ford Foundation.* Patricia Wald and Peter Hutt, co-chairpersons. Foreword by McGeorge Bundy. New York: Praeger Publishers, 1972.

EVANS, WAYNE O., and KLINE, NATHAN S., eds. *Psychotropic Drugs in the Year 2000: Use by Normal Humans.* Springfield, Ill.: Charles C. Thomas, 1971. Based on the meeting of the Study Group for the Effects of Psychotropic Drugs on Normal Humans held at the annual meeting of the American College of Neuropsychopharmacology, Puerto Rico, 1967.

FORT, JOEL. *The Pleasure Seekers: The Drug Crisis, Youth and Society.* New York: Bobbs-Merrill Co., 1969.

GOSHEN, CHARLES E. *Drinks, Drugs, and Do-Gooders.* New York: Free Press; London: Collier-Macmillan Publishers, 1973.

ISBELL, H., and CRUŚCIEL, T. L. "Dependence Liability of 'Non-Narcotic Drugs." *Bulletin of the World Health Organization* 43, supp. (1970), pp. 1–111.

KLERMAN, GERALD L. "Psychotropic Hedonism *vs.* Pharmacological Calvinism." *Hastings Center Report* 2, no. 4 (1972), pp. 1–3.

LENNARD, HENRY L. *Mystification and Drug Abuse. Hazards in Using Psychoactive Drugs.* Jossey-Bass Behavioral Science Series. San Francisco: Jossey-Bass, 1971.

LINDESMITH, ALFRED RAY. *The Addict and the Law.* Bloomington: Indiana University Press, 1965.

MANDELL, WALLACE, and GOLDSCHMIDT, PETER. *Interdrug: An Evaluation of Treatment Programs for Drug Abusers.* Baltimore: Johns Hopkins University School of Hygiene and Public Health, 1973.

PEELE, STANTON, with BRODSKY, ARCHIE. *Love and Addiction.* New York: Taplinger Publishing Co., 1975.

RADÓ, SÁNDOR. "The Psychoanalysis of Pharmacothymia." *Psychoanalytic Quarterly* 2 (1933): 1–23.

ROSENTHAL, MICHAEL P. "Legal Controls on Mind-and Mood-Altering Drugs." *Journal of Social Issues* 27, no. 3 (1971), pp. 53–72.

SZASZ, THOMAS S. "The Ethics of Addiction." *American Journal of Psychiatry* 128 (1971): 541–546.

VEATCH, ROBERT M. "Drugs & Competing Drug Ethics." *Hastings Center Studies* 2, no. 1 (1974), pp. 68–80.

WEIL, ANDREW. *The Natural Mind: A New Way of Looking at Drugs and the Higher Consciousness.* Boston: Houghton Mifflin, 1972.

WEST, LOUIS JOLYON. "Hallucinogenic Drugs: Perils & Possibilities." *Hastings Center Studies* 2, no. 1 (1974), pp. 103–112.

WITTERS, WELDON L., and JONES-WITTERS, PATRICIA. *Drugs and Sex.* New York: Macmillan Co., 1975.

World Health Organization, Expert Committee on Drug Dependence. *Sixteenth Report.* World Health Organization Technical Report Series, no. 407. Geneva: 1969.

YABLONSKY, LEWIS. *Synanon: The Tunnel Back.* Baltimore: Penguin, 1967. Originally published as *The Tunnel Back: Synanon.*

II
DRUG USE FOR PLEASURE AND TRANSCENDENT EXPERIENCE

Introduction

When youthful recreational drug users are asked why they consume their chosen chemical, the most frequent response is some variation of "to feel better." Their response has two implied meanings. One is the relief of some noxious physical or mental condition—relief from dysphoria. The other is the achievement of a euphoric feeling-tone—a "high." A surprising number of chronic drug abusers are actually treating themselves for some distressing psychological ailment. The disorder may be excessive shyness, boredom, depression, or frustration. Just as common, though, is the eternal search for euphoria, the willingness to explore a variety of chemical configurations for some transient feeling of gladness, joy, elation, or simply a relaxation of the tensions of the day. This article deals with the use of drugs for purposes of pleasure, self-transcendence, and religion, as conceived in a continuum, highlighting the principal ethical and social issues involved.

The value issues

The quest for chemically induced euphoria raises a number of ethical issues, including whether the achievement of gratuitous satisfaction is in itself morally objectionable, and whether the price paid for enjoyment enters into the transaction, affecting the quality of that enjoyment. Further, supposing that an inexpensive, nontoxic euphoriant could be produced, socioethical issues arise regarding its permissible use, its control and dispensation, and the general effect on society of the availability of "instant happiness" in pill form.

With the relaxation of the Western view that pleasure exacts a price and that gratification should be delayed, chemically induced pleasure per se is losing its pejorative connotations and becoming a positive value. Balanced against this burgeoning value are a number of disvalues, both to others and to oneself. In relation to others, indulgence in chemical pleasures can render the user a public charge, and the current system of illegalities involved can force the user into transgressions against others in order to support his own dependence on illegal chemicals. Personally, in addition to the loss of their freedom of choice in their exercise of "freedom of action," users incur neurophysiological penalties: repetitive stimulation of the nonspecific reward centers by chemical or electrical means results in a diminution of the pleasurable feeling-tone, so that more and more stimuli are needed to augment a waning emotional response. Ordinary pleasurable activities hardly register after vigorous electrochemical stimulation, and the biphasic quality of the central nervous system manifests itself—e.g., for every amphetamine "high" there is a subsequent postamphetamine depression. Learning may also be impaired, for learning involves the aversive and reward centers of the brain; where the reward is "for nothing," then nothing is learned. Pleasure is thus no longer a source of value in learning, for the learning and the pleasure have become dissociated.

The acceptable euphoriants

The detailed stories of alcohol, tobacco, and the caffeinated beverages need no retelling here

They are culturally accepted and widely used. The choice of ethanol and tobacco as pleasure-giving agents has been, in retrospect, not entirely wise. Their hazards have become international concerns, but like all items that have become ingrained into the cultural matrix they can hardly be eliminated. When culturally approved euphoriants are used, society adopts fairly lenient attitudes toward them. Unfortunately, the acceptable pleasure-giving drugs are neither invariably mood-elevating nor nontoxic.

Alcohol, although consumed for good cheer and fellowship, provokes aggression more than all psychochemicals. When consumed heavily, its psycho- and physiopathology involve every organ system. Many heavy drinkers drink to allay anxiety and tension; strangely enough, they are measurably more anxious while under the influence. Besides the relaxation that does occur at low doses, the well-known disinhibiting effects are sought after. They make the user more vivacious and gregarious and facilitate social interaction. However, a lingering reservation remains: Could those social graces have been better achieved by learning them?

The dilemma of alcohol is that, while lesser doses provide surcease and group well-being, chronic, higher intake levels can result in physical dependence and a multitude of personal, economic, and social disasters. About ten percent of all who drink for pleasure and good fellowship end up with addiction or an assortment of disabilities.

Tobacco is a puzzling substance. It is hardly a euphoriant, and it is clearly productive of varied disabilities. When cigarette users are asked why they persist in their smoking ritual, they are hard pressed to describe clearly the rewards of smoking. Some will mention mild feelings of relaxation, others slight stimulation, but most notice no mood alteration at all. Smoking seems like a minimally rewarding activity. The joys of inhaling the pyrolytic products of tobacco can hardly be a justification for its entrenched use. Instead, we should wonder whether it is the reinforcement of interminably repeated oral–manual behaviors that produces the reward, just as a fair part of the reward of a two percent bag of heroin is in the "fixing." Furthermore, nicotine has been shown to produce a withdrawal syndrome in laboratory animals when its administration is suddenly discontinued. This has also been amply confirmed in humans whose accounts of "kicking" cigarettes are commonplace.

The stimulants

Turning to those drugs used for pleasure under other than legal conditions, a number of oddities are encountered. "Highs" occur not only with stimulants but also with depressants. Attempts to stay "high" continuously are never successful. Although the initial period of use may be delightful, continued substantial usage can result in a transformation into greater dysphoria than ever. The individual may become locked into the habitual requirement that increasing amounts of the drug be procured and injected or swallowed. Most heroin addicts will say that they no longer use the drug to get "high"; rather, it is needed to avoid the withdrawal sickness. What was once a euphoriant experience has become a losing struggle to feel normal.

The stimulants are chosen for hyperphoric purposes because of their mood-elevating, energizing properties. Cocaine must be considered the supreme euphoriant. The "rush" comes within moments of "snorting" or injecting intravenously, and it is very intense. The effects dissipate quickly, and the process can be repeated dozens of times a day. The various amphetamines behave like a long-acting cocaine. They, and the amphetamine-related anorectics, provide a lift to the tired and a bit of brightness for the sad. A decade ago a wave of intravenous amphetamine users, the "speed freaks," demonstrated once again that indescribable pleasure infinitely prolonged was an impossible goal.

The hallucinogens are listed with the stimulants because they produce a state of sympathetic dominance with dilated pupils, hyperthermia, tachycardia, and a hyperaroused tracing on the electroencephalogram. The use of so potent a drug as LSD for pleasure needs to be explained (Cohen, pp. 45–63). In average doses (50–150 mcg) it induces an intensification of sensory awareness—particularly, but not exclusively, visual. Colors are more saturated. The perceived object has greater depth and luminosity and seems enormously meaningful. Immobile objects move. Time is slowed down. Synesthesias are noted: The scent of music can be detected and colors are tasted. Thought, emotion, and sensation seem to fuse into some primordial mental process. The critical function of the ego is obliterated along with the ego's boundaries. The LSD "trip," then, is an intense, novel esthetic experience made more so by one's inability to be critical of its effects.

Western societies are not the only ones that employ stimulants for conviviality. Caffeine-containing plants have a worldwide market, and there are others. Khat (*Catha edulis*) is a mildly euphoriant plant containing pseudo-norephedrine. It is chewed in a social setting and is a well-established stimulant in the Arabian peninsula, enjoyed by all classes and sold in the market place of every town. Originally it was imported from Ethiopia, where the authorities are quite permissive about khat use despite the interdiction against alcohol and drug use by the prevailing religion. The chewing of pituri leaves (*Dubosia hopwoodii*)—a mild stimulant that fostered animation and well-being—was a part of the culture of the Australian aborigines long ago.

The depressants

Chemical enjoyment is not merely a matter of procuring stimulation and exhilaration. Drugs that provide relaxation, withdrawal, stupor, and even coma are valued for those effects. For that reason, narcotics, hypnosedatives, and minor tranquilizers are also popular recreational agents. Anesthetics like ether, chloroform, and nitrous oxide have had their periods of popularity. These substances were used for ether frolics, chloroform jags, and laughing gas soirées even before their usefulness as anesthetics became known. Certain chemicals not ordinarily thought of as suitable for human consumption like gasoline, paint thinner, spray paint aerosols, and other volatile solvents are favored by some juveniles to induce a rapid, intoxicated "high."

Marijuana (*Cannabis sativa*) is second only to alcohol in worldwide popularity as a pleasure-producing drug. Typically, it has been the recourse of rural or tribal populations or of the urban poor, but with the recent indulgence of middle-class youths in drugs that alter consciousness, its use has become widespread. Cannabis, like LSD, is an example of a substance that has been used for both pleasure and self-transcendence. Yogis have, in the past, employed it as an aid in their meditations, and it has been used as a religious ceremonial drug in a number of cultures.

The antipathy toward marijuana in the United States is difficult to understand. As commonly used, it has a rather trivial effect upon consciousness and behavior. The stereotypes of sex-crazed dope fiends presented in the earlier popular literature can scarcely be confirmed by field studies and pharmacological investigations. Perhaps the excessive reaction to the introduction of cannabis occurred because it was a culture-alien drug introduced by strangers. Meanwhile, however, established attitudes and legislation toward cannabis are changing in a reasonable direction. Although a new intoxicant is far from needed, the public health hazards of marijuana require moderate, rather than draconian, controls.

The transcendental experience

The use of botanicals to achieve a transcendental experience may well have occurred early in man's history, even before plants were sought for their medicinal properties. It has been speculated that some primitive concepts of God could have been derived from the ingestion of natural hallucinogenic materials.

A definition is needed for the word "transcendental" because many transitional states between intense pleasure and the transcendent event exist. The transcendental experience (also called peak, mystical, religious, cosmic, Satori, etc.) is one in which most of the following phenomena are apperceived (adapted from Stace):

1. A feeling of oneness with the universe to the point where the boundaries between Me and Not Me have completely dissolved.

2. A feeling that this state is the real reality, much more valid than sober reality.

3. A sense of timelessness and of spatial nonexistence (the "Now Moment" of Meister Eckhart) pervades the experience.

4. A sense of sacredness, awesomeness, and significance is felt by the person in the throes of such an experience.

5. The perceptual component may be a blazing white light or a vision of surpassing beauty.

6. A deeply felt positive mood, be it joy, ecstacy, bliss, peace, or love, is reported.

7. A common comment of those who have undergone such a state is that it is indescribable, ineffable.

8. In this condition paradoxes become resolved, and opposites are seen simply as two aspects of the same thing.

9. Sometimes (by no means invariably) abrupt, dramatic alterations of values and belief systems occur. The changes may last for a lifetime or for a day. If the changes are transient, the awesome experience may leave the person worse off than ever. The load of guilt and despair may be greater because he had "seen the Light" and failed.

A critical issue is whether the hallucinogen-induced transcendental state is the same as the spontaneously occurring one. All of the qualities described above have been encountered after the ingestion of large amounts of hallucinogens by some people under certain conditions. Nevertheless, there are differences. The nonchemical state is likely to be more highly valued and more impressive since it takes place without evident cause. Mystical states of this sort have been instrumental in the founding of religions, have changed people's lives dramatically, and have altered whole social systems. The chemical transcendental state that is purchased for a few dollars is less apt to transform the individual but has been known to do so in a few instances. Perhaps the greatest difference in the two conditions is that the spontaneous state comes forth following meditations, vigils, strenuous exercises, severe deprivation, suffering, or similar stressful events. The person involved is more likely to be prepared for the strange, out-of-the-body experience and is apt to use it as a constructive turning point in his existence. The LSD-induced experience often takes place in unprepared individuals, and they may undergo a disintegrating rather than an integrating outcome of such a cataclysmic event.

It should not be assumed that the transcendent experience cannot be induced by other pharmacologic classes of drugs. William James considered that "the sway of alcohol over mankind is unquestionably due to its power to stimulate the mystical faculties of human nature usually crushed to earth by cold facts and dry criticisms of the sober hour" (p. 72). DeQuincy's *Confessions of an English Opium Eater* contains passages indicating that he experienced transcendent experiences, on occasion, under laudanum. Nitrous oxide has evoked similar subjective responses. It may be that any drug that can produce a dissociation state is capable of evoking a transcendent experience under favorable personality and environmental conditions.

Cultural justification for peak experiences

The use of pleasure-giving chemicals has long been approved: Each society appears to have its own approved substances for this purpose. New euphoriants arouse concern, but if they become culturally approved hedonic materials, the moral issues are relegated to such questions as under what circumstances they should be sold, to whom, or what portion of the tax load they should bear. Since the condoned euphoriants in industrialized countries are at least as harmful as the illegal ones, the morality of interdicting certain substances while permitting others becomes obscure. Traditional usage and familiarity appear to be the major grounds of justification.

Can sociopolitical systems survive without some natural or synthetic euphoriant? Usually it is the religious sector of society that prohibits these items: among others, the Muslims, Latter Day Saints, and Seventh Day Adventists, for example. Clearly, the devout subsist quite well without chemicals that alter mood, but the popularity of mood-elevating materials indicates that most people are unwilling to relinquish them. Although no perceptible biological need for these substances exists, large numbers of humankind insist that they be available.

Religions have been based upon the use of theochemicals (usually as theobotanicals). These religions hold either that a religious experience can be induced by the use of chemicals or that chemicals are necessary for sacramental ritual. The Native American Church of North America uses the peyote cactus in the context of a communal, ritualized, direct experience of God. During the 1960s churches were formed by people who had religious experiences with LSD or mescaline: the Neo-American Church and the League for Spiritual Discovery, to name only two groups in the United States. Efforts to obtain recognition for the use of the latter-day psychedelics as sacramental agents were unsuccessful, and the advocates of an "acid" religion appear to have faded away. The residual mark upon the dominant culture is evident. It is likely that the interest in Eastern mystical religions and in meditative techniques in the Western world stems from the upsurge in the taking of LSD and related agents during the 1960s. Perhaps episodic recrudescences of psychedelic-induced sectarian fervor will occur in the future.

Our understanding of paranormal experience, including the transcendental state, requires revision. Traditionally, our culture has employed a sanity–insanity continuum. The phenomenology of the mystical state would then require that it be placed at the insanity end of the continuum since it was obviously not a sane event. In other societies, and increasingly in North America, the mystical state is becoming highly regarded as a superlative state of human awareness. Perhaps the time has come to consider that peak and cosmic experiences are forms of a new category: "unsanity." Unsanity would be a marked alteration of consciousness that brings about an integration of oneself and one's universe. Then the continuum would consist of insanity at one end—a disorganized altered state of consciousness in which the meaning, organization, and significance of existence have disintegrated. Sanity would occupy a middle position, and at the other end would be unsanity. It could not be a straight-line continuum; rather it would have to be bent into a circular alignment until only a gap separated the insane from the unsane state because of the ability of some people to slip between the two mental conditions, disintegration and integration. The reawakened interest in the direct experience of altered states of consciousness, however obtained, indicates that the simple insanity–unsanity polarity is being abandoned. Alterations of consciousness that can be called unsane are held to be of value either for themselves or as opportunities to learn from such unusual changes in mental functioning.

Conclusion

The hope for euphoria and relief from dysphoria are common motivations for nonmedical drug taking. Chemical hedonism is becoming more acceptable as groups endeavor to increase freedom of action by individuals. Whether drug-induced joy is qualitatively identical with the naturally occurring emotion is problematic because of the nature of the functions of the nervous system. The conflicts between personal freedom and social responsibility are apparent in the issues of illicit drug use.

The available culturally acceptable euphoriants vary from the relatively harmless (whether to the individual or to society) to the definitely harmful. The same can be said of the illegal euphoriants sold in the black market. It would seem reasonable to attempt to reduce the personal and social morbidity and mortality wherever possible.

The hallucinogens are the pharmacological class capable of evoking both the hedonic and transcendental states more precisely than other drug classes. The chemical transcendental experience is similar to, but not identical with, the spontaneous religious experience. Efforts to establish a psychedelic religion based upon LSD have failed because of the lack of a philosophy, an ethic, and an ability to integrate the psychedelic experience into daily life, as well as the assumption that the experience was something for everyone.

The chemical transcendental state has provided us with two opportunities: (1) to study the phenomenology of transcendent experience and (2) to revise our incorrect notions about altered states of awareness that cannot be understood by being subsumed under the word "insane."

SIDNEY COHEN

[*For further discussion of topics mentioned in this article, see the entries:* ALCOHOL, USE OF; PAIN AND SUFFERING; *and* SMOKING. *Also directly related are* HEALTH AS AN OBLIGATION; *and* MENTAL ILLNESS, *article on* CONCEPTIONS OF MENTAL ILLNESS.]

BIBLIOGRAPHY

CLARK, WALTER HOUSTON. *Chemical Ecstasy: Psychedelic Drugs and Religion.* New York: Sheed & Ward, 1969.
COHEN, SIDNEY. *The Beyond Within: The LSD Story.* 2d ed. Foreword by Gardner Murphy. New York: Atheneum, 1967.
HUXLEY, ALDOUS LEONARD. *The Doors of Perception.* New York: Harper, 1954.
JAMES, WILLIAM. *The Varieties of Religious Experience: A Study in Human Nature.* Gifford Lectures on Natural Religion, 1901–1902. New York: Modern Library, 1902.
MASLOW, ABRAHAM HAROLD. *Religions, Values and Peak-Experiences.* The Kappa Delta Pi Lecture series. Columbus: Ohio State University Press, 1964.
MASTERS, ROBERT E. L., and HOUSTON, JEAN. *The Varieties of Psychedelic Experience.* New York: Holt, Rinehart & Winston, 1966.
PAHNKE, WALTER N., and RICHARDS, WILLIAM A. "Implications of LSD and Experimental Mysticism." *Journal of Religion and Health* 5 (1966): 175–208.
SMITH, HUSTON. "Do Drugs Have Religious Import?" *LSD: The Consciousness-Expanding Drug.* Edited by David Solomon. Introduction by Timothy Leary. New York: G. P. Putnam's Sons, 1964, chap. 8, pp. 152–167.
STACE, WALTER TERENCE. *Mysticism and Philosophy.* Philadelphia: Lippincott, 1960.
WATTS, ALAN WILSON. *The Joyous Cosmology: Adventures in the Chemistry of Consciousness.* Foreword by Timothy Leary and Richard Alpert. New York: Pantheon Books, 1962.
ZAEHNER, ROBERT CHARLES. *Mysticism, Sacred and Profane: An Inquiry into Some Varieties of Praeter-Natural Experience.* Oxford: Clarendon Press, 1957.

DYNAMIC THERAPIES

Concepts and principles underlying the ethical issues discussed in this entry can be found in the entry BEHAVIOR CONTROL.

Introduction

The term "dynamic therapies" refers to both psychoanalysis and psychotherapy. In psychoanalysis, the analyst and patient undertake a general examination of the patient's personality, feelings, and social behavior for the purpose of changing disturbed or unsatisfactory patterns of feeling and action. Typically they meet several times a week for a fifty-minute session over a period of several years. The techniques of analysis, as of therapy, are verbal. Psychotherapy is a more general term than psychoanalysis. It sometimes refers to a course of treatment in which the therapist and patient meet over a relatively short period of time with specific goals, for example, the treatment of particular symptoms of distress. More generally, it refers to any course of treatment that employs psychoanalytical assumptions about personality and behavior even when the techniques of treatment vary. In this discussion, the term "therapist" is used for therapists and analysts alike, and the term "therapeutic relationship" refers as well to the analytic relationship (but not, of course, to medical relationships, which are also in one obvious sense therapeutic).

A neurotic condition is one in which a patient's feelings and behavior are disturbed by patterns of anxiety and internal conflict but in which he or she can respond relatively well to everyday demands. Recently, dynamic therapy has come to be used more and more effectively with psychotic patients, who are more seriously disturbed and incapacitated.

The patient who undertakes treatment with a psychotherapist or psychoanalyst commits himself to an extended interaction that involves characteristic goals, values, and responsibilities. The relationship between patient and therapist may be compared with the medical (doctor–patient) relationship and the teacher–student relationship, and it may be distinguished from both of them in the following ways.

The goal of psychotherapy, like the goal of medicine, is the health of the patient. Physical health is, however, a much less controversial notion than emotional or mental health. For medicine, the body can be seen as a mechanism, and the job of the physician is to intervene to the best of his limited ability to put the mechanism right when some part malfunctions. The patient's body is the more or less passive object of the doctor's ministrations, which may be medical or surgical. The disturbances treated by psychotherapy, on the other hand, are disturbances in the patient's relations to other persons, in his feelings about himself, and in his self-understanding—usually all three at once. Therefore, the aim of therapy is not restoration of bodily functions but a change in social behavior and in the patient's attitudes toward himself. At best, the therapist provides a context or situation in which the patient can act to achieve these aims. Thus, the goals of the therapeutic relationship and the roles of the participants stand in contrast to the goals and roles of the medical relationship. There are of course situations in which the two relationships intersect. A physician will have to be alert to the psychosomatic aspects of physical malfunction, as in hysteria, and a therapist must be prepared to find organic causes for emotional disturbance in some cases.

The therapeutic relationship can be compared with the mutual relationship of teacher and student. One model of the teaching relationship is the Socratic model set forth in Plato's writings. The teacher is like a "midwife" who leads students to use capacities and reveal knowledge that they possess latently. Paradoxically, the therapeutic relationship is more Socratic than teaching itself. In many teaching situations, the student cannot really be said to know "unconsciously" what he is learning, but in every therapeutic situation the patient is seen as trying to make conscious the unconscious attitudes, fears, and conflicts that shape his behavior.

Basic values

Self-examination. In psychoanalytical theory the patient and therapist are assumed to share certain values that are inherent in their mutual activity. The patient must share with the therapist the conviction that self-examination and self-discovery are the essential means of treatment. In this way, psychotherapy and psychoanalysis are distinguished from other ways of treating emotional and mental disturbance, e.g., behavioral therapy and drug treatment. Some theoreticians claim not only that self-examination is the chosen means of effecting change, but that the cultivation of self-knowledge is an end in itself. This view echoes the philosophical commitment, derived from Socrates, that the unexamined life is not worth living. Accordingly, self-examination not only brings about behavioral change and some resolution of the patient's problems but remains a continuing activity that enriches the patient's life. In this sense, the successfully treated patient is quite unlike the untreated "healthy" person, for he is trained to maintain special strategies of self-perception.

In treatment itself, the patient can achieve self-knowledge only indirectly. Because his anxiety blocks direct admission of his deepest fears and conflicts, he is encouraged to give the therapist clues to his emotional expectations and thought processes by saying whatever "comes into his head," the stratagem of free association. To the extent that the self-ascribed task of introspection involves structuring, editing, and thus censoring of his output by the patient, it is from a psychoanalytical point of view self-defeating.

Autonomy. Freud referred to the inherent value of self-examination in saying about the goals of psychoanalysis, "where id was, there ego shall be." This means in part that behavior which carries out understood and integrated purposes is to take the place of unconsciously motivated and therefore compulsive behavior. This is not to say that psychoanalysis values unspontaneous action. Rather, it recognizes that the spontaneous actions of a child are largely unavailable to adults and that the compulsive behavior of disturbed patients is not spontaneous at all but the product of inhibition and repressed conflict. Therefore, a second value in psychoanalytical theory, one also suggested in Freud's slogan, is autonomy.

According to the theory, all persons deal with childhood fears and crises by learning patterns of response. When such fears are particularly overwhelming and such crises particularly traumatic, the learned pattern is not so much one of coping as one of escaping. The person learns to shut off certain possibilities of action and achievement when the threat of trying and failing is, again unconsciously, felt to be too great. The disturbances produced in this way preempt some social and personal achievements: The patient, far from acting spontaneously, is the prisoner of inflexible patterns of feeling and action, which he uses undiscriminatingly and often inappropriately in his mature life. He is literally the prisoner of his past, paradoxically the prisoner of himself. The goal of therapy is invariably to free the patient, to allow him to build a more flexible set of emotional responses and actions to achieve self-worth and well-being. Like the value of self-examination, the value of autonomy is achieved only as an ongoing process, not as a stopping place.

Implications of the dominant values. The commitment of patient and therapist to the twin values of self-examination and autonomy has several implications. A comparison with medicine is again relevant. In medicine, it is often assumed that the patient submits himself voluntarily for treatment. This is important but relatively unproblematic: The patient must be informed of his disorder and of the planned treatment and its attendant risks, and must consent.

In psychotherapy, voluntariness is also important and much more problematic. First, the patient's reasons for seeking therapy and his conception of personal goals are to some extent shaped by his emotional and social expectations. The first difficult job of the analyst is to see that the choice of therapy is made as freely and realistically as possible. Second, the patient resists expressing his conflicts because to express them is to experience them, i.e., to do what he most fears, whether it is to stand up to a feared father, separate himself from an overprotective mother, or make some other move. The voluntary decision to proceed with therapy is one that must be remade continually; the relatively uncensored expression of conflict is itself an expression of autonomy.

There are other implications. The preeminent value given to self-examination and autonomy implies that all other values are to be seen in their light. For example, altruism and kindness have value not in themselves but only if they emanate from the actor's free choices and not from his fears and conflicts. Self-sacrificing generosity may be a symptom of unconscious patterns of self-destruction. This "transvaluation of values" is far-reaching; the determinant of value of action is not the traditional interpersonal one, whether the act benefits or harms those affected by it, but an intrapersonal one, whether the act is genuinely an autonomous response to the needs of others.

Certain other characteristic attitudes proceed from the choice of self-examination as the mode of therapy (in contrast, for example, to drugs). The therapeutic process involves repeated encounters with emotional pain and suffering—not the magnified (and therefore intolerable) pain that the patient unconsciously expects, but the real pain of suffering everyday frustrations and of accepting one's own limitations. The acceptance of pain and suffering is therefore a basic value in the psychoanalytical picture of the well-lived life. A related aspect of such a life is that it will involve gratification. The person will be able to delay gratification and control impulses, but also to achieve gratification in its time. In psychoanalytical theory and practice, disturbance is ordinarily traceable to fears about sexual activity and conflicts in attitudes toward sex; it follows that symptoms of disturbance will be found in adult sexual practices and fantasies. The capacity for vigorous heterosexual activity is traditionally held to be a mark of health. Some recent writers use a more subjective criterion for sexual health, the satisfaction of the individual and his capacity to give satisfaction to his sexual partners. Disagreement here turns on the question whether non-heterosexual preferences are clearly a symptom of neurotic conflict and of aborted emotional growth.

Responsibilities

Responsibilities of the therapist to the patient. The involvement of the therapist in the patient's life is intimate. Although they meet only at regularly scheduled times in a controlled setting, the patient is expected to trust the therapist with his seemingly most irrational fantasies and his most embarrassing fears. The more unguarded the patient is, the more the therapist can help. The patient, vulnerable to shame and disappointment, must trust the therapist, and the therapist must show that he deserves such trust.

Countertransference. The characteristic mode of response by the patient is called transference. This means that the patient acts out with the therapist his personal ways of dealing with other persons; he projects or transfers onto the therapist his expectations about others. The therapist will play many different roles as the patient relives and reconstructs different relationships. As that occurs, the therapist has two major responsibilities. He must allow the patient to proceed with transference by maintaining a basic situation in which the patient will not feel vulnerable or ashamed, and he must prod the patient into discussing and understanding the patterns revealed in the transference.

The demands on the therapist are very high. While an ordinary physician or teacher may allow his personal spontaneity to express itself in his role, the therapist's expressions of personality will be likely to impede transference. One responsibility of the therapist is to guard against such intrusions with self-awareness. Accordingly, therapists and analysts are usually required to be psychoanalyzed themselves to bring their own conflicts to some resolution and to become aware of their personal predilections for abusing the therapeutic relationship. For example, the therapist may unconsciously cultivate the patient's dependence for the satisfaction that this gives, and furthermore he may rationalize doing so as therapy even if it frustrates the long-term goals of the patient. In other words, the responsibility of the therapist is to minimize, if not avoid altogether, what is called "counter-transference."

Reality-testing. One way of describing the patient's problem is to say that he acts unreal-istically in his disturbed everyday behavior. The paranoiac patient attributes malevolent purposes to persons who do not have them; a sexually unresponsive woman patient may fear the violence of men who in reality will not be violent. In helping the patient to see and understand such patterns, the therapist aids the patient to test his or her expectations against reality.

This responsibility of therapists becomes controversial when therapists are accused of imposing their own notion about reality on their patients. A way of examining the controversy is by asking whether the relevant sense of the term "reality" is one about which different therapists may have their own ideas. On one hand, it is clear in our examples that the absence of malevolent intentions or of the prospect of violence may be objective facts. That is not to say that a mistaken expectation of violence is always a symptom of neurotic conflict; there is a burden on the therapist to measure the patient's expectations by what is reasonable (even if mistaken) in the circumstances. This comment, however, reintroduces the controversy, since it will be said that therapists impose on patients their own idea of what is reasonable.

To this, there are two responses. The first is an admission that abuse *is* always possible. A therapist *may,* in contravention of his responsibilities, shape a patient's attitudes to fit his own political, ethical, or other beliefs. There are obvious cases of abuse as there are obvious cases of nonabuse in which the patient's fears and expectations, typically by his own admission, are "unreal." There is a gray area as well. Debates about whether all sexual inversion is derived from unreal perceptions and fears of the opposite sex, and is therefore neurotic, are one illustration of the controversial or gray area. The second response is that the therapist's responsibility is to help the patient to test his expectations against reality in those areas in which the nature of reality is to the highest degree uncontroversial.

"Arm's-length" aspects. For reasons which have been discussed, the therapist must be especially careful to minimize the patient's dependence on him. The therapist must allow the patient to bring about the transference and not collaborate, so that the patient may in time see the transference as the product of his expectations and fears. Moreover, dependence of any sort during therapy undercuts or makes more remote the goal of autonomy.

There are various opinions and practices with regard to implementing this responsibility. According to some theories the therapist is allowed or even encouraged to touch, advise, or otherwise guide the patient if this will serve the ultimate ends of therapy. Therapists of this kind are expected to exercise wide discretion in meeting patients' perceived needs. An extreme minority view sanctions sexual activity with patients in suitable situations. Such practitioners reject many of the strictures of orthodox Freudian practice as outlined above.

The traditional practice of therapists trained in methods set by Freud is to interfere as little as possible with patients' free associations and yet guide them to speak freely and reflect on the significance of those associations. This explains many formal constraints in psychoanalysis. The patient usually lies on a couch so that he will not be influenced by the therapist's facial expressions and gestures. Sessions are strictly limited to fifty minutes and are scheduled as regularly as possible. The therapist usually insists on making the patient's financial responsibilities as unambiguous as possible and on holding the patient financially liable for missed appointments. The patient is expected to make and adhere to a long-term commitment to therapy with brief vacations scheduled at the therapist's convenience. The rationale for these features of therapy/analysis is that they help the therapist maintain an arm's-length relationship within which the patient's own projections are most clearly distinguishable from the idiosyncratic contributions of the therapist. Even within these constraints, of course, there will be subtle differences among therapists and these will be reflected in their minute-by-minute decisions about whether and how to intervene in the patient's presentations.

The controversy between the relatively austere Freudian procedures and those of so-called revisionists can be seen as a controversy about the relation of methods to goals. On one side, it may be said that orthodox Freudian therapists set rigorous goals for patients and that the patient is so thoroughly "on his own" that the prospects of succeeding are minimized. The patient needs the active support of the therapist to change his conception of himself as fearful and rejected. On the other side, the argument is that such support achieves short-term gains at the cost of aggravating the patient's dependence and frustrating transference by changing a projected into an actual relationship. On one side, the goals are called too high and unreachable; on the other, they are called too

transitory and limited. A therapist will shape his own conceptions of his responsibility in forming an opinion about this debate.

Responsibilities of the patient. Since the relationship of therapist and patient involves reciprocal roles, each has responsibilities defined by his role. The responsibility of the therapist is to the patient, but the patient's responsibilities are to himself, since his benefit is the object of the activity. Therefore, one tends to think of the therapist's responsibilities as ethical responsibilities; by comparison, the patient's responsibilities are not ethical ones unless a person can be said to have ethical responsibilities to oneself, e.g., to improve one's condition. Whether or not one calls them ethical, the patient's responsibilities reciprocate those of the therapist.

First of all, the patient has a responsibility to be honest. In ordinary cases it may be hard or easy to be honest; in therapy it is always hard, because one is asked to be honest in just those cases where one is most tempted to evade because the truth is inherently painful. As patient, one must question and reassess one's picture of oneself, one's goals, and the bases of one's most intimate relationships. One must also stand ready to entertain and tolerate paradoxical beliefs, for example the awareness of loving and hating the same person at the same time. Finally, one must be ready to entertain and admit irrational feelings of anger, aggression, and guilt even when this entails feeling altogether vulnerable.

A commitment of this kind to honesty is a commitment to spontaneity. One must say what "comes into one's mind," censoring it as little as possible, however nonsensical it seems and shameful it feels. The most important clues for a therapist will characteristically seem nonsensical or shameful to the patient: nonsensical when the patient as self-censor denies their possible importance, shameful when they intimate unconscious fantasies of danger.

The so-called arm's-length aspects of therapy impose discrete and unambiguous responsibilities on the patient. Part of the patient's early "work" is to examine his response to these constraints. He must assume a long-term schedule, appear at appointments, and take on what is typically a considerable financial burden.

Responsibilities of the therapist outside the therapeutic setting. In obvious ways the therapist plays a uniquely intimate role in the patient's life and has ethical responsibilities that extend beyond the work of the therapeutic appointments. However austere the therapist's way of proceeding may be, the patient at some point during treatment feels dependent on the therapist. This is not simply the result of the patient's transference; it is also a recognition of the fact that the therapist becomes an important and powerful person in the patient's life when the analysis is successful.

The patient's trust of the therapist rests on the assurance that his communications will be confidential. The therapist has an obvious duty to protect confidentiality as much as possible. While the therapeutic relationship shares this feature with the medical relationship, the need for confidentiality in the former is more pervasive since the patient in therapy typically sees his remarks as revelations about his own vulnerability and about what is most embarrassing to him. In this respect it is more closely comparable to the relationship of lawyer and client, where a breach of confidentiality is likely to endanger the client and frustrate the purposes for which the relationship exists.

The responsibility to protect patients' confidentiality is a negative one, viz., to refrain from certain actions. Does the therapist have a positive responsibility to be available to the patient outside fixed appointments? That would be like any physician's responsibility to respond in emergencies, but there are special complications. The long-term interests of the patient, autonomy and self-reliance, are undercut if the therapist encourages dependence and is seen as too readily available in periods of crisis. The job of the patient is to acquire his own strategies for crises. At the same time, the patient who is in genuine danger from himself (from suicidal wishes, for example) or from others may not survive to achieve these long-term goals. The therapist's role must be to guide him through such situations in such a way as to minimize both their recurrence *and* dependence.

So far, the discussion of the therapist's responsibilities has been about responsibilities to the patient. There are obvious situations in which these responsibilities will come into conflict with responsibilities to others. Suppose, for example, that the patient reveals plans to harm his family. (To simplify matters, imagine that the contemplated actions are legal.) Suppose also that the therapist believes the patient has the capacity to carry out his plans, intends to do so, and will do so. Does the therapist have a responsibility to warn intended victims or otherwise prevent harm? Theorists disagree. All em-

phasize that the therapist's primary obligation is to the patient, and intervention is justified only if the harm is particularly severe or irreversible. Beyond this, some say that the obligation to the patient is absolute and emphasize that the therapist must try to prevent such actions only through his work with the patient.

The most serious problems of this kind arise when the patient intends to do something harmful that is forbidden by law, in the most extreme kind of case when he intends to take a human life. In such cases one may say that even if the therapist's responsibilities *as therapist* extend only to the patient, he will usually believe on good grounds that the patient's interests cannot be advanced by letting him proceed. Decisions to intervene will be difficult, because the therapist must assess the likelihood that the patient will act and the impact of his intervention on the patient, both on continued treatment and on the patient's social and legal status. In any case, it cannot be said that such hard cases can be made easy because the obligation to protect confidentiality is absolute.

There are really two kinds of moral argument for intervention. The therapist *as therapist* has obligations to the patient, and this will precipitate moral dilemmas about the effects of intervention. But the therapist also has responsibilities as a person. A second kind of moral argument is that his responsibilities to potential victims will in serious cases override his responsibilities as therapist. There are in other words acute dilemmas in which the therapist must weigh his responsibilities as therapist and as a person, dilemmas that cannot be resolved by appealing to rules and general formulas.

Therapists are often asked to give so-called expert testimony about the competence of defendants to stand trial or face legal hearings. This does not involve a breach of confidentiality where the examinee is not the therapist's patient and where there has been no intimation of confidentiality. Even so, there is a moral dilemma since the therapist's role as therapist is in conflict with his legal role in two ways. First, he is accustomed by training to consider the needs of examinees (or patients) without having to balance those needs against the needs of other persons like potential victims. In testimony he is usually asked to make just such a judgment. Second, he is not ordinarily expected to decide between responsibility or nonresponsibility (sanity or insanity) but to see all persons as relatively autonomous in personally idiosyncratic ways. To be sure, his expertise allows him to predict with some confidence how certain persons will act in certain situations, but this is only one ingredient of the morally relevant determinations that the law asks of him.

There is another complicating feature of the therapist's role as expert witness. He is, by training, an expert on the effect on the subject (usually the defendant) of imprisoning him, of returning him to his home or the street, and so forth. As witness he is asked to leave these insights aside and make a judgment only about what the subject is likely to do. But at the same time he knows that his testimony is a determinant of what happens to the subject. He is therefore asked to do two things which are antithetical to his training: to disregard the welfare and interests of the subject and to intervene directly in the subject's life. The demand that he participate thus generates a moral dilemma.

Therapy in its social setting

The dilemmas of the therapist as expert witness are one kind of illustration of general conflicts between the values of dynamic therapy as an institution and other values. In most roles in daily life—as friend, parent, worker, teacher, student, political participant, etc.—the values of self-examination and autonomy are not treated as absolute but are qualified by other values. Ordinarily, the well-functioning individual is socially defined by such communal purposes as his contribution to the joint external enterprise rather than by such self-regarding goals as freedom from fear, conflict, and anxiety. To some extent, of course, there is no conflict insofar as psychological health allows one to be a full participant in other roles. At the same time, the pursuit of psychological health will also lead to the rejection of overdemanding friends or overprotective parents or to mitigation of an obsessive commitment to one's job. One may respond to this clash of values in several ways. One may employ the notion of autonomy to criticize those institutional practices that seem to impede self-determination. Or one may say that the claims of friendship, work, and political goals should in many instances override self-regarding claims.

The social role of psychotherapy and psychoanalysis comes under attack in another way. Because they involve great investments of time by the therapist and time and money by patients, they are available to few persons and involve, even for those few, an uncertain prognosis.

These features provoke the criticism that dynamic therapy involves an inefficient and wasteful allocation of society's resources. The political questions here involve hard moral questions about what sorts of economic allocations are just and justifiable.

THOMAS H. MORAWETZ

[*Directly related are the entries* BEHAVIOR CONTROL; MENTAL HEALTH THERAPIES; MENTAL ILLNESS; SELF-REALIZATION THERAPIES; *and* THERAPEUTIC RELATIONSHIP. *Other relevant material may be found under* CONFIDENTIALITY; HEALTH AS AN OBLIGATION; INFORMED CONSENT IN MENTAL HEALTH; MENTAL HEALTH, *article on* MENTAL HEALTH IN COMPETITION WITH OTHER VALUES; *and* SEX THERAPY AND SEX RESEARCH, *article on* SCIENTIFIC AND CLINICAL PERSPECTIVES. *See* APPENDIX, SECTION IV, AMERICAN PSYCHIATRIC ASSOCIATION, *and* AMERICAN PSYCHOLOGICAL ASSOCIATION.]

BIBLIOGRAPHY

EDELSON, MARSHALL. *The Idea of a Mental Illness.* New Haven: Yale University Press, 1971.

ERIKSON, ERIK H. *Insight and Responsibility: Lectures on the Ethical Implications of Psychoanalytic Insight.* New York: W. W. Norton & Co., 1964.

FREUD, SIGMUND. *The Standard Edition of the Complete Psychological Works of Sigmund Freud.* 23 vols. Translated under the editorship of James Strachey. London: Hogarth Press, 1954–1964. See especially: "The Dynamics of Transference," vol. 12, pp. 99–108; "Remembering, Repeating, and Working-through," vol. 12, pp. 147–156; "Introductory Lectures on Psycho-Analysis," vol. 15, pp. 15–239 and vol. 16, pp. 243–463; "The Ego and the Id," vol. 19, pp. 13–66; "Civilization and Its Discontents," vol. 21, pp. 64–145; "New Introductory Lectures on Psycho-Analysis," vol. 22, pp. 7-182; and "Analysis Terminable and Interminable," vol. 23, pp. 216–253.

FROMM-REICHMANN, FRIEDA. *Principles of Intensive Psychotherapy.* Chicago: University of Chicago Press, 1950.

GOLDSTEIN, KURT. *Human Nature in the Light of Psychopathology.* The William James Lectures Delivered at Harvard University, 1937–1938. Cambridge: Harvard University Press, 1940.

Group for the Advancement of Psychiatry, Committee on Psychiatry and Law. *Criminal Responsibility and Psychiatric Expert Testimony.* Report, no. 26 (May 1954). Topeka, Kans.: 1954.

GUREVITZ, HOWARD. "Tarasoff: Protective Privilege versus Public Peril." *American Journal of Psychiatry* 134 (1977): 289–292.

HAMPSHIRE, STUART. *Thought and Action.* London: Chatto & Windus; New York: Viking Press, 1960.

HARTMANN, HEINZ. *Essays on Ego Psychology: Selected Problems in Psychoanalytic Theory.* New York: International Universities Press, 1964.

HORNEY, KAREN. *Neurosis and Human Growth: The Struggle toward Self-Realization.* New York: W. W. Norton & Co., 1950.

REDLICH, FREDERICK C., and FREEDMAN, DANIEL X. *The*

Theory and Practice of Psychiatry. New York: Basic Books, 1966.

RIEFF, PHILIP. *Freud: The Mind of the Moralist.* New York: Viking Press, 1959.

———. *The Triumph of the Therapeutic: Uses of Faith after Freud.* New York: Harper & Row, 1966.

ROGERS, CARL RANSON. *On Becoming a Person: A Therapist's View of Psychotherapy.* Boston: Houghton Mifflin, 1961.

SCHAFER, ROY. *A New Language for Psychoanalysis.* New Haven: Yale University Press, 1976.

SULLIVAN, HARRY STACK. *The Interpersonal Theory of Psychiatry.* Edited by Helen Swick Perry and Mary Ladd Gawel. New York: W. W. Norton & Co., 1953.

SZASZ, THOMAS STEPHEN. *The Ethics of Psychoanalysis: The Theory and Method of Autonomous Psychotherapy.* New York: Basic Books; Dell Publishing Co., 1965.

———. "Psychiatry, Ethics, and the Criminal Law." *Columbia Law Review* 58 (1958): 182–198.

WAELDER, ROBERT. "Psychiatry and the Problem of Criminal Responsibility." *University of Pennsylvania Law Review* 101 (1952): 378–390.

WINNICOTT, DONALD WOODS. *Collected Papers: Through Paediatrics to Psycho-Analysis.* New York: Basic Books, 1958.

E

EASTERN EUROPE
See Medical Ethics, History of, *section on* europe and the americas, *article on* eastern europe in the twentieth century.

EASTERN ORTHODOX CHRISTIANITY

Eastern Orthodox Christian ethics bases its ethical judgments on Holy Scripture and Holy Tradition. Holy Tradition consists of the "mind of the Church" and is discerned in the decisions of ecumenical and local councils, the writings of the Fathers of the Church, canon law, and the penitentials (guides for the administration of the sacrament of Penance).

Issues not directly treated in the ancient sources are dealt with by modern Orthodox ethicists by seeking to express ethical judgments that are in harmony with the "mind of the Church." Thus, their writings have a certain provisional character and are always subject to episcopal, synodical, or general ecclesial critique. There are occasionally differences of substance in the writings of modern Orthodox Christian ethicists. By and large, however, responsible Orthodox ethicists maintain a common ethical stance. Modern issues in bioethics often require of ethicists that they find parallels in the tradition and, with the help of reason, deduce new ethical applications from established doctrinal, historical, and pastoral positions.

Basic doctrine and ethical affirmations

The Eastern Christian doctrinal position tends to be cautious in defining positively the central affirmations of its faith. It prefers the *via negativa,* or "apophatic" method (i.e., saying what is not the case). In ethics, a practice may be proscribed as not in harmony with the ethos of the faith, but often no positive solution is offered other than the need for patience and acceptance of the situation.

Nevertheless, Eastern Orthodox Christianity does avail itself of positive or "kataphatic" doctrinal and ethical statements. These are taken seriously when they are normative in character, but not in a rigid, legalistic, or absolute fashion. All positive statements regarding divine revelation—the Tradition—are seen as limited and subject to mystery as a necessary dimension of all human understandings of the divine. In canon law and in ethics this has led to the practice of "economia," which authorizes exceptions to the rule without considering the exception a precedent or abrogating the rule. In most cases the justification for the application of "economia" is the avoidance of greater harm in the case of the strict application of the rule (Kotsonis). Several key doctrinal teachings have immediate ethical application with specific reference to bioethical issues.

Theological anthropology. The *humanum* of our existence is both a given and a potential. Some of the patristic authorities distinguish between the creation of human beings in the "image" of God, and in his "likeness." "Image" is the *donatum* of intellect, emotion, ethical judgment, and self-determination. In fallen humanity these remain part of human nature, albeit darkened, wounded, and weakened. The "likeness" is the human potential to become like

347

God, to achieve an ever expanding, never completed perfection. This fulfillment of our humanity is traditionally referred to as *theosis* or "divinization." Human beings are in fact "less than fully human." To achieve *theosis* means to realize our full human potential. Ethically, this teaching leads to the acceptance, on the one hand, of the existence of a "human nature," but, on the other, it clearly does not restrict our "humanum" to conformity to that nature. The "image" provides a firm foundation for ethical reasoning. The "likeness" prohibits the absolutizing of any rule, law, or formulation (Maloney).

Divine energies and human self-determination. Though God's essence is totally incomprehensible to the human mind, God's energies are present in every human experience. To speak of divine energies is to speak of God's actions in relation to the created world. The relationship of God's energies to human freedom and self-determination has obvious ethical implications. Orthodox Christianity teaches that, though God is Lord of history, he does not coerce or force obedience and conformity to his will. Coerced conformity is dehumanization, whereas fulfilled humanity—which is the divinization of human life—must be free, since God is free. This raises the question of Divine Providence and Human Responsibility. Orthodox Christianity holds these two in paradoxical tension: man is responsible and must act, but God accomplishes his will, either with or in spite of man's actions. Ideally, human actions are harmoniously integrated with divine purposes in a perfect synergy of divine and human wills. This belief is but an extension and application of the Orthodox doctrine of the divine and human natures in the one person of Jesus Christ. Ethically, this means that we are not permitted simply to wait upon God. Rather, we are committed to the exercise of self-determination and responsibility in conformity with both human reality and divine purpose (Florovsky, pp. 113–120).

Body–spirit. God is seen as the creator of both the material and the spiritual dimensions of reality. Eastern Orthodox Christianity sees these aspects of existence as closely bound together. The icon is an example of this belief. At first sight, the icon appears to be a stylized artistic representation of a holy figure. Yet the iconographer's purpose is to capture in form, line, color, and symbol both the spiritual and the physical reality of the figure. The sacramental use of material means (such as water, oil, bread, wine, etc.) for spiritual purposes also illustrates Eastern Orthodoxy's comprehension of the intimate relationship of matter and spirit. For bioethics, this key concept is important because it leads to a serious affirmation of the psychosomatic unity of human life. "Body" and "soul" are the constituents of human existence; the Orthodox emphasis on the Resurrection confirms its view that human life and human fulfillment are inextricably bound to both the physical and the spiritual dimensions of human existence. In more contemporary terms, body and personhood are essential for the fulfillment of human potential (Antoniades, 1: 204–208).

Law, motive, intent. Based on the above, ethical reasoning in Orthodoxy is a balanced combination of law, motive, and intent. Moral law is based in large part on the *donatum* of human nature. For Eastern Orthodoxy, natural law refers primarily to the elementary relationships that are necessary for the constitution and maintenance of human society. For the Fathers of the Church, the Decalogue is an excellent expression of the natural law common to all men (Harakas, 1964). In a similar yet more flexible pattern, there are modes of behavior that are either prescribed or proscribed for the lives of Christians growing in the image and likeness of God toward *theosis* or full humanity. These positive and negative injunctions are found in the Holy Scriptures, in the writings of the Fathers and in the canons of the Church. For the Orthodox these statements are normative in the sense that they embody the mind of the Church and reflect standards of behavior that are appropriate and fitting for the members of the Church and, potentially, for all human beings growing in the image and likeness of God for the full realization of personhood.

This first level of ethical direction is saved from legalism and rigid prescriptivism by the fundamental emphasis on love as a motive of action. Grounded thoroughly on a Trinitarian theology that understands the Holy Trinity first as a community of persons united in love, the Church teaches that being God-like means being loving. In general, the commandments of the moral law are embodiments of loving concern for the welfare of others. Consequently, in most situations the loving action is in conformity with the guidelines provided by the commandments (Harakas, 1970).

The possibility remains open, however, for the exception, i.e., for the exercise of "economia" when conformity to the prescribed action is perceived as detracting from the basic intent of all reasoning—the advancement of each person in community toward the fulfillment of the image and likeness of God. Thus, both order and compassion are harmonized in an approach to Christian ethics that seeks to avoid the extremes of legalism and relativism.

Bioethics

It is convenient to treat the Eastern Orthodox approach to bioethics under two major rubrics: the protection of life and the transmission of life. Implicit in the treatment of each of the bioethical issues are the affirmations implied in the doctrines of the image and likeness, *theosis*, human self-determination and responsibility, the intimate bond of body and personhood, and the interpenetrating relationship of commandment, love, and the realization of true human potential.

The protection of life. Orthodox Christian ethical thought universally holds that life is a gift of God and as such is the necessary prerequisite of all other physical, spiritual, and moral values. As a gift of God it is a moral good held by the individual and by societies in trust, and over which they do not have absolute control. Both the individual and societies, however, are charged with the moral responsibility of protecting, transmitting, and enhancing life. The concerns of bioethics relate primarily to the first two of these concerns. Generally speaking, human responsibility for the preservation of life means that we are not given the right to terminate human life. Even the exceptions to this rule are understood as arising when conflicting claims to life become mutually exclusive, and a choice must be made. The preservation and protection of life are thus seen as crucial in ethical decision making. Since life is the prerequisite of all other this-worldly goods such as education, intelligence, social worth, and service to humanity, it has an intrinsic value that may not be violated under normal circumstances.

Health care. It follows quite logically that the care of one's own health and societal concern for public health are moral imperatives (Androutsos, pp. 191–195, 250). Throughout its history, Eastern Orthodox Christianity has concerned itself sacramentally with the physical health of the faithful. The Sacrament of Holy Unction has not been conducted as a service of the "last rites." Rather, it is a healing service conducted both publicly and privately for the faithful. One of the constituents of the condition of original sin in which man actually finds himself is sickness. Total harmony of the creation with God would in fact eliminate sickness and ill health. The spiritual and physical dimensions of health are closely bound together in Orthodox thought. Thus, it was natural for the priest and the physician often to be one and the same person (Constantelos, 1967).

The issue of the allocation of scarce medical resources demands a general principle of distribution. Neither the ability to pay nor an aristocratic criterion of greater human value or worth is acceptable. Eastern Christianity has always distinguished between the essential value of human life and social worth. In spite of the enormous difficulties involved, the ethical imperative from the Orthodox perspective calls for the widest possible distribution of health care and life-protecting facilities and resources, rather than a concentration of such resources for the select few. The famous health care center established by Saint Basil in the fourth century in Cappadocia of Asia Minor was designed to reach as many people as possible. It and similar institutions embodied the Eastern Christian view on health distribution (Constantelos, 1968, chap. 11).

Rights of patients. The understanding that each person is created in the image and likeness of God with the personal destiny of achieving *theosis* implies that each patient has an essential and inviolate dignity as a person. The fact that individuals can achieve personhood only in community (*Unus Christianus, nullus Christianus*), requires the concern of the healthy for the ill. Those who deliver health care, therefore, do not morally discharge their responsibility by the mere mechanical application of healing methods and practices. Underlying every medical procedure ought to be a basic respect for the patient as God's image and likeness. The patient is never a thing. Consequently, medical practitioners are obligated, within reason and in the light of the patient's well-being, to maintain confidentiality and to obtain informed consent for procedures that entail excessive risk. Exceptions and restrictions on this obligation should be made in the light of the patient's welfare and whenever possible in consultation with those having immediate responsibility for the patient, e.g., his or her family.

Human experimentation. For the same reasons articulated in the previous section, the Eastern Orthodox Christians take a very hesitant stance vis-à-vis human experimentation.

Medical trial and error conducted for the well-being of the patient himself is often required and necessary. However, the submission of a patient to experimental procedures without significant regard for his or her direct personal benefit is wrong. There is no moral obligation of any person to be used by another for the benefit of a third party. Human self-determination requires that the patient decide. Such a decision must be based on adequate information regarding the procedures, ends to be achieved, and risks involved. The patient does not have the right to inflict harm upon himself unnecessarily. The researcher should use human experimentation procedures only after all other means of testing have been exhausted and there is every reasonable expectation of the avoidance of harm to the subject. In every case, experimenter and subject are morally obligated to exercise great caution. The hope of benefiting mankind in general does not outweigh the moral obligation of the protection of the individual life.

Abortion. Eastern Christianity has a long history of opposition to abortion. Its ethical teachings as embodied in canon law and in the penitential books, as well as in more formal ethical instruction, condemn abortion as a form of murder. Because our humanity is a psychosomatic unity and because Orthodox Christians see all of life as a continuous and never ending development of the image and likeness toward *theosis* and full humanity, the achievement of particular stages of development of the conceptus is not ethically relevant to the question of abortion.

In his second canon, St. Basil specifically rules out the artificial distinction between the "formed" and "unformed" conceptus (*The Rudder*, pp. 789–790). Thus, any abortion is seen as an evil. Since the physical and the personal aspects of human existence are understood as essential constitutive elements of our humanity, the conceptus—unfulfilled and incomplete as it may be—may not be destroyed under normal circumstances. Eastern Orthodox ethicists reject as unworthy those counterarguments which appeal to economic and social reasons and so hold life to be less valuable than money, pride, or convenience. Armed with modern genetic information, they also reject the argument that an abortion may be justified because a woman is entitled to control her own body. That basic affirmation of self-determination is not rejected; what is rejected is the claim that the conceptus is a part of the mother's tissue. It is not her body; it is the body and life of another human being entrusted to her for care and nurture.

Only in the case in which the life of the mother is endangered by the conceptus is it morally appropriate to consider the possibility of abortion. Yet, even here, the main operative value is the preservation of life. Numerous prudential considerations will be taken into account, though it is likely that the preservation of the mother's life will most often be chosen. In any case, it falls into the class of "involuntary sin" in which the evil of the event is recognized, while the personal guilt is mitigated (Papacostas, pp. 9–13, 83–105).

Organ transplants. In the case of organ transplants, the crucial ethical considerations are two: the potential harm inflicted upon the donor and the need of the recipient. Historically, the Orthodox Church has not objected to similar, though not identical, procedures, such as blood transfusions and skin grafts. In both cases, no radical threat to the life of the donor is perceived, and the lifesaving consequences for the recipient are substantial. Similar considerations affect the Orthodox Christian judgment of organ transplants. In no case should a person ignore or make light of the ethical implications of organ donation. Donating an organ whose loss will impair or threaten the life of the potential donor is never required and is never a moral obligation of any person. If the condition of health and the physical well-being of the donor permits, some transplants are not objectionable. Renal transplants are a case in point. A healthy person may consent to donate a kidney knowing that his or her health is not thereby impaired.

The recipient of an organ transplant ought to be in otherwise good health, and there should be a substantial expectation of restoration to normal living in order to warrant the risk to the donor.

Heart transplants present a special case. Objectively they are different from other sorts of organ transplants because they presuppose the death of the donor. Though some Orthodox hierarchs have objected to heart transplants because the "heart" is often designated in the devotional literature of the Church as the seat of the soul, most have not responded negatively to heart transplants in principle. However, caution has been expressed regarding the temptation to hasten the death of the donor for the sake of the recipient. Also, so long as this procedure does not yet have a high success rate, it is morally questionable to continue its practice until the phenomenon of tissue rejection is better understood.

Drug addiction. The *use* of stimulants, depressants, and hallucinogens for any purpose other than the restoration of health or the alleviation of abnormal pain, when properly and legitimately prescribed by a physician, is condemned; but Orthodox ethics, because of its teaching on "involuntary sin," is able to recognize the evil of the condition of drug addiction and yet also recognize that the essence of the evil is that personal self-determination has been lost, and with it a large measure of personal responsibility. Orthodox texts often refer to sinful conditions as "sickness" and "illness." In the case of drug addiction the cure is the restoration of self-determination. In the Orthodox view, the judgment that drug addiction and alcoholism are evil and sinful, on the one hand, and the judgment that they are illnesses, on the other hand, are not mutually exclusive. This is not to say, of course, that every sickness is the result of individual voluntary sins, a position specifically denied by the Orthodox doctrine of original sin.

Mental health: values, therapies, institutions. At the heart of the Eastern Orthodox Christian approach to mental health is the understanding of human wholesomeness in the doctrine of *theosis.* True and full human well-being is the consequence of our proper relationship with God (Demetropoulos, pp. 155–157). Mental health is one dimension of this total relationship. Since no individual human being perfectly achieves this relationship, it may be noted that, just as we are all in some measure "less than fully human," in the same manner we are all in some measure lacking in full mental health. The Orthodox concept of repentance or *metanoia* implies a change of mind, a transfiguration and transformation of the human mind. What is significant is that the teaching of the spiritual Fathers of the Eastern Church emphasizes the need for constant repentance on the part of every human being in the direction of his human goal and destiny.

Some recent studies have related traditional spiritual methodologies to standard psychotherapeutic theories, methods, and approaches (Faros). There are differences, of course, but there is also a remarkable number of parallels to be found between the ancient spiritual disciplines and modern schools of psychology.

Orthodox ethics sees the mentally ill as fellow human beings who need compassionate assistance. Therapies that degrade their essential humanity and attitudes that dehumanize the mentally ill in the eyes of society and deny assistance, relationship, and therapeutic support are in themselves immoral and dehumanizing.

Aging. In the ethical consciousness of the Church, respect and deference for the elderly, and especially for elderly parents, is an important moral responsibility. There is a strong feeling that children ought personally to care for their aged parents. It is only when circumstances are such that it is truly impossible for children to care for their aged parents that they may be placed in appropriate institutions for care. Such institutions have long been a part of the Eastern Orthodox Church's social mission (Constantelos, 1968, chap. 13).

Death, dying, and euthanasia. The traditional definition of physical death is "the separation of soul and body." Such a definition is not subject to objective observation. Thus it is not within the province of theology to determine the medical indications of death and the onset of the dying process. However, in reference to the terminally ill person, certain distinctions can be made. Physical life is generally understood to imply the ability of the person to sustain his or her vital activities. Physical death begins when interrelated systems of the body begin to break down. Death occurs when the systemic breakdown becomes irreversible. It may well be that physical life and death are events in a continuum in which it is impossible to discern when the dying process actually begins. Nevertheless, the bias of the Church and the traditional bias of the medical practitioner (cf. Oath of Hippocrates) is to do everything possible to maintain life and hinder the onset of dying and death. The medical use of drugs, surgical operations, and even artificial organs (mechanical kidneys, lungs, hearts, etc.) are considered legitimately used when there is a reasonable expectation that they will aid the return in due time to normal or close to normal functioning of the whole organic system.

The special case arises in that it is now medically possible to keep the body "alive" with a complex array of artificial organs, medications, transfusions, and the like. Under these conditions it may not be feasible to expect, with any degree of probability, the restoration of the organic functioning of the body. When, especially, there is no evidence of brain activity in conjunction with the systemic breakdown, we can safely say that the patient is no longer alive in any religiously significant way, and that, in fact, only certain organs are functioning. In such a case there is no moral responsibility to continue the use of artificial means. It is of interest that the Prayerbook of the Eastern Orthodox Church includes a whole service devoted to those in the process of dying. In the case of the individual whose death is prolonged and attended by much "struggling to die," the key sentence in the prayer calls upon God to separate the soul from the body, thus giving rest to the dying person. It asks God "to release your servant (name) from this unbearable suffering and this continuing bitter illness and grant rest to him" (*Mikron Euchologion*, p. 192).

However, it must be emphasized that this is a prayer directed to God, who, for the Orthodox, has ultimate dominion over life and death. Consequently, the preceding discussion in no way supports the practice of euthanasia. Euthanasia is held by some to be morally justified and/or morally required to terminate the life of an incurably sick person. To permit a dying person to die, when there is no real expectation that life can sustain itself, and even to pray to the Author of Life to take the life of one "struggling to die" is one thing; euthanasia is another, i.e., the active intervention to terminate the life of another. Orthodox Christian ethics rejects the alternative of the willful termination of dying patients, regarding it as a special case of murder if done without the knowledge and consent of the patient, and suicide if it is permitted by the patient (Antoniades, II, pp. 125–127). One of the most serious criticisms of euthanasia is the grave difficulty in drawing the line between "bearable suffering" and "unbearable suffering," especially from an Eastern Orthodox perspective, which has taken seriously the spiritual growth that may take place through suffering (Rom. 8:17–39).

Ethical decision making is never precise and absolute. The principles that govern it are in a measure fluid and subject to interpretation. But to elevate euthanasia to a right or an obligation would bring it into direct conflict with the fundamental ethical affirmation that as human beings we are custodians of life, which comes from a source other than ourselves. Furthermore, the immense possibilities, not only for error but also for decision making based on self-serving ends, which may disregard the fundamental principle of the sanctity of human life, argue against euthanasia.

Generally speaking, the Orthodox Church teaches that it is the duty of both physician and family to make the patient as comfortable as possible, to provide the opportunity for the exercise of patience, courage, repentance, and prayer. The Church has always rejected inflicted and unnecessary voluntary suffering and pain as immoral; but at the same time, the Church also has perceived in suffering a positive value that often goes unrecognized in the "logic of the world."

The only "eu-thanasia" (Greek for "a good death") recognized in Orthodox ethics is that death in which the human person accepts the end of his or her life in the spirit of moral and spiritual purity, in hope and trust in God, and as a member of his kingdom. True humanity may be achieved even on a deathbed.

The transmission of life. Orthodox Christian ethical thought considers that the transmission of human life is no less a fundamental responsibility of mankind than its protection. The Church sees this aspect of its concern as the divinely chosen means by which human beings contribute cooperatively in God's creative work. The transmission of human life is thus a holy and sacred moral responsibility. This responsibility is a generally human one and is taken up, sanctified, and made a part of the corporate life of the body of Christ in the Sacrament of Holy Matrimony. Though not the only purpose of marriage, the transmission of human life is an important duty and moral responsibility. This is readily seen in the fact that if each and every person now alive failed to contribute to the transmission of human life, it would be only a matter of time until human life would be extinguished from the face of the earth. The divine injunction "to be fruitful and multiply" (Genesis 1:28) is a fundamental moral imperative in the teaching of the Orthodox Christian Church. It is within this larger framework that we approach the specific issues of human sexuality, fertility control, population, artificial insemination, in vitro fertilization, and genetic screening and counseling.

Human sexuality. The Church teaches that human sexuality is a divinely given dimension of human life that finds its fulfillment in the marital relationship. This is also supported by empirical observation, for at their very biological basis, sexual differences clearly exist for reproductive purposes. Because of the fact that human reproduction requires a long period of time for the newly born child to achieve a level of development permitting physical self-care, and increasingly long periods for social, educational, emotional, and economic maturity, the human race long ago recognized the need for some kind of permanent relationship of the sexes for the purpose of serving the reproductive purpose. That permanent relationship is marriage.

However, the purpose of marriage is not limited or restricted to this aspect alone. The purposes of marriage and their ranking in importance are a point of difference among Orthodox authorities (both patristic and contemporary), but scriptural and patristic evidence argue for at least four purposes for marriage, without ranking them in order of primacy: (1) the birth and care of children, (2) the mutual aid of the couple, (3) the satisfaction of the sexual drive, (4) growth in mutuality and oneness, i.e., love. In the mixture of these purposes, the whole purpose of human sexuality is fulfilled and completed, ethically and humanly (Constantelos, 1975).

Ethical corollaries of this position are: (1) all the dimensions of human sexuality are properly fulfilled in marriage, and the married have the moral obligation to seek the enrichment and fulfillment of their marriage in all of its aspects, as indicated above; (2) premarital sexual relations between unmarried persons are sinful and as such are labeled fornication; (3) sexual relations between two persons, at least one of whom is married to a third person, are morally evil and as such are labeled adultery; (4) sexual relations between persons for payment is sinful and is labeled prostitution; (5) sexual relations between brothers and sisters, parents and children, and other close relatives are morally wrong and as such are labeled incestuous; (6) sexual relations between persons of the same sex are immoral and as such are labeled as acts of homosexuality in the case of males, and lesbianism in the case of females; (7) sexual relations between a human being and animals are condemned as immoral, being labeled acts of bestiality; (8) autoerotic activity is adjudged as an improper expression of human sexuality, and as such is labeled masturbation.

Fertility control. Fertility control, or contraception, is the practice by which mechanical, chemical, or other means are used, either before or after a sexual act, in order to prevent fertilization of the ovum by the sperm, thus circum-

venting the possible consequences of the sexual act—the conception and ultimate birth of a child.

General agreement exists among Orthodox writers on the following two points: (1) since at least one of the purposes of marriage is the birth of children, a couple acts immorally when it consistently uses contraceptive methods to avoid the birth of any children, if there are not extenuating circumstances; (2) contraception is also immoral when used to encourage the practice of fornication and adultery.

Less agreement exists among Eastern Orthodox authors on the issue of contraception within marriage for the spacing of children or for the limitation of the number of children. Some authors take a negative view and count any use of contraceptive methods within or outside of marriage as immoral (Papacostas, pp. 13–18; Gabriel Dionysiatou). These authors tend to emphasize as the primary and almost exclusive purpose of marriage the birth of children and their upbringing. They tend to consider any other exercise of the sexual function as the submission of this holy act to unworthy purposes, i.e., pleasure-seeking, passion, and bodily gratification, which are held to be inappropriate for the Christian growing in spiritual perfection. These teachers hold that the only alternative is sexual abstinence in marriage, which, though difficult, is both desirable and possible through the aid of the grace of God. It must be noted also that, for these writers, abortion and contraception are closely tied together, and often little or no distinction is made between the two. Further, it is hard to discern in their writings any difference in judgment between those who use contraceptive methods so as to have no children and those who use them to space and limit the number of children.

Other Orthodox writers have challenged this view by seriously questioning the Orthodoxy of the exclusive and all-controlling role of the procreative purpose of marriage (Zaphiris; Constantelos, 1975). Some note the inconsistency of the advocacy of sexual continence in marriage with the scriptural teaching that one of the purposes of marriage is to permit the ethical fulfillment of sexual drives, so as to avoid fornication and adultery (1 Cor. 7:1–7). Most authors, however, emphasize the sacramental nature of marriage and its place within the framework of Christian anthropology, seeing the sexual relationship of husband and wife as one aspect of the mutual growth of the couple in love and unity. This approach readily adapts itself to an ethical position that would not only permit but also enjoin sexual relationships of husband and wife for their own sake as expressions of mutual love. Such a view clearly would support the use of contraceptive practices for the purpose of spacing and limiting children so as to permit greater freedom of the couple in the expression of their mutual love.

Population. There would appear to be a direct contradiction between the ethical imperative to "be fruitful and multiply" and the need to respond ethically to the "population explosion."

Those few Orthodox writers who have addressed themselves to this question ask if the issue is not so much a question of population as it is one of the fair and just distribution of the world's resources. (Papacostas; Gabriel Dionysiatou; Evdokimov, pp. 163–174). However, in the light of strong evidence that food and mineral resources are limited, population control is, without question, of ethical significance. This is not necessarily in conflict with the Orthodox teaching on marriage. Of interest in this instance is a fourth-century quotation from St. John Chrysostom, made in reference to the purpose of marriage, which the saint considered to be primarily the satisfaction of the sexual drive:

It was for two reasons that marriage was introduced; so that we may live in chastity [*sophrosyne*] and so that we might become parents. Of these the most important reason is chastity . . . especially today when the whole inhabited world [*he oikoumene*] is full of our race [John Chrysostom].

If overpopulation in the saint's eyes was a fact of the fourth century providing an argument to support his views on marriage, it implies that today the fact of overpopulation continues to have ethical significance. If it is true that humanity has in fact been obedient to the divine command and has been "fruitful" and has "multiplied" and has "filled the earth" (Gen. 1:28), then it would appear that this has ethical significance.

Thus, it seems valid to raise the question, within the context of Orthodox ethics, of the appropriate means of population control. Orthodox ethics disapproves of any means of population control that would violate and coerce the individual couple's choice regarding their obligation to procreate. It opposes the use of those means on a large scale that it opposes in individual cases, i.e., abortion. Those Orthodox teachers who oppose contraceptive practices of any nature, when faced with the facts of population pressures, are placed in the position of proposing widespread abstinence from sexual relations by huge numbers of people. Those who hold to the legitimacy of a reasonable use of contraceptives within marriages that have produced some offspring are prepared to accept the need and propriety of population control through educational methods, encouraging smaller families through contraceptive methods. All Orthodox ethicists, however, would hold that respect for the freedom of each couple to decide must be considered an important and significant factor of population control policy.

Artificial insemination. For obvious reasons, artificial insemination of unmarried women, or of married women without the consent and cooperation of the husband, is rejected by the Orthodox, in the first instance as a form of fornication, and in the second as duplicity and a form of adultery (Galanopoulos, pp. 455–456). What of the cases in which the husband gives his permission or urges the procedure upon his wife? In this situation, when a donor's semen is used, Orthodox ethicists readily view it as the intrusion of a third person into the sacred marital relationship and reject it as a form of adultery not ethically appropriate. In the instances in which the couple is not able to bear their own children, the other purposes of marriage remain in effect, and the marriage of the couple continues to be both valid and fulfilling. Such a couple may decide to adopt children.

In the case of insemination with the husband's sperm (AIH), there are differing opinions. Some ethicists hold that AIH is also improper because the child is not conceived as a result of natural sexual intercourse (Constantinides). This position, however, does not prohibit medical treatment of the husband for the correction of some medical defect that may be the cause of the failure to achieve conception. This view is countered by the consideration that the integrity of the marital relationship is not attacked by AIH. Rather, one of its main purposes is permitted to be fulfilled. It is questionable if the ethical argumentation connecting AIH with the requirement for the physical act of sexual intercourse is drawn from Eastern Orthodox sources.

Orthodox writers have not dealt with artificial inovulation and in vitro fertilization procedures.

It would seem consistent, though, to hold that, so long as the sperm and ovum are those of the husband and wife, and the wife carried the child to term, such procedures would not in themselves be objectionable. However, egg grafts from anonymous donors and the transplantation of a fertilized ovum to a foster mother who would then carry the conceptus to term would attack the integrity of the marriage and the mother-child relationship.

Another topic that has received little treatment from Orthodox writers is sterilization: vasectomy in the case of the male and tubal ligation in the case of the female. It would appear that the irreversible character of these procedures would cause most Orthodox to see them as a violation of one of the purposes of marriage, though it is conceivable that some cases involving serious threat to the life of the wife might justify the procedures. Obviously, the use of the operation to permit promiscuous sexual living would be rejected out of hand by Orthodox ethicists (Zozos).

Genetic counseling and genetic screening. At first glance it may appear that the Eastern Orthodox Church has little or nothing to say on genetic counseling and screening. Yet genetic counseling, which seeks to provide information to prospective parents before a child is conceived, simply makes more precise that which the Church has sought to do through its canon law, which prohibits marriages between closely related persons (*The Rudder*, pp. 977–999). This ancient compendium of prohibitions to inbreeding clearly has its historical antecedents in the observation that genetic defects tend to multiply when inbreeding takes place. Consequently, it would appear that genetic counseling most appropriately should take place before marriage. It seems equally clear that for the Orthodox the option of abortion is not ethically appropriate when amniocentesis indicates some genetic deformation.

Genetic screening of whole groups or populations to determine carriers of genetic disease would also be encouraged by Orthodox ethics, so as to provide as much information as possible to persons before marriage. Ethical prudence would cause two persons who are carriers of the same genetic disease not to marry, thus avoiding the high probability that deformed children would be born to them.

In this way, what is more or less crudely effected through the Church's rules regarding prohibited marriages because of consanguinity would be accomplished more accurately through scientific genetic screening. In the same spirit, it would be possible to support legislation prohibiting marriage between two carriers of the same genetic disease, especially in the case of a disease that is widespread and a threat to the total human genetic pool.

Conclusion

The common denominator of all the issues discussed is the high regard and concern of the Church for human life as a gift of God. Orthodoxy tends to take a conservative approach to these issues, seeing in them a dimension of the holy and relating them to transcendent values and concerns. An intense respect for human life is needed to hold the reins upon those who would attack it. The human person, from the very moment of conception, is dependent upon others for life and sustenance. It is in the community of the living, especially as it relates to the source of life, God in Trinity, that life is conceived, nurtured, developed, and fulfilled. The trust we have in others for the continued well-being of our own lives forms a basis for generalization. Eastern Orthodox ethics, consequently, functions with a pro-life bias that honors and respects the life of each person as a divine gift, which requires development and enhancement.

STANLEY S. HARAKAS

[*For further discussion of topics mentioned in this article, see the entries:* ABORTION; CONTRACEPTION; DEATH AND DYING: EUTHANASIA AND SUSTAINING LIFE; DOUBLE EFFECT; ETHICS, *article on* THEOLOGICAL ETHICS; GENETIC DIAGNOSIS AND COUNSELING; GENETIC SCREENING; MENTAL HEALTH, *article on* RELIGION AND MENTAL HEALTH; MENTAL ILLNESS, *article on* CONCEPTIONS OF MENTAL ILLNESS; ORGAN TRANSPLANTATION, *article on* ETHICAL PRINCIPLES; POPULATION ETHICS: RELIGIOUS TRADITIONS, *article on* EASTERN ORTHODOX CHRISTIAN PERSPECTIVES; *and* SEXUAL ETHICS. *Also directly related are the entries* DEATH; EMBODIMENT; HUMAN EXPERIMENTATION; INFORMED CONSENT IN HUMAN RESEARCH; LIFE; NATURAL LAW; *and* RATIONING OF MEDICAL TREATMENT. *See also:* REPRODUCTIVE TECHNOLOGIES, *article on* ETHICAL ISSUES; *and* STERILIZATION, *article on* ETHICAL ASPECTS.]

BIBLIOGRAPHY

ANDROUSTOS, CHRISTOS. *Systema ethikes* [Ethical system]. 2d ed. Thessalonike, Greece: Basil Regopoulos Publishing House, 1964.

ANTONIADES, VASILEIOS. *Encheiridion kata Christon ethikes* [Handbook of Christian ethics]. Constantinople: Fazilet Press, 1927.

BASIL, SAINT; RALLE, G. A.; and POTLE, M. *Syntagma ieron kanonon* [Compendium of sacred canons]. Athens: Hartophylakos Press, 1854, vol. 4, pp. 88–294.

CONSTANTELOS, DEMETRIOS J. *Byzantine Philanthropy and Social Welfare.* New Brunswick, N.J.: Rutgers University Press, 1968.

————. *Marriage, Sexuality and Celibacy: A Greek Orthodox Perspective.* Minneapolis, Minn: Light and Life Publishing Co., 1975.

————. "Physician-Priests in the Medieval Greek Church." *Greek Orthodox Theological Review,* Winter 1966–1967, pp. 141–153.

CONSTANTINIDES, CHRYSOSTOM. "Technike gonimopoiesis kai theologia." [Artificial insemination and theology]. *Orthodoxia* 33 (1958): 66–79; and 34 (1959): 36–52.

DEMETROPOULOS, PANAGIOTES. *Orthodoxos Christianike ethike* [Orthodox Christian ethics]. Athens: 1970.

EVDOKIMOV [EVDOKIMOFF], PAUL. *Sacrement de l'amour: Le Mystère conjugal à la lumière de la tradition orthodoxe.* Paris: Éditions de l'Épi, 1962. Greek ed. *Mysterion tes agapes* [Mystery of love]. Translated by Serapheim Orphanos. Athens: 1967.

FAROS, PHILOTHEOS. "Mental Patients and Verbal Communication of the Religious Message." *Theologia* 42 (1971): 602–606.

FLOROVSKY, GEORGES. *Bible, Church, Tradition: An Eastern Orthodox View.* Belmont, Mass.: Nordland Publishing Co., 1972.

GABRIEL DIONYSIATOU. *Malthousianismos: To englema tes genoktonias* [Malthusianism: The crime of genocide]. Volos: Holy Mountain Library, 1957.

GALANOPOULOS, MELETIOS. *Systema ieras exomologetikes* [A study of penitential practice]. Athens: Orthodox Source Books, 1954.

HARAKAS, STANLEY S. "The Natural Law Teaching of the Eastern Orthodox Church." *Greek Orthodox Theological Review,* Winter 1963–1964, pp. 215–224.

————. "An Orthodox Christian Approach to the 'New Morality'." *Greek Orthodox Theological Review,* Spring 1970, pp. 107–139.

JOHN CHRYSOSTOM. "Eis to apostolikon reton: Dia de tas porneias ekastos ten heautou gynaika echeto" [On the words of the apostle: Concerning the fornication each has with his own wife]. *Patrologiae cursus completus: Series graeca* [*Patrologia Graeca*]. 161 vols. Paris: Apud Garnier Fratres, editores & J.-P. Migne successors, 1857–1894, vol. 51, cols. 207–218, at col. 213.

KOTSONIS, JEROME. "Fundamental Principles of Orthodox Morality." *The Orthodox Ethos: Studies in Orthodoxy.* Edited by A. J. Philippou. Oxford: Holywell Press, 1964.

MALONEY, GEORGE A. *Man, The Divine Icon: The Patristic Doctrine of Man Made According to the Image of God.* Pecos, N.M.: Dove Publications, 1973.

MANTZARIDES, GEORGE. *Christianike Ethike: University Lectures.* Thessalonike, Greece, 1975.

Mikron euchologion, e aghiasmatarion [Shorter prayer book]. Athens: Apostolike diakonia tes ekklesias tes Ellados, 1956.

PAPAKOSTAS, SERAPHEIM. *To zetema tes teknogonias: To demographikon problema apo Christianikes apopseos* [Question of the procreation of children: The demographic problem from a Christian viewpoint]. Athens: Brotherhood of Theologians "Zoe," 1933, 1947.

The Rudder. Translated by D. Cummings. Chicago: Orthodox Christian Educational Society, 1957.

WARE, TIMOTHY. *The Orthodox Church.* Baltimore: Penguin Books, 1972.

ZAPHIRIS, CHRYSOSTOM. "The Morality of Contraception: An Eastern Orthodox Opinion." *Journal of Ecumenical Studies* 11 (1974): 677–690.

ZOZOS, CONSTANTINE. "The Medical, Legal, and Moral Aspects of Sterilization." *Ekfrasis,* Spring 1974, pp. 33–54.

EASTERN ORTHODOX ETHICS
See EASTERN ORTHODOX CHRISTIANITY.

ECOLOGY
See ENVIRONMENT AND MAN; ENVIRONMENTAL ETHICS.

EDUCATION
See MEDICAL EDUCATION; MEDICAL ETHICS EDUCATION; NURSING; POPULATION POLICY PROPOSALS, *article on* POPULATION EDUCATION.

EGYPT
See MEDICAL ETHICS, HISTORY OF, *section on* NEAR AND MIDDLE EAST AND AFRICA, *articles on* ANCIENT NEAR EAST, CONTEMPORARY ARAB WORLD, *and* CONTEMPORARY MUSLIM PERSPECTIVE. *See also* ISLAM.

ELDERLY
See AGING AND THE AGED.

ELECTRICAL STIMULATION OF THE BRAIN

Concepts and principles underlying the ethical issues discussed in this entry can be found in the entry BEHAVIOR CONTROL.

Electrical stimulation of the brain (ESB) was developed primarily as a research technique with therapeutic potential. Stimulation of areas deep within the brain can contribute parts of a functional "map" by making it possible to correlate observed behavioral responses with specific brain sites. ESB is therapeutically valuable both in its own right and as a diagnostic procedure. It can, for example, be used to locate the precise point at which the neurosurgeon will make a therapeutic lesion in order to relieve a variety of symptoms.

The technique typically involves the introduction within cerebral tissue of fine metallic conductors, which are insulated except at their tips, and with terminals located outside the scalp for making connections with instrumentation, including transmitting and receiving equipment and quite possibly a computer for processing incoming signals and selecting appropriate signals for transmission to the brain.

State of the art

The modern era of experimental work was initiated by the discovery of the motivational effects of electrical stimulation and of its effectiveness as a conditioned stimulus. This development was facilitated technically by the development of stereotaxic surgery, by means of which depthelectrodes may be implanted deep in the brain with a very high degree of accuracy. The fine metallic conductors cause minimal and functionally undetectable damage to brain tissue. There is every indication that the conductors may remain in place indefinitely with no untoward effects. The problem of using cumbersome wiring between subject and instrumentation has been solved by development of miniaturized, multichannel radiostimulators, which may be implanted beneath the skin of the subject. ESB may now be administered in a variety of settings by remote control.

Clinical applications have been or are being developed for inhibition of epileptic seizures, sensory prostheses, and treatment of some types of psychopathology. ESB has already been used experimentally in primates to influence the following functions: motor activity, food intake, aggressive behavior, maternal relations, sexual functions, motivation, learning, anxiety, pleasure, and friendliness. ESB is clearly impressive as a behavior control technology, but it still leaves scientific problems unsolved and a large array of ethical issues to be considered.

Although ESB has established correlations between brain sites and behavioral functions, the details of the physiological response to ESB and the nature of the neural changes associated with the conditioning process are not well understood. ESB does not reveal the mode of action of a particular brain site, nor does it provide an integrated understanding of brain functions or of mediating processes in the brain at the time of stimulation.

Direct manipulation of the brain for purposes of controlling behavior raises serious questions for psychiatry. The nature of psychopathology, the relation between organic and functional concepts in the etiology of mental illness, and the choice of appropriate methods of treatment may all need revision in light of these new techniques. The relative simplicity and effectiveness of ESB may lead to its widespread use before its secondary and indirect effects on personality are well enough understood, and before social and ethical implications have been carefully considered.

Ethical issues

ESB presents ethical issues by virtue of its status as a major clinical procedure; because it must be considered an experimental rather than a standard therapy; because of its potential for placing the control of one's behavior in the hands of others who may or may not be of one's choosing, and for ends not necessarily one's own; and because it controls behavior by directly manipulating the brain.

So long as the procedure is requested or agreed to by a competent individual who understands the nature and consequences of the procedure and who elects the procedure for reasons that appear reasonable and medically justifiable, there need be only the assurance that the patient is well protected as a subject of human experimentation and that the patient is competent to give consent. In this ideal situation, however, all parties must still determine whether the risks are justified and whether the consent to those risks is both voluntary and informed.

It is in the nature of ESB that the ideal of the competent, rational patient may be difficult to fulfill, since it is precisely the organ of consent and reason which is "ill" or functioning improperly. Thus, the locus of decision and control is likely to shift radically to others, and with this shift the dangers of control by others must be taken into account. What criteria of normalcy are employed in diagnosing behavioral dysfunction; and what behavior is to be controlled? Who will make these decisions, and to what extent are the controllers accountable to the patient, his representatives, and the public?

One must weigh the costs and benefits of ESB relative to other modes of treatment or to no treatment at all. Should one alter the brain directly or the environment in order to change behavior? If treatment is imposed on the patient by others can this intrusion on the patient's freedom and dignity be balanced by the expansion of freedom and self-control to be gained as a result of treatment? If treatment were to be undertaken not in the individual's best interests but to protect society (as in the case of an assaultive prisoner), does the gain in protection of others warrant the denial of the freedom and dignity of the person who is subjected to the treatment? How best may these decisions regarding legitimacy and evaluation be made?

These questions take on special importance because they deal with the direct manipulation of the brain. No other organ is so intimately associated with our conceptions of personhood, identity, and self-control. The brain is the locus of mind and "agent" of behavior, and presumably modification of the brain will affect personality more than other kinds of manipulation. Thus the intrusiveness of ESB procedures may be a high cost to pay for the benefits. The very directness of ESB, the lack of mediation by consciousness, may have consequences for humans that ought to be avoided, if those consequences include a reductive, mechanistic, and manipulative image of man.

If ethical problems arise in the medical context, where relief of suffering is the object, and the expected benefits of ESB are therefore relatively easy to specify and widely perceived to be legitimate, how much more difficult it will be to decide whether and to what ends to use ESB to program the experiences and behavior of the well. The social history of psychotropic drugs is suggestive. The question remains of how best to weigh all considerations—the possible costs to personal dignity and individual liberty and the possible gains in happiness and knowledge.

JOEL MEISTER

[Directly related are the entries BEHAVIOR CONTROL; and MENTAL HEALTH THERAPIES. See also: INFORMED CONSENT IN MENTAL HEALTH; MENTAL HEALTH, article on MENTAL HEALTH IN COMPETITION WITH OTHER VALUES; PERSON; and RESEARCH, BEHAVIORAL. For discussion of related ideas, see the entries: ELECTROCONVULSIVE THERAPY; PSYCHOPHARMACOLOGY; and PSYCHOSURGERY.]

BIBLIOGRAPHY

COOPER, I. S.; CRIGHEL, E.; and AMIN, I. "Clinical and Physiological Effects of Stimulation of the Paleocerebellum in Humans." Journal of the American Geriatrics Society 21 (1973): 40–43.

DELGADO, JOSÉ M. R. Evolution of Physical Control of the Brain. New York: American Museum of Natural History, 1965.

———; MARK, V.; SWEET, W.; ERVIN, F.; WEISS, A.; BACH-Y-RITA, A.; and HAGIWARA, R. "Intracerebral Radio Stimulation and Recording in Completely Free Patients." Journal of Nervous and Mental Disease 147 (1968): 329–340.

———; ROBERTS, W. W.; and MILLER, N. E. "Learning Motivated by Electrical Stimulation of the Brain." American Journal of Physiology 179 (1954): 587–593.

ERVIN, FRANK R.; MARK, VERNON H.; and STEVENS, JANICE. "Behavioral and Affective Responses to Brain Stimulation in Man." Neurobiological Aspects of Psychopathology. Edited by Joseph Zubin and Charles Shagass. New York: Grune & Stratton, 1969, pp. 54–65.

GAYLIN, WILLARD; MEISTER, JOEL; and NEVILLE, ROBERT, eds. Operating on the Mind: The Psychosurgery Conflict. New York: Basic Books, 1975.

GILMAN, S.; AMIN, I.; and COOPER, I. S. "The Effect of Chronic Cerebellar Stimulation upon Epilepsy in Man." Transactions of the American Neurological Association 98 (1973): 192–196.

HEATH, R. G. "Electrical Self-Stimulation of the Brain in Man." American Journal of Psychiatry 120 (1963): 571–577.

INGRAHAM, BARTON L., and SMITH, GERALD W. "The Use of Electronics on the Observation and Control of Human Behavior and Its Possible Use in Rehabilitation and Parole." Issues in Criminology 7, no. 2 (1972), pp. 35–53.

LONG, DONLIN M. "Electrical Stimulation for Relief of Pain From Chronic Nerve Injury." Journal of Neurosurgery 38 (1973): 718–722.

MARK, VERNON H. "The Relief of Chronic Severe Pain by Stereotactic Surgery." Pain and the Neurosurgeon: A Forty Years' Experience. Edited by J. C. White and W. H. Sweet. Springfield, Ill.: Charles C Thomas, 1969, pp. 843–887.

———, and ERVIN, FRANK R. Violence and the Brain. New York: Harper & Row, 1970.

NEVILLE, ROBERT. "Zalmoxis, or The Morals of ESB and Psychosurgery." Gaylin, Operating on the Mind, pp. 87–116.

OLDS, JAMES, and MILNER, PETER. "Positive Reinforcement Produced by Electrical Stimulation of Septal Area and Other Regions of Rat Brain." Journal of Comparative and Physiological Psychology 47 (1954): 419–427.

"Physical Manipulation of the Brain." Hastings Center Report, special supp., May 1973.

SCHWITZGEBEL, ROBERT, and SCHWITZGEBEL, RALPH K. Psychotechnology: Electronic Control of Mind and Behavior. New York: Holt, Rinehart & Winston, 1973.

SHEER, DANIEL E., ed. Electrical Stimulation of the Brain. Austin: University of Texas Press, 1961.

VALENSTEIN, ELIOT S. Brain Control: A Critical Examination of Brain Stimulation and Psychosurgery. New York: Wiley-Interscience, 1973.

VAUGHAN, HERBERT G., JR. "Some Reflections on Stimulation of the Human Brain." Neurobiological Aspects of Psychopathology. Edited by Joseph Zubin and Charles Shagass. New York: Grune & Stratton, 1969, pp. 66–77.

ZUCKER, MITCHELL H. Electronic Circuits for the Behavioral and Biomedical Sciences. San Francisco: W. H. Freeman, 1969.

ELECTROCONVULSIVE THERAPY

Concepts and principles underlying the ethical issues discussed in this entry can be found in the entry BEHAVIOR CONTROL.

Nature and effect of the treatment

Electroconvulsive therapy (ECT) is a method of psychiatric treatment using an electric current to induce a convulsion. Much confusion has arisen over the years through the use of the misnomer "shock treatment" as synonymous with ECT. In fact, ECT has nothing to do with surgical or physiological shock (acute progressive circulatory failure), nor is it accompanied by "shock" in the usual psychological sense of the term.

The stimulus for the development of convulsive therapy was the ancient observation that some mental patients temporarily improved after a spontaneous seizure. Allied to this was the belief, now recognized as erroneous, that epilepsy and psychosis, particularly schizophrenia, never occurred together. In actuality, certain forms of epilepsy (temporal lobe) are often indistinguishable clinically from schizophrenia, while certain types of schizophrenic psychoses are thought to form a continuum with epilepsy, the so-called borderlands of epilepsy.

In 1938 two Italian psychiatrists, Drs. U. Cerletti and L. Bini, first induced a convulsion in a patient by a simple electrical apparatus using an alternating current (Cerletti and Bini). Up until that time convulsions had been induced by the intravenous injection of a mixture of camphor and oil, or subsequently by the use of inhalants such as aliphatic fluorinated ethers, which were administered through a vaporizer to a completely anesthetized patient. Although still in use, inhalation-induced convulsions have been largely replaced by ECT.

Despite many modifications in technique since Cerletti and Bini, the basic method of ECT has changed very little. Electrodes are applied to one side of the head (unilateral ECT) or to both (bilateral ECT) temples. The patient is prepared with a muscle relaxant and anesthetized with a short-acting barbiturate. The electric current is then applied for 0.1 to 0.5 seconds, resulting in a two-stage or tonic-clonic convulsion. (If the degree of muscle relaxation is sufficient the visible signs of convulsions—the tonic-clonic movements—may be entirely absent; an EEG recording, however, will demonstrate evidence of a cerebral seizure.) Afterward the patient regains consciousness in five to ten minutes but remains lethargic and mildly confused from anywhere from fifteen minutes to an hour (Kalinowsky and Hippius).

The number of treatments given during a course of ECT varies from patient to patient and from psychiatrist to psychiatrist, but in general two or three a week for a period of two to four weeks is standard, varying with diagnosis and age of patient. Although originally used for inpatients, it is now frequently given on an outpatient basis, with the patient returning home a few hours after the ECT.

The safety of ECT appears to be reasonably well established with only brain tumors serving as absolute contraindications. Relative contraindications include coronary artery disease or a recent heart attack. Nor does age seem to be a limiting factor in its use since elderly patients have undergone courses of ECT without adverse reactions. In all age groups, however, there is a transient loss of memory that varies with the age of the patient, the number of treatments received, and the method (unilateral ECT causes less memory impairment than does bilateral ECT) (Squire and Chace; Harper and Wiens). Innovations and techniques such as the administration of high concentrates of oxygen or the use of unilateral electrodes have lessened the memory loss considerably (Harper and Wiens).

Originally introduced as a treatment for schizophrenia, ECT is now generally recognized as more effective in the treatment of affect or mood disorders, particularly depression. The indications for its use are involutional depression, psychotic depression, and the depressive phase of manic–depressive psychosis. Although more controversial, its use has been advocated by some in the control of mania and certain forms of acute schizophrenia (acute catatonic excitement). Its value in behavior or personality disorders as well as neurosis has not been established. Its foremost indication remains the imminent probability of suicide. Data exist, however, to indicate that ECT can decrease the mortality of depression quite apart from any consideration of suicide. The total morbidity for depression is not limited to suicide but includes death from infection, malnutrition, and cardiovascular problems (Avery and Winokur).

Bioethical problems associated with ECT

The bioethical issues associated with ECT are similar to those involving psychosurgery and certain forms of drug treatment.

The consent issue. In most instances patients referred for ECT have severe restrictions on the consent process secondary to their illness, which is usually depression, often of a psychotic degree. Since the patient's decision-making powers are affected and other persons often decide on the use of ECT, the treatment demands little in the form of a therapeutic alliance. The patient consequently is "objectified" and "controlled" rather than persuaded to be a willing participant in the treatment. The same, however, could be said of any alternative treatment.

The question of brain damage. Most authorities state that ECT is not associated with permanent changes in brain tissue. In addition there are no autopsy findings that prove ECT causes "brain damage." Despite this, it is the impression of many clinicians that frequent and extended courses of ECT result in a blunted or "burnt out" personality. Since depression is a self-limiting illness whose natural history, at least for any acute episode, is toward improvement or suicide, the question of risk versus benefit assumes critical proportions. The resolution of this important therapeutic and ethical dilemma must await further studies of the basic pathophysiology of natural and induced seizure states, and of depressive illnesses.

Unpleasant psychological effects. It has been recognized for years that patients often demonstrate fears regarding ECT that seem out of proportion to the treatment risks (Kalinowsky and Hippius). These "psychopathological phenomena" can be quite disabling and difficult to manage although they usually terminate after the beginning of the treatment. When present, however, such phenomena greatly complicate the consent issue since the patient may, as a result of these fears, reject ECT on grounds that may appear "unreasonable" to the treating psychiatrist, thus leading to further manipulation and control.

The empiricism of ECT. Despite an impressive body of knowledge on the electrochemical and physiological accompaniments of ECT, the treatment remains largely an empirical one, similar to all treatments for illnesses of unknown etiology. Such a state of affairs is particularly unsatisfactory in behavior control technologies since the patient obviously cannot be adequately informed regarding all the implications of a treatment if the basis for the treatment's efficacy remains mysterious. It should be recalled, however, that ECT has been in use since 1938—a longer experience than we have had with either behavior or drug therapies—and that the patient can therefore be offered reasonable reassurance that treatment, when indicated, will be safe and free of known long-term permanent side effects. It remains to be seen whether or not more subtle consequences to nervous system functioning may be discovered.

Societal factors in the use of ECT. There are indications that in at least one state (Massachusetts) ECT is overutilized in private psychiatric hospitals, while the treatment is underutilized in public state mental hospitals (Dietz). Although the exact reason for the disparity in its use is controversial, it may be at least partly due to economic considerations: ECT is covered by many private health insurance policies. Most of the inmates of private psychiatric hospitals have some form of private health insurance, whereas public mental hospital patients rarely possess private insurance. There is also the question of the availability of anesthetists or anesthesiologists, who are more available for financial reasons at private rather than state hospitals. (There are no rigid requirements that ECT be administered with an anesthetist present, but such an arrangement is frequent enough to constitute "standard medical practice.")

An additional bioethical problem under the "societal factors" heading is the use of ECT to accelerate recovery from depression. If a depressed patient is protected from suicide he eventually will recover; with the use of selective antidepressant drugs he will recover more quickly; finally, improvement may be further accelerated in certain selected cases with the use of ECT. It is not unusual, therefore, in private psychiatric facilities for "productive" or "creative" individuals to receive ECT so that they may sooner resume busy professional careers. This poses an ethical problem of considerable magnitude if depression is considered to be at least partly the result of environmental circumstances, in addition to biological bases and perhaps even genetic predisposition. Is the ECT serving to return a patient to a professional or social situation that is responsible for the development of his depression in the first place?

Conclusion

The bioethical issues raised by ECT are of overriding importance in the light of the treatment's proven effectiveness when intelligently applied. The storm of controversy accompanying its use has led some to advocate its discontinuation altogether. This is surely an over-reaction: ECT as a treatment procedure has great potential either for therapeutic benefit or for abuse. Specific challenges include a greater understanding of the physiological mechanisms underlying its effectiveness and increased integration with other treatment methods leading to greater cooperation between the patient and the treating physician.

RICHARD M. RESTAK

[*Directly related are the entries* BEHAVIOR CONTROL; *and* MENTAL HEALTH THERAPIES. *For discussion of related ideas, see the entries:* ELECTRICAL STIMULATION OF THE BRAIN; PSYCHOPHARMACOLOGY; *and* PSYCHOSURGERY. *Other relevant material may be found under* GENETIC ASPECTS OF HUMAN BEHAVIOR, *article on* GENETICS AND MENTAL DISORDERS; INFORMED CONSENT IN MENTAL HEALTH; *and* MENTAL HEALTH SERVICES, *article on* SOCIAL INSTITUTIONS OF MENTAL HEALTH.]

BIBLIOGRAPHY

ABRAMS, RICHARD. "Recent Clinical Studies of ECT." *Seminars in Psychiatry* 4 (1972): 3–12.

AVERY, DAVID, and WINOKUR, GEORGE. "Mortality in Depressed Patients Treated with Electroconvulsive Therapy and Anti-Depressants." *Archives of General Psychiatry* 33 (1976): 1029–1037.

BLACHLEY, P. H., and GOWING, D. "Multiple Monitored Electro-convulsive Treatment." *Comprehensive Psychiatry* 7 (1966): 100–109.

CERLETTI, U., and BINI, L. "L'Elettroshock." *Archives of General Neurology, Psychiatry and Psychoanalysis* 19 (1938): 266–268.

CRONHOLM, BORJE, and OTTOSSON, JAN-OTTO. "The Experience of Memory Function after Electroconvulsive Therapy." *British Journal of Psychiatry* 109 (1963): 251 ff. Special issue.

DIETZ, JEAN. "ECT Study Reveals Disparity between Public, Private Units." *Psychiatric News* 10, no. 15 (1975), pp. 1, 14–15.

ESSMAN, WALTER B. "Neurochemical Changes in ECS and ECT." *Seminars in Psychiatry* 4 (1972): 67–79.

FINK, MAX. "The Mode of Action of Convulsive Therapy: The Neurophysiologic-Adaptive View." *Journal of Neuropsychiatry* 3 (1962): 231–233.

————. "The Therapeutic Process in ECT." *Seminars in Psychiatry* 4 (1972): 39–46.

FURLONG, F. W. "The Mythology of Electroconvulsive Therapy." *Comprehensive Psychiatry* 13 (1972): 235–239.

GIAMARTINO, GARY A. "Electroconvulsive Therapy and the Illusion of Treatment." *Psychological Reports* 35 (1974): 1127–1131.

HARPER, ROBERT G., and WIENS, ARTHUR N. "Electroconvulsive Therapy and Memory." *Journal of Nervous and Mental Disease* 161, no. 4 (1975), pp. 245–254.

HURWITZ, THOMAS D. "Electroconvulsive Therapy: A Review." *Comprehensive Psychiatry* 15 (1974): 303–314.

KALINOWSKY, LOTHAR B. "The Convulsive Therapies." *Comprehensive Textbook of Psychiatry*. 2d ed. Edited by Alfred M. Freedman, Harold I. Kaplan, and Benjamin J. Sadock. Baltimore: Williams & Wilkins, 1975, vol. 2, pp. 1969–1976.

————, and HIPPIUS, HANS. *Pharmacological, Convulsive, and Other Somatic Treatments in Psychiatry.* New York: Grune & Stratton, 1969.

SQUIRE, LARRY R., and CHACE, PAUL M. "Memory Functions Six to Nine Months after Electroconvulsive Therapy." *Archives of General Psychiatry* 32 (1975): 1557–1564.

VOLAVKA, JAN. "Neurophysiology of ECT." *Seminars in Psychiatry* 4 (1972): 55–65.

EMBODIMENT

For a discussion of an important parallel topic basic to many ethical issues in bioethics, see the entry MIND–BODY PROBLEM.

"Embodiment" as used herein designates a specific phenomenon inherent to human life and experience which, although touched upon periodically in the history of thought, has been studied only in recent times as a focal issue. As thus used, embodiment refers to a distinctively different range of issues from those traditionally associated with the "mind–body" problem. One way to make this difference prominent would be to point out that, whether or not what has been called "mind" is or is not ultimately or metaphysically explainable by or reducible to "body," or vice versa, persons nevertheless experience their own bodies in specific ways which can be studied as such. Embodiment as a philosophical and bioethical phenomenon designates a fundamentally different range of issues from those entailed in any of the variety of positions adopted as regards the so-called mind–body problem.

Perhaps a better way of eliciting this phenomenon would be to note one striking peculiarity of Descartes's (1596–1650) efforts. On the one hand, he argued that mind (*res cogitans*) and matter (*res extensa*) are "substances": mutually exclusive, self-subsistent, and ontologically distinct entities, neither of which requires the other *to be* or to be *known*. This metaphysical bifurcation of reality (dualism) led Descartes to the view that, somehow, mind and body "interact," although specifying that "somehow" proved to be inordinately difficult if not impossible. However that may be, his reflections on the mind–body complex, *especially in his own case*, showed him that, as he put it, the mind is not "in" the body in the way a boatman is "in" a boat—that is, not contingently or accidentally. To the contrary, he discovered and reiterated often (Descartes, vol. 1, pp. 118, 255, 345, and *passim*), my mind is "intimately" connected to my body, and this "intimate union" itself constitutes a major problem. The difficulty he faced was, in one sense, that his metaphysical view could not provide the grounds for understanding that "intimacy": if everything must be *either* mind *or* body and nothing can be both, how can the one be "united" or "interact" with the other? In another sense, the difficulty is, as Gilbert Ryle pointed out (p. 22), that Descartes's efforts incorporate a "category mistake." Both "interactionists" and "reductivists" are guilty of the "dogma of the ghost in the machine": Since "the phrase 'there occur mental processes' does not mean the same sort of thing as 'there occur physical processes,' . . . it makes no sense to conjoin or disjoin the two" (ibid.).

Correct in its way though Ryle's point is, it raises very much the same problem, since he wants to say that "one and the same activity" (e.g., raising my arm) can be described and explained in more than one way (ibid., pp. 50–51). This, however, leaves obscure how logically *different* order statements can yet pertain to "one and the same thing."

More important, such an argument in effect obfuscates Descartes's insight—which is genuine, however much he and others tended to confuse it: *that one does in truth experience one's own body* as profoundly "intimate." The problem is that one must be able to account for this sense of "intimacy." Several philosophers immediately after Descartes saw this issue, and thereby pointed the way to the phenomenon of embodiment. Blaise Pascal (1623–1662) noted with marked irony that if one, like Descartes, composes all things of mind and body, surely that mixture would itself be intelligible. Yet, he insisted, not only do we not understand the body, and even less the mind, least of all do we know "how a body could be united to a mind. This is the consummation of [our] difficulties, and yet it is [our] very being" (Pascal, pp. 27–28). That is, whether or not there are two, or more, substances in reality, and however one may try to explain them, that we are *both* mind *and* body and do not comprehend their "intimate union," is thus "[our] very being." It is this "intimacy" which calls for attention, regardless of one's particular metaphysical point of view on mind and matter.

Benedict de Spinoza (1631–1677) saw, too, that Descartes's bifurcation created insuperable difficulties in understanding that union. While he focused his principal argument in metaphysical terms (arguing that neither mind nor matter could possibly be genuine "substances," but only the "attributes" of the one unitary substance which is reality itself), Spinoza nevertheless saw the importance of accounting for what Descartes had identified merely as a "union." Both mind and body are essential to one another, for Spinoza, and he came to conceive the one, body, as mirrored in the other, mind, as its "idea" (Spinoza, pp. 82–107). Although, to be sure, Spinoza's theory is far more complex, the point of major emphasis here is that by rejecting the Cartesian dualism he was enabled to come to a clearer understanding of that very "intimate union" which had impressed Descartes.

But it was not until relatively recently, in the early writings of Henri Bergson (1859–1941), that this sense of intimacy became a specifically focal issue on its own (although, it is true, Bergson did not fully explore this insight). The human body itself must be viewed as that whereby any person has a locus, a placement, in the world, and this is a unique and *sui generis* phenomenon (Bergson, pp. 11, 14–16, 57). What makes the body not simply an object like other objects in the world (that is, its "intimacy") is that it is fundamentally *"mine."* Thus, although it is indeed physical, it is not simply that—for it is the only one uniquely singled out as *mine,* and as a "center." The field of physical objects and events is spatially organized around *my* body as its center of reference. In the second place, when my body is viewed as such it is clear that its functioning as center is not at all limited to such matters as spatial location—it is as well that by means of which I am able to engage in activities of any sort. Thus spatial location and the familiar sense-qualities pertaining to physical things are *never* experienced independently of specific contexts of *action.* My body is an "actional center." For the perceiver, things are not first of all conglomerations of data, and only later taken up into contexts of bodily action; even being aware of such sensa, where possible, requires highly specialized and technical means and equipment—i.e., specific contexts of specialized action are present even here. Perception is thus not a matter of "data reception" ("input") followed by "internal neural translation" and then by "externalization" ("output"). *For the perceiver,* "things" are "menacing," "helpful," "handy," "obstacles,"—in short are, as Piaget also recognized, experientially organized as "poles of action" (Piaget, chap. 1) appearing only in and through specific activities directed toward them. As such, "things" of all sorts are *essentially* tied to these actional contexts.

My body is thus uniquely singled out for, and experienced by, me as *mine* (i.e., as "intimate"). It is as well a "center," *that by means of which* I am in the world, in the midst of objects, people, language, culture, etc., and is that by means of which the surrounding milieu is presented to me for my thought and action. These points, which had impressed Bergson, turn out to be fundamental to the phenomenon of embodiment, and are crucial for understanding the subsequent discussions of it.

As Edmund Husserl (1859–1938) showed in his many writings, the primary phenomenon is the experiential relation of consciousness to its own embodying organism (Husserl, 1950, pp. 130–131). Granted that *this* organism is uniquely singled out (Husserl, 1959, p. 97), the problem of embodiment is to determine in *what sense* this organism is "mine" or *how it becomes experienced* as "mine," and thus enables the experiencing of surrounding things (ibid., pp. 60–61).

What had so impressed and troubled Descartes—the "intimate union"—Husserl calls the experiential relation to the body as mine. But it was just this that Descartes and many others following him had obscured in the interest of trying to resolve the very different metaphysical question concerning the "mind–body" relation. It is to the embodiment phenomenon that Gabriel Marcel's analysis of the fundamental opacity at the heart of personal experience, my *body-qua-mine*, is addressed (Marcel, 1940, p. 40); it is here that Maurice Merleau-Ponty locates an essential ambiguity intrinsic to the body itself (Merleau-Ponty, 1962, pp. 237 ff., 269 ff., 350 f.). So "intimate" is this "union" that one is tempted to say, with Jean-Paul Sartre, "I *am* my body" (Sartre, pp. 368–427). So profound is the experiential connection to my animate organism that it is necessary to say that there *are* no other things in the world, no experienced world at all, except on condition of my having this body experienced by me as mine (Straus, 1966, pp. 38–58, 137–165). Thus, the sense in which things "belong" to me is a sense ultimately derived from the ways in which I experience my own body as "belonging" to me; the latter is the condition for the former (Marcel, 1935, pp. 223–225). This phenomenon becomes especially manifest in instances where mental disturbances occur, and the sense of "mineness" becomes severely compromised, or never develops (Bosch, pp. 61–112).

One central problem is this: In virtue of what is this one animate organism uniquely singled out for and in my experience? Which specific experiences are there, without which this organism would cease to be experienced by me as mine, or which give it its sense as mine (Straus, 1958)?

The issue is by no means a settled one (Zaner, 1964, pp. 198–261) but is exceedingly complex and subtle. In one way or another, however, it seems generally agreed that the animate organism becomes and remains an embodying organism solely to the extent that (1) it is not just a body (*Körper*) but an animate organism (*Leibkörper*), the sole object within which belong my own fields of sensation; (2) it is the only object "in" which I "rule and govern" immediately, within each of its "organs" and the total organism itself; (3) it enacts most immediately my "I can" (go, perceive, move, turn, grasp, and the like); (4) it is that "by means of which" I perceive and otherwise experience the field of objects in the world and thus is my access to the world and the focus of the world's actions on me; and (5) it is not only that whereby I experience other things, but is itself experienced by me at the same time as I experience other things (that is, the organism is essentially reflexively related to itself) (Husserl, 1959, p. 97).

In short, embodiment is fundamentally connected with various levels and modalities of bodily attitudes, stances, and movements (Buytendijk, pp. 238–275, 285–344, 401–488), personal striving or willing, and perceptual awareness of things. Solely to the extent that wishes, desires, advertences, movements, etc., are or can be actualized or embodied by means of corporeal kinaesthetic flow-patterns, which are functionally determinative of the several perceptual fields and of what appears therein, can one sensibly say that this organism is "uniquely singled out as 'mine.'" Processes of sensory "feeling" (coenesthetic, kinaesthetic, proprioceptive, etc.), elementary strivings (reaching, squinting, locomoting, etc.), and the consequent achievement of an actional/perceptual field of objects in the surrounding environs—all these, and doubtless still others, go to constitute the phenomenon of embodiment.

But it needs to be stressed that there is quite another dimension to this theme, to which surprisingly little attention has been devoted, but which turns out to be just as essential to embodiment. However tempting it is to say "I am my body" (as when, for example, someone strikes one in the face: "Don't hit *me!*" we say), many cases in psychopathology (Binswanger), literature, and even situations of daily life, show that the temptation is deceptive. The situation is far more complex, for the human self's relation to its own body is *not only one of "mineness" but also of radical "otherness."* However intimate and profound is the relation between me and my body, it is equally the case that this body is experienced as strange and alien, and in specific ways.

I *am* my body; but in another sense I am *not* my body—or *not just* that. Indeed, this otherness is so profound that we inevitably feel forced to qualify the "am": It is not identity, equality, or inclusion. It is "mine," but this means that I am in a way distanced from it, for otherwise there would be no sense to "belonging"; it would not be characterizable in any sense as "mine." So "close" is the union that the experience of my body's otherness can be psychically shattering (whether it be my body's happy obedience which I notice for the first time, or its hateful refusal to obey my desires to do something). So intimate is it that I have moments in which I genuinely feel "at one" with it. Yet, so other is it that there are times when I treat it as a mere thing *other than* me (for instance, obsessively stuffing it with food, or otherwise mistreating it; or as when I encounter it as "having a life of its own" to which I must willy-nilly attend—like it or not, "my" hair grows and must be trimmed for action in certain contexts, "my" hands cleaned, "my" bowels moved, "my" cold cured, and so on and on) (Zaner, 1966, pp. 85–87).

I find myself, in short, as a creature who is embodied by an animate organism whose connections to me (and I to it) *are themselves an experiential impasse*—an *aporia* in Plato's sense. Nothing so much as me my*self* is at once so utterly familiar and usual (Who else could I be?), yet so completely foreign and alien (Who, indeed, am I?). This unique complex, it seems, is not indicative of a mere inability to make up one's own mind, but is rather the disclosure of the essence of embodiment. And, what seems so distinctive is just this "mineness/otherness" dialectic which is the core of the human body-as-experienced (Engelhardt, pp. 28–60, 89–119, 130–168).

In these terms, to speak of embodiment is to speak of something *which I am,* and not something which can be placed over against me as a sort of object (*ob-jectum*). I am myself, as embodied, my own most fundamental problem, as Pascal had already perceived with remarkable insight. What is expressed by the "problem of embodiment" is precisely my *being as embodied* —i.e., the very context, setting, and meaning of human life itself. The self–body problem *is thus enacted* at every moment in the ongoing life of the human person.

Recognizing this embodiment/enactment contexture makes it possible to appreciate that the human body is essentially an *expressive* phenomenon. While the particular ways in which wishes, feelings, desires, strivings, and so on are expressed, doubtless vary from culture to culture, in the life of a particular individual to some extent, as well as historically, this does not deny but in fact goes to show that embodiment is expressive (Merleau-Ponty, pp. 174–199). Nor does the fact that people can and do dissemble and deceive themselves and others belie the expressiveness of the body; indeed, these are themselves expressive phenomena, however difficult it may be to discover and then to interpret them (Burrell and Hauerwas).

This expressiveness signifies that embodiment is essentially a *value phenomenon.* In simplest terms, precisely because this one specific organism is uniquely singled out as embodying me, and thus is most intimately "mine" (me-yet-not-me), whatever can happen to it happens to me. Though my body is that wherein I "rule and govern," I am as well subject to *its conditions.* Hence, it is fundamental to the experience of embodiment that "it matters" what can and does happen to my body. Its value character can also be made clear if one considers, quite apart from bioethical issues, what one thinks of someone who is "loose" with his or her body. Indeed, embodiment as "intimate union" seems clearly to lie at the heart of the prominent sense of "inviolability" of the person. Thus, too, is it more understandable that persons have a sense of their own "privacy" (i.e., with the basic desire to maintain one's *integrity,* as expressed in the traditional "principle of totality"), and that there are constraints felt as regards unwanted intrusions (as in psychosurgery) into the lived-body; that is, the life of the embodied person.

It is also clearer why current discussions of bioethical issues—abortion, psychosurgery, euthanasia, etc.—are so highly charged. On the one hand, medical practices (and much biomedical experimentation) are ways of intervening or intruding into that most intimate and integral of spheres—the embodied person. On the other hand, every person is embodied, enacts himself through that specific animate organism which is "his own" and is thus expressive of that very person. Bodily schemata, attitudes, movements, actions, as well as perceptual abilities are all value-modalities by which one articulates and expresses one's character, personality, habits, goals—in short, one's life as a totality.

From the perspective of embodiment, then, medical practice and biomedical research are planned or potential interventions into the sphere of intimacy—whether this sphere be only initial (as in infancy) or more developed. And, whether such interventions be mainly directed to the body or to the mind, all of them unavoidably have their impact on the other; that is, a person's *life as a whole* is necessarily affected. *Psyche* and *soma* are inextricably bound together as constituents of an integral context in all living humans (Zaner, 1975). So, because embodiment is necessarily expressive, and therefore a value phenomenon, *every medical intervention is by nature of the case ethical in character*—although this is obviously not in any way to settle the specific issues inherent to any specific intervention.

In these terms, attempting to settle such specific issues requires that the fundamentally ethical nature of any intervention be explicitly brought out and appreciated and, second, that the specific details of the particular case be determined as far as possible. That is to say, of course, that respect for the person—his/her values, goals, etc., in short, *integrity*—is not a value brought in extraneously, *but is inherent to the very nature of medical interchanges*. In different terms, an appreciation of embodiment as expressive and valuational *requires* respect for the perspective, concerns, values—integral, embodied life—of the patient himself. It might be added here that, in the event that adopting that point of view is not possible—as when one confronts an unconscious patient, e.g.,—the decision to intervene in ways which do not include the perspective of the patient requires *other* ethical grounds, and must thus be subject to critical assessment as such. Other exceptional cases can also be thought of—mental retardates,

neonates, etc.—but these, too, do not escape the requirement to respect the patient's integrity, though they do require special ways of taking it into account (e.g., consulting relatives) as well as the additional ethical issues for decision making.

Accordingly, every medical issue is not only *ethical* but highly *context-specific. There is thus no way of settling any bioethical issue in the abstract* (e.g., "Should a life-threatening tumor be removed at the cost of memory?" Or "Is it morally good to cure emotional disorders by cutting the brain?"). Every medical practice, no matter how trivial, is *to begin with* value-laden, which means that each one either explicitly or (most often) implicitly is expressive of some vision of what is or is thought to be morally good. As Hauerwas effectively argues, furthermore, moral notions are such that they *construe the world* in a certain way as opposed to other ways of construing it (Hauerwas). In addition, it is suggested here that the primary issue for bioethics—given the perspective of an embodied person, and recognizing that moral notions are neither simply descriptive nor simply normative—is to educe, to make explicit, the "ways of construing the world" found in ongoing medical interventions and patient-responses. Only subsequently does it become possible to make informed judgments about the particular context-specific practices and issues facing medicine. How one can come to such truly informed judgments is an obvious problem, but it is not within the scope of this article; it is hopefully enough to have delineated the phenomenon of embodiment, its expressive and value character, and the ethical nature of medicine itself—its incorporation of ethical notions in each of its practices, and the necessity of having to assess these in their own terms as such.

RICHARD M. ZANER

[*Directly related are the entries* MAN, IMAGES OF; MIND–BODY PROBLEM; *and* PERSON.]

BIBLIOGRAPHY

BERGSON, HENRI. *Matière et mémoire.* 54th ed. Paris: Presses Universitaires de France, 1953. Translated as *Matter and Memory* by Nancy Margaret Paul and W. Scott Palmer. London: G. Allen Unwin; New York: Humanities Press, 1970.

BINSWANGER, LUDWIG. "The Case of Ellen West." *Existence: A New Dimension in Psychiatry and Psychology.* Edited by Rollo May, Ernest Angel, and Henri F. Ellenberger. New York: Basic Books, 1958, pp. 237–364.

Bosch, Gerhard. *Infantile Autism*. Translated by D. Jordan and I. Jordan. New York: Springer-Verlag, 1970.

Burrell, David, and Hauerwas, Stanley. "Self-Deception and Autobiography: Theological and Ethical Reflections on Speer's *Inside the Third Reich*." *Journal of Religious Ethics* 2 (1974): 99–117.

Buytendijk, Frederik J. J. *Attitudes et mouvements: Étude fonctionelle du mouvement humain*. Paris: Desclée de Brouwer, 1957.

Descartes, Réne. *Philosophical Writings*, 2 vols. Translated by Elizabeth S. Haldane and G. R. T. Ross. New York: Dover Books, 1955. See especially "Discourse on Method," "Principles of Philosophy," and "Passions of the Soul" (all vol. 1).

Engelhardt, H. Tristram, Jr. *Mind–Body: A Categorial Relation*. The Hague: Martinus Nijhoff, 1973.

Gurwitsch, Aron. *Field of Consciousness*. Pittsburgh: Duquesne University Press, 1964.

Hauerwas, Stanley. "The Self as Story: Religion and Morality from the Agent's Perspective." *Journal of Religious Ethics* 1 (1973): 73–85.

Husserl, Edmund. *Erste Philosophie (1923/24)*. (*Husserliana*, vol. VIII.) Den Haag: Martinus Nijhoff, 1959. Pt. 2.

————. *Ideen zu einer reinen Phänomenologie und phänomenologischen Philosophie*. Vol. 1: *Allgemeine Einführung in die reine Phänomenologie (Husserliana*, vol. III). Vol. 2: *Phänomenologische Untersuchungen zur Konstitution (Husserliana*, vol. IV). Den Haag: Martinus Nijhoff, 1950, 1952. English paperback translation by W. R. Boyce Gibson as *Ideas*. New York: Macmillan, 1962.

Marcel, Gabriel. *Du refus à l'invocation*. Paris: Gallimard, 1940.

————. *Etre et avoir*. Paris: F. Aubier, 1935.

Merleau-Ponty, Maurice. *Phénoménologie de la perception*. Paris: Gallimard, 1945. Translated by Colin Smith as *Phenomenology of Perception*. Atlantic Highlands, N.J.: Humanities Press; London: Routledge & Kegan Paul, 1962.

Pascal, Blaise. *Pensées*. New York: Modern Library, 1941.

Piaget, Jean. *The Origins of Intelligence in Children*. Translated by Margaret Cook. New York: International Universities Press, 1952.

Ryle, Gilbert. *The Concept of Mind*. New York: Barnes & Noble, 1949.

Sartre, Jean-Paul. *L'Être et le néant*. Paris: Librairie Gallimard, 1943. Translated by Hazel E. Barnes as *Being and Nothingness*. Buffalo, N.Y.: Washington Square Press, 1966.

Spinoza, Benedict de. "Ethics." *Chief Works*. Translated by R. H. M. Elwes. New York: Dover Publications, 1951, vol. 2.

Straus, Erwin. "Aesthesiology and Hallucinations." *Existence: A New Dimension in Psychiatry and Psychology*. Edited by Rollo May, Ernest Angel, and Henri F. Ellenberger. New York: Basic Books, 1958, pp. 139–169.

————. *Phenomenological Psychology*. New York: Basic Books, 1966.

Zaner, Richard M. "Context and Reflexivity: The Genealogy of Self." *Evaluation and Explanation in the Biomedical Sciences*. Edited by H. Tristram Engelhardt, Jr. and Stuart F. Spicker. Dordrecht, Holland: D. Reidel Publishing Co., 1975, pp. 153–174.

————. *The Problem of Embodiment*. Phaenomenologica, no. 17. The Hague: Martinus Nijhoff, 1964. 2d ed. 1971.

————. "The Radical Reality of the Human Body." *Humanitas* 2 (1966): 73–87.

EMBRYO TRANSFER

See Reproductive Technologies, *articles on* in vitro fertilization, ethical issues, *and* legal aspects.

EMOTIVIST ETHICS

See Ethics, *article on* non-descriptivism.

ENVIRONMENT AND GENETICS

See Genetic Constitution and Environmental Conditioning.

ENVIRONMENT AND MAN

This entry does not discuss concrete ethical dilemmas concerning the quality of human life in the biosphere. Rather, it examines those underlying concepts, attitudes, and ideals involved in the relationship between humans and their environment that tend to give shape to conflicting ethical views in many areas of bioethics, particularly those discussed in the next entry, Environmental Ethics.

| I. western thought | Ian G. Barbour |
| II. eastern thought | Hajime Nakamura |

I
WESTERN THOUGHT

In the history of Western thought, views of the relation of human life to the environment have been diverse. To simplify the representation of this diversity within a brief article, some of these views have been grouped under three headings: (1) man's dominion over nature; (2) man's participation in nature; and, intermediate between these extremes, (3) man's stewardship of nature. Each motif has characteristic implications for the way one treats the environment. A final section discusses the crucial ethical issues today. The generic terms "man" and "mankind" refer throughout to both men and women, and the term "nature" is an abbreviation for "nonhuman nature."

Man's dominion over nature

Biblical and classical roots. The first chapter of Genesis (1:28) includes the commission to "have dominion over the fish of the sea and over the birds of the air and over every living thing." Man alone is created "in the image of God" (Gen. 1:26) and set apart from all other creatures. Moreover, nature is desacralized in biblical religion. Ancient Israel believed that God had revealed himself primarily in historical events rather than in the sphere of nature. Such assumptions contributed to the Western cultural outlook within which science and technology could eventually arise; for if nature is orderly, but not divine or demonic, it can be understood and used by human beings.

A number of recent authors have claimed that this biblical idea of dominion was the main historical root of exploitative attitudes in the West. In a widely quoted article, Lynn White points to the separation of man and nature and the assertion of the rights of man over nature in biblical thought. Holding that ideas and attitudes are significant influences in history, White concludes that, because of its anthropocentrism and "arrogance toward nature," Christianity "bears a huge burden of guilt" for the environmental crisis (White, p. 1206). However, such an account seems to neglect the complexity of Western thought. To be sure, the Genesis passage about dominion was used in later centuries to justify exploitative practices. But we shall note that (1) several nonbiblical sources of the dominion theme can be identified in the West; (2) the stewardship theme in the Bible itself sets limits on dominion, which were subsequently ignored; (3) environmental destruction has been common in nonbiblical cultures of both East and West since antiquity; and (4) institutions as well as ideas must be examined as determinants of environmental behavior, even if institutions are themselves partly the product of ideas.

From the many strands of Greek thought, Plato, Aristotle, and the Stoics may be singled out for their influence on the West. Their writings portrayed a gulf between man and all other beings, based on the unique human capacity for reason. Aristotle stated that other creatures are devoid of the contemplative activity in which man is most akin to God; plant and animal life exist simply for the sake of human life. Cicero, drawing upon Stoic writings, insisted that we have no obligation to respect animals because they are not rational beings (Glacken, chap. 1). To the neo-Platonists of the Hellenistic era, the eternal forms are only imperfectly embodied in the world of nature. To the Gnostics and Mani-

cheans, nature is the realm of evil from which the human soul seeks to escape. Greek and Roman views were indeed extraordinarily diverse, and we shall mention later some pantheistic authors who were more appreciative of the natural world. But the classical sources that were most influential on the early Church, the Middle Ages, and subsequent Western thought seem to have stressed the separation of man and nature.

The growth of science and technology. With the rise of the scientific world view in the seventeenth century, the dominion theme assumed increasing prominence. To Francis Bacon (1561–1626), the conquest of nature is the goal of science, for "knowledge is power." "Let the human race recover the right over nature which belongs to it by divine bequest." Bacon's *New Atlantis* called for a state-funded research establishment and a scientific elite through which man's rightful supremacy would be systematically extended. René Descartes (1596–1650) similarly extolled practical knowledge that would make us "the lords and masters of nature." Like the Stoics, he thought that man's unique rationality justified such sovereignty. Descartes elaborated a sharp dualism of matter and mind. Apart from human life, the world consists of particles in motion, and mathematics is the key to understanding it. Animals, he asserted, are machines without minds or feelings. The gap between mind and matter in Descartes's anthropocentric outlook posed the central problems for modern philosophy.

The mechanistic interpretation of nature was further developed by Isaac Newton (1642–1727). In earlier centuries the world had been viewed as a hierarchy of organisms, each with its place and purpose in an overall plan. For Newton and his followers, nature was taken to be constituted by impersonal masses and forces, operating according to deterministic laws. The measurable "primary" qualities, such as mass and velocity, were said to be objective characteristics of the real world; all other "secondary" qualities, such as color and temperature, were relegated to subjective responses in the observer's mind. Here was the "objectification" of nature as a realm essentially alien to man, and the detachment of the observer from the world he is observing. While Newton himself respected the cosmic watch as the product of the Divine Watchmaker, it is not surprising that his more secular successors had no scruples about exploiting it. If nature is a machine, it has no inherent rights, and man need not hesitate to manipulate and use it.

John Locke (1632–1704) provided the political philosophy within which such dominion could be justified and encouraged. Locke maintained that the political order is necessary primarily to protect the natural rights of the individual to "life, liberty, and property." Unfettered private ownership and use of resources, he said, would lead to economic and technological growth. By protecting the property rights of the rising middle class, the state would be encouraging industrial development and prosperity. Locke's influential writings thus endorsed individualism, the accumulation of wealth, technological development, and the subjugation of nature, all of which were to be promoted by the structures of government.

In the emerging industrial technology of the eighteenth century, man's dominion was increasingly achieved in practice as well as in theory. To the leaders of the industrial revolution, the environment was primarily a source of raw materials. In the new capitalism, the private ownership of resources encouraged treatment of the natural world as a source of commercial profit. Along with rising standards of living came increasing burdens on the environment. Since antiquity there had been deforestation, overgrazing, and soil erosion; but the technologies that developed in the last two centuries produced pollution and consumed natural resources at unprecedented rates. Here were combined the influences of biblical religion, dualistic philosophy, mechanistic science, and, above all, capitalist economics and industrial technology.

The American experience. For the New England Puritans, the new surroundings were strange and threatening, and their writings often refer to nature as an enemy to be subjugated. As the pioneers moved progressively westward, much that they encountered was hostile, a threat to survival, an obstacle to be overcome. Forests were cleared and wilderness destroyed to make way for civilization. The advancing frontier was interpreted in the light of the nation's "manifest destiny" to "conquer a continent." The New World offered apparently endless stretches of good land and seemingly unlimited natural resources. Air, water, and land appeared ample to absorb the waste products of a burgeoning civilization.

In the early days of the nation, there was considerable support for Thomas Jefferson's ideal of a nation of farmers. The agrarian, pastoral vision, which stressed the virtues of a rural society, contrasted with Alexander Hamilton's goal of an urban, mercantile nation in which commerce and manufacturing would thrive. The tensions between these two ideals continued, but it was clearly the industrial vision that prevailed. The steam locomotive, the "iron horse," had by the Civil War become a symbol of both technology and the conquest of nature in the growth of the nation. As industry thrived, urbanization accelerated, and the United States changed from a rural and small-town nation to a predominantly urban one. The new technologies and the private ownership of land and resources led to the concentration of economic power, the amassing of personal fortunes, and the rise of giant corporations for which the environment was a source of wealth.

To these geographic and economic factors may be added some characteristic American values that encouraged exploitative attitudes. Faith in technology and confidence in the expert have been pervasive. An optimistic belief in inevitable progress has until recently been shared by all levels of society. America has also been obsessed by the goal of growth, the assumption that "bigger is better." Impressive increases in productivity and gross national product have certainly occurred, but at social and environmental costs that have only slowly been recognized. It can also be argued that a male-dominated society has admired in public life the aggressive, active qualities that it calls "masculine," rather than the nurturing, conserving, sensitive qualities it has associated with women and family life. For a variety of reasons, then, the dominion theme has been even more prevalent in America than in the rest of the Western world.

Man's participation in nature

The opposing theme of man's participation in nature also has diverse religious and scientific roots.

Religious versions of participation. The religions of the ancient Near East sought the harmonious integration of man's life within the life of nature. Their rituals and festivals celebrated the annual cycle of the seasons and the fertility of nature rather than historical events. In nations around the Mediterranean, the earth-mother figure assumed differing forms: Athene, Artemis, Demeter, Isis, etc. Myths of dying and rising gods (e.g., Adonis, Osiris) were associated with the rebirth of life in the spring, and other gods and goddesses represented the power of a variety of natural forces.

Greek popular religion often made reference to the sacred in nature: the sacred grove or mountain, the spirit of the river or rock. Other versions of man's interconnectedness with nature is found in such Greek thinkers as the Epicureans. Lucretius, for example, held that the world was not designed for human use; in his nature poetry he reflected on the beauty and interdependence of the world as a natural process. But neither the nature religions of Asia Minor nor the naturalistic or pantheistic philosophies of Greece were as influential on later Western thought as the biblical and Greek themes previously mentioned. The theme of participation is of course strongly represented in Eastern thought, especially in Taoism in China and Zen Buddhism in Japan.

St. Francis's deep love of the natural world and his sense of union with it were far from typical of medieval thought, and yet they have continued to appeal to the popular imagination. He saw nature as a living whole and all creatures as objects of God's love, and hence as significant in their own right. He spoke of our sister the earth and greeted the birds as brothers, extending the family relationship and the circle of God's love to include all created beings sharing a common dignity and equality under God. Humanity is part of a wider community, and each creature has its own integrity, which must be respected.

Nineteenth-century Romanticism. Apart from several of the Christian mystics, the participation motif found few defenders in the early modern period. Only after the industrial revolution—and largely as a reaction to it—did this theme come into prominence. For such poets as Blake, Wordsworth, and Goethe, nature is not an impersonal machine but an organic process with which man is united. God is not the remote watchmaker but a vital force immanent in the natural world. Not rational analysis but feeling and imagination are the highest human capacities. Intuition grasps the unity of organic wholes, the interrelatedness of life. In natural settings a person can find a healing power, a sacramental presence, a bond with the human soul, an experience of peace and joy. Other Romantic authors extolled wild, sublime, untouched landscapes and forests. They idealized the "noble savage," uncorrupted by civilization, and exalted the "natural" and the "primitive."

The New England Transcendentalists referred in similar terms to the presence of the sacred in the realm of nature. Henry David Thoreau (1817–1862) held that nature is a source of inspiration, vitality, and spiritual renewal; it can teach us humility and simplicity. "In Wildness is the preservation of the World," he wrote. Thoreau criticized the frantic pursuit of progress and affluence, the growth of technological industrialism, and the pressures of an impersonal urban life. His year and a half of living alone at Walden Pond made him more aware of the interrelationships among creatures and the natural stability upset by humans; in solitude he found serenity and freedom. But he did not advocate giving up civilization. He sought rather a simplification of life and an alternation and balance between life with nature and life with civilization.

Starting in the 1870s, the writings of John Muir gave wide circulation to a philosophy of wilderness preservation. With the disappearance of the frontier, wilderness areas can be saved only by deliberate national policy. Muir, like Thoreau, found a divine harmony in nature, a freedom not possible in the artificial constraints of civilization, a source of serenity in a decadent society. He was founder of the Sierra Club (1892), and through his writing he campaigned tirelessly for legislation to protect wild areas of the American West.

George Perkins Marsh's *Man and Nature* (1864) was the first detailed study of the destructive influence of man on his environment. Marsh was an accomplished linguist familiar with ancient history and literature. As ambassador to Italy he traveled in Mediterranean countries and saw barren deserts where great cities and civilizations had once flourished. He traced the effects of deforestation and overgrazing on soil erosion, and the destruction of land by salination from excessive irrigation. He provided careful documentation of the fragility of the environment and the disruptive and often irreversible effects of civilization in disturbing the natural equilibrium.

The ecology movement. The scientific version of the participation theme received its first systematic expression in Darwin's *The Origin of Species* (1859) and *The Descent of Man* (1871), in which man was presented as a part of nature, in continuity with other forms of life. No sharp discontinuities separated human from animal life, either in evolutionary history or in present morphology and behavior. The theory of evolution seemed to undermine man's unique status, and close parallels to most human capacities could be found among lower forms. Moreover, Darwin's studies brought out the interconnectedness of the web of life and the complex balance of interactions in the biological world. Subsequent research in population dynamics has underscored the importance of the relation of organisms to their environment (habitat, food sources, predator–prey relationships, etc.). Recognition of the interdependence, diversity, and vulnerability of biological species prepared the way for ecology.

Within the twentieth-century science of ecology two concepts in particular have significant implications concerning man's relation to the environment: (1) The ecosystem concept emphasizes the interdependence of all forms of life in biotic communities and the far-reaching repercussions of thoughtless human intervention. Ecologists have traced the complex reciprocities and mutualities among organisms, the food chains linking diverse species, the interlocking cycles of elements and compounds, and the delicate balances that are easily upset. (2) There are limits to the growth of populations, and every environment has a finite carrying capacity. Human life, too, is dependent on limited resources —land, air, water, plant life, oil reserves, mineral ores, etc.—whose uses can be extended by technology, but not without new environmental costs. Writing in the 1930s, Aldo Leopold was one of the first ecologists to suggest that our ethical concern must be extended to apply to the land and nonhuman life as well as to human beings. Since Rachel Carson's *Silent Spring* (1962), the call for an ecological conscience has been repeated with increasing urgency, coupled often with a critique of the short-sightedness of most technological solutions.

In recent years, many biologists have focused on growth as the crucial problem. For Paul Ehrlich and Garrett Hardin, the control of population overshadows all other issues. Gains in agricultural and industrial production in developing countries cannot keep up with exponential population growth. In the Club of Rome study, *Limits to Growth* (1972), and the British *Blueprint for Survival* (1972), attention is directed also to the limits of industrial growth which are set by resource reserves and pollution levels. These studies advocate policies of "no growth" for industrial production as well as population. In opposing growth and in underscoring the finite carrying capacity of the environment, these authors adopt an ecological

viewpoint, even if at times their outlook seems more anthropocentric than the views of other authors mentioned previously.

The youth counterculture since the late 1960s has been influenced by the ecology movement, but its approach has had more in common with Romanticism. Like the latter, it has valued feeling, imagination, and immediacy of experience more than intellect and rationality. The counterculture has been disenchanted with technology, holding that preoccupation with efficiency, productivity, and rational control has alienated industrial man from nature and from his fellow man. Some young people have dropped out of society to form communes in rural settings within which they hope to recover harmony with nature and with each other. Other youths have sought alternative life-styles that might encourage personal, social, and environmental harmony without a radical break from the prevailing social order.

Finally, process philosophy should be mentioned as an intellectual system influenced by evolutionary biology and consistent with an ecological outlook. Much of twentieth-century philosophy, especially in Europe, has perpetuated the Kantian separation of the human realm of freedom and history from the realm of nature. Existentialism, for example, emphasizes the distinction between the sphere of personal selfhood and the objective world of impersonal nature. In phenomenology this split is partially overcome in the analysis of "being in the world." But in the thought of Alfred North Whitehead (1861–1947) and his more recent followers the realms of selfhood and nature are more systematically brought together again. Nature is a creative process, a community of interacting organisms, not a deterministic machine. Every being is constituted by its relationships and dependent on its environment, but each is at the same time in its own way a center of experience. Process thought rejects matter–mind dualism (as in Descartes), the subordination of matter to mind (idealism), and the reduction of mind to matter (materialism). Mind and matter are not two opposing substances, but two aspects of events in systems having many levels of organization. Thus all beings are intrinsically valuable and worthy of respect as centers of at least rudimentary experience. In process thought, man is to be understood in the same categories as other beings. There are no metaphysical discontinuities, though the importance of any given category will vary widely among different levels of being. God transcends nature but is also immanent in the creative process; he does not intervene coercively from outside, but participates throughout cosmic history. Process thought thus avoids the separation of man and nature and of God and nature, which have in the past encouraged environmentally destructive attitudes.

Man's stewardship of nature

Stewardship in biblical thought. The third motif in Western thought, stewardship or responsible use, represents a middle ground between dominion and participation. In the story of Adam and Eve, man is put in the garden "to till it and keep it" (Gen. 2:15), and throughout the Bible, man does not have absolute and unlimited dominion, for he is responsible to God. "The earth is the Lord's" because he created it. The land belongs ultimately to God; man is only a trustee, caretaker, or steward, responsible for the welfare of that which is entrusted to him and accountable for his treatment of it. The biblical outlook is, in the last analysis, theocentric rather than either anthropocentric or biocentric.

Whereas dominion implies that the environment has no reason for existence except for our use, stewardship affirms the intrinsic value of nature. In the biblical view, the created world is valued in itself, not simply as an instrument of human purposes. In several of the Psalms (19, 89, 104, etc.) God is said to delight in the earth and the manifold variety of life quite apart from man. Even in the first chapter of Genesis, each form of life is pronounced good before mankind is on the scene. The Sabbath is a day of rest for the earth and living things as well as for man. Human life and nature stand together as jointly God's creation.

Many biblical passages express appreciation and wonder in response to nature. Job is overwhelmed by the majesty of natural phenomena. Jesus spoke of the lilies of the field and the sparrow's fall. Value pervades all life, not just human life. Furthermore, nature is part of the drama of redemption and will share in the ultimate harmony, as portrayed in the symbolic vision of the coming kingdom when "the wolf shall dwell with the lamb, and the leopard shall lie down with the kid" (Isa. 11:6). Paul imagines that "the whole creation has been groaning in travail together until now," but it will all take part in the final fulfillment (Rom. 8:22). Although the focus of attention was on man and human history, the world of nature was not neglected within the Bible as it was in much of later Christian thought.

St. Benedict might be taken as an early model of the stewardship perspective. Compared with St. Francis's deep feeling and sense of union with the natural world, St. Benedict's response was more practical, using nature but using it with care and respect. The Benedictine monasteries combined work and contemplation. They developed such sound agricultural practices as crop rotation and care for the soil, drained swamps, and husbanded timber all over Europe; they were creative in the practical arts related to nature.

There has also been a continuing literary tradition that has extolled the pastoral ideal of "cultivated nature," intermediate between the expanding city and the inhospitable wilderness. The pastoral poems of Theocritus, Virgil, and Horace celebrated the beauties of the country landscape and the virtues of the simple rural life in contrast to the growing urbanization of Greek and Roman life. The pastoral motif continued through the history of literature and was prominent in eighteenth-century Europe. Leo Marx has traced the importance of the "middle landscape," which combines the values of civilization and nature, in a number of nineteenth-century American novels.

The conservationist outlook. From more recent times Gifford Pinchot might serve as an example of a conservationist rather than preservationist viewpoint. Whereas John Muir campaigned for the preservation of untouched wilderness, Pinchot advocated "wise use" and "scientific management" of federal lands and eventually secured Theodore Roosevelt's support. In 1905 the U.S. Forest Service was established, with Pinchot at its head. Its policy was intermediate between unlimited exploitation and absolute protection: the maximum sustained timber yield that would conserve forests for the future. And if the Forest Service can be criticized for opening up federal lands too rapidly to mining, grazing, and lumber interests, it can also be appreciated for the dedicated service of the new professional foresters. A similar conservationist viewpoint prevailed in other government agencies.

The biologist René Dubos gives a contemporary rendition of a philosophy of "respectful use" and "creative intervention." He advocates managing and transforming the earth, but with awareness of the consequences and limitations of human activity. Man has unique capacities and potentialities, yet he is dependent on the biotic community, and there is no radical disjunction of man and nature. Dubos writes:

We certainly must reject the attitude which asserts that man is the only value of importance and that the rest of nature can be sacrificed to his welfare and whims. But we cannot escape, I believe, an anthropocentric attitude which puts man at the summit of creation while still a part of it [Dubos in Barbour, p. 53].

Barry Commoner considers the relative roles of population, affluence, and technology in environmental pollution. He rejects the thesis of Ehrlich and others that population is the main problem, and instead lays the blame on heavily polluting technologies (especially plastics, detergents, fertilizers, and pesticides). He argues that continued growth is possible with ecologically sound agriculture and technology. But Commoner's rejection of a no-growth policy is based also on his concern for social justice. Improvement of living standards of the poor at home and abroad requires the growth of technologies that are not so environmentally destructive. While Commoner gives insufficient attention to the population question, he does look at issues of distributive justice and at the political and economic structures that perpetuate inequalities, which are ignored by many environmentalists (Commoner, chaps. 10–12).

Social justice and environmental preservation. Issues of justice and environment are intertwined, because exploitation of man and of nature arises from the same institutions and attitudes, such as the concentration of economic power, the pursuit of profit, and the manipulative mentality. In the words of C. S. Lewis, "What we call Man's power over Nature turns out to be a power exercised by some men over other men with Nature as its instrument." Karl Marx was keenly aware of the importance of economic institutions and technology in the exercise of power, but he shared the dominant Western view of "mastery over nature," though with some concern to conserve nature as an object of aesthetic satisfaction. The environmental records of the Soviet Union and the Chinese People's Republic seem to have been no better than those under capitalism.

Like the exponents of dominion, the environmental movement has in the past tended to neglect the issue of justice. From Thoreau to Muir to countercultural communes, the retreat to nature has often involved turning one's back on the city and "the dirty institutions of men."

(To be sure, Thoreau advocated the abolition of slavery, and Muir campaigned for wilderness legislation, but the areas of their political activity were limited.) The political viewpoint of environmentalists has reflected their predominantly middle-class background and interests. Today, with widespread recognition of limited global resources, there is among environmentalists a greater concern for inequalities within and between nations. There is awareness that the United States, with six percent of the world's population, accounts for thirty to forty percent of the world's annual resource consumption. As the gap between rich and poor countries increases, questions of distribution, and hence of political and economic power, assume high priority.

Advocates of this third ("stewardship") position will thus often join those in the second ("participation") group in political action to protect the environment. Together they recognize that, by treating air and water as free commodities, the market economy has not charged industry for the true costs. Any "public goods" or unrestricted "commons" will be overused. These indirect costs ("externalities") can only be acknowledged by legislative action (e.g., effluent standards, taxes, or subsidies). Those in this third group differ from the second group in practice mainly by putting more emphasis on the human consequences of legislation. Who pays for and who benefits from a particular law? What happens to the men who lose their jobs in the rare cases when a factory closes because it cannot meet strict standards? Concrete decisions involve the agonizing balance of conflicting values: technological progress, environmental preservation, and social justice.

Continuing issues

The above classification of viewpoints into three groups is an oversimplification. On any issue there is a continuum of intermediate gradations. Moreover, a person might be closer to group two on some topics, and to group three, say, on other topics. As presented above the third view seems to be a compromise between two extreme positions, whereas its proponents claim that it can be defended in its own right. Let us summarize some of the underlying issues today:

1. God's relation to nature. The "dominion" theme has been associated historically with an emphasis on the transcendence of God. The religious versions of "participation," on the other hand, have stressed divine immanence, understood in terms of nature gods, or a pantheistic principle, or a mystical unity known by intuition. The "stewardship" view usually combines transcendence and immanence. Nature is to be neither exploited nor worshiped. Contemporary religious thought has explored this option in the liturgical celebration of nature and in sacramental, incarnational, or evolutionary theologies of nature.

2. Man's status in nature. Classical thought portrayed a radical disjunction, an absolute gulf, between man and nature. The ancient Near East, at the opposite extreme, incorporated man into nature, and Darwin in his day contended that any differences between humans and animals are minimal. Today it is more common to acknowledge the evolutionary continuity of human life with lower forms and the presence of structural and behavioral similarities, while insisting that there are significant differences in degree—which amount to qualitative distinctiveness—in human language, culture, and personal and interpersonal life. Priority can be given to human needs and the value of persons without ignoring the welfare of the nonhuman world. "Stewardship" implies the cooperation and partnership of man and nature for the fulfillment of the highest potentialities of both.

3. Man's attitude to nature. The attitudes of mastery, subjugation, control, and manipulation have been predominant in the modern West, especially in recent decades in the United States. Technological man since Bacon has often expressed in word and deed a Promethean or Faustian arrogance. In this cultural situation, and with economic and political pressures exerted by institutions having a vested interest in exploiting nature, the "stewardship" position can easily be co-opted or pushed in the direction of "dominion." This is a point at which the scientific version of the "participation" motif—the ecological recognition of finitude, limits, and interdependence—needs to be strongly stressed. Awareness of the far-reaching repercussions of human actions can encourage humility and caution in seeking to impose technological solutions.

4. The role of technology. If those in the first group have great confidence in technology, many of those in the second are ready to curtail or even abandon it because of its environmental and human costs. But the rejection of technology today would condemn most of the world to continued poverty, hunger, and disease. A middle position seeks through political processes the reduction of environmental degradation and a more equal distribution of the benefits of technology. One can be realistic about the exercise of economic power by affluent nations and by polluting industries and yet believe that legislation expressing new national priorities can effect change. There are also unexplored possibilities of intermediate technologies scaled to local needs and resources, which may offer a path between large-scale industrial technology and primitive agrarian conditions in both developed and developing countries.

5. The problem of growth. Between the options of "pro-growth" and "no growth" lies a policy that asks "Whose growth?" and "What kind of growth?" Global justice requires that in developed nations economic growth be channeled toward services that are not resource-intensive. Ecological wisdom requires research on technologies for recycling and waste reduction, in addition to effective birth control measures, which have not been discussed here. Both justice and ecology require that affluent nations practice restraint in consumption, for which changes in personal values and life-styles, and in national priorities and policies, will be necessary. But the "pro-growth" mentality is so deeply ingrained that those who favor "selective growth" will have to devote most of their efforts to limiting the inequitable demands that the industrial West places on the world's resources and environment. The path of responsible stewardship leads to individual action and institutional change to combine environmental preservation and social justice.

IAN G. BARBOUR

[*For further discussion of topics mentioned in this article, see the entries:* EVOLUTION; *and* LIFE. *Also directly related are the entries* ENVIRONMENTAL ETHICS; MAN, IMAGES OF; SCIENCE: ETHICAL IMPLICATIONS; *and* TECHNOLOGY. *See also:* FUTURE GENERATIONS, OBLIGATIONS TO; JUSTICE; MIND–BODY PROBLEM; *and* REDUCTIONISM.]

BIBLIOGRAPHY

BARBOUR, IAN G., ed. *Western Man and Environmental Ethics.* Reading, Mass.: Addison-Wesley Publishing Co., 1973.

BLACK, JOHN. *The Dominion of Man.* Edinburgh: Edinburgh University Press, 1970.

COMMONER, BARRY. *The Closing Circle.* New York: Alfred A. Knopf, 1971.

DUBOS, RENÉ. *A God Within.* New York: Charles Scribner's Sons, 1972.

GLACKEN, CLARENCE. *Traces on the Rhodian Shore.* Berkeley: University of California Press, 1967.

LEISS, WILLIAM. *The Domination of Nature.* New York: George Braziller, 1972.

MARX, LEO. *The Machine in the Garden.* New York: Oxford University Press, 1964.

NASH, RODERICK. *Wilderness and the American Mind.* New Haven: Yale University Press, 1967. Rev. ed. 1973.

PASSMORE, JOHN. *Man's Responsibility for Nature.* New York: Charles Scribner's Sons, 1974.

SANTMIRE, H. PAUL. *Brother Earth.* New York: Thomas Nelson, 1970.

TUAN YI-FU. *Topophilia: A Study of Environmental Perception, Attitudes, and Values.* Englewood Cliffs, N.J.: Prentice-Hall, 1974.

WHITE, LYNN, JR. "The Historical Roots of Our Ecologic Crisis." *Science* 155 (1967): 1203–1207. Reprinted in Barbour, *Western Man*, pp. 18–30.

II

EASTERN THOUGHT

Conformity to nature. Chinese thought traditionally tended to consider that all things could exist only insofar as they were in conformity with human nature. This gave rise to the attitude of esteem for the principle of nature that exists in the human mind. Since ancient times, the idea of Heaven (*T'ien*) was conceived by the Chinese in close relation with human life. According to a poem composed in the ancient period of the early Chou dynasty, Heaven created all human beings, and therefore Heaven, as the ancestor of man, handed down moral precepts which humans must observe. This idea was inherited by Confucius. He recommended acknowledging "the order of Heaven," which meant that "one should follow the morality given by Heaven." There was a general assumption that politics should follow laws based upon natural law.

The opinion that "man should follow his true nature" was also stated by other scholars in ancient China, but their interpretation was different from that of Confucius. Mo-tzu taught that the ruler should follow only what Heaven wished. Lao-tzu insisted that the correct way for man is to follow the way of Heaven; therefore, the basis of the correct way is *T'ien-tao* (the Way of Heaven). Yang-chu (who lived between the times of Mo-tzu and Mencius) stated: "Original human nature desires only sex and food. Therefore, it is better for one not to have relations with others but only to satisfy one's own desires. It is a natural law that one does what he wants." Mencius taught that "the true character of man is good; however, the evil mind arises by the temptation of material desires. Therefore, one should cultivate one's own mind and exhibit one's own true character."

An exception to Chinese thought was Hsü-tzu, who maintained that the true character of man tends to evil. Nevertheless, he recognized the possibilities in man of becoming good. Chuang-tzu taught that one should perfect one's true character, and his followers came to teach the theory that "one should return to his true character." In the San-kuo dynasty, Wang-pi (A.D. 226–249) also taught the doctrine of "return to one's true character." This thought was developed greatly in the Sung philosophy, where the central theme was the concept of a person's true character. The traditional current of thought in Chinese history is "to return to the true and natural human character." This idea was shared by the Japanese also, probably under the influence of Chinese thought.

Buddhism was also influenced by this current of thought. Buddhists did not look for truth in the phenomenal world but explored the inner thought as expressed in a peculiarly Chinese way: "If one realizes the truth that all existences are the same, one immediately returns to one's true nature." Both illusion and enlightenment of people were understood to be derived from the natural character of humanity:

The mind is the ground and nature is the king. Where there is nature there is the king, and where there is no nature, there is no king. Where there is nature, there are body and mind. Where no nature exists, there is neither body nor mind. Buddha is created by knowledge of self-nature; therefore, one must not look for the Buddha through the body. If self-nature comes by enlightenment, then the self-enlightened being is namely the Buddha.

There was, in India, no such idea of self-nature as the principle that maintains the body and mind as ignorant or enlightened. Some Chinese scholars have recognized a Taoist influence in this conception of self-nature. However, this concept could have appeared from the traditional ideas of the Chinese.

Medieval Confucians said that the whole of nature is to be found in any single item, which theory seems originally to have been due to the influence of Buddhist philosophy, especially the Buddhist Hua-yen school.

Nature as the absolute. Taoism taught that nature is the absolute. Chinese Buddhist Pure Land teachings adopted the ideas of Taoism. Chinese Buddhists had to pass through a process of complicated thought before they acknowledged a Chinese type of naturalism. In this connection, Chi-tsang reasoned as follows: Chinese philosophical thought, especially in Lao-tzu and Chuang-tzu, regarded existence as phenomena, and void (*Sunyata*) as a substance other than existence. Therefore, void was not identifiable with existence. Buddhism, on the contrary, taught that phenomena are actually the manifestation of the Absolute. Therefore, the absolute significance of the phenomenal world cannot be recognized in actual life in the philosophy of Lao-tzu and Chuang-tzu. In Buddhism, however, one can accept this phenomenal world as absolute states of existence, because actual life in this world is identical with absolute existence. Although this criticism by Chi-tsang may not be correct, at least he tried to recognize a significance in life in this world.

The T'ien-t'ai and Hua-yen sects further expanded on this thought. According to the T'ien-t'ai sect, appearance and actuality are not different kinds of substances because appearance is identical with reality. Therefore, they taught that "each existence in this world is the middle way." Each of the phenomenal forms of this world is a form of absolute existence. The Hua-yen sect developed this thought even further and taught the theory of "mutual penetration and identification of all things with one another." The supreme meaning emerges when all phenomena are perfectly identified by their harmonious interrelationships. Therefore, nothing exists outside of phenomena and their diverse forms of manifestation.

As a result, the actual natural world was acknowledged as absolute existence. In Zen Buddhism, for example, this naturalistic tendency led to the conclusion that each one of the existences of this world is, just as it appears, a manifestation of truth. Zen monks, of course, opposed and rejected any merely superficial naturalism. Nevertheless, the Chinese generally accepted the view that nature is the absolute. Finally, the T'ien-t'ai sect taught the theory that "all existences and even grass, trees, and earth can attain Buddhahood." That is to say, even physical matter existing in nature can realize enlightenment and become Buddha. Generally speaking, the tendency was to regard nature as the most beautiful and highest existence, on an equal plane with humans. Therefore, the Chinese Buddhists (especially Zen monks) tried to seek absolute significance in everyday life. Every-

day life, just as it truly is, is identical with enlightenment. Zen masters also made much of natural beauty, as in the words of Master Ryō-kan:

> In spring, the flowers;
>   and in autumn the moon;
> In summer a refreshing breeze,
>   and in winter the snow;
> What else do I need?

Zen Buddhists also endeavored to take the surroundings in the natural world as they are.

As the result of the tendency to regard nature or actuality as absolute existence, the Chinese came to adopt an attitude of optimism. Thus, they regarded this world as a good place in which to live; they finally came to believe that perfect existence must exist in this world. Here, the idea of the *Sheng-jen* (sage) was established. He was the perfect person such as the Chou King or Confucius. The sage is not a god but a man.

The Chinese identified nature with human life. The harmony of all existences is necessary in order to harmonize with nature and live in peace. Thus, they asserted the idea of "moderation." As the Chinese regarded man as a part of nature or the universe, they did not regard nature as opposed to man. Since they seldom thought nature needed to be transformed by experimental manipulation in order to master her ways or laws, natural science did not develop quickly in China. This fact is perhaps the chief reason why China lagged scientifically behind other countries in the modern world. Leaders of the People's Republic of China recognize this fact and are trying to improve and develop natural science, although this may lead to a conflict with traditional values maintained by Taoist-minded people.

Throughout all modern Eastern countries, Eastern thought has found an accommodation to technology and its manipulation of nature. In many Eastern countries studies of natural sciences and technology are strongly encouraged by governments and big businesses. Traditionalists also admit this line of development, which is unavoidable in modern civilization.

However, in some cases conflict with traditional values prevents the development of technology. This is most conspicuous with the Jains, who prohibit killing animals and the use of any insecticide, owing to the spirit of compassion towards all living creatures. They may not use animals for experiments; they may not exploit marshes, for the enterprise will kill many small living creatures living there. With the Sikhs and

Parsis there are no such prohibitions, and that is why they have been ahead of others in the modernization of India. For Chinese, Japanese, and Koreans who profess Mahāyāna Buddhism there is no problem of this kind.

Relationship between Heaven and man. The Chinese elaborated an organic theory of a "reciprocal relationship between Heaven and man." In the period of the Chan-kuo (Warring States period, 480–222 B.C.), "scholars of the positive and negative principle" advocated a kind of nature worship, which was carried into the Early Han period. According to this principle, natural phenomena and man-made institutions are mutually interrelated, and therefore if the King, who was the representative of man, governed the country well, then the phenomena of nature—such as weather, wind, and rain—would be favorable to man. If the reign of the King was poor, on the other hand, then natural calamities would arise. This idea was most strongly stressed by Tung Chung-shu (179?–104? B.C.) of the Early Han dynasty, who thought that disasters were sent from Heaven in order to admonish the King. The thought of *Ko-ming* (revolution) which means, literally, "to cut off (or take away) the mandate of Heaven from some particular ruler" played a role in checking or correcting the tyranny of aristocrats. This thought was influential in later periods in China. Some Indian Buddhists also held the theory that "disasters arise through poor government by the King."

Buddhism had sutras which stated the theory of disaster and which were highly regarded by the Chinese. A typical example of these sutras is the *Chin-kuang-ming* (*Suvarnaprabhasa*, Golden Splendor) sutra, which states in detail in the thirteenth chapter that, if the King does not protect the *dharma* (religion, law) well, a terrible calamity will arise. That is to say, as the result of maladministration on the part of the Emperor, falsehood and struggle will increase in his country, and the ministers and subjects will rise against him. Furthermore, the deities will become angry; wars will break out; the enemy will overrun the country; family members will fight each other; nothing will be pleasant or comfortable for man. Natural phenomena will at the same time become worse. Living beings will lack vigor, plagues will arise, and pestilence will sweep the land. Therefore, the Emperor should attempt his best in governing the country by the *dharma* (law).

Naturalized Buddhist monks from India propagated Buddhism in conformity with this organic way of Chinese thinking. Gunavarman, for example, taught Buddhism to Emperor Wen of the Sung dynasty in the following way:

The four seas are your land and all existences are your subjects. One pleasant word and all your subjects are happy. One act of a good ruler brings harmony to the people. If you only punish wrongdoers without killing and do not impose heavy taxes, then nature will harmonize with man, and fruits and crops will ripen well.

This organic form of ethical thought continued in China for a long time. Pure Land teachings of China also explained this ethical theory in terms of the relationship between the Buddha's grace and nature (Nakamura, p. 283).

Action and change as reality. The inclination to live contentedly in this given phenomenal world appears in ancient Shintoism as well as in modern sectarian Shintoism. The founder of the Konkō sect, for instance, teaches, "Whether alive or dead, you should regard the heaven and earth as your own habitation." The process of the phenomenal world is activity—mighty, self-maintaining, and procreative with the creative power and freedom of sublime wonder. Master Dōgen says, "Being is time, and time is being. Everything in the world is time at each moment." He said quite radically, "Birth and death is the life of Buddha."

In the long history of Japanese thought it was traditional to seek for the Absolute in the phenomenal (physical) world, and this way of thinking has played an effective role in the assimilation of Zen as well. For Master Dōgen, impermanence is itself the absolute state, and this impermanence is not to be rejected but to be valued. "Impermanence of grass, trees, and forests is verily the Buddhahood. The impermanence of the person's body and mind is verily the Buddhahood. The impermanence of the country and scenery is verily the Buddhahood."

Jinsai Itō (1627–1705), the Japanese Confucianist, regards heaven and earth as the evolution of great activity in which nothing but eternal development occurs, and hence he completely denies what is called death. According to Itō, the world of reality is nothing but change and action, and action is in itself good. All of the characteristically Japanese scholars believe in phenomena as the fundamental mode of existence. They unanimously reject the passivity of the neo-Confucianists of the Sung period.

Love of natural beauty. The way of thinking that recognizes absolute significance in the phenomenal world seems to be culturally associated with the Japanese traditional love of nature, which has been characteristic of the Japanese since ancient times. The Japanese in general love mountains, rivers, flowers, birds, grass, and trees, and represent them in the patterns of their kimono, and they are fond of the delicacies of the season, keeping their edibles in natural forms as much as possible in cooking. Within the house, flowers are arranged in a vase and dwarf trees placed in the alcove, flowers and birds are engraved in the transom, simple flowers and birds are also painted on the sliding screen, and in the garden miniature mountains are built and water is drawn. The literature is also closely tied up with warm affection for nature. *Makura no Sōshi* (Pillow Books) begins with general remarks about the four seasons and then goes into the description of the scenic beauties of the seasons and human affairs. There are many essays of this kind. If the poems on nature should be removed from the collections of Japanese poems, few poems would be left.

The love of nature, in the case of the Japanese, is tied up with their tendencies to cherish minute things and treasure delicate things. Contrast the Japanese love of individual flowers, birds, grass, and trees with the British enjoyment of the spacious view of the sea, the Dover Cliffs, and the countryside. Such aesthetic preferences of various nations are culturally significant traits of their respective peoples.

The Japanese enjoy nature as it is reflected in their compact range of vision, which is particularly evident in the following poem:

In my garden fall the plum blossoms—
  Are they indeed snowflakes
Whirling from the sky? [*Maunyōshū*, V, 822.]
The nightingale sings
Playing at the lower branches
Lamenting the fall of the plum blossoms [ibid., 824].

In this respect the Japanese love of nature differs somewhat from the Chinese attachment to the rivers and mountains. The point may be best illustrated by the comparison of the following two poems. Dōgen, the Japanese Zen master (thirteenth century A.D.), writes:

   Flowers are in Spring, Cuckoos in Summer,
   In Autumn is the moon, and in Winter,
   The pallid glimmer of snow.

The meaning of the above poem coincides with what is intended by the Chinese verse of *Wu-men-kuan* (Gateless Gate, by Wu-men Hui-k'ai).

   A hundred flowers are in Spring, in Autumn
      is the moon,

In Summer is the cool wind, the snow is in
   Winter;
If nothing is on the mind to afflict a man,
That is the best season for the man.

The word "cuckoos" of the Japanese is replaced in the Chinese by the "cool wind," which gives an entirely different effect. The cool wind and cuckoos are both sensible objects, but while the former gives the sense of indefinite, remote boundlessness, the latter gives a limited and familiar, homely impression.

The Indians also love nature and construct gardens (*udyana*, *arama*)—where they plant grass and trees and lay out wells and springs—but they rarely try to imitate natural rivers and mountains on a small scale. The Indian ascetics also composed poems in praise of nature. They enjoy and extol nature as the sanctuary beyond worldly sensuous attachments, afflictions, and bondages. In their case nature is conceived to be something opposed to human vicissitudes, and at a distance from human feeling.

In the case of the Japanese, however, priests and laymen alike are attached to nature, which is at one with human beings. They esteem the sensible beauties of nature, in which they seek revelations of the absolute world.

   Cherry blossoms, falling in vain,
   Remind me of the Treasure plants,
   That adorn paradise [Emperor Kazan].

There is no inkling of a view that regards the natural world as cursed or gruesome.

Love of animals.   The tender love of animals traditionally runs in the veins of the Japanese, but that love is concentrated on minute, lovable living things.

   A copper pheasant warbles out.
   Listening to its voice I thought,
   Could it be the father calling?
   Could it be the mother calling? [Master Gyōki.]

The image of the "copper pheasant" is very Japanese. In contrast, the people of India and the South Asiatic countries are often fond of a story such as willingly abandoning oneself to a hungry tiger who attacks one. Such a story is not quite congenial to the poetic sentiments of the Japanese, although both peoples wanted to express the idea of benevolence toward living creatures.

Surroundings are sentient.   The conception was prevalent in medieval Japan that even grass and trees have spirits and consequently are eligible for salvation. The idea that even the things of "no-mind" (the objects of nature that have no spirits) can become Buddhas, based upon the

Tendai doctrines, was particularly emphasized in Japan. This constituted an important theme for study in the Japanese Tendai sect, and the idea was inherited also by the Nichiren sect. Nichiren (1222–1282) sought the superiority of the *Hokke* (Lotus) *Sūtra* in its recognition of the eligibility of the grass and the trees to become Buddhas. There appear time and again among the Japanese Buddhist writings the following lines: "When a Buddha, who has attained enlightenment, looks around the universe, the grass, trees, and lands, all become Buddhas." In "Noh" songs we often come across such an idea, which was taken for granted socially and religiously in those days. There is a story of a willow tree's becoming a Buddha, based upon the religious faith of the Jōdo-shin sect. The oral tradition of the medieval Tendai sect of Japan pushed the idea of grass and trees that become Buddhas so far as to preach "the non-becoming Buddhas of the grass and trees" (for they are already Buddhas). According to this theory, everything is by nature a Buddha—that is to say, to attain enlightenment through ascetic practice is one and the same thing as being a Buddha without recourse to ascetic practice. Not only the grass and trees but also rivers, mountains, and the earth are themselves Buddhahood, already possessed intact. There is no becoming a Buddha in the sense of coming to be something separate and different in nature. That is the reason why the nonbecoming of Buddhahood was preached. The logical conclusion of the idea of the acceptance of the given reality is here definitely and clearly crystallized.

Some Indian Buddhists also admit the spirituality of grass and trees, along with certain schools of Indian philosophy that also adopt such a view. However, most Indian philosophies maintain that all living things attain the state of deliverance through enlightened intelligence (*vidyā*), and that grass and trees do not become Buddhas in their actual state as they are. Such a tendency of thinking as discussed above still seems to be effective among the Japanese even in these days, when the knowledge of natural science prevails. In fact, there is probably no other nation on earth that uses an honorific expression prefixed to the names of everyday objects such as tea and water. This is not merely a question of an honorific expression, but a manifestation of a way of thinking that seeks a raison d'être and sacredness in everything that exists.

Exploitation of nature. Monks of Southern Asia did not want to be involved in productive work of any kind. They just practiced meditation without working physically. This attitude has been preserved throughout Asiatic countries except in China and Japan. In China, Zen priests began to cultivate fields attached to their own temples in the eighth century A.D. in order to secure a permanent supply of food. The reason for the transformation of the monks' activities is as follows. Originally, the monks lived on alms, begging food from lay believers; but because of the devastation caused by many wars, Zen monks escaped from the confusion in cities and towns and settled deep in the mountains, where they could not beg for alms. At this point they began cultivating the land and building their own lodgings by manual labor. Thus physical labor came to be cherished. The motto, "If one did not work a day, one should not eat on that day" became their favorite saying. This motto has also been greatly encouraged by the Communist government under Mao Tse-tung.

In Japan monks of many sects went so far as to engage in such economic activity as constructing roads, rest houses, hospitals, ponds, and harbors, and exploiting fields. Philanthropic works were encouraged in Japan: Rendering service to others was said to be the essence of Mahāyāna. For laymen all sorts of productive work except slaying animals and selling wines, weapons, and so on were encouraged.

Harmony with nature. One of the most prominent features of Buddhist thought is its zest for harmony with nature. The joy of enjoying natural beauty and of living comfortably in natural surroundings was expressed by monks and nuns in *The Poems of the Elders* (*Theragāthā* and *Therigāthās*). This attitude was inherited from the ancient Indian hermit-sages (*ṛṣis*) as described in the *Mahābhārata* and the *Rāmāyana*. This attitude is most clearly reflected in Japanese gardening. Japanese gardens, which were developed after those in ·China, differ greatly from the Western and Islamic ones, which concentrate on geometrical patterns and symmetry. Japanese gardens, although artificially made by adept gardeners, give us the impression of reproducing natural beauty as such, inducing us to imagine ourselves as living in real nature: Artifice and nature are not separate. Harmonious union with nature is the ideal of the Buddhists' view of the environment.

Contemporary implications. According to Buddhist philosophy, humans constitute just one class of living beings and have no right to an unlimited dissipation of natural resources. Also, humans have no right of unlimited exploitation of animal and plant life, which form part of nature. Hitherto, Westerners or moderns too often tended to think of themselves as quite separate and different from the natural world and to believe that they were qualified for the exclusive use of the natural world, for they were created by, and in the image of, God. But this assumption of dominion over nature by humans is ungrounded and unreasonable. The modern Western view has brought devastation to the environment. Now we are incurring nature's retaliation. In order to deal with the difficult situation in which we are now placed, we must find a solution. Solution can be approached in two ways: objectively and subjectively.

On the objective side, the views reported above would suggest that we should discard the arrogant attitude that we are entitled to exploit the natural world at our own will, without limit and regardless of the consequences. If nature is to be met with affection, we can scarcely afford to maintain the attitude of "conquerors of nature." The entire world of nature, rather than being monopolized by a limited number of countries, should be shared by all mankind. Just as individual egoism should be curtailed and placed under control, so national and ethnic egoism should be restrained in the name of justice and respect for nature.

On the subjective side, there is need for a corrective factor against the opinion of moderns that the progress of mankind consists in the unlimited satisfaction of human desires for material objects. Buddhism taught satisfaction with what is given to men. "To know what it is to be truly satisfied" was thought to mean knowing the way of spiritual happiness. The key to the relationship between man and environment may very well lie in the control of our desires according to this concept of satisfaction.

HAJIME NAKAMURA

[For further discussion of topics mentioned in this article, see the entries: BUDDHISM; CONFUCIANISM; DEATH, article on EASTERN THOUGHT; HINDUISM; TAOISM; and MEDICAL ETHICS, HISTORY OF, section on SOUTH AND EAST ASIA, articles on INDIA, PREREPUBLICAN CHINA, and JAPAN THROUGH THE NINETEENTH CENTURY. See also: ENVIRONMENTAL ETHICS; ISLAM; PURPOSE IN THE UNIVERSE; SCIENCE: ETHICAL IMPLICATIONS; and TECHNOLOGY.]

BIBLIOGRAPHY

BOSE, D. M.; SEN, S. N.; and SUBBARAYAPPA, B. V., eds. *A Concise History of Science in India.* New Delhi: Indian National Science Academy, 1971.

DE BARY, WILLIAM THEODORE; CHAN, WING-TSIT; and WATSON, BURTON, eds. *Sources of Chinese Tradition.* New York: Columbia University Press, 1960.

———; HAY, STEPHEN; WEILER, ROYAL; and YARROW, ANDREW, eds. *Sources of Indian Tradition.* New York: Columbia University Press, 1958.

JAGGI, OM PRAKASH. *Scientists of Ancient India and Their Achievements.* Delhi: Atma Ram & Sons, 1966.

LESLIE, CHARLES, ed. *Asian Medical Systems: A Comparative Study.* Berkeley: University of California Press, 1976.

NAKAMURA, HAJIME. *Ways of Thinking of Eastern Peoples: India, China, Tibet, Japan.* Rev. English trans. Edited by Philip P. Wiener. Honolulu: East–West Center Press, 1964.

RIEPE, DALE. *The Naturalistic Tradition in Indian Thought.* Seattle: University of Washington Press, 1961.

TSUNODA, RYŪSAKU; DE BARY, WILLIAM THEODORE; and KEENE, DONALD, eds. *Sources of Japanese Tradition.* New York: Columbia University Press, 1958.

ZIMMER, HEINRICH ROBERT. *Hindu Medicine.* Edited with a foreword and preface by Ludwig Edelstein. Publications of the Institute of the History of Medicine, The Johns Hopkins University. 3d ser.: The Hideyo Noguchi Lectures, vol. 6. Baltimore: Johns Hopkins Press, 1948.

ENVIRONMENTAL ETHICS

I. ENVIRONMENTAL HEALTH AND HUMAN DISEASE
    Samuel S. Epstein
II. QUESTIONS OF SOCIAL JUSTICE
    Norman J. Faramelli
    and Charles W. Powers
III. THE PROBLEM OF GROWTH   *C. P. Wolf and*
    Drew Christiansen

I
ENVIRONMENTAL HEALTH AND HUMAN DISEASE

This article will deal with the moral and ethical aspects of the relationship between environmental pollution and disease in the general and working populations. First, the scope and extent of environmentally induced disease is discussed. Second, the problem is analyzed with respect to the cost-benefit considerations of modern technology. Third, problems of biased data are described, including how these may impact on regulatory decisions. Finally, the need for a greater role of ethical consideration in decision-making processes is emphasized. Although the themes considered are universal, particular reference is made to problems in the United States.

Human disease

There is now growing evidence that much human disease hitherto regarded as spontaneous, including cancer, is caused by environmental pollutants. The contributory role of air pollution in chronic respiratory disease is also well recognized. Additionally, there is a growing body of evidence relating specific pollutants to psychobehavioral disorders and birth defects. Finally, emerging data incriminate specific pollutants with mutations and mental deficiency.

This realization of a relationship between pollution and disease is heightened by the exponential increase in human exposure to new synthetic chemicals and to their degradation and combustion products in air, water, and soil. In general, these new chemicals are not adequately characterized, either toxicologically or ecologically.

Chronic respiratory disease. Chronic respiratory disease, including bronchitis, emphysema, and asthma, is widely prevalent in the general population. Air pollution, especially particulates and sulfates from stationary sources, such as municipal incinerators and utility plants, and automobile emissions, are major causes of chronic respiratory disease. For example, it has been estimated that failure to meet current sulfur dioxide standards, which are exceeded in most U.S. cities, is responsible annually for six thousand premature deaths, six million to ten million avoidable asthma attacks, and twenty million to thirty million days of exacerbation of cardiovascular and respiratory disease. It is further estimated that automobile emissions contribute ten to fifteen percent of health hazards from air pollution. Additionally, many kinds of dust present in the work environment cause debilitating lung diseases, called pneumoconioses. About 125,000 U.S. coal miners suffer from coal workers' pneumoconiosis, and the disease is estimated to cause three thousand to four thousand deaths each year. Other pneumoconioses include asbestosis, as well as various cancers, from asbestos; byssinosis from cotton dust; bagassosis from sugar cane dust; and silicosis from various silica-containing dusts. Over all, nine thousand annual deaths in the United States are attributed to these occupational dust diseases.

Cancer. Cancer is now a major killing and disabling disease of epidemic proportions. More than 53 million of the 210 million U.S. population (twenty-five percent) will develop some form of cancer, and approximately twenty percent of Americans now die from cancer (Epstein, "Environmental Determinants"). It is estimated that 665,000 new cancer cases were diagnosed and that there were 365,000 cancer deaths in 1975. Thus, cancer deaths in 1975 alone were approximately five times higher than the total U.S. military deaths in the Vietnam and Korean war years combined.

Human misery apart, the total economic impact of cancer is massive. Estimates indicate that in 1969 the direct costs for hospitalization and medical care for cancer exceeded $500 million. The direct and indirect costs of cancer, including loss of earnings during illness and during the balance of normal life expectancy, were estimated in 1971 as $15 billion (ibid.); estimates for 1976 are about $18 billion.

The rate of recent increase of cancer deaths in the United States and other industrialized countries is more rapid than the rate of increase in population. It is of interest to note that besides cancer only two other major causes of death—homicide and cirrhosis of the liver—have significantly increased in the recent past. The increase in new cancer cases is real and over and above any increase due to age alone.

There is now a growing consensus that the majority of human cancers (some estimates go from seventy to ninety percent) are environmental in origin and that they are hence ultimately preventable. Prevention, however, demands vigorous legislative and regulatory initiatives, which have not yet been forthcoming. The basis for such estimates largely derives from epidemiological studies, in large community populations over extended periods, which have revealed wide geographic variations in the incidence of cancer of various organs. It should be noted, however, that the role of specific environmental carcinogens has been so far implicated or identified in only relatively few of the studies (ibid.).

It is of particular interest that a recent National Cancer Institute (NCI) atlas has demonstrated marked geographical clustering of high mortality rates from cancers of various organs in the United States among white male and female populations in heavily industrialized counties (Mason et al.). Such data are presumptive of associations between cancer rates in the general community and the proximity of residence to certain industries, in addition to exposure of workers in these industries. There are growing analytic data on the spillover of carcinogens from industry into the adjacent community by routes including air, water, and clothing of workers.

Apart from the importance of occupational factors in the incidence of "neighborhood" or community cancer in the population at large, specific occupational exposures are an important cause of cancer deaths, particularly in males. Various estimates have suggested that five to fifteen percent of all current cancer deaths in males are occupational in origin. These include lung and other cancers in insulation workers and others, such as construction workers, exposed to asbestos; bladder cancer in the aniline dye and rubber industry, induced by such chemicals as 2-naphthylamine, benzidine, 2-aminobiphenyl and 2-nitrobiphenyl; lung cancer in uranium miners of Colorado, in coke oven workers, and in workers even briefly exposed to bischloromethylether; skin cancer in shale oil workers; nasal sinus cancer in wood workers; cancer of the pancreas and lymphomas in organic chemists; and angiosarcoma of the liver, besides other cancers, in workers involved in the manufacture and fabrication of polyvinyl chloride (PVC).

The toll of cancer related to particular occupational exposures is overwhelming. For instance, it has been estimated that approximately twenty percent of all of the long-term asbestos workers die of lung cancer. Approximately thirty percent of all premature deaths in uranium miners are due to lung cancer. Many other occupational groups are at high cancer risk, including steelworkers, miners and smelters, rubber workers, and workers in a wide range of petrochemical industries (Epstein, 1976).

Birth defects. There is also growing recognition of the importance of environmental pollutants as causes of birth defects. The incidence of gross congenital malformations in the United States, although unknown in the absence of a comprehensive national registry, has been estimated at from three to four percent of total live births. Three major categories of human teratogens have so far been identified: viral infections, X-irradiation, and chemicals and drugs, such as mercurials, thalidomide, and diethylstilbestrol.

Thalidomide is a drug that was widely marketed in Europe in the late 1950s and early 1960s for "morning sickness." An alert medical practitioner associated the drug with the birth of thousands of babies with unusually malformed limbs. It should be noted that the teratogenicity of thalidomide was detected only because of the unusual birth defects it produced; had it induced a similar incidence of more common defects, in all likelihood, it would still be

in use as a "safe" drug to this date. The phenoxy herbicide 2,4,5-T and related compounds, including their dioxin contaminants, have also aroused concern because of their widespread and increasing use and because of their teratogenicity in mice and rats; their incrimination in human birth defects is not yet clearly established.

Mutations. The first evidence that environmental pollutants may influence the genetic constitution of future populations resulted in the 1930s from the discovery that high-energy radiation induces mutations. The subsequent development of nuclear energy added a new dimension and enhanced awareness of the problem of genetic hazards. Once radiation-induced mutagenesis was discovered, there were reasons to suspect that some chemicals would act similarly, but proof of this was delayed until World War II, when mustard gas was shown to induce mutations in fruit flies. Many and varied types of chemicals have subsequently been shown to be mutagenic in various systems, including mammals. The likelihood that some highly mutagenic chemicals may come into wide use or indeed may already be in wide use is now of serious concern.

Psychobehavioral defects. Emerging data are establishing clear relationships between exposure to a wide range of environmental and occupational pollutants and acute and delayed psychobehavioral or neurotoxic effects, ranging from disturbances in fine judgment and discrimination and mild alterations in personality and behavior to advanced dementia. Illustrative of a common pollutant producing acute psychobehavioral effects is carbon monoxide, which, at concentrations found in common traffic conditions, produces disturbances in reflexes, judgment, and orientation. Further examples are the delayed effects of lead, which, at exposure levels and body burdens now considered to be relatively low, induce disturbances in personality and nerve conduction in workers, and mental deficiency and psychobehavioral disorders in young children.

Cost-benefit analysis

There is considerable controversy today over whether narrow "cost-benefit" language is truly adequate for arriving at sound environmental policies, since that kind of calculus does not in itself account for such ethical considerations as justice, human rights, and personal preferences. Furthermore, when a policy is determined by cost-benefit analysis, it is important to take into account what kind of benefit and what kind of risk are involved, who enjoys the benefit, who suffers the risk, and how those benefits and risks are evaluated and perceived by the parties involved. Thus, for example, it is sometimes difficult to know what conclusion to draw when the health risk is significant to a very small portion of the population and the benefits are minimal (perhaps esthetic) yet desirable to almost the entire nation.

Chemical products and processes. Since World War II there has been an exponential and largely unregulated increase in the numbers and quantities of synthetic organic chemicals manufactured and used in industrialized countries. The claimed need, generally in the absence of supportive documentation, to use increasing numbers of new synthetic chemicals makes it essential to recognize and evaluate carcinogenic and other human hazards with regard to the real or alleged matching benefits they confer; similar considerations extend to direct and indirect environmental degradations. Such costs must be balanced by factors including the persistence and environmental mobility of the chemical, the size of the general or occupational population exposed, and the reversibility of the adverse effects. The costs must be viewed realistically: The total annual U.S. costs of approximately $15 billion due to cancer have hitherto been largely discounted ("externalized," in the language of the economist). As the majority of human cancers, in both the general and the working population, are now considered to be due to environmental carcinogens, and hence preventable, there should be clear economic and other incentives to reduce this environmental and occupational burden. Yet, strangely enough, there has been a low fiscal allocation (less than ten percent of the $830 million budget in 1976) to environmental and chemical carcinogenesis in the budget of the National Cancer Institute (NCI).

The criterion of broad societal efficacy, once extended from therapeutic drugs to other synthetic chemicals, such as food and feed additives, pesticides, and industrial chemicals, may further simplify the cost-benefit calculus. As an illustration of this argument, food additives would have to be excluded from products unless they are both safe and either significantly improve the quality of the nutritive value of the food or lower its costs. Food dyes and other such "cosmetic" food additives do not meet the criterion of efficacy, let alone safety (further societal reflection is needed to determine what

extent of risk if any is reasonable in achieving a purely cosmetic effect in foods).

Similarly, claims that occupational carcinogens serve industrially unique purposes must be examined openly by experts representing a broad range of viewpoints and interests, with particular recognition of the attendant and generally externalized or discounted human costs and of the lack of economic incentives to develop similarly efficacious and less hazardous product or process alternatives. In the absence of such alternatives, consideration should be directed to the possible banning of the manufacture and use of the carcinogen or to restricting its use to large industrial facilities willing and able to use closed systems that are continuously monitored with instrumentation of maximum sensitivity, with the results made accessible to exposed workers.

Inherent in toxicological and regulatory practice is acceptance, in principle, of the concept of balancing benefit—benefit to the general public rather than to industry—against cost to public health and the environment rather than cost or risk to industry. If this standard is to be taken seriously, one might ask: If the chemical product or process in question does not demonstrably serve a broad social and economically useful purpose for the general population, why introduce it and force the public at large to accept potential costs without general matching benefits? The concept of matching benefits against costs has generally been employed in practice to maximize short-term benefits to industry, even though this may entail minimal benefits and maximal costs to the general public. While such an approach is detrimental to the general public, it is also often detrimental to the long-term interests of industry, which may suffer major economic dislocation when hazardous products and processes, to which it has improperly developed premature major commitments, are belatedly banned from commerce.

Nuclear energy. It has been argued that conventional cost-benefit considerations cannot be applied to policy questions in the development of a national, large-scale, fission-based economy, since such questions are largely ethical rather than technological. These questions, relating to whether society should strike a Faustian bargain with atomic physicists and engineers, have been posed, for example, as the burden of requiring continuous monitoring in order to avoid unparalleled disaster (Kneese).

It appears that the immediate environmental

impact of the routine operation of the nuclear fuel cycle can be reduced to lower levels than is possible with fuel-fired plants. The attendant problems include strip-mine land reclamation, pneumoconioses, and community air pollution, especially from acid sulfates. However, such an immediate superiority of nuclear technologies does not necessarily exclude other potential alternatives, including solar and geothermal energy, on which very small research and development efforts have so far been expended, and on which the U.S. and other governments appear reluctant to increase their commitments. Furthermore, the technologies for controlling adverse environmental and public health impacts of fossil fuel utilization have been developed and are being used without major economic perturbations. Such alternatives apart, the advantages of fission are more easily stated in terms of cost-benefit analysis than are the hazards, particularly those associated with operation of the fuel cycle and with long-term waste storage. Estimates on the probability and consequences of major accidents at a nuclear facility vary. A not unfamiliar association of estimates of low consequence with direct or indirect economic interest, and of estimates of higher probability and higher consequences with the absence of such interest, appears to exist. Property damage apart, critiques by the Union of Concerned Scientists (1974) and the American Physical Society (1975) have indicated that a report contracted by the then Atomic Energy Commission (AEC), underestimated the health consequences of a power plant accident by a factor of sixteen to fifty. Furthermore, it is clear that the probability of accident rises with increasing numbers of nuclear facilities and is increased by sabotage, terrorism, and warfare. The continued insistence of the nuclear industry on subsidies, such as the limited liability conferred (in the United States) by the Price–Anderson Act, indicates that the industry itself is concerned about the probability and financial consequences of accidents.

Of equal concern is the problem of storage of high-level radioactive wastes. Unequivocal assurances by the then AEC that the Lyons, Kansas, salt formations were the best site for waste storage were shortly followed by disclosures that the site was a "leaky sieve" (Metzger, p. 158). Current emphasis on the design of surface storage facilities, intended to last a hundred years or so pending development of more permanent storage sites, will necessitate development of sophisticated automated monitoring and elaborate safeguards against accidents, terrorism, and theft.

The costs and hazards from nuclear technology are of utmost gravity and clearly extend to mankind many generations hence. It is clear that decisions on the benefits and costs of nuclear technologies must be shifted from the narrow and constrained arena of the private sector and technology to the wider domain of the public interest and representative government.

Burden of proof. The concept of the burden of proof in public policymaking and in cost-benefit analysis is somewhat unfamiliar to the scientific and technological communities. The absence of comprehensive and definitive data on a particular problem too often results in an unwillingness of scientists and technologists to express opinions or accept a role in the decision-making process. However, a lack of information or the presence of certain levels of uncertainty are key elements in the appropriate reallocation of the burden of proof from the public and the federal government to any party initiating the risk (Karstadt). In administrative conflicts and, increasingly, in judicial decisions, "the burden of proof rests on the party that *initiates* the risk, that *profits* from the risk, and that has the greatest resources to *do* something about the risk" (Nader). Thus, the absence of data on any particular adverse effect would indicate that policies should be developed on the basis of "worst possible case" assumptions about safety to public health and the environment. Subsequent development of such data would allow appropriate policy modifications.

Generation and interpretation of the data base

The data base. Decisions on costs and benefits can be only as good as their underlying data base. There is growing evidence to confirm and document the long-held suspicion that data generated by an interested party, whether by in-house industrial scientists, commercial testing organizations, or universities under contract, may exhibit constraints ranging from biased interpretation to frank manipulation; charges of biased interpretation have also been directed against public advocacy groups. Such constrained data can no longer be regarded as exceptional; for example, in common consumer products such as drugs, there have been the criminal conviction of a drug company's officials for fraudulent manipulation of data on the drug MER/29; the conviction for submission of false data by another company on the drug Dornwall; the nolo contendere plea of a laboratory for concealing information on Flexin; the withdrawal of Panalba from the market after its producer had been found to conceal data on its lack of efficacy ("Introduction of a Bill"); and the testimony by Food and Drug Administration (FDA) Commissioner Schmidt before Senator Kennedy on 20 January 1976 that a commercial testing laboratory under contract to a pharmaceutical company reported on nonexistent slides on animals under carcinogenicity tests with Aldactone. Deputy Administrator Quarles of the Environmental Protection Agency (EPA) also testified on 20 January 1976 on the manipulation of toxicological and carcinogenicity data on pesticides, including Chlordane and Heptachlor, tested by a commercial testing laboratory under contract to a pesticide manufacturer. A later report based on preliminary analysis of chronic toxicity data submitted before 1971 by industry to one of EPA's predecessor organizations (FDA) in support of tolerances for twenty-three pesticides and accepted for this purpose revealed that the data on only one of these pesticides were satisfactory; the twenty-three pesticides were selected for analysis since tolerances on a particularly large number of food commodities had been established for most of them. The other data were so flawed and biased as to invalidate any possible inferences as to carcinogenicity (Reuber). On the basis of such reports, the policy of the EPA is to have an extensive audit of data, in its files, previously submitted by industry in successful support of petitions for pesticide tolerances.

Turning to another class of consumer products, the automobile, the following examples provide further illustrations: In 1972 a well-known automobile company falsified emission control certification tests; however, it was able to ward off a criminal prosecution by paying a $7 million fine. During the first EPA suspension hearing in April 1972, the automobile manufacturers claimed that installation of emission controls in 1975 cars would induce a five to ten percent fuel penalty over 1972 cars. However, by April 1973, at the second EPA suspension hearing, the manufacturers admitted that there would be no fuel penalty. Finally, by June 1973 another automobile company publicly announced and then informed Congress that there would be a sales-weighted fuel economy of thirteen percent due to catalytic converters (Epstein, "The Public Interest").

Examples in the field of occupational disease abound. The seriousness and extent of the problem cannot be exaggerated. The chronology of the development of data, from 1972 to 1975, on the carcinogenicity of vinyl chloride, used in the production of PVC, has recently been reviewed in a report of the AAAS Committee on Scientific Freedom and Responsibility. The report documents the suppression of carcinogenicity data by the Manufacturing Chemists Association (MCA), allowing continued exposure, without warning, of tens of thousands of workers to high concentrations of vinyl chloride (Edsall).

Blatant examples of constrained data are also evident in recent analyses of the economic impact of proposed regulations. A now apparently standard response by certain sectors of industry to attempts by regulatory agencies to promulgate standards limiting environmental and occupational exposure to chemical carcinogens is to forecast major economic disruption and unemployment attendant on compliance. Apart from the questionable economic validity of such forecasts, they do not appear to address themselves to the unrecognized ("externalized") costs, economic and otherwise, of carcinogenic and other toxic effects due to human exposure to carcinogens (Epstein, 1976).

Inflated economic analyses have also been used by industry to discourage "Toxic Substances" legislation, which mandates the requirements for premarket notification to the EPA and in some cases toxicological testing of new chemical agents prior to their introduction to commerce and the workplace.

Policies for improving data base. It is now clear that there is a critical need to ensure impartial and competent testing of all products to which human exposure is anticipated. The present system of direct, closed-contract negotiations between manufacturing industries and commercial and other testing laboratories, including universities, is open to potential abuse and creates obvious mutual constraints. One possible remedy would be the introduction of a disinterested advisory group or agency as an intermediary between manufacturers and commercial or other testing laboratories. Proper legal and other safeguards could be developed to minimize potential abuses and conflicts of interest. Manufacturers could notify the intermediary group when safety evaluation was required for a particular product. The advisory group would then solicit contract bids on the open market. Bids would be awarded on the basis of economics, quality of protocols, and technical competence. The progress of testing would be monitored by periodic reports and site visits, as with federal contracts. At the conclusion of the studies, the advisory group would comment on the quality of the data, make appropriate recommendations, and forward these to the concerned regulatory agency for routine action.

This approach appears preferable to the secret award of unbid contracts. Additionally, quality checks during testing would ensure the high quality and reliability of data and minimize the need to repeat studies, thus reducing pressure on federal agencies to accept unsatisfactory data on an ex post facto basis. This approach not only would minimize constraints due to special interests but would also upgrade the quality of testing in commercial and other testing laboratories (Epstein, "Public Health Hazards").

Major constraints in the field of occupational health and safety would be reduced by the future employment of physicians and hygienists by joint management–labor groups or committees, rather than exclusively by management, as is the current practice.

Interpretation of the data base. The significant influence of economic and related constraints on expert advisory committees, both federal and nongovernmental, is being increasingly appreciated. In addition to constraints on the generation of objective data, constraints on the evaluation and interpretation of these data by regulatory agencies may also influence resulting policy decisions.

A major scandal in regulatory agencies is the personnel "revolving door." Agencies recruit directly from industry significant numbers of senior administrative staff, who often tend to perpetuate philosophies and practices consistent with interests of industry and not of the broader public. More seriously, a significant number of senior agency officials leave for industry positions during their active careers or after retirement. This creates a potential conflict of interest and an apparent inducement to agency officials to interpret data in a manner consistent with their future interests and not to take action possibly detrimental to future employers. As of January 1977, one-year restricted employment mobility clauses have been introduced in agency–employee contracts; such clauses are long-standing and commonplace in industry. Furthermore, a major mitigating factor would be development of an enhanced economic and professional status for regulatory employees and of third party testing and other measures that would re-

strict the discretionary power of senior agency officials, especially those eligible for early retirement.

In this connection, equally serious potential conflicts of interest and a source of pressure on agency scientists arise with the senior science advisers to agencies, generally university scientists, who may receive substantial contracts and grants from the agency and who may also be consultants to industries regulated by the agency and receive research contracts from these industries. These senior science advisers may play a key role, and one that is largely hidden from Congress, in major decision making in agencies (Epstein, 1977).

The public interest movement as an ethical renaissance

The "public interest" movement. The "public interest" movement, as a modern expression of social ethics and as an instrument of political change, is now less than one decade old. Public interest groups embrace a wide spectrum of heterogeneous styles and objectives, from conservationists and environmentalists, some of whom are traditionalist and conservative, to more activist consumer and citizen groups. Some contemporary concerns of a few public interest groups dealing with occupational health and safety issues present a potential for ad hoc alliances between labor and the public interest.

The public interest movement expresses the conviction that the "common good" is inadequately represented in the brokerage of decision making at the federal and local levels, where narrow and concentrated economic and political interests are joined and where considerations of social equity are largely precluded. The movement also expresses convictions that public health and environmental costs are poorly perceived and too readily discounted in regulatory decision making, and that the burden of proof for such costs is too readily accepted by government or inappropriately shifted from the private to the public sector. Specifically, these public interest convictions have been aroused because of considerations such as the following: restrictions in public access to regulatory data; the unwillingness of agencies to accept qualified citizen and consumer representatives in their decision-making processes; and the legislative failure to create formal mechanisms for representation of the public interest in the regulatory process.

Public access to data. Public interest groups are pressing for further legislation concerning open access to data. Formal and informal discussions among agencies, industry, and federal and nongovernment expert committees on all issues relating to human safety and environmental quality, and data relevant to such discussions, properly belong to the public domain. Indeed, under the 1967 Freedom of Information Act (U.S. Public Law 89–487, 80 Stat. 250), all federal records are intended to be open to the public except for specified and validated exemptions, such as trade secrets. Demands for access to internal data and working papers are being extended to agency memoranda and to quasi-governmental bodies in the United States, such as the National Academy of Sciences (NAS), which has successfully claimed exemption from the requirements of the Freedom of Information and Federal Advisory Committee Acts (Boffey).

Impetus to demands for routine access to internal agency memoranda is periodically reinforced by "leaks" of confidential agency documents, which make it clear that an agency is seriously derelict. In some instances, such "leaks" have resulted in congressional investigations and major policy shifts. There is no evidence to suggest that unrestricted access to agency data, excluding security and validated proprietary documentation, would in any way impede regulatory practice.

Public involvement in decision making. It is important that the citizen and consumer be adequately represented at the earliest stages of the decision-making process and of agency–industry discussions on the widest range of issues concerning the public interest. Decisions by agencies on setting standards, in areas including technological innovations and new products after closed discussions of data that have been treated confidentially, are no longer acceptable; similar considerations obtain for products already established in commerce with relation to data on safety and efficacy. Such methods of decision making are contrary to the long-term interests of industry, quite apart from the best interests of the public: The possibility of legal penalties and of third party suits and class actions further point to the need for citizen participation. While there is a growing acceptance by industry of the legitimacy of demands for representation by public interest groups, formal mechanisms for this purpose have not yet been adequately developed.

Federal advisory committees, as stipulated by the 1972 U.S. Federal Advisory Committee Act (FACA), are required to be a "means of furnishing expert advice, ideas and diverse opinions to the Federal government." While many committees are not particularly effective and meet only infrequently, others wield great power, and their recommendations provide important input into government actions. While the FACA made important strides in opening up deliberations of advisory committees to the public, there are still major problems in making the system responsive to broader interests. Most agencies exclude public interest representatives, whether technically qualified or not, and also qualified experts nominated by public interest groups, from their advisory committees. The lack of fair balance on committees hinges on the contention by government that industry members should be designated "public" representatives. Of equal concern is the increasingly common device, particularly in EPA, of appointing fact-finding "panels," in contrast to recommendation-making advisory committees, as the panels are alleged to be exempt from the requirements of the FACA for balance and openness (Epstein, 1977).

Need for an agency for consumer protection. While numerous agencies in the United States, particularly the Department of Commerce and the Small Business Administration, already support the positions and interest of industry, as of March 1977 no government agency was charged with the advocacy and protection of consumer and citizen interests. Whether these interests relate to concerns such as clean air, auto safety, meat inspection, or land use, there was no currently adequate mechanism for presenting the public interest.

It is freely recognized that business representatives outnumber consumer representatives by over one hundred to one in appearances before federal agencies (Epstein, "Statement"). The offices of consumer affairs of the various U.S. federal agencies are small and relatively ineffectual, reflecting as they do overall agency policies and pressure, and are clearly no substitute for an independent agency, uniquely and solely charged with representing the public interest. This is a critical deficiency in regulatory practice, especially as the health, safety, and other interests of the public have been and can be massively influenced by the decisions and actions of a wide range of federal agencies.

Summary

While problems of environmental pollution and human disease are long-standing, they have been greatly magnified by the accelerated utilization of natural resources and the progressive development of new technologies. The historical causes date from the industrial revolution, the petrochemical era of the 1930s, and the nuclear technologies since World War II.

Although "pollutant" is often pejoratively applied to synthetic industrial chemicals and to nuclear fission products, there is a wide range of other chemical pollutants comprised in four broad categories. The first group consists of natural chemicals in excess, such as nitrates and arsenic. Natural fungal or plant toxins in crops constitute the second group. The third group consists of complex organic and inorganic mixtures, such as community air and water pollutants and occupational pollutants, including coal tar pitch volatiles, which comprise a wide range of undefined as well as partially defined chemical components. Finally, there is the group of synthetic chemicals: agricultural chemicals, notably pesticides and fertilizers; food additives, which may be intentional, such as antioxidants and dyes, or accidental, such as pesticides, heavy metals, and plasticizers; fuel additives; household chemicals; and industrial chemicals. Most of these chemicals are derived from petroleum, which is now the basic stock for the synthesis of the majority of organic chemicals.

Pollutants may induce a wide range of adverse or toxic effects. Acute or chronic toxicity per se may appear in the growing embryo, infant, child, or adult with effects ranging from slight impairment of health and fitness to disabling disease and death. More specific manifestations of chronic toxicity include the induction of cancer (carcinogenicity), birth defects (teratogenicity) and genetic abnormalities (mutagenicity). That chronic toxicity may also impair immunity or produce psychobehavioral disorders has become increasingly evident. Some pollutants may induce more than one type of toxicity. Pollutants, or their precursors, may also interact outside (in vitro) or inside the body (in vivo) with other chemicals to produce otherwise unanticipated cumulative effects. Such effects can also result from interactions between otherwise harmless and common environmental chemicals, such as nitrites in vegetables and secondary amines in meat and fish, to produce a class of chemicals known as nitrosamines, which are usually potent carcinogens, mutagens, and teratogens.

The need to use increasing numbers of synthetic industrial chemicals makes it essential to recognize and estimate the human and ecological hazards they pose and their societal acceptability with regard to the real or alleged matching benefits they confer. Hazards from particular products or processes, or from particular synthetic chemicals, whether in consumer products or in the workplace, need not necessarily be accepted even when their matching benefits are, or are alleged to be, high. Equally efficacious but less hazardous alternative chemicals, processes, and products are generally available. The imposition of mandatory criteria such as broad societal utility, efficacy, or other characteristics prior to the introduction of synthetic chemicals into commerce may well simplify such equations (Epstein, "Public Health Hazards").

Rational judgments on the benefits of technological innovations and on the risks of environmental pollution are critically dependent on the availability of a comprehensive, unbiased, and valid data base to competent decision makers who represent a broad range of balancing interests. However, growing evidence has demonstrated that data on both risks and benefits, generated directly or indirectly by economically interested parties, frequently suffer from constraints ranging from biased interpretation to frank manipulation. Moreover, critical analysis of major current problem areas in environmental pollution demonstrates that, while these problems are frequently presented in a technological or scientific guise, their primary determinants are economic, political, and evaluative. As a corollary, the prevention of such problems requires sensitivity to social equity and justice—a calculus not sufficiently represented in contemporary policymaking, which is currently based, with rather excessive emphasis, on the narrower perspectives and interests of regulatory agencies, industry, and the technological or scientific communities.

SAMUEL S. EPSTEIN

[For further discussion of topics mentioned in this article, see the entries: DRUG INDUSTRY AND MEDICINE; JUSTICE; and RISK. For discussion of related ideas, see the entries: DECISION MAKING, MEDICAL; ENVIRONMENT AND MAN; FUTURE GENERATIONS, OBLIGATIONS TO; HEALTH AND DISEASE; HEALTH POLICY; PUBLIC HEALTH; SOCIAL MEDICINE; and TECHNOLOGY. See also: MEDICAL ETHICS, HISTORY OF, section on EUROPE AND THE AMERICAS, article on EASTERN EUROPE IN THE TWENTIETH CENTURY; and SMOKING.]

BIBLIOGRAPHY

American Physical Society. "Report on Light Water Reactor Safety." *Reviews of Modern Physics* 47, supp. 1 (1975), pp. S1–S123.

BOFFEY, PHILLIP M. *The Brain Bank of America: An Inquiry into the Politics of Science.* Introduction by Ralph Nader. New York: McGraw-Hill Book Co., 1975.

EDSALL, JOHN T. "Scientific Freedom and Responsibility: A Report of the AAAS Committee on Scientific Freedom and Responsibility." *Science* 188 (1975): 687–693.

EPSTEIN, SAMUEL S. "Environmental Determinants of Human Cancer." *Cancer Research* 34 (1974): 2425–2435.

————. "The Political and Economic Basis of Cancer." *Technology Review* 78, no. 8 (1976), pp. 34–43.

————. "Public Health Hazards from Chemicals in Consumer Products." *Consumer Health and Product Hazards—Chemicals, Electronic Products, Radiation.* The Legislation of Public Safety, vol. 1. Edited by Samuel S. Epstein and Richard D. Grundy. Cambridge: MIT Press, 1974, pp. 45–99.

————. "The Public Interest: Overview." *Environmental Health Perspectives* 10 (1975): 173–179.

————. "Statement in Support of Legislation to Create the Agency for Consumer Protection." Committee on Government Operations, House of Representatives. *Establishing an Agency for Consumer Protection.* Hearings on H.R. 7575 before a subcommittee. 94th Cong., 1st sess., 17–20 June 1975. Washington: Government Printing Office, 1975, pp. 378–381.

————, and GAGE, KIT. "The Federal Advisory Committee System: An Assessment." *Environmental Law Reporter* 7 (1977): 50001–50012.

"Introduction of a Bill Establishing a National Drug Testing Center." United States, Congress, Senate, *Congressional Record,* 91st Cong., 1st sess., 1969, 115, pt. 16: 21360–21370. Remarks and items supporting Senator Nelson's Bill S. 2729, dealing with problems and needed reforms in the pharmaceutical industry. No hearings held; the bill died in the Committee on Labor and Public Welfare.

Joint Review Committee of the Sierra Club and the Union of Concerned Scientists. "Preliminary Review of the AEC Reactor Safety Study." Washington, November 1974, p. 95. Unpublished study.

KARSTADT, MYRA L. "Protecting Public Health from Hazardous Substances: Federal Regulation of Environmental Contaminants." *Environmental Law Reporter* 5 (1975): 50165–50178.

KNEESE, ALLEN V. "Benefit-Cost Analysis and Unscheduled Events in the Nuclear Fuel Cycle." *Resources* (A Newsletter of Resources for the Future, Washington), no. 44 (1973), pp. 1–5.

MASON, THOMAS J.; MCKAY, FRANK W.; HOOVER, ROBERT; BLOT, WILLIAM J.; and FRAUMENI, JOSEPH F. *Atlas of Cancer Mortality for U.S. Counties: 1950–1969.* DHEW Publication no. (NIH) 75–780. Bethesda, Md.: National Institutes of Health, 1975.

METZGER, H. PETER. *The Atomic Establishment.* New York: Simon & Schuster, 1972.

NADER, RALPH. "Professional Responsibility Revisited." Proceedings of the Conference on Science, Technology, and the Public Interest. The Brookings Institution, Washington, D.C., 8 October 1973. The proceedings are available from the Commission for the Advancement of Public Interest Organizations, Suite 1013, 1975 Connecticut Avenue, Washington, D.C. 20009.

REUBER, MELVIN D. *Review of Toxicity Test Results Submitted in Support of Pesticide Tolerance Petitions.* Report for the Office of Pesticide Programs, United States Environmental Protection Agency, 9 April 1976. Available from the EPA in photoreduplicated form.

II
QUESTIONS OF SOCIAL JUSTICE

An increasing concern with the natural environment has developed recently throughout the world. Many factors have contributed to this, for example, the growth in global population with its attendant demands upon the biosphere, the depletion of many natural resources and threat of extinction of many forms of plant and animal life, and the realization that human life and welfare are interrelated with the life and welfare of other organisms within the biosphere.

Concomitant with the victories of the environmental movement has been the apprehension of some social critics that the effort to protect the environment would place the "rights of nature" above the "rights of humanity," and especially the rights of poor people (Neuhaus; Faramelli). Many worry, for example, that in the name of conservation or of ecological balance justification would be found for exclusionary policies (e.g., zoning) that would ensure the preservation of unjust enclaves of privilege. There is also apprehension about the possibility that strong environmental legislation might cripple economic growth and increase unemployment. Those who are pessimistic about securing any redistribution of goods and services from the existing economic order frequently see in the environmental movement a threat to efforts to secure more benefits for the poor from increasing economic activity. These people have not been reassured by arguments that in a stationary-state economy redistribution would *have* to occur (Daly).

Although this view, which pits the environment against people, can be and has been seriously challenged by responsible critics, e.g., Leonard Woodcock and Congressmen Rangel, Dellums, and Conyers of the Black Congressional Caucus, it brings to the fore important theoretical questions that demand the attention of ethicists. Among the major issues that it raises are the following: (1) How do the rights of human beings and the rights of the environment come into conflict? (2) If, in justice, we are required to protect the environment, can we also adequately protect people and meet their just demands? (3) What assumptions about justice and the social order led to the perception that there is a conflict between the rights of persons and the rights of the environment?

Justice, the rights of human beings, and the rights of the environment

There are, of course, competing views of justice. Differing definitions of justice are generally differing proposals as to the means by which persons may legitimate and adjudicate among or reconcile the various *claims* made upon a society. Put differently, conceptions of justice represent different ways of evaluating or reconciling competing claims that someone or some group has a "right."

For people to make a rights claim is for them to voice "the conviction that what they are demanding is both legitimate and necessary" (Jenkins). The claims that people articulate as "rights" are incredibly variegated. They are, moreover, becoming more, not less, complicated as we move from a tradition wherein rights were seen primarily as negative ("freedom from" various intrusions) to a situation where rights lay claim "to" or "for" particular goods and services. The danger in this shift lies in a propensity to claim as a basic "right" that merits social recognition all kinds of desires of individuals and groups (ibid.), with the consequent difficulty, made ever more hazardous by the mere fact of proliferation, of determining when these claims are indeed grounded in justice. The adjudication between conflicting rights claims demands a theory of justice by which to distinguish genuine rights from arbitrary claims. But just such a theory of justice is precluded by the liberal tradition's inclination to identify rights and interests and, as we shall see, by its rejection of rational discrimination of rights and its belief in the identity of interests.

Rights for nonhuman beings and things?

Environmentalists have argued that it is erroneous to assume that only human beings have rights. These authors (Stone; Cobb) propose that nonhuman beings and things, indeed the natural environment as a whole, have rights that demand, in justice, recognition and protection by society. In developing this argument Stone, Cobb, and others have made explicit what has been implicit in much of the environmental movement for some time. So long as nonhuman natural things were considered simply "of value,"

it was unclear whether they were valuable in themselves or valuable simply because they were instrumental in achieving some *human* purpose or in meeting some *human* need. By claiming that nonhuman things have rights, environmentalists impute an intrinsic worth to natural systems independently of human purposes and needs. This eco-ethic is frequently accompanied by a rejection of the "homocentrism" of traditional Western thought.

There are two other aspects to the proposal that natural systems have rights. These aspects, if accepted, would have revolutionary implications for our concepts of rights and of justice. First, the rights at issue are less those of individuals than those of classes or species of things, and difficult to define natural units, such as landscapes and ecologies. Second, when it is species and natural systems that have rights, then one is concerned not just with adjudicating claims made in the present, but with the preservation and protection of those classes of things in the future. For instance, one of the issues in the controversy over the use of nuclear power is the legacy of radioactive wastes that are generated to serve present energy needs but at the same time pose problems for the future of the ecosystem.

All these propositions (that nonhuman entities have rights, that these rights pertain more to classes than to individuals, and that these rights belong to future and not just present entities) compel clarification of the concept of justice and its role in prioritizing rights claims.

Rights, duties, and the concern for social justice

Earlier it was noted that the proliferation of claims for "human rights" brings with it the great difficulty of judging which claims are authentic and which are not. Not only are more and more claims being made—and to the claims made in behalf of human subjects of rights must now be added claims made in behalf of the environment—there is also an uncertainty about our personal relationship to those claims. If we are responsible not only for ensuring the rights of those who make direct claims upon us but also for taking into consideration *future* claims by future persons and things, it becomes more and more difficult to determine just what our responsibilities are. In the resulting confusion, there is the tendency to give merely rhetorical allegiance to any one of the vast array of possible rights that could be affected by our choices and actions. When this happens, normative discourse can easily serve as the rationalization for any personal predilection. This indeed is to a large extent what is happening today.

The proliferation of rights claims results in a weakening of the moral binding power of all rights language by sheer reiteration. Moreover, the expansion of positive demands upon scarce social resources dilutes the imperative for social justice, with dire consequences for the welfare of the poor, who have relied on rights claims to make up for the failures of social policy. Let us see how this process takes place.

First, it has long been recognized that if rights are to be protected and ensured, there must be a duty correlative to each right. That is, it must be possible to specify an action that is definitely required by specifiable persons in situations in which rights are in jeopardy. Yet this is no easy task (Macklin), especially where there are competing rights claims.

Second, claims made on behalf of the environment are structurally similar to the more traditional protective or "natural rights" claims made on behalf of human subjects rather than to the more contemporary assertive "human rights" claims central to discourse concerning issues of social justice.

From this we can see how the claims of environmentalists can come to have a standing that would threaten the claims for action made in the name of social justice ("human rights" claims). In the social policy area, these concerns surface when we consider who pays for pollution control costs. For instance, will expenditures for environmental quality increase unemployment and thus foster poverty? In other words, do the claims made for clean streams take precedence over the claims made for human welfare?

Here we are either caught in a genuine cul de sac or need to rethink our notions of rights and of justice. The latter is, in our judgment, the case, and the *apparent* conflict pitting human welfare *against* the rights of the environment is rooted in an inadequate theory of justice.

The need for an adequate theory of justice

Central to the apparent conflict between human rights and environmental rights are two assumptions about the meaning of justice that have been bequeathed to us by eighteenth-century rationalism. The first assumption was that there is a body of self-evident and delimited "natural rights," which, if protected, will provide sufficient basis for the establishment of an acceptable human community. The second was that there is a "natural identity of interests," that is, that if all participants in politico-economic processes are given the chance to pursue their self-interest, the resultant distribution of goods, services, or political decisions will magically orchestrate themselves to the optimum welfare of all. This, for instance, is the "invisible hand" ordering economic life. The use of rights claims as a moral and legal tool of self-interest has led to the abandonment of the belief that rights are limited and self-evident. In the subsequent confusion, all that anyone knows in the presence of a rights claim is that its adherents feel that the claim is "legitimate and necessary." Similarly, the natural identity of interests assumption has created confusion in public policy, because it provides no rational ground for the adjudication of claims. The abandonment of the principle of limited and self-evident rights, the identification of rights with interests, and the assumed identity of interests have all contributed to the "misplaced debate" that pits the rights of human beings against the rights of the environment. It has also created anarchy in public policy and has led to the view that governmental intervention, whether to advance the "human rights" of poor people or to protect the environment, is seen as an illegitimate intrusion into the "natural order" of things.

If systematic judgments about the relative position of competing rights claims and duties can be made in any coherent and intelligent fashion, it is necessary to develop a coherent theory of justice (Macklin). Such a theory has either not yet evolved or has not yet been recognized, nor do we propose to develop one here. But it is possible to state what characteristics it would have if it were to help adjudicate concerns about the environment and the concerns of social justice:

1. It would provide persons and communities with the capacity to validate moral claims, including rights claims, and to order them hierarchically.
2. In order to have such a capability, the theory would reject the assertion that rights are "unanalyzable primitives" (Feinberg) and instead would disentangle instrumental from substantive rights (Cobb).
3. It would have the capacity to reformulate rights claims so as to protect and evaluate the concern expressed and to do so in such a way that potential reconciliation with other claims would be possible.

4. It would provide criteria for the identification of which agents are responsible for actions in which kinds of situations to ensure that validated concerns of claims are met. Among the kinds of criteria necessary would be, for example, those which enable an agent to know what degree of probability about future events would be required to establish an obligation from need-meeting action now in order to avoid an adverse consequence to future generations.

The kind of moral theory suggested would provide the missing link between general exhortations to rid the world of poverty or to reconceive the relationship between nature and history and the cacaphony of rights claims we have discussed.

People and the environment in public policy

Up to this point discussion has focused on characteristics of the state of normative discourse that help explain why the tension between the environment and social justice is so strongly felt. The proposed remedy for this situation is the development and legal implementation of a widely shared normative theory of justice. This cannot be expected to occur in the near future. Hence, for the foreseeable future the perception that concern for the environment and concern for people will be inimical will continue. In the meantime, public policy and its implementation must still go on. The question is, How shall this be carried out?

A partial answer may be found by extending a concept pioneered in the 1970 National Environmental Policy Act in the United States. As a result of that legislation, the responsible public official must "include in every recommendation or report on proposals for legislation and other major Federal actions" an environmental impact statement setting forth not only the expected environmental consequences of the proposed action but an assessment of the alternative to it. What this environmental legislation recognizes is that "at stake" in every federal action is its environmental impact. But if we are to make headway in developing policies relating synergistically the impacts they will have, *all* the impacts of those policies should be analyzed. Put differently, even if we do not yet have the conceptual tools or the normative consensus necessary to order our priorities among various claims, we can insist that a good faith effort is made both to determine who or what has a "stake" in what is proposed and to forecast what the consequences of those policies will be on those who will be affected. Viewed in this way, policy formation is an active and self-conscious reconciliation of the competing claims of the "stakeholders" in every policy. It would be possible to require that all parties, public or private, advocating legislation, administrative regulations, or public action, be put under the discipline of seriously attempting to assess all the consequences of thir proposals. Such a requirement would tend to discourage the advocacy of proposals that seriously ignore any major affected interest; it might even encourage creativity and innovation in policy development. And an indirect benefit might be slow inductive progress toward the ordering of normative priorities to correspond with the conceptual ordering of priorities through the more theoretical process suggested earlier. For example, social policies designed to foster both environmental equality and social justice are not impossible to conceive or even implement, if a broader range of alternatives are considered differently and a society moves beyond the dead-end of ecology versus human rights.

Conclusion

The contemporary debate about the environment and social justice is understandable but misplaced. It is understandable because, in the absence of a commonly shared theory of justice and in the midst of rhetorically inflated claims about policy effects, battle lines tend to form along the environment-versus-social-justice axes. As noted above, this polarization is the result of considering too few public policy alternatives and the implications of those alternatives. But it is misplaced because the debate, when posed this way, reinforces patterns of discussion that shut off more constructive efforts to discover precisely what most needs protection or support in the human community and in nature. And it is also misplaced because it tends to discourage a more imaginative search for policy approaches that will relate concern for people to concern for the environment. Until a consensus can be reached on a normative theory of justice, and in order to avoid anarchic and rhetorical approaches, we should place the participants in the political process under the pedagogy of assessing what the consequences for everyone and everything of "value"—that is, for all the "stakeholders"—will be as a result of every formal policy proposal. Such a consideration will result in a better understanding of "Who pays the costs?" and "Who receives the benefits?" of each policy proposal.

Until those questions are answered the misplaced debate will continue.

NORMAN J. FARAMELLI
AND CHARLES W. POWERS

[See the following article: THE PROBLEM OF GROWTH. For further discussion of topics mentioned in this article, see the entries: ANIMAL EXPERIMENTATION, article on PHILOSOPHICAL PERSPECTIVES; FOOD POLICY; FUTURE GENERATIONS, OBLIGATIONS TO; JUSTICE; POPULATION ETHICS: ELEMENTS OF THE FIELD, articles on DEFINITION OF POPULATION ETHICS and ETHICAL PERSPECTIVES ON POPULATION; and RIGHTS. For discussion of related ideas, see the entries: ENVIRONMENT AND MAN; and TECHNOLOGY, article on TECHNOLOGY AND THE LAW.]

BIBLIOGRAPHY

BURCH, WILLIAM R. Daydreams and Nightmares: A Sociological Essay on the American Environment. Harper & Row Monograph Series in Sociology. New York: 1971.

CALLAHAN, DANIEL J. The Tyranny of Survival, and Other Pathologies of Civilized Life. New York: Macmillan Co., 1973.

COBB, JOHN B., JR. "The Population Explosion and Rights of the Subhuman World." IDOC International (North American Edition), no. 9 (12 September 1970), pp. 41–62. Published by IDOC (International Documentation on the Contemporary Church), 432 Park Ave. S., New York, N.Y. 10016. In a collection of documents on "A Theology of Survival."

DALY, HERMAN E. "Toward a Stationary-state Economy." Patient Earth. Edited by John Harte and Robert H. Socolow. New York: Holt, Rinehart & Winston, 1971, chap. 14, pp. 226–244.

Ethics 85, no. 1 (October 1974), pp. 1–66. Issue on John Rawls, A Theory of Justice.

FARAMELLI, NORMAN J. "Ecological Responsibility and Economic Justice: The Perilous Links between Ecology and Poverty." Andover Newton Quarterly 11, no. 1 (1970), pp. 81–93.

FEINBERG, JOEL. "The Nature and Value of Rights." Journal of Value Inquiry 4 (1970): 243–260.

JENKINS, IREDELL. "From Natural to Legal to Human Rights." Human Rights: Initial Publication of the American Section of the International Association for the Philosophy of Law and Social Philosophy, Consisting of the Papers Prepared for Its Second Plenary Meeting. AMINTAPHIL 1. Edited by Ervin Harold Pollack. Buffalo: Jay Stewart Publications, 1971, pp. 203–218.

KRIEGER, MARTIN H. "Six Propositions on the Poor and Pollution." Policy Sciences 1 (1970): 311–324.

———. "What's Wrong with Plastic Trees?" Science 179 (1973): 446–455.

LONGWOOD, MERLE. "The Common Good: An Ethical Framework for Evaluating Environmental Issues." Theological Studies 34 (1974): 468–480.

MACKLIN, RUTH. "Moral Concerns Appeals to Rights and Duties: Grounding Claims in a Theory of Justice." Hastings Center Report 5 (1976): 31–32, 34–38.

National Environmental Policy Act of 1969. Pub. L. No. 91-190. 83 Stat. 852. 42 U.S.C. sec. 4321 et seq. (1970).

NELL, ONORA. "Lifeboat Earth." Philosophy and Public Affairs 4 (1975): 273–292.

NEUHAUS, RICHARD JOHN. In Defense of People: Ecology and the Seduction of Radicalism. New York: Macmillan Co., 1971.

"The No-Growth Society." Daedalus 102, no. 4 (Fall 1973), pp. 1–245. Entire issue.

PASSMORE, JOHN ARTHUR. Man's Responsibility for Nature: Ecological Problems and Western Traditions. New York: Charles Scribner's Sons, 1974.

POWERS, CHARLES W. "Growth as an American Value: An Ethicist's Point of View." Growth in America. Edited by Chester L. Cooper. Woodrow Wilson International Center for Scholars, Contributions in American Studies, no. 21. Edited by Robert H. Walker. Westport, Conn.: Greenwood Press, 1976, chap. 3, pp. 26–38.

RAWLS, JOHN. A Theory of Justice. Cambridge: Harvard University Press, Belknap Press, 1971.

SILLS, DAVID L. "The Environmental Movement and Its Critics." Human Ecology 3 (1975): 1–41.

SMITH, JAMES N., ed. Environmental Quality and Social Justice in Urban America. Washington: Conservation Foundation, 1974.

STONE, CHRISTOPHER D. "Should Trees Have Standing? —Toward Legal Rights for Natural Objects." Southern California Law Review 45 (1972): 450–501. Reprint. Foreword by Garrett Hardin. Los Altos, Calif.: W. Kaufmann, 1974.

Yale Task Force on Population Ethics. "Moral Claims, Human Rights, and Population Policies." Theological Studies 35 (1974): 83–113.

III

THE PROBLEM OF GROWTH

Introduction

The term "environmental ethics" refers to a broad range of considerations about mankind's relationship to the physical environment. Among these are cultural attitudes toward the non-human world, proposals for resymbolizing humanity's relation to nature and to its own technology, and examination of normative guidelines for assessing human interventions in the physical environment. A special set of problems is raised by studies showing the projected consequences of exponential rates of economic growth and population expansion. This article will be concerned with those problems caused by economic growth and with the broader ethical questions that they raise. The problems can be summarized in the following way: (1) Anticipation of unprecedented natural and economic catastrophes through the depletion of natural resources, pollution of the environment, and the increasing demands of an expanding population raises serious doubts about the long-term survival of the human species and of the earth's ecosystem. (2) Proposals for the revision of economic life in the interest of global survival threaten to exacerbate difference over distribution of wealth and political power. (3) Related schemes for review of human attitudes toward the natural world with an eye to long-term survival question the appropriateness of Western values, as found in Judaism, Christianity, and secular, scientific rationalism for preventing global environmental catastrophes. (4) Questions arise as to whether an environmental ethics can succeed in providing social guidance without a radical change of ethos or a shift in religious outlook.

The growth problem

When human technologies were less extensive, humanity lived in relative balance with nature. Natural systems continued the rhythm of growth and decay in a process of dynamic compensation (Commoner). The expansion and transformation of technologies since the Second World War brought a break in this circle and introduced linear, noncompensating forces into the physical economy. Many products of late industrialization are not biodegradable and so become pure waste rather than recyclable matter. Other substances set up dangerous interactions with basic ecological processes. Phosphates, for example, lead to the eutrophication of water sources, and there is some evidence that fluorocarbons break down the earth's protective ozone layer.

Articulation of the problem. The potential in human technology for inflicting long-term and cumulative damage on the environment was first noted by George P. Marsh in his 1864 book *Man and Nature* (Glacken). In defining this problem, Marsh formulated the modern concept of natural equilibrium. He believed that even in the face of natural disasters nature is a self-compensating system. But human interventions in the environment, he thought, were uncontrolled disturbances with irreversible consequences. He even considered it possible that the earth would become uninhabitable due to human disruption of natural systems.

Such concerns have been voiced by the environmental movement, beginning with the 1962 publication of Rachel Carson's *Silent Spring*. The most notable of these cautionary studies was *The Limits to Growth* (Meadows et al.). Marsh had considered only the damage done the environment by simple people—shepherds, for example, working with primitive tools as they eked out a livelihood, very often at near-subsistence levels. The authors of *Limits*, however, studied the impact of advanced technology in meeting the growing demands of expanding populations for higher and higher material standards of living. They found that exponential growth in population, production, and consumption was accompanied by similar exponential increases in pollution and in depletion of natural resources, especially nonrenewable mineral reserves. They also noted that many of these trends were resistant to immediate change because of time lags. Certain pollutants, for example, would continue to accumulate at higher levels of the food chain, even after they were no longer produced and once fertility rates declined to replacement levels, populations would still continue to grow for some years before stabilizing. If these trends continued unchanged, the authors forecast sudden and uncontrollable collapses in ecological and economic systems.

Nature of the problem. The problem of growth, therefore, consists in the rapid increase in strains—in the form of pollution and resource depletion—which modern industrial economies place on the finite capacity of the globe. It emphasizes the cumulative and systemic effects of economic activity on the global environment which jeopardize the survival of the human species and of the biosphere which sustains it. The notion of limits to growth places in doubt the efficacy of material progress in both capitalist and socialist economies.

The debate among economists. Despite these problems, growth has many defenders. In conventional economic thinking it has been upheld as a cardinal economic value (Rostow; Barnett and Morse). It has a peculiar fascination in the United States, where national character and institutions have been shaped by material abundance (Potter). It is defended as the best—possibly the only way—to improve conditions of life for the poor (Rostow; Passell and Ross; Kahn et al.).

For a short time prior to the appearance of *Limits*, a few economists had questioned the ecological and social costs of economic growth. The standard economic measures of Gross National Product were criticized for neglecting the costs of production borne by third parties and future generations (Kapp). The assumed connection between social welfare and economic growth was also scrutinized in view of the disamenities (e.g., lack of privacy, quiet and clean air) and diseconomies (e.g., increased transportation time and costs, increased solid waste generation) associated with growth economics (Mishan). An economic policy based on the pursuit of growth was also thought to diminish consumer choice and social welfare, and the costs of growth were seen as regressive, diminishing the choices of the poor before those of the middle and upper classes (ibid.).

While some economists have begun to "internalize the externalities" of industrial production in their measurements (Schurr), the usefulness of these indices will depend on correct analysis of the social and environmental costs, the assignment of responsibility for them, and the effectiveness of the mechanisms employed to overcome them (Kapp). Mishan's work in challenging the assumption that growth increases choice and that social welfare is synonymous with choice has been extended by Hirsch (1976) to a general critique of the moral basis of growth economics.

Since *Limits*, debate has focused on three issues: whether economic policy should shift to a no-growth model, what the components of a no-growth economy should be, and what social mechanisms can be relied upon to produce the shift to a less hazardous economic system. The authors of *Limits* argued that an "equilibrium society" must supplant one based on exponential growth. In the sequel to *Limits*, entitled *Mankind at the Turning Point*, Mesarović and Pestel condemn not growth per se but "unbalanced and undifferentiated growth." They advocate an "organic growth" in which differentiated regional economies are kept in balance with the demands of basic human welfare and biological integrity. Thus, in certain developing areas of the world economic growth with attendant pollution and resource depletion might be permissible, while in industrial regions negative growth would be required to bring the economy within sustainable limits.

Among classical economists, J. S. Mill stands out for his perception of the potential benefits of a "stationary state" economy. For Mill, increased production was a desirable goal only in backward countries; in industrial countries the need was for better distribution of wealth for the sake of greater enjoyment of life. John Maynard Keynes also foresaw a point in economic development where essential needs would be satisfied and people would prefer to devote themselves to noneconomic purposes.

These speculations have their modern counterparts in the notions of "steady-state" economics and a shift from "quantitative" to "qualitative" growth. A frequent prescription is to reorient economic activity from capital- to labor-intensive production and to divert those energies from exploitation of nonrenewable resources toward expansion of the service sector—health, education, recreation, and the like.

Types of limits. Four main types of "limits" have been distinguished: physical, environmental or biological, social, and scientific or technological. Physical limits are said to be given in the First and Second Laws of Thermodynamics, the First in regard to the conservation of matter—waste or recycling must equal processed material resources (Olson, p. 3), the Second in respect to depletion of "low entropy" sources of materials and energy. Environmental limits are indicated in the concept of "carrying capacity" —the ability of a habitat to sustain particular numbers of particular species—and the biological limits of degradability, or "ecological resiliency." Social limits (Miles; Hirsch; Heilbroner) include political and economic limits as major subtypes. Political limits are expressed in terms of institutional arrangements and political "will." Economic limits are set at the point where rising marginal costs of physical growth exceed falling marginal benefits, thus reducing welfare rather than increasing it (Daly). Finally, scientific and technological limits concern the possible future knowledge and applications that may raise or remove the limits to growth. Space colonization as the ultimate evasion of the Malthusian trap is an example of what economist Charles Cicchetti terms the "Apollo syndrome"— the faith that technology, like God, will provide. Along with technological optimism (or pessimism), a second issue is the limits to substitutability. According to conventional economic wisdom, these appear indefinitely expansionable. "The reservation of particular resources for later use, therefore, may contribute little to the welfare of future generations" (Barnett and Morse, p. 11).

These types of limits interact and interpenetrate with one another. For example, physical limits are transferred and translated to social limits, so that physical density reveals itself symptomatically in forms of social stress such as crowding. In a manner reminiscent of Thomas Malthus's "positive" and "preventive checks,"

Forrester declares that the question of social choice regarding growth is one between physical and social limits, with the availability of choice resting largely on the social side. If those choices are not exercised wisely, he contends, the outcome will be imposed and enforced by physical necessity.

Criticisms of such "limits" emphasize the potency of both technological and value change. For example, the authors of *Limits* are criticized for taking an unduly pessimistic view of human values as resources for change (Cole et al.; Mesarović and Pestel). Values were "swept up" into the aggregation of economic trends and given no independent valence. Moreover, they were regarded as conservative and so yet another obstacle to establishing timely restraints on growth. Whatever the truth of these judgments, whether society can muster the political will to alter economies of growth remains one of the basic questions of the growth debate. It has also been charged that *Limits* underestimated the problem-solving potential of science and technology, and that technological solutions can be found to technologically created problems (Cole et al.; Kahn et al.).

The broader ethical issues

Global survival. The "limits to growth" debates raises the stakes for environmental ethics by widening the scope of concern from a local to a global context and by shifting the normative issue from quality of life to planetary survival. The nature of global survival, the characteristics of possible survivors, the allocation of costs exacted for the sake of survival, and moral limits on the irrational strength of claims made in the name of survival constitute one primary set of ethical issues raised by the growth debate.

The meaning of survival. From the time of the Greeks, philosophers extended moral credit to the notion that children represent a sort of personal continuity for mortal human beings. Only with the Enlightenment, however, did a generalized notion of posterity as a sort of symbolic immortality appear as an important motivating factor in the Western ethos. The fear of widespread ecological catastrophe has broadened the notion of survival to refer not only to the continuation of the human species but also to the maintenance of the basic biological conditions of terrestrial life as well.

For some thinkers, the preservation of the earth's biosphere alone—without humanity—would be sufficient to count as survival and even

to make moral claims against human persons. This judgment is based on appeals to the beauty, order, and variety of forms of life other than humanity. More often, however, planetary survival is taken to include preservation of human life, with some admixture of other values defining the level of civilization thought to constitute a minimal threshold for a worthwhile human life beyond mere subsistence. The debate over survival as a value, therefore, centers on the definition of civilized life.

Searching for a standard. Definitions of survival are especially difficult to formulate in technological societies, where there is a tendency to confuse survival with material comfort (Callahan, 1973; Mishan). One approach to global survival, which tries to avoid the ideological deceptions inherent in allowing survival to be defined in terms of the preservation of a particular way of life, is the attempt to establish "basic human needs" as a baseline for international cooperation (Aspen Institute). This approach assumes that planetary survival depends on the sacrifices of many groups and that the costs and benefits of a global survival pact must seem reasonable to all parties.

An opposite line of argument contends that the provision of basic needs, in the form of relief and development assistance to the poor, is counterproductive, increasing suffering in the long term and hastening economic and environmental catastrophe. In this view, what is required is a system of incentives to stimulate conservation, and benign neglect of marginal groups who drain the economy without appreciably contributing to the social product (Forrester). Proposals for allocation of food assistance (triage) to starving peoples on the basis of the recipients' proven capacity to curb demand through population limitation frequently share the latter view. Recent economic studies of fertility decline, however, indicate that income distribution and the satisfaction of basic needs are preconditions of couples' limiting their family size (Rich).

At the extreme, survival is taken to exclude all other right-making considerations, so that a given group's claim to survival rests on its exclusive possession of a stock of resources, which it is obliged to manage only in its own interest and that of its own descendants (Hardin, 1974). Neither this "lifeboat" mentality nor the milder liberal economic view tries to set a standard of living compatible with global survival. Both demonstrate a preference for protection of future generations matched by a readiness to exclude marginal groups from use of the present store of resources.

Speculation about imaginable standards of survival is found in discussions of the "stationary-state economy" and the "equilibrium society" (Daly; Meadows et al.). There is some agreement among proponents of equilibrium that the needs of future generations should be taken into account so that long-term needs prevail over short-term ones (Meadows et al.; Forrester; Daly). But there is also considerable support for meeting basic human needs in the short run, especially in the area of food (Mesarović and Pestel; Aspen Institute). Other factors in setting a standard of civilized survival would include the ethics of production and distribution, the philosophy of community or human sociality, and notions of human fulfillment.

Survivors. Who should survive? Conceivably, species survival is consistent with the continued existence of a small remnant—a band of aborigines, say, living at a very low level of civilization. That prospect may seem unsatisfactory, because the meaningfulness of human survival is tied to "progress" and more generally to the values of civilized life. This objection gives rise to the notion that those entitled to survive are the bearers of civilization: long-term rational economizers, people who are scientifically inventive, latter-day ascetics, self-reliant organic gardeners, or nature mystics. Claims made for these groups are often nationalistic and sometimes racist and elitist (e.g., the presumption that procreation by the poor presents the greatest threat to survival). The difficulty in adjudicating the claims of competing groups to represent civilization and the apparent self-interest and prejudice in some such claims suggest that a more universal standard is necessary in deciding who shall survive. While not every group may expect to perdure indefinitely and, once comparable sacrifices are made on all sides, no group can demand exceptional protection for itself on historical grounds, one could reasonably argue that no group should be sacrificed for the sake of planetary survival under a standard that is less than universal.

Sacrifices. Because planetary survival will place different burdens on various groups, specification of any universal standard of survival implies at least rough comparability among the sacrifices exacted from different groups (Yale Task Force). Where large families are the only insurance parents have against neglect in their

old age, for example, it would be unfair to see sterilization of poor couples in less developed countries as standing on parity with a shift to energy-efficient automobiles by affluent individuals in the industrialized countries. Distinctions are required between enjoyments and needs, between secondary (status) needs and the basic requirements of survival, and between limits on the exercise of fundamental rights and the blanket denial of such rights. Enjoyments should always be sacrificed before limits are imposed on the satisfaction of basic needs. Such limitations do not abrogate the rights they restrict, however; they only circumscribe their proper exercise. Hence an enjoyment such as eating steak twice a week would be surrendered before asking any group to ration its food; and meatless days might be imposed without infringing the right to food.

Moral limits. Survival is a strong value, and frequently its invocation signals a readiness to take exceptionally strong measures to protect the interest of one group against others. For the sake of survival men and women are willing to sacrifice many other values. The need for moral strictures on appeals to survival is motivated by the fear that this imperative may destroy "everything in human beings that makes them worth survival" (Callahan).

Building on what has already been said, there are at least five criteria for determining the prima facie moral acceptability of appeals to global survival: universality, just distribution of differential burdens, a common material standard of sufficiency, the constellation of values for civilized life that accompany the appeal and the disinterestedness of the proponents. (1) Universality requires that no human group be excluded from the class of potential survivors. (2) The norm of justice requires that the sacrifices asked of each group be truly comparable. (3) The norm of sufficiency asks whether the level of material well-being envisaged by the proponents is reasonable, distinguishing between surfeit and basic need, and defining a common standard of what is required to live a dignified human life. (4) A concern for civilized life demands clarity about the values that define human dignity and worthwhile survival. Are values we cherish threatened or only reasonably curbed? What is it we sacrifice for the sake of survival: freedom, justice, compassion, artistic expression, trust between persons? And what will replace them? (5) Disinterestedness is a common norm of all moral judgments. Thus, one can ask, does the person invoking survival, his nation, or class have anything to gain from adoption of proposed measures? Does the survivalist or his/her group sacrifice anything of comparable value to what is asked of others?

Obligations to future generations. Duties to posterity are postulated on a variety of grounds: justice as fairness, love implying care for the future of what we love, gratitude for life, responsibility to the God of all being. Though obligations to the future are widely recognized, the extent of the obligation of the present generation to provide for the future is much disputed. Where biological survival functions as the dominant value, there is a tendency to extend the obligation to remote generations (Forrester; Hardin, 1972; Callahan). Such temporalizing of universal moral standards has been criticized as unreasonable and unworkable. Ignorance of the future and lack of control over the long-term consequences of our action are seen as possible grounds for limiting the temporal scope of these obligations. Perhaps we are obliged to avoid worsening the world posterity receives from us and especially to avoid actions that have irreversibly harmful consequences (Callahan), but we cannot be expected to calculate the effect of our actions on very distant generations. The inclusion of the remote future in our moral calculus, moreover, may lead to avoidance of proximate obligations to our contemporaries and immediate descendants. Two proposed norms that limit obligations to proximate future generations are the extent to which persons can expect to share a common moral ideal with the future generations (Golding) and the extent to which parental love can imagine taking responsibility (Passmore).

A new ethics and a new ethos

Criticism of the traditional ethos and its ethics. In discussions of environmental problems, the ideas of ethos and ethics are frequently conflated. We can distinguish the two this way: An ethos is a set of beliefs characteristic of a particular culture and exemplified by its dominant institutions; an ethics is a system of moral action guides employed to adjudicate conflicts within a given ethos. Thus, the medieval Christian church's ban against usury regulated commercial transactions as long as ecclesiastical life gave shape to social institutions. But when the church was replaced by commerce as the dominant institution of European society the con-

trols on usury were whittled away in keeping with the new ethos.

If a shift in ethos is indeed required to respond to the potential dangers of growth, then the elaboration of ecological ethics in the absence of a new world view may prove an empty exercise. An ethics developed in the context of the present technico-economic structure, for example, may already cede priority to the growth mentality in such a way that normative principles would provide only a neat casuistry for minor problems instead of the radical criticism and imaginative speculation which are needed to establish a stable-state economy.

Many environmentalists have questioned the adequacy of traditional Western moral ideas in treating ecological problems. At least three sorts of criticism are made: (1) The anthropocentrism of Judeo-Christian thought is incapable of dealing with ecological problems because it gives precedence to human needs rather than to the whole of nature of which humanity is only a part. (2) Ethical principles alone are inadequate to the crisis; only a change in world view on a par with religious conversion will guarantee survival. (3) Global survival is too grave a matter to be left to individual conscience and democratic decision-making processes; support must be given to knowledgeable elites to direct society's future.

Anthropocentrism. The charge that Judaism and Christianity are responsible for the evil consequences of the growth ethic rests on the claim that the biblical notion of man's dominion over the earth was the origin of the West's utilitarian indifference to nature. Whether or not the notion of dominion is to be interpreted as such critics suggest, the biblical tradition and the Western tradition more broadly contain many strands with quite distinct attitudes toward nature (Passmore). Monastic Christianity, for example, first in its Benedictine and later in its Cluniac form, showed considerable respect for nature and found in created things an avenue to contemplation of the Creator (Glacken; Dubos). It has been argued, moreover, that scientific rationalism, not religious anthropocentrism, is the true precursor of the present ecological crisis (Passmore). Another source of growth mania may be the anthropology of liberal economics, which excludes any common definition of essential human needs, opposes asceticism and self-examination, and encourages economic activity as a means of allaying psychological insecurity (Wolin).

Perhaps *homo economicus* is at fault; but that does not provide grounds for concluding that all person-centered ethical systems are incapable of constructive responses to problems of global ecology. Where essential human needs are distinguished from artificial ones and asceticism is understood as a beneficial form of behavior, a person-centered ethic might very well uphold ecological values. Similarly there may well be a convergence between protection of the biosphere and prevention of harm to human persons such that there is no need to resort to sacralization of nature to protect the environment.

Moral conversion. The fear that codes of moral rules, especially those built on traditional principles, will be insufficient to redirect the juggernaut of technological supergrowth has led to proposals to resacralize nature, especially on Oriental or Amerindian models. To form a culture that shows respect for nature, it is argued, changes are required in the deeper levels of society's affective response to the environment. This kind of shift, it is assumed, can be brought about only by a change in religious outlook.

A more moderate position argues that profound reverence for nature need not imply resacralization and that sound ecology is compatible even with uses of nature that alter the traditional ecology of a place (Dubos). The "land ethic" proposed by Aldo Leopold takes a stronger position, but one still short of mystification of the environment. "A thing is right," Leopold wrote, "when it tends to preserve the integrity, stability, and beauty of a biotic community." On the other side, the philosopher John Passmore considers that all schemes to deal with the environment as a religious problem are "rubbish," and that scientific rationalism and existing categories of ethical analysis are adequate to the task.

Taking a pragmatic view, Jay Forrester argues that religion is the domain of humanity's long-range intentions and so a primary instrument of social change. Organized religion should use its resources to support a future-oriented, meritocratic, and nature-oriented conservation ethic that will assure the preservation of scarce resources for future generations and should forgo a traditional commitment to altruism, egalitarianism, and humanitarianism, which will only create worse conditions in the future.

Political ethics. Like the authors of *Limits*, some environmentalists view the present crisis as refuting the false hope that economic growth alone will solve such obdurate problems as poverty and racial discrimination (Commoner), or that the wealth of a nation can replace the well-being of its people. Taken seriously, the admission of limits to growth may place in jeopardy the power structure which has encouraged unlimited productivity as the basis of political harmony and "progress" (Commoner).

Instead of the diffusion of power Commoner advocates, others argue for greater concentrations of power in the interest of timely response to unprecedented crises. The "systems dynamics" school (Forrester; Meadows et al.) contends that ordinary political judgments in a democratic society are counterproductive because of the counterintuitive behavior of complex social systems. Hence they would vest responsibility for societal guidance in an elite of computer experts. Forrester argues that in the interest of future generations power must be left to those who will use resources wisely. More crassly, Hardin proposes that those nations which have the resources for self-sufficient survival have no obligations to share with those who have less, and he supports coercive measures to encourage no-growth. A moderate solution, which may help to balance the need for control in the interest of future generations with respect for freedom and basic human rights, is to apply coercion, when it is needed, only on the macroeconomic level (Pirages and Ehrlich). Thus, by applying pressure to large economic institutions, freedom can be preserved for the individual human beings to whom it properly belongs.

DREW CHRISTIANSEN AND C. P. WOLF

[*Directly related is the entry* ENVIRONMENT AND MAN. *For further discussion of topics mentioned in this article, see the entries:* FOOD POLICY; FUTURE GENERATIONS, OBLIGATIONS TO; JUSTICE; *and* RATIONING OF MEDICAL TREATMENT. *Other relevant material may be found under* POPULATION ETHICS: ELEMENTS OF THE FIELD, *articles on* ETHICAL PERSPECTIVES ON POPULATION *and* NORMATIVE ASPECTS OF POPULATION POLICY.]

BIBLIOGRAPHY

Aspen Institute for Humanistic Studies. *The Planetary Bargain: Proposals for a New Economic Order to Meet Human Needs: Report of an International Workshop Convened in Aspen, Colorado, July 7– August 1, 1975.* Aspen Institute for Humanistic Studies, Program on International Affairs, Occasional Paper. Palo Alto, Calif.: 1976.

BARNETT, HAROLD J., and MORSE, CHANDLER. *Scarcity and Growth: The Economics of Natural Resource Availability.* Baltimore: Resources for the Future, Johns Hopkins Press, 1963.

CALLAHAN, DANIEL J. *The Tyranny of Survival and Other Pathologies of Civilized Life.* New York: Macmillan Publishing Co., 1973.

——. "What Obligations Do We Have to Future Generations?" *American Ecclesiastical Review* 164 (1971): 265–280.

CHEN, KAN, et al. *Growth Policy: Population, Environment, and Beyond.* Ann Arbor: University of Michigan Press, 1974.

COLE, H. S. D.; FREEMAN, CHRISTOPHER; JAHODA, MARIE; and PAVITT, K. L. R., eds. *Models of Doom: A Critique of "The Limits to Growth."* With a reply by the authors of *The Limits to Growth.* New York: Universe Books, 1973. Papers by members of the Science Policy Research Unit, University of Sussex, Brighton, England. Published in England as *Thinking about the Future: A Critique of "The Limits to Growth."* London: Chatto & Windus, Sussex University Press, 1973.

COMMONER, BARRY. *The Closing Circle: Nature, Man and Technology.* A Borzoi Book. New York: Alfred A. Knopf, 1971.

DALY, HERMAN E., ed. *Toward a Steady-State Economy.* San Francisco: W. H. Freeman & Co., 1973.

DUBOS, RENÉ. *A God Within.* New York: Charles Scribner's Sons, 1972.

FORRESTER, JAY W. "Churches at the Transition between Growth and World Equilibrium." *Zygon* 7 (1972): 145–167.

GLACKEN, CLARENCE J. "Man's Place in Nature in Recent Western Thought." *This Little Planet.* Edited by Michael Hamilton. Introduction by Edmund S. Muskie. New York: Charles Scribner's Sons, 1970, pp. 163–201. Cooperative project of the National Presbyterian Center and the Episcopal Cathedral in Washington.

GOLDING, M. P. "Obligations to Future Generations." *Monist* 56 (1972): 85–99.

HARDIN, GARRETT. *Exploring New Ethics for Survival: The Voyage of the Spaceship 'Beagle'.* New York: Viking Press, 1972.

——. "Lifeboat Ethics: The Case against Helping the Poor." *Psychology Today,* September 1974, pp. 38–43, 123–124, 126.

HEILBRONER, ROBERT L. *An Inquiry into the Human Prospect.* New York: W. W. Norton, 1974.

HENDERSON, HAZEL. "Redefining Economic Growth." *Environmental Quality and Social Justice in Urban America.* Edited by James Noel Smith. Washington: Conservation Foundation, 1974, chap. 8, pp. 123–145.

HIRSCH, FRED. *Social Limits to Growth.* Twentieth Century Fund Study. Cambridge: Harvard University Press, 1976.

ILLICH, IVAN. *Tools for Conviviality.* World Perspectives, vol. 47. Edited by Ruth Nanda Anshen. New York: Harper & Row, 1973.

JONAS, HANS. "Technology and Responsibility: Reflections on the New Task of Ethics." *Religion and the Humanizing of Man.* 2d rev. ed. Edited by James M. Robinson. Waterloo, Ont.: Council on the Study of Religion, 1973, pp. 3–20. Plenary Addresses, International Congress of Learned Societies in the Field of Religion, Los Angeles, 1–5 September 1972.

KAHN, HERMAN; BROWN, WILLIAM; MARTEL, LEON; and the Hudson Institute Staff. *The Next 200 Years: A Scenario for America and the World.* New York: Morrow, 1976.

KAPP, KARL WILLIAM. *The Social Costs of Private Enterprise.* New York: Schocken Books, 1971.

LEOPOLD, ALDO. *A Sand County Almanac.* New York: Oxford University Press, 1949. Enl. ed. 1966.

MEADOWS, DONELLA H.; MEADOWS, DENNIS L.; RANDERS, JØRGEN; and BEHRENS, WILLIAM W., III. *The Limits to Growth: A Report for the Club of Rome's Project on the Predicament of Mankind.* New York: Universe Books, 1972.

MESAROVIĆ, MIHAJLO, and PESTEL, EDUARD. *Mankind at the Turning Point: The Second Report to the Club of Rome.* New York: E. P. Dutton & Co./Reader's Digest Press, 1974.

MILES, RUFUS E., JR. *Awakening from the American Dream: The Social and Political Limits to Growth.* New York: Universe Books, 1976.

MISHAN, EZRA J. [EDWARD J.] *The Costs of Economic Growth.* New York: Praeger Publishers, 1967.

OLSON, MANCUR. "Introduction." *Daedalus* 102, no. 4 (1973), pp. 1–13. Introduction to an issue entitled "The No-Growth Society."

PASSELL, PETER, and ROSS, LEONARD. *The Retreat from Riches: Affluence and Its Enemies.* Foreword by Paul A. Samuelson. New York: Viking Press, 1973.

PASSMORE, JOHN. *Man's Responsibility for Nature: Ecological Problems and Western Traditions.* New York: Charles Scribner's Sons, 1974.

PIRAGES, DENNIS C., and EHRLICH, PAUL R. *Ark II: Social Response to Environmental Imperatives.* San Francisco: W. H. Freeman & Co., 1974.

POTTER, DAVID M. *People of Plenty: Economic Abundance and the American Character.* Charles R. Walgreen Foundation Lectures. Chicago: University of Chicago Press, 1954.

RICH, WILLIAM. *Smaller Families through Social and Economic Progress.* Overseas Development Council Monograph, no. 7. Washington: 1973.

ROSTOW, WALT WHITMAN. *The Stages of Economic Growth: A Non-Communist Manifesto.* Cambridge: University Press, 1960. 2d ed. 1971.

SCHUMACHER, ERNST FRIEDRICH. *Small is Beautiful: Economics as if People Mattered.* New York: Harper & Row; London: Blond & Briggs, 1973.

SCHURR, SAM H., ed. *Energy, Economic Growth, and the Environment.* Baltimore: Resources for the Future, Johns Hopkins University Press, 1972. Papers presented at a forum conducted by Resources for the Future, Washington, D.C., 20–21 April 1971.

TINBERGEN, JAN, coordinator. *RIO: Reshaping the International Order: A Report to the Club of Rome.* New York: E. P. Dutton & Co., 1976.

WOLIN, SHELDON S. *Politics and Vision: Continuity and Innovation in Western Political Thought.* Boston: Little, Brown & Co., 1960.

Yale Task Force on Population Ethics. "Moral Claims, Human Rights, and Population Policies." *Theological Studies* 35 (1974): 83–113.

ENVIRONMENTAL HAZARDS

See ENVIRONMENTAL ETHICS, *articles on* ENVIRONMENTAL HEALTH AND HUMAN DISEASE *and* QUESTIONS OF SOCIAL JUSTICE.

ETHICAL THEORY

See ETHICS.

ETHICS

In this twelve-part entry the first article, THE TASK OF ETHICS, *is intended as an introduction to the meanings, methods, and questions of ethics. It also serves as a guide to the remaining eleven articles, which explain in detail the varieties of ethical theories upon which bioethics is built.* RULES AND PRINCIPLES *describes various ways of distinguishing moral from nonmoral rules and some of the problems connected with the moral justification of rules and the appeal of moral principles.* DEONTOLOGICAL THEORIES *is concerned with theories founded on the notion of duty and contrasts them with consequentialist theories in general.* TELEOLOGICAL THEORIES *discusses theories founded on the notion of good. Some of the conceptions of good are described and some general objections to teleological theories are discussed.* SITUATION ETHICS *defends one type of teleological ethics, i.e., act-utilitarianism. The article on* UTILITARIANISM *sets forth the general features of utilitarianism as a consequentialist type of ethics, and discusses the distinction between act-utilitarianism and rule-utilitarianism.* THEOLOGICAL ETHICS *distinguishes three basic theistic orientations and then uses them to show the relationship of religion to the issues of normative ethics.* OBJECTIVISM IN ETHICS *deals with theories of ethical knowledge and other conceptions of ethical rationality.* NATURALISM *describes three types of naturalism in ethics, examines critically the "naturalistic fallacy," and explains some of the problems concerning the relation of science to ethics.* NON-DESCRIPTIVISM *distinguishes between two types of metaethical theory: descriptivism, which includes naturalism and intuitionism, and non-descriptivism, which includes emotivism and prescriptivism.* MORAL REASONING *discusses an important philosophical problem concerning the nature of moral reasoning, namely, the problem of showing how moral reasoning can be practical, by motivating and guiding action, and yet be universally applicable in the sense that it involves universally valid criteria of evidence. The final article,* RELATIVISM, *distinguishes among descriptive, normative, and metaethical relativism and relates each to the problem of medical ethics.*

I
THE TASK OF ETHICS

Remarks on terminology

In this article "ethics" will be taken to mean the philosophical inquiry into the principles of morality, of right and wrong conduct, of virtue and vice, and of good and evil as they relate to conduct. The term "ethics" has a number of other meanings. For example, "ethics" is often used to mean professional ethics as it is incorporated into ethical codes for professional conduct set forth, say, by medical associations. "Ethics" is also sometimes used to refer to the beliefs or practices of a particular sect or group, as in Christian or Jewish ethics, or to describe the values or conduct of a particular individual, as in Hitler's ethics. The subject matter of this article, however, is ethics in the traditional sense in which it has been a subject of investigation by Western philosophers since the time of Plato and Aristotle.

It should be noted that there is no standard distinction of meaning between "ethics" and "morality" (or "morals"). The most that can be said with certainty is that "ethics" comes from Greek, whereas "moral" comes from Latin. Individual philosophers often use the words to make a distinction that they feel is important; other philosophers use them synonymously.

Finally, a word of warning about *labels*. It is easy to overestimate the importance of labels. A label is merely a convenient device designed for a very limited purpose; making labels or learning about labels is not itself a philosophical activity. Again, there is no standard use among philosophers of labels like "naturalism," "utilitarianism," "descriptivism," "intuitionism," "subjectivism," "relativism," and "skepticism." Each individual writer employs such labels for his own particular purposes. Indeed, many philosophers refuse to provide labels for their own positions, although they are not at all reluctant to assign labels to positions with which they disagree.

One of the most mischievous consequences of

excessive preoccupation with labels is that it lends credence to the erroneous opinion that every theory comes in a hermetically sealed package that can be accepted or rejected only as a whole. It is also inconsistent with the idea that ethical theories can be and ought to be open-ended and capable of assimilation and differentiation as well as of change and development.

The distinctive nature of ethics

Ethics, law, custom, institutional practices, and positive morality.   It is important to distinguish ethics from law, custom, institutional practices, and positive morality (i.e., the body of accepted popular beliefs of a society about morality). Ethics is logically prior to all of these in that it comprises principles and standards that can be used to criticize and evaluate those other norms. Thus, ethics is not directly concerned with what law is, or what custom is, or what institutions are, or what positive morality is; rather, it is concerned with what they *ought* to be. It is therefore fallacious to argue in any simple or direct way from the fact that certain laws, certain practices, or certain beliefs exist to the conclusion that a certain kind of conduct is right or wrong. Law, in particular, differs from ethics in that sanctions play a crucial, perhaps even an essential, role in law and legal decisions, and norms depend for their definition and determination on the actions of specific institutional organs such as the courts and the legislature. To argue directly from the illegality of a certain form of behavior, e.g., euthanasia, to its immorality is therefore to commit a kind of fallacy. Americans, as Tocqueville pointed out, tend to construe ethical (and political) questions as if they were legal questions. It is important constantly to be on one's guard against approaching medical ethics in that way. In this regard, considerable confusion results from the indiscriminate use of the concept of "right" to solve any and every moral problem in medical ethics, as in the "right to life," the "right to die," or the "right to medical treatment." When these supposed rights are discussed, hardly any effort is made to explain what kind of right is intended, e.g., whether or not it can be waived, who has the corresponding duty, and what kind of conduct it calls for.

Although ethics is logically independent of law, custom, practices, and positive morality, it does not follow that there are no ethically significant connections between them. We cannot avoid such moral questions as: Ought we always to obey the law, and ought we to conform to custom, to conventional medical practice, and to positive morality? And what are the limits to the obligation to obey and to conform?

The controversial character of ethics.   In order to understand what philosophical ethics is all about it is necessary to begin by recognizing that ethics, by its very nature, is controversial. That is, like philosophy in general, it is essentially disputatious, while at the same time it must deal with issues that are both urgent and inescapable. In this regard, ethics is very much like politics and law, with which it is frequently compared.

The controversial character of ethics is best understood by noting three essential conditions of a genuine controversy as contrasted with, say, a simple clash of interests or tastes: (1) There must be a real inconsistency, rather than a merely verbal disagreement, between the two positions, that is, they must be logically incompatible in some sense. (2) Each of the opposing positions must be reasonable (i.e., nonarbitrary) and capable of being supported by argument. (3) A meeting of minds must, in principle at least, be possible; for an issue would not be controversial if it is taken for granted that arguing over it will inevitably and necessarily be futile.

It should be clear that in all three respects ethical disagreements are quite unlike mere differences of subjective preference or differences of taste. *De gustibus non est disputandum* —there is no disputing over tastes. Ethical issues, on the other hand, are eminently disputable in the three ways just mentioned; hence, it is a mistake to think that one can or ought to choose an ethical theory as one chooses foods from a menu.

In view of the controversial character of ethics, one should not expect moral philosophers to provide definitive answers to all of our moral problems, that is, answers of the kind that would be acceptable to any rational being at any possible time. But, although philosophers cannot in good conscience claim infallibility, it does not follow that what they say can be ignored. Why this is so should become clear presently.

Dogmatic skepticism and skeptical dogmatism. Broadly speaking an ethical theory is a theory about reasons—reasons for doing or refraining from doing something, reasons for approving or disapproving of something, or reasons for believing or asserting something about morality, virtuous or vicious conduct, good and evil rules, practices, institutions, policies and goals. The rightness or wrongness of an action may itself be regarded as a reason for performing or not performing that action. In this broad sense, then, the task of ethics may be described as the search for and establishment of reasons for various sorts of things connected with conduct, including such things as actions, motives, attitudes, judgments, rules, ideals, and goals. This general concern with reasons explains why ethics is commonly taken to be a rational activity and a matter of practical reason.

There is a prevailing opinion to the effect that there are no good reasons for any of the things just mentioned, that is, reasons that could in any serious way be regarded as objectively or intersubjectively valid. This position may be called *ethical skepticism* (like other philosophical labels, "ethical skepticism" is used differently by different philosophers). Ethical skepticism, in the sense intended here, entails the denial of the distinction between right and wrong; for, if there can be no good reason or at least no good moral reason for preferring one sort of conduct over another, then it follows that everything is permitted. The obverse of ethical skepticism is *ethical dogmatism*, the position that no reasons need be given for one's ethical views. Skepticism holds that no reason is possible, whereas dogmatism holds that no reason is necessary. It should be obvious that ethical skepticism, as depicted here, is itself a dogmatic position, and that ethical dogmatism, as depicted here, is essentially skeptical. Hence, the two positions may also be called "dogmatic skepticism" and "skeptical dogmatism," respectively. Persons who have not studied or thought very much about ethics as such often take for granted that those two positions are the only alternatives. Since it is not easy for anyone to remain completely morally neutral about *everything*, it is difficult, if not impossible, to find persons who are consistent skeptics in actual practice. On the other hand, practicing ethical dogmatists are unfortunately much too common—unfortunately, perhaps even tragically, because in practice a stubbornly dogmatic attitude on ethical issues inevitably results in a breakdown of communication between dissenting parties and, in the end, sanctions the use of coercive measures and violence. However, neither of the two doctrinaire positions, absolute skepticism and dogmatism, is accepted by any reputable philosopher, whatever else he may believe. It is easy to see why, for it is self-defeating to hold either that it is impossible or that it is unnecessary to give reasons for one's assertions: Anyone who openly advocates either position cannot, at risk of self-contradiction, attempt to give any reasons to anyone else for accepting what he says.

The methods of ethics

A brief discussion of the methods of argumentation that are likely to be encountered in ethical discussions will be helpful. The discussion presented here will be patterned after Peirce's article, "The Fixation of Belief" (Peirce), although there are some obvious differences between the view of ethics presented here and Peirce's view.

The first method is the *appeal to authority*. In the development of Western moral notions, the method of authority has had widespread use as the basis for morality. Much of Judaic as well as of Christian ethics illustrates this, although there are also authoritarian elements in Greek and even in Egyptian ethics. The appeal to authority seeks to establish a proposition on the ground that a particular authority declares it to be so. In ethics, for example, it is held that one ought or ought not to do something, to approve or disapprove of something, or to believe something to be right or wrong on the ground that the authority tells us to do so. The authority may be a human or a supernatural person, a group of persons, an institution (e.g., a church or a government), or a collection of writings: it may even be a fictitious person (e.g., society or the ideal observer). In order to validate the reported pronouncements of the authority, it is necessary to show (1) why the supposed authority is an authority, that is, it is necessary to establish its credentials, and (2) that the alleged pronouncements truly emanate from the authority, that is, it is necessary to establish the authenticity of the reports of its pronouncements. Various types of religious ethics amply illustrate how these two questions might be answered. With regard to ethics, the credentials of the authority are generally based on the authority's superior knowledge and moral superiority (e.g., the supreme love, benevolence, solicitude, or disinterestedness found in the authority). Thus, theologians usually ascribe these qualities to God and then use them to vindicate his ethical authority; the authenticity of the reports of God's commands depends on a variety of other assumptions that need not be detailed here. Insofar as religious systems depend on faith or revelation to establish the credentials of the authority, or the authenticity of what is attributed to it (e.g., in the Scriptures), this use of the method of authority has only a very limited appeal; it has cogency only for believers.

Philosophical ethics, in contrast to faith-based religious ethics, is directed to a universal audience rather than to a particular subgroup. As such, it does not require an act of faith. In this connection, it should be mentioned that not all versions of the natural law theory are fideistic or authoritarian. Aristotle's version, for example, is neither. Locke's version is authoritarian but not fideistic. By the same token not all theological ethics is fideistic or authoritarian [*see article* VII *below on* THEOLOGICAL ETHICS].

From what has been said about the method of authority it should not be concluded that it is never a valid form of argument. Of course it is, provided satisfactory answers are given to the two questions. We often use the method of authority to settle questions outside of ethics, for example, questions of law or of medicine.

A second method of argument often used in ethics is the appeal to *consensus hominum*, that is, the citing of the alleged agreement of people in general or of particular groups of people concerning an issue to establish a particular ethical contention. In arguments of this sort, essentially the same two kinds of question are relevant as were asked concerning the use of the appeal to authority, namely: (1) Is there any reason to believe that the people cited are especially wise and ethically competent? and (2) Do they, as a matter of fact, actually subscribe to the beliefs attributed to them?

A third method of argument is the appeal to "intuition," "self-evidence," or "gut feelings." The use of the concept of intuition by philosophers should be carefully distinguished from its more general use by nonphilosophers, say, physicians and patients. Philosophers, particularly those known as intuitionists (e.g., G. E. Moore), have developed theoretical arguments to the effect that ethical knowledge is ultimately founded on intuition; "intuition" is a technical concept in their system [*see article* VIII *below on* OBJECTIV- ISM IN ETHICS]. The use of the method of in- tuition in practice, however, has certain draw- backs; for one thing it carries no conviction for persons who have not already had the intuition, or what they think is an intuition. Thus it is very difficult, if not impossible, to persuade someone who is not already convinced that euthanasia is wrong on the grounds that it is self-evident that killing is wrong. More generally, something that may seem incontrovertibly self-evident to you today may not seem so tomorrow or to someone else. Particularly in the field of medical ethics, conditions and categories are changing so rapidly that a person's intuitions are apt to become out of date as quickly as the medical technologies that give rise to the ethical problems in the first place.

Finally, the method par excellence of the moral philosopher in both his theoretical and his practical investigations is what may be called the method of argumentation or the dialectical or Socratic method, that is, the method of asking questions and looking for answers backed up by good reasons. In philosophy, and ethics in par- ticular, no position, theory, or answer is sacro- sanct; it is acceptable only if it can be supported by argument. It is important, therefore, to pay close attention to the arguments and reasons that philosophers give for their various conten- tions, for without them what they say would simply be dogmatic and boring.

The subject matter of ethics: normative ethics and metaethics

The subject matter of ethics may be divided into two parts, which are generally called "nor- mative ethics" and "metaethics." *Normative ethics* asks questions directly related to the crite- ria and standards of right and wrong action, what things are good and evil, and questions about moral conduct in general. *Metaethics*, on the other hand, is a second-order inquiry into the nature of ethical discourse itself. Normative ethics gives us ethical theories about what we ought to do, while metaethics gives us theories about what ethics is all about.

As a second-order type of inquiry, metaethics is related to normative ethics as philosophy of science is to the sciences, or philosophy of art is to the arts. It is often called "analytical ethics" or sometimes simply "moral philosophy." His- torically, the distinction between normative ethics and metaethics is probably due to G. E. Moore, who differentiated between the ques- tions: "What kinds of thing are good?" and "What is the definition (or meaning) of good?" (Moore). Accordingly, it is sometimes held that metaethics and normative ethics employ differ- ent methods; metaethics, for example, is said to use the method of conceptual, logical, or linguis- tic analysis; on an older view, that meant searching for definitions. At one time it was held (e.g., by Ayer) that metaethics is ethically neutral (i.e., non-normative), and that the moral philosopher ought to concern himself only with metaethics, leaving normative ethics to others. Today, this view of metaethics is re- pudiated by many moral philosophers. Perhaps the only essential distinction that remains between normative ethics and metaethics is a difference of levels or orders, the subject matter of normative ethics being moral conduct and the subject matter of metaethics being ethics itself (i.e., ethical discourse, judgments, concepts, and reasoning). Although the questions of normative ethics and metaethics often overlap or even merge, it will be convenient to discuss them separately.

The questions of normative ethics

As in other areas of ethics, what the basic questions of normative ethics are is a matter of dispute. It will become clear as we proceed that the particular questions selected for investigation already reflect a prior ethical commitment as to what is important and urgent. In order to understand what is at issue, therefore, it is extremely important that we take these biases into account.

In general terms, normative ethics may be said to concern itself with the problem: *What ought I (or we) to do?* This question may be very general—i.e., By what principle ought I (or we) to order my life (our lives)? Or, on the other hand, it may be very specific—i.e., What ought I to do here and now about this particular thing? In most ethical theories, the question is taken at the intermediate level: It is assumed to be about the rules, principles, or standards of right and wrong conduct.

One ramification that is of particular relevance in problems of bioethics is that the ought question is asked in a variety of different contexts. Consider the question: What ought to be done with an infant with a hopelessly incurable genetic disease, e.g., spina bifida? It is clear that this question might be asked by a particular physician with regard to a particular infant, or it might be asked by the governing board of a hospital trying to decide on a general policy, or it might be asked by the general public as a question of public policy. Considerations that are relevant to the ought question at one level may not be identical with those that are relevant at another level, although they are obviously interconnected.

Questions like, "What ought I (or we) to do?" reflect a number of different practical predicaments, which, in turn, generate several different categories of moral problems. Here we shall examine four of these categories.

1. Ought questions arising out of conflicts of interest. Let us begin with moral problems that arise out of conflicts of interests. Basically the same kinds of problem are found in connection with conflicts of wants, desires, needs, preferences, pleasures, or other types of "subjective value." The moral perplexity, the ought question with which we are concerned here, is due to the fact that in certain instances it is impossible to satisfy one interest (or "value") without sacrificing other interests. Consequently, we are forced to choose between interests. Which one ought to be preferred?

Philosophers who take conflict of interest problems to be the most basic category of moral problem usually claim that the chief function of ethics is to provide an objective procedure for adjudicating between conflicting interests (Rawls, 1951).

When conceived in this way, the task of ethics is to develop a way of ordering interests. The best known theory of ordering is utilitarianism, which uses the maximization principle to order interests [see article VI *below* on UTILITARIANISM]. Rawls's theory of justice provides another, rather sophisticated method of ordering interests (or goods) (Rawls, 1971). The kind of ought questions that are involved here are usually taken to be questions of distributive justice.

The basic assumption underlying this particular conception of ethics is that every interest (or "value") has, as such, a prima facie claim to be satisfied. That is, other things being equal (i.e., ideally), one ought to try to satisfy all the interests of everyone. Of course, almost all of the time other things are not equal, so that one interest has to give way to other more pressing interests. According to this approach it is the simple fact of being an interest that constitutes its claim to be satisfied rather than the quality of the interest itself, e.g., its object or its rationality. This assumption is rejected categorically by philosophers like Kant, who would not agree that it is the function of ethics to settle conflicts of interest (or "values").

2. Ought questions arising out of moral dilemmas. Another set of ought questions comprises those that arise from a conflict of moral demands, e.g., conflicts of duty. Such a conflict occurs when in a particular situation it is impossible for a person to do one of his duties without failing to do one of his other duties. Unlike conflicts of interests, conflicts of this kind presuppose the antecedent moral quality of the actions or activities that conflict and so should be called *moral dilemmas*.

Moral dilemmas are, of course, a common occurrence in the medical world; for example, doctors often have to choose between duties to different patients. Philosophers have generally adopted the (unfortunate) terminology of W. D. Ross and now refer to such conflicting duties as prima facie duties (Ross). The term "prima facie" is unfortunate because it suggests that the duty in question is only apparently a duty; for Ross and others who accept the distinction, on the other hand, a so-called prima facie duty is simply a real duty that is overridden by another duty. A prima facie duty is one that, other things being equal, is binding; however, if other things are not equal, one prima facie duty may be overridden by another prima facie duty. The overriding duty may be called "the absolute duty" [see article III below on DEONTOLOGICAL THEORIES]. Thus, a doctor's prima facie duty to save the baby might be overridden by his duty to save the mother. Depending on what the writer takes as his basic ethical framework, moral dilemmas may be regarded as conflicts of duties, of obligations, of loyalties, of rights, of moral rules, or of "morally relevant facts" [see article VIII below on OBJECTIVISM IN ETHICS].

The ought question in the case of moral dilemmas is: Which of my prima facie duties ought I to perform when it is impossible to perform all of them? Some philosophers have offered the principle of utility as a deciding principle in case of a conflict of duties. Others have offered a "sense of urgency (or importance)" as a deciding principle. Ross himself described the selection of an absolute duty from among a set of prima facie duties as a "fortunate" act. Many would agree with Gert that two impartial persons might reach different conclusions concerning a decision in a particular case [see article VIII below on OBJECTIVISM IN ETHICS].

Again, it should be observed that moral dilemmas come into existence only when all of the acts in question are in fact prima facie duties. Hence, ought questions arising out of dilemmas make sense only if the prima facie duties, rules, or other "morally relevant considerations" are not in dispute. This assumption about prima facie duties is not shared by some philosophers, e.g., by act-utilitarians and situationalists, who maintain that in principle there are no moral dilemmas and hence that ought questions of this type can be easily eliminated [see articles V and VI below on SITUATION ETHICS and UTILITARIANISM].

3. **Ought questions arising out of ethical disagreements.**   In a pluralistic society such as ours and in a world divided by different ideologies, religions, and cultures, it is inevitable that people should disagree over the rightness or wrongness of various kinds of conduct. An act that is regarded as right in one group is regarded as wrong in another group and as morally neutral in still another. The differences in question here do not call for ordering or weighting as in the case of conflicts of interest or of moral dilemmas; here we are dealing with black and white, as it were—that is, positions that are incompatible in the sense that they are mutually exclusive logically. Solutions to problems of this type depend on the deployment of a complete ethical theory, the refutation of alternatives to it, and, in general, a theory of ethical reasoning.

It is unnecessary to point out that differences of opinion about right and wrong like those being considered here create moral problems for the medical practitioner. They cannot be avoided, however, by a simple resort to dogmatic skepticism or skeptical dogmatism. It should be obvious that the ought question can take different forms depending on how it is construed and what one's purposes are. If a doctor wants (or has the time) to try to change the other person's mind, then we are dealing with an ought question of the third type, i.e., an ethical disagreement; but if he has to act at once on the basis of what he thinks to be right, then he is faced with a moral dilemma: Does his duty to respect the ethical beliefs of others that he knows to be wrong override his duty to save the patient's life?

4. **Ought questions turning on the distinction between duties and other oughts.**   Finally, there is a set of problems relating to the distinction between duties and other things that one ought to do for nonmoral reasons [see article II below on RULES AND PRINCIPLES]. It would be absurd to say that a doctor either has a duty to play golf on his day off or a duty not to do so, although it might be perfectly correct to say that he ought to play because he enjoys it. There are many issues relating to the scope of morality; some philosophers regard the scope as very large, so that almost everything that a person might do is either right or wrong. (This kind of moral rigorism is a consequence of certain versions of act-utilitarianism.) Most philosophers, however, narrow the scope; some do so very radically and hold, for example, that a person can have duties only to others and not to himself. This view raises interesting questions for medical ethics, for it automatically excludes the duty to oneself to take care of one's own body: Why should a patient take pills prescribed by a doctor if he has no duty to try to get well?

Metaethical questions

It should be pointed out at once that all of the preceding discussion concerning normative ethics properly comes under metaethics, since it is *about* normative ethics rather than being part of normative ethics. Five of the articles in this entry are directly concerned with metaethical issues. The issues of metaethics are, however, quite technical and so may not appear to be as directly relevant to medical ethics as are the issues of normative ethics. Nevertheless, it is impossible to deal with normative problems intelligently without entering into the field of metaethics, as should be evident from the foregoing discussion of ought questions.

Metaethics encompasses three broad categories of questions. The first group of questions concerns the connection between ethics (morality) and conduct. How can the belief that a certain action is right or wrong move a person to do or refrain from doing an action? On the other hand, how can a person ever fail to do his duty? (Mortimore). Traditionally, the problem has been formulated: How can ethics and moral reasoning be practical? [*See articles* x *and* xi *below on* NON-DESCRIPTIVISM *and* MORAL REASONING.]

The second group of questions concerns the connection between ethics (e.g., beliefs about right and wrong) and facts about the real world. What is the relationship of "value" to "fact," of "ought" to "is," or of "normative" to "descriptive"? (Hudson, 1969). This kind of issue might be important for medical ethics in establishing, for example, the connection between "normative" concepts like health and physiological conditions specifiable in purely scientific terms (Kovesi) [*see article* IX *below on* NATURALISM].

The third kind of question covered by metaethics concerns the logical relationship between ethical propositions of various degrees of generality, e.g., (1) all-embracing super-principles like the principle of utility or the categorical imperative, (2) moral rules and practices, and (3) individual, here-and-now moral decisions. Is one of these types logically more basic than the others? Are they linked deductively or inductively, conductively, constructively, or in some other way? [*See article* II *below on* RULES AND PRINCIPLES.]

One answer is that the rightness or wrongness of a particular action can be derived deductively from a super-principle, e.g., the principle of utility, with the aid of intermediate factual premises of an empirical nature. There are numerous objections to this kind of "mechanical" model of ethical reasoning. Another answer, which is adopted by the so-called rule-utilitarians, offers a two-tier model in terms of which the rightness or wrongness of particular actions is justified by appeal to a rule or practice, and the rules or practices are in turn justified by appeal to the super-principle, e.g., the principle of utility (Rawls, 1955). Yet another answer is to interpret the different kinds of ethical propositions as serving different functions in ethical discourse, that is, as providing answers to different categories of ought questions mentioned earlier. On this view, the super-principle may be taken as an answer to the question: How is a moral rule distinguished from a nonmoral rule?

In conclusion, it is important to realize that all of the questions outlined here are interconnected; one cannot satisfactorily answer one of them without addressing oneself to the others, and it should become clear as one probes into them that the problems of ethics are both complicated and subtle.

The following articles on ethics

In reading the articles on ethics that follow, it may be helpful to bear these three points in mind. First, while the articles as a group offer a comprehensive survey of the principal theories of ethics, one should not expect the articles to be entirely consistent with each other: each article reflects, to some extent, its author's own philosophical perspective. Second, philosophers prefer to organize their discussions around a problem or a set of problems; hence, the title of each article might be more accurate if it were prefaced by the words: "Problems concerning . . . " (e.g., rules, utilitarianism, etc.). Finally, it is important to recall the remarks made earlier about labels and to note that in almost every article the author takes pains to point out that the label in question is used in a number of different ways.

The first five articles (II-VI) are primarily concerned with questions of normative ethics. The next article (VII) describes some of the ways in which religious beliefs are connected with ethics. The last five articles (VIII-XII) deal with questions of metaethics; the last two of them discuss special problems that are particularly important for an understanding of the nature of ethics in general.

JOHN LADD

[*While all the articles in this entry are relevant, see especially the articles* RULES AND PRINCIPLES *and* MORAL REASONING. *For further discussion of topics mentioned in this article, see the entries:* HEALTH AS AN OBLIGATION; LAW AND MORALITY; NATURAL LAW; *and* OBLIGATION AND SUPEREROGATION. *This article will find application in the entries* ACTING AND REFRAINING; BIOETHICS; DECISION MAKING, MEDICAL; DOUBLE EFFECT; JUSTICE; *and* SEXUAL ETHICS. *For discussion of related ideas, see:* PRAGMATISM.]

BIBLIOGRAPHY

ARISTOTLE. *Nichomachean Ethics.*
AYER, ALFRED JULES. "On the Analysis of Moral Judgments." *Philosophical Essays.* New York: St. Martin's Press; London: Macmillan & Co., 1954, pp. 231–249, esp. p. 245.
HUDSON, WILLIAM D. *Modern Moral Philosophy.* Garden City, N.Y.: Anchor Books, Doubleday & Co., 1970. A lucid, critical exposition of contemporary metaethical theories.
————, ed. *The Is–Ought Question: A Collection of Papers on the Central Problem in Moral Philosophy.* Controversies in Philosophy. Edited by A. G. N. Flew. London: Macmillan & Co., New York: St. Martin's Press, 1969.
KOVESI, JULIUS. *Moral Notions.* Studies in Philosophical Psychology. Edited by R. F. Holland. New York: Humanities Press, 1967.
McCLOSKEY, J. *Meta-ethics and Normative Ethics.* The Hague: Martinus Nijhoff, 1969. A defense of ethical intuitionism, including an explanation of the concept of prima facie duties.
MacINTYRE, ALASDAIR. *A Short History of Ethics.* Fields of Philosophy. Edited by Paul Edwards and John Hospers. New York: Macmillan Co., 1966.
MELDEN, ABRAHAM IRVING. *Ethical Theories.* 2d ed., rev. Englewood Cliffs, N.J.: Prentice-Hall, 1967. A standard collection.
MOORE, GEORGE EDWARD. *Principia Ethica.* Cambridge: At the University Press, 1903, pp. 3–6.
MORTIMORE, GEOFFREY, ed. *Weakness of Will.* London: Macmillan & Co.; New York: St. Martin's Press, 1971.
PEIRCE, CHARLES SANTIAGO SANDERS. "The Fixation of Belief." *Popular Science Monthly* 12 (1877): 1–15. Reprint. Charles S. Peirce. *Essays in the Philosophy of Science.* Edited by Vincent Tomas. New York: Liberal Arts Press, 1957, pp. 3–30. Reprint. *Collected Papers of Charles Sanders Peirce.* 8 vols. Vol. 5: *Pragmatism and Pragmaticism.* Edited by Charles Hartshorne and Paul Weiss. Cambridge: Harvard University Press, 1960, pp. 223–247.
PLATO. *Apology.*
————. *Protagoras.*
————. *Republic.*
RAWLS, JOHN. "Outline of a Decision Procedure for Ethics." *Philosophical Review* 60 (1951): 177–197, esp. 186–187.
————. *A Theory of Justice.* Cambridge: Belknap Press, Harvard University Press, 1971.
————. "Two Concepts of Rules." *Philosophical Review* 64 (1955): 3–32.
ROSS, W. D. *The Right and the Good.* Oxford: At the Clarendon Press, 1930, pp. 19–32.
SELLARS, WILFRED, and HOSPERS, JOHN, eds. *Readings in Ethical Theory.* 2d ed. Century Philosophy Series. Edited by Justus Buchler. New York: Appleton-Century-Crofts, 1970. A collection of important recent writings in metaethics.
TAYLOR, PAUL W. *Principles of Ethics: An Introduction.* Belmont, Calif.: Dickenson Publishing Co., 1975.

II
RULES AND PRINCIPLES

Questions about the role of rules and principles in ethics have a special relevance for many discussions in bioethics. First, it has been true historically that the ethical positions associated with the profession of medicine have almost always been articulated in sets of rules. Even when the form in which the ethical position is presented is an oath or a prayer, the substantive content is usually embodied in a set of more or less specific rules laid down for the conduct of those in the medical profession.

Second, it is clear that any adequate response to the ethical quandaries that beset the biomedical sciences today must take the form of a set of general action guides: rules or principles. Most of the prominent ethical dilemmas in modern biomedicine—e.g., the design of experiments involving human subjects, the distribution of scarce medical resources, and questions surrounding the issue of when exotic lifesaving technology is to be employed—arise in areas where medicine is most socially complex and highly organized. The difficulties involve crucial decisions to be made by individual agents; but primarily they demand policies that must be made at a high level of the organizational pyramid and that will affect different persons in different ways.

It is of course possible that the policies actually adopted will be overly rigid and insensitive to subtle differences among the various cases to which they apply. To acknowledge this danger, however, is hardly fatal to the argument in favor of rules. To suggest that the *possibility* of the promulgation of overly rigid rules in this area provides good reason for jettisoning rules and principles altogether—in favor, perhaps, of immersion in the particular aspects of individual cases—is surely mistaken. Persons whose lives are affected by the institutions and agencies within modern biomedicine are entitled to reliable expectations about the stance of medical professionals toward certain basic ethical issues. The only way to provide for such expectations is through the formulation of general policies, i.e., sets of rules and principles, that guide the conduct of those who work within the institutions. The policies need not, of course, be so rigid as to eliminate all discretionary decision making on the part of those to whom they apply.

General features of rules

In the context of moral discussions, both rules and principles are best conceived as general action guides specifying that some type of action is prohibited, required, or permitted in certain circumstances. The distinction between a moral rule and a moral principle is difficult to draw with precision, but principles are generally distinguished from rules by being both more general and more foundational.

The most obvious feature of rules is their diversity (Wittgenstein, pp. 56–88). Rules are important for a wide variety of human activities, and the features they have in one area may be completely lacking in another. To be convinced of this, one need only reflect on the roles played by rules in morality, games, language, scientific investigation, etiquette, legal procedure, religious ceremonies, and love affairs, not to mention the practice of medicine. In all these areas, rules surely exist in that they both guide an agent's own actions and provide a basis on which the action of others may be evaluated. It is difficult, however, to find a single model that will characterize the nature and function of rules in all those areas.

The force of rules. Consider first how the force of rules may vary in different areas. Some rules have the force of restrictions, while others have the force of regulations, permissions, or prescriptions. More important, there may be great variation in the point of having rules in an area at all. Sometimes rules are required to coordinate the activity of large groups of persons. In such cases it may be unimportant which particular rules are adopted as long as everyone follows the same ones. The rule of driving in the United States that all drivers must stay on the right except when passing is often cited as an example of a rule with this purpose. Rules by which different uniforms are assigned to a hospital staff in order to allow easy identification constitute another example. Other rules have as their point the efficient achievement of some particular goal. Rules that govern the monitoring procedures in an intensive care unit would be an example here. There are yet other rules the point of which is to create situations

of stress where mental or physical dexterity can be demonstrated, such as the rules of games.

The sanctions of rules. Rules can also vary with regard to the sanctions attached to them. An almost limitless variety of rewards and punishments can be distributed in accord with conformity to or breach of rules. There is also significant diversity in the possible sources of such distributions. Sometimes the appropriate sanctions are applied by the actions of other persons, such as policemen. At other times, as in the case of rules like "Don't be exposed to too many X-rays," there are "natural" sanctions attached to a rule. At still other times it is alleged that the sanctions are in the hands of some supernatural agent to be distributed in either this world or the next.

The existence of rules. Conditions for the existence of rules also vary across different areas of their operation (Warnock, pp. 43–52). In some areas, a particular rule is said to exist only if it is the result of legislation by some "official" body. The official rules of such highly organized games as football and baseball exist only on this condition. Other rules are said to exist if a sufficiently large group of persons recognize them in their practical decisions and in their appraisal of the behavior of others. Linguistic rules and the rules of etiquette would be examples here. The rules of medical etiquette, which regulate referral, consultation, fee-splitting, etc., are in a somewhat ambiguous position with regard to the grounds for their existence. Such rules are partially grounded in traditional practices, partly in legislation by professional bodies (e.g., the American Medical Association), and partly in governmental regulation. The often acrimonious disagreements among health-care workers about these matters may very well be explained by a lack of agreement on the conditions for the existence of such rules.

The scope of rules. Rules also vary in their scope of application, with regard to both the persons to whom they apply and the locations within which they have application. Some rules apply to all persons in all places, e.g., moral rules, in some views. Some rules apply to some persons in all places, e.g., rules concerning physician advertising. Some rules apply to all persons in some places, e.g., rules forbidding smoking when oxygen is in use. Some rules apply to some persons in some places, e.g., rules for the maintenance of sterility in operating rooms. There is some dispute about the significance of these distinctions of scope, since by manipulation of the particular formulation of a rule it is possible to change its scope without changing its substantive content (Kovesi, pp. 73–85). There is nevertheless a difference in the generality of rules that is at least partially captured by these distinctions.

The concreteness of rules. One final way in which rules may vary is in concreteness. All rules associated with practical contexts will mention an action, but the description involved can vary in its concreteness. Thus, within traditional medical ethics one finds rules as abstract as "Do no harm," and as concrete as "Do not engage in fee-splitting." One would expect the relative concreteness of a rule to be reflected in the manner in which it regulates action. Thus, relatively abstract rules function primarily to set goals or parameters for action, while more concrete rules normally invoke prohibitions or requirements.

It is important to keep the diversity of rules in mind when discussing the nature of moral rules. Without such an awareness, one is likely to fasten upon some particular model for the function of rules drawn from a single area of human activity and to treat moral rules as if they must fit that model. If one supposes that moral rules must have the precision and concreteness of the rules of chess, or that they must be the result of explicit legislation like the rules of tournament golf, one is likely to despair of finding any moral rules at all. Once one recognizes, however, that rules function differently in the different areas of human life where they play significant roles, it is possible to appreciate the distinctive features of moral rules.

Moral rules in classical ethical theory

The diverse ways in which the nature and function of moral rules and principles can be understood is also illustrated in their treatment by classical moral philosophers. Most classical moral philosophers have agreed that rules and principles play a central role in moral deliberation and justification; there has also been agreement for the most part on the content of the correct moral rules. Moral philosophers as otherwise diverse as Kant and Mill or Plato and Hume have agreed that moral rules requiring, for example, fidelity, veracity, justice, and beneficence should be observed. Alongside this agreement, however, deep disagreement has existed about the nature and function of moral rules.

For Plato and Aristotle moral rules are requirements on action necessary for each person to achieve a satisfying and fulfilling life. The penalty for failure to abide by moral rules is the disintegration of the personality of the wrongdoer. In Immanuel Kant's ethical theory, moral rules play a quite different role. Kant argues that in all action by rational creatures a maxim, or general rule of action, is implied. Some maxims or rules of action are incumbent on an agent because of the particular projects he may be pursuing or because of his rational concern for his own happiness. Other maxims, however, which Kant called moral laws, are requirements on the actions of every rational agent no matter what his particular aims might be. The binding force of these rules, which give rise to what Kant called categorical imperatives, derives from what Kant took to be certain universal features of human rationality. Unlike Plato, Kant did not think there was any necessary connection between an agent's observance of moral rules and his achievement of happiness. Indeed, Kant felt that the parity between virtue and happiness, which is at the heart of Plato's doctrine, can be ensured only if there is some supernatural agent to distribute appropriate rewards and penalties in an afterlife.

J. S. Mill's conception of the role and nature of moral rules differs importantly from those of both Plato and Kant. Mill holds that moral rules are rules of thumb based on our experience of the general tendencies of actions to promote certain ends, which should be observed if the utilitarian goal of the greatest happiness is to be achieved (Cunningham, pp. 168–196). Rules are necessary since it is not usually possible, because of insufficient time or insufficient information, to plot the consequences of particular actions when an occasion for action arises. Moral rules for Mill, then, are necessary because of certain limitations inherent in human deliberation; they could be dispensed with in the practical deliberation of a creature with perfect knowledge.

Underneath the surface agreement on the part of classical moral philosophers about the importance of moral rules and about the content of these rules, there remained, then, large areas of disagreement. They disagreed about (1) the point of having moral rules at all; (2) the sanctions attached to the rules; (3) the techniques of argument required to support the particular rules they accepted; and (4) the conditions under which an agent might be required to make an exception to one of the rules.

All of these areas of controversy within classical ethical theory also make their appearance in recent discussions within bioethics. Thus, there are disputes about the point of having rules in bioethics at all. Some have argued that rules are necessary in order to ensure coordinated activity within biomedicine, which will lead to some overarching end, such as the greatest happiness of the greatest number. Others have argued that rules are required so that the practice of medicine will approximate some abstract model of justice or rational human conduct.

There are also disputed questions about the sanctions appropriate to rules in bioethics. Should the ultimate sanctions for the rules be located in the professional bodies to which health-care professionals belong, or in some governmental body more attentive, perhaps, to the desires of the general public? Or again, should external sanctions be rejected altogether in favor of making adherence to the rules a matter of individual integrity?

There are endless disputes within bioethics, of course, about the techniques of argument appropriate to establishing a specific moral rule. According to a familiar view, such arguments must rest on ultimate premises that direct the medical profession to promote some broadly teleological goal. Others have argued to the contrary that the premises should be of the sort that specify certain types of action as absolutely forbidden.

Finally, there are many questions within bioethics that turn on decisions about how to treat alleged exceptions to moral rules. On some views a rule that admits of exceptions is really no rule at all. According to other views, rules are primarily designed to handle "normal" cases and will always admit of exceptions in extraordinary cases. There clearly are extraordinary cases where a physician, for example, is justified in revealing confidential information gained in a medical encounter with a patient—where, say, prevention of some great disaster is in question. Such cases, some argue, demonstrate that it is misleading to speak of a rule enjoining confidentiality in the doctor–patient relationship. They further argue that such cases show that questions about when one is justified in breaching medical confidentiality are to be settled on a case-by-case basis. Others, taking a different view of rules and their exceptions, contend that such cases merely show that the applicability

of any rule is called into question by extraordinary circumstances.

It is of some importance to recognize that many of the most recalcitrant problems within bioethics merely reflect disputes within classical ethical theory about the nature and function of moral rules and principles. To recognize this is to acknowledge the importance for bioethics of an adequate account of such rules and principles.

Moral rules and moral justification

Three explanations of moral justification.   Rules have come into ethical theory primarily through a theory of justification. A common picture of the moral justification of actions is one that relies on the following principle:

> An action A is morally justified if it is in accord with the relevant moral rules, where these rules have been derived from a set of adequate moral principles.

According to the view of justification associated with this principle, questions about the moral justification of an action are typically raised at the level of rules. When the morality of a particular action is brought into question, the discussion is shifted to the justification of the relevant moral rules and eventually to the adequacy of those moral principles on which the rules rest. This model is usually taken to be thoroughly deductive, where the transitions from principle to rule and from rule to action are criticized from the standpoint of deductive logic. The moral rules would normally be seen as derivable from the moral principles together with some empirical data.

This scheme of justification is not unfamiliar in bioethics. Thus, in order to defend a particular experimental procedure against the charge that it unjustifiably puts experimental subjects at risk, someone might claim that informed consent has been obtained from the subjects. He could then appeal to the generally recognized rule that it is morally permissible to put experimental subjects at risk if their informed consent has been obtained. (Of course, other conditions must also be met.) If he is challenged further to support this rule, he may then turn to some higher-level principle from which it can be derived. For example, he might point out that the moral principle requiring us to treat others as ends, and not merely as means, supports the rule of informed consent.

Even though this model of justification may

be familiar, however, it has been criticized for a number of reasons. First, it has been argued that it can give no adequate account of justification, since it merely puts off the really difficult questions. One such question, how the adequacy of a particular principle or set of principles is to be determined, has seemed to many moral philosophers to admit of only two possible answers: Either the principles must be derived from yet more abstract principles, which themselves would then need to be justified, or the principles are in some sense self-evident. It is further pointed out that certain well-known difficulties confront those who adopt either of the two options.

Some recent existentialist moral philosophers, e.g., Sartre, and noncognitivist moral philosophers, e.g., Hare, have suggested, however, a third possibility: Ultimate principles are neither derivative nor self-evident, but are rather the objects of free and creative choice. According to this view, the moral principles that ultimately support the superstructure of an agent's morality are chosen by him. Any attempt to deny this essentially voluntaristic account of the foundations of morality is, it is claimed, bound to be shot through with self-deception or, in Sartre's terminology, "bad faith." These views, of course, do not answer questions about the justification of ultimate moral principles, but rather rule them irrelevant. Such questions are regarded as inappropriate at the level of such foundational practical principles.

Resistance to rules and principles. Some moral philosophers have found the difficulties of justification discussed above so formidable that they have suggested that the model that engenders them must itself be faulty. They have argued that justification, instead of flowing from principles to rules to action, rather moves in the opposite direction. According to their view, it is actions that are seen quite directly as justified or not, and rules and principles are adequate only insofar as they summarize correct moral perceptions. The function of rules and principles, thus, would not be to ground or support particular judgments about the moral character of individual actions, but rather to sum up in the manner of rules of thumb our particular perceptions about the moral character of particular actions. Rules and principles that play this role may nevertheless be important in the moral life, particularly in moral pedagogy, but they lack the foundational character that they have in the more traditional picture.

A second source for much of the resistance to rules and principles as playing an important role in morality is found in the feeling on the part of many that if rules and principles are given such a role, decision making will inevitably become rigid, legalistic, and insensitive to the nuances of particular cases. The rather ill-defined contemporary view, situation ethics, has attempted to develop this criticism (Fletcher, pp. 18–22). Proponents of situation ethics characteristically emphasize the complexity of particular moral dilemmas and conclude from this that any general action guide, whether rule or principle, will either be useless in coming to a reasoned decision or force the problem into a preconceived mold that may leave out the very features that demanded our moral attention. Situation ethics, then, proposes that we make moral decisions by immersing ourselves in the particular features of a problematic situation, and by freeing ourselves as much as possible from the influence of general action guides. Our decision making must, of course, be guided by some goals or ends, and situation ethics has opted here for a concern for the welfare of others. Ultimately, situation ethics seems to be coincident with act-utilitarianism, inheriting its weaknesses as well as its strengths.

The summary conception and the practice conception of rules. Both of these objections to the centrality of rules in morality can be illuminated by considering recent discussions of two distinct conceptions of how rules relate to the actions that they regulate (Rawls; Searle). First, according to what has been called *the summary conception*, rules function to summarize our perceptions about the permissibility or obligatoriness of a certain range of actions. In this view, we suppose that the possibility of performing a certain action exists prior to the adoption or recognition of a rule regulating that action. The rule arises out of an attempt to summarize our particular perceptions of when it is permissible, obligatory, or prohibited to perform the action. A rule that regulates smoking in certain areas— e.g., where oxygen is in use—is an example of such a rule. Smoking is an action possible prior to and independently of any rules regulating or specifying the activity. For various reasons, persons might come to recognize that smoking in certain places or situations, in unventilated rooms or around asthmatic children, should be forbidden. As a result of such recognition, rules prohibiting smoking in those situations could be formulated. Here the rule functions to regulate an activity that was possible independently of the rules, and can be said to summarize our perception of the inappropriateness of a number of individual acts of smoking.

This conception of the process by which rules come to be formulated and of the relation of such rules to the actions they regulate has been contrasted with a quite different view, the *practice conception of rules*. According to this view, rules do not function to regulate independently existing actions but rather serve to create the possibility of new forms of action. Actions within the context of games are often pointed to in this regard. Within baseball, for example, the actions of striking out, walking, and stealing a base are not possible prior to the rule-governed structure that gives a special significance to movements on the baseball field. The rules of baseball do not regulate actions that were possible prior to those rules, but rather create the possibility of performing those actions. The rules of baseball both make it possible to strike out and attach sanctions to striking out.

The distinction between the two conceptions has a special significance for any discussion of ethical rules within biomedicine. While the practice of medicine is not a game with health-care workers and patients playing according to well-defined rules, there is nevertheless a large part of medicine that is highly conventional. The standard doctor–patient encounter is not unlike a stylized performance where parties on both sides have a clear notion of the parts they are expected to play. A doctor is not just someone to whom we *happen* to turn for help, as we might turn to a friend or a neighbor. The doctor is rather certified as having a certain competence and the patient's encounter with him is guided by certain clear-cut conventions. The moral rule that enjoins confidentiality on the doctor–patient relationship, for example, is not based on our recognition that for the most part medical confidentiality has better overall results than its opposite. Rather, confidentiality is one of the constituents of the doctor–patient relationship. If we removed the requirement of confidentiality, we would not have the same relationship somewhat damaged, but another relationship altogether. In this sense, the rule of confidentiality seems to fit more closely the practice conception of rules rather than the summary conception. Other rules, such as that which enjoins the doctor to be truthful to the patient or that which invokes the notion of fairness in the allocation of scarce medical resources, also seem

to approximate the practice conception. There are other rules in medicine, however, that would seem to fit more closely the summary conception. Consider, for example, a rule physicians might adopt specifying the conditions under which placebos would be prescribed.

These two conceptions of rules are not intended, of course, to be competing accounts of the nature of all rules. Clearly, some rules fit the practice conception and others fit the summary conception. The central question for ethical theorists has been which conception most nearly captures the nature of moral rules, and about the answer to this question there has been little agreement. If one focuses on moral rules dealing with such highly conventional activities as promise keeping and truth-telling, or such institutionally complex areas as punishment and social justice, one is inclined to understand moral rules in accord with the practice conception. Moral rules associated with beneficence, however, would seem to push one toward the summary conception. What is clear is that those who have objected most strenuously to giving rules a central role in the processes of practical deliberation and moral justification (e.g., act-utilitarians and situationists) have also held that moral rules fit the summary conception; their opponents have emphasized the similarity of moral rules to the rules of practices. The most plausible view would seem to be that some moral rules fit one conception and others another.

Conclusion

There is no doubt that many of the most difficult problems within bioethics resist solution partly at least because of disagreement about relatively abstract issues about the nature and function of moral rules and moral principles. Recent discussions within ethical theory have provided powerful analytical tools for approaching some of these issues, but a consensus on them does not appear to be at hand. The primary lesson to be learned from much of the recent work would seem to be that one should avoid applying some simple model of the nature and function of moral rules and principles to all the contexts in which they play a role. An ultimately satisfying account of these issues can surely be given only within the framework of a comprehensive ethical theory.

WM. DAVID SOLOMON

[*For further discussion of topics mentioned in this article, see the entries:* BIOETHICS; CODES OF MEDICAL ETHICS; DECISION MAKING, MEDICAL;

LAW AND MORALITY; *and* PRAGMATISM. *While all the articles in this entry are relevant, see especially the article* SITUATION ETHICS, *which offers a different perspective on the same topic, as well as the following:* THE TASK OF ETHICS, DEONTOLOGICAL THEORIES, TELEOLOGICAL THEORIES, UTILITARIANISM, NON-DESCRIPTIVISM, MORAL REASONING, *and* RELATIVISM. *This article will find application in the entries* DOUBLE EFFECT; HEALTH POLICY; THERAPEUTIC RELATIONSHIP; *and* TRUTH-TELLING. *For discussion of related ideas, see the entries:* ACTING AND REFRAINING; JUSTICE; NATURAL LAW; *and* OBLIGATION AND SUPEREROGATION.]

BIBLIOGRAPHY

CUNNINGHAM, ROBERT L. *Situationism and the New Morality.* Contemporary Problems in Philosophy. New York: Appleton-Century-Crofts, 1970. A collection of articles surveying issues raised by the contemporary attack on moral rules.

FLETCHER, JOSEPH FRANCIS. *Situation Ethics: The New Morality.* Philadelphia: Westminster Press, 1966. A popular defense of situation ethics.

KOVESI, JULIUS. *Moral Notions.* Studies in Philosophical Psychology. London: Routledge & Kegan Paul; New York: Humanities Press, 1967. Develops idea that moral rules are involved in the application of moral concepts.

RAWLS, JOHN. "Two Concepts of Rules." *Philosophical Review* 64 (1955): 3–32. The classic discussion of the distinction between the summary and practice conception of rules.

SEARLE, JOHN R. *Speech Acts: An Essay in the Philosophy of Language.* London: Cambridge University Press, 1969. A development of Rawls's earlier discussion of the two concepts of rules, with special application to linguistic rules.

WARNOCK, GEOFFREY JAMES. *The Object of Morality.* London: Methuen & Co., 1971. A defense of the moral centrality of virtue, as opposed to rules.

WITTGENSTEIN, LUDWIG. *Philosophical Investigations.* Translated by G. E. M. Anscombe. Oxford: B. Blackwell, 1953. Reprint. New York: Macmillan Co., 1958, 1973. An important philosophical work in which the notion of rule-governed activity is one of the major explanatory tools. It has had enormous influence on contemporary philosophical discussions of rules.

III
DEONTOLOGICAL THEORIES

The diversity and complexity of ethical opinions and theories invite classification. Dichotomies are especially popular, because they promise to organize a multitude of disagreements around a fundamental one from which they are derived. One of these dichotomies, teleology/deontology, introduced in 1930 by C. D. Broad, was an improvement on Sidgwick's confusing trichotomy (into intuitionism, egoism, and utilitarianism), and caught on during the subsequent decades. It is perhaps worth noting

that deontology was not always contrasted with teleology. Ironically, deontology (from Greek, *deon*, duty, and *logos*, discourse) was first introduced, as the title of one of his books, by the archteleologist Jeremy Bentham. He used the word to suggest that his work had turned the art of determining what is one's duty, into a quantifiable discipline, based on the hedonic (pleasure) calculus: "the science of morality." The current use of "deontological ethics" strongly suggests a very different conception of ethical theory.

Even its current use as one-half of a classificatory pair has not been uniformly the same. Some use the two terms as a mutually exclusive and jointly exhaustive pair, others merely as coupled names for interestingly different types of theory. Some aim primarily at satisfying the canons of dichotomous classification, others at bringing to light the profoundly important difference between two groups of ethical theories, some of which are paradigms of deontological, others of teleological, ethics.

The Hebrew–Christian paradigm

The oldest of the four major paradigms of deontology, Hebrew–Christian ethics, conceives of the ideal life for man as obedience to the will of God, or to some positive law or rule believed to express that will, whatever may be the individual's own plans or desires. The central idea here is that, while the conception of the ideal life does indeed determine what is the right thing for one to do, such determination is independent of what one would oneself desire or choose to do, or what would maximize satisfaction all round. Of course, many ethical theorists, from Kant to the present day, also stress that what one actually desires may differ from what is the right thing for one to do but nevertheless maintain that the right thing is what one would choose to do if only one were in some way idealized, e.g., if one followed one's rational part, had full information about all the consequences of the alternatives, or did not suffer from weakness of will. By contrast, in the Hebrew–Christian ideal under discussion there is no necessary connection between the right thing for one to do and what even such idealized human dispositions would dispose one to do, because the right thing for one to do is to *submit* to someone else's will. And while that will is necessarily an ideal will, not all strands in the Hebrew–Christian tradition tie that ideal to rationality.

Another idea, closely related to the previous

one, is that there are certain absolute prohibitions which the morally good person will never disobey, whatever the consequences of obedience may be. In the Hebrew–Christian tradition these absolute prohibitions comprise the deliberate killing of the innocent (including abortion), suicide, adultery, and, a favorite of recent philosophical discussions, procuring the judicial punishment of the innocent. In this view, if one were moved by the contemplation of the disastrous consequences of obeying and of the favorable consequences of disobeying, one would not be following reason or morality but would necessarily be yielding to temptation or fear. A corollary sometimes extracted is that to advocate the systematic study of what a person should do if, in certain rather special circumstances, the consequences of obeying would be particularly disastrous, is to advocate systematically corroding people's moral fiber. For by such routine thinking about the "unthinkable" one is led to construe *disobedience* not as wickedness or even weakness, but as the rational thing to do, as when someone performs an act of euthanasia because he cannot endure the suffering of a terminally ill person or kills a deformed baby because he wants to spare it the physical and mental torments it will have to suffer.

Immanuel Kant

A second paradigm of deontology is Kant's ethics. At the cost of greatly oversimplifying it, its main theses can be summarized as follows: the requirements of morality always override all other kinds of reasons for doing something when they run counter to them. Therefore, these moral requirements, expressed by the imperatives of duty, cannot be explained as merely "hypothetical imperatives," i.e., as what we ought to do because it is the means to certain ends that our psychological makeup and the circumstances in which we find ourselves cause us to have. For, since men are only partly rational and partly desiring creatures, the merely hypothetical imperatives that are based on desire always can and often do come into conflict with the imperatives of duty. In order, therefore, that these imperatives of duty should always override incompatible nonmoral (hypothetical) imperatives, men would have to be—and as partly rational creatures they actually are—subject to a desire-independent or categorical imperative, an imperative based solely on the formal nature of the law, its universality; an imperative, therefore, which unconditionally requires of every

rational being that it act only on maxims it can will to become universal laws of nature and that it follow these maxims whatever the consequences of doing so. Therefore a morally upright person cannot be one who assiduously and conscientiously does what, as reason tells him, is the best means to his ends whatever they happen to be but, rather, someone with a good will, i.e., someone always prepared to do *whatever* moral duty requires. And the good life for man cannot consist in the maximal satisfaction of desires and the attainment of merely desire-determined ends. It must, rather, be a life in which people form moral communities where everyone obeys the Categorical Imperative, and everyone therefore regards everyone else as "an end in himself," and so acts on the principle of never treating anyone merely as a means to his own desire-determined ends. It must, therefore, be a life in which individual rights, freedom, dignity, self-respect, and justice are maintained.

There are in Kant's ethics at least four importantly different emphases, the first two continuous with the Hebrew–Christian conception of the ideal life, the second two incompatible with it: (1) the insistence that the ideal life for man consists in submission to a certain will or command expressed in universal imperatives that hold for everyone and contain no exceptions; (2) the insistence that unlike hypothetical imperatives moral imperatives are unconditional, and so inescapable, containing no exceptions, and therefore absolute, i.e., binding whatever the consequences, and supreme, i.e., overriding all others with which they come into conflict; (3) the insistence that the will to which a morally good person submits is not the will of another, but his own will, insofar as he is rational and so respects law; and (4) the stress on certain liberal values, such as autonomy, freedom, dignity, self-respect, and the respect for individual rights.

Broad's definition of deontology attempts to do justice to these two paradigms. In his definition, deontological ethical theories are those maintaining that there are certain types of acts—and it is known what types these are—that are "absolutely wrong," i.e., such that every particular act of these types is wrong whatever else may be true of it, in particular, whatever its consequences or those of any of the alternative acts open to the agent. If a physician is such an "absolutist" deontologist then he may believe, for instance, that killing a fetus is wrong whatever its consequences, even if the mother were to die without the operation. He must, therefore, let the mother die rather than save her life by killing the fetus, for that would be using a human being as a means only. If he is a teleologist, then he will believe that performing an abortion is the right thing to do, if and only if in the circumstances it is the act with the best consequences.

The absolutist account has two serious weaknesses. One is that it identifies deontology with absolutism, a view that many philosophers, including some who want to call themselves deontologists, regard as irrational. But deontology should not be so defined, using the name for an extreme and widely unacceptable type of ethical theory. A second weakness is that it excludes a group of philosophers, namely, the Oxford Intuitionists of the 1930s and 1940s—H. A. Prichard and his followers, W. D. Ross, and E. F. Carritt—all of whom would want to be included among deontologists and are often treated as deontologists par excellence, but who reject absolutism as well as all forms of consequentialism.

The Oxford Intuitionists

The main theses of the Oxford Intuitionists are as follows. The determination of the moral rightness or wrongness of a particular act depends on its intrinsic nature. This intrinsic nature is composed of the many intrinsic properties of an act. Some of these are "right-making," others "wrong-making," and still others morally neutral. If an act involves killing a fetus, then it has a wrong-making property. If it is also an act of saving the life of a human being, then it has a right-making property. In that it is an act of performing a surgical operation, it is morally neutral. Determining the rightness or wrongness of an act must proceed through two stages. The first is the determination of all of its right/wrong-making properties. As soon as one such property is ascertained, the act is classified as "prima facie right," "right other things equal" (say, the act of saving the life of the mother), or "prima facie wrong," "wrong other things equal" (say, the act of killing a fetus). The second stage involves determining the relative "weights" of the various right/wrong-making properties, and the corresponding "stringencies" of the "prima facie duties" of a person who is contemplating performing an act with this set of right/wrong-making properties. Determining the relative stringency of these prima facie duties establishes the "final duty," "duty sans phrase," or "duty all things considered." In answer to how someone knows what are right-

making and what are wrong-making properties of an act, and which are the more stringent, Prichard and his followers claim that he knows this by intuition, that is, in a manner comparable to that in which he knows the basic truths of mathematics. If a physician intuits the wrongness of killing a fetus as being weightier than the rightness (obligatoriness) of doing whatever will save the life of his patient (and if he does not detect any other right/wrong-making property in the act), he will judge killing the fetus to be wrong, all things considered, and will regard it as his final duty not to perform the operation. If he intuits the obligatoriness of saving his patient's life to be more stringent than the obligatoriness of not killing the fetus (and if he does not detect any other right/wrong-making property in the act) then he will think it his final duty to perform the abortion.

This theory of the Oxford Intuitionists shares with the two paradigms of deontological theories already discussed the acceptance of "intrinsicalism" (as it might be called), i.e., the view that acts are right/wrong on account of their intrinsic nature. However, this theory rejects absolutism on the ground that, however horrible the intrinsic nature of an act may be, the alternatives available in the circumstances in which it is performed may be still more horrible. The question cannot be answered a priori. The considerations must be weighed when *all* the procurable information about the nature of the act is in. For this reason, intrinsicalism can reject the absolutist's denial of the relevance of the consequences either of refusing to do or of doing an intrinsically (i.e., prima facie) wrong act. But while intrinsicalism can affirm the relevance of the consequences of any act to the determination of its rightness, it must do so in one of two ways, which distinguish it from the consequentialist and the teleologist in general. Consequentialists maintain that the rightness/wrongness of an act depends solely on its consequences. They need not thereby deny the intrinsicalist's claim that the rightness/wrongness of an act depends solely on its intrinsic nature, but must insist, against the intrinsicalists, that there is only one right-making property, "optimificity," i.e., being among the acts open to the agent the one with the best consequences, and only one wrong-making property, nonoptimificity. Now, the intrinsicalist may assert merely that in addition to optimificity there are other right-making properties, and that the consequences of an act bring such other properties to light. Suppose it is discovered that the consequences of killing a certain fetus include the preservation of the mother's life and that no other course of action has this consequence. Then this information about the consequences of this act may show, not, perhaps, that it is the optimific act, but rather something else, namely, that this act has the right- (or even obligatory-) making property of being the only way of discharging a physician's duty to look after the health and life of a patient. A physician may well regard this duty as his most stringent, more stringent even than his duty not to kill the fetus or the duty to do what has the best possible consequences.

An intrinsicalist could, however, deny that optimificity is a right-making property at all, on the grounds that optimificity is not an intrinsic property of an act, since whether an act is optimific depends not solely on *its* nature and consequences but also on the nature and consequences of the *other* acts open to the agent.

Lastly, the intrinsicalist differs from the consequentialist in a third way, in that he maintains that the intrinsic nature of an act is not determined solely by its consequences but also by its relation to the past. Unlike a consequentialist, an intrinsicalist can admit, as relevant to the question of whether the mother has a right to terminate her unwanted pregnancy, the fact that the pregnancy was the result of rape.

To avoid absolutism, the Oxford Intuitionists would have to reject Broad's definition, but could define as deontological any ethical theory which holds that an act is finally right if its right-making properties are weightier than its wrong-making ones, where right- and wrong-making properties are those on account of any single one of which an act would be prima facie right (or wrong), and if it were its only such property, also finally right (or wrong). This definition retains the intrinsicalism rejected by consequentialists but does not imply absolutism, since it allows that the consequences of an act are always relevant to its rightness, though not of course the only thing relevant. This still leaves open the question, on which deontologists might disagree, whether among the right/wrong-making properties to which the consequences of an act are relevant, its optimificity is or is not to be included. In this account of the distinction, an ethical theory can contain teleological and deontological elements and so can be classified as being both. Thus, rule-utilitarianism, the theory that an act is right if it conforms to rules that pass the test of utility, can be thought of as a utilitarian modification of intrinsicalism. For it retains the intrinsicalist claim that an act is right if and only if it conforms to universal principles or rules. But it replaces the deontological claim that these principles are known by intuition by the teleological claim that they are those which satisfy the criterion of utility. Thus a "pure" teleological theory, e.g., act-utilitarianism, might hold that a given act of euthanasia was right because it was the act, of all those open to the physician, that produced the greatest happiness or least unhappiness of all those affected. A pure deontologist, e.g., a Kantian, would reject this on the ground that this was to treat the patient merely as a means to the end of maximizing happiness. But a mixed theory, e.g., rule-utilitarianism, might reject the act if it is of a kind whose general performance or permissibility would not maximize the happiness of those affected by or engaging in the practice of euthanasia.

Recent contract theories

There is a fourth group of moral theorists who want to be and usually are thought of as typical deontologists. Their work, a revival of classical contract theory, has been much discussed recently, above all that of their most distinguished member, John Rawls. These contract theories differ from their prototypes, Hobbes, Locke, and Rousseau, in at least two important respects. They use the conceptual machinery of the classical contract philosophers, but not to justify political obligation, the claim that all those subject to a municipal legal order have a moral obligation to abide by it. They use it, rather, to derive with the help of this conceptual machinery whatever they take to be the principles that obligate us, above all the principles of justice. Nor do they rest their claims about what it is right for a person to do on the existence of a basic contractual obligation to do this thing, either because he is somehow bound by an actual original contract by which the contractors have bound themselves and their heirs or because he has himself actually consented to do this thing, although perhaps only tacitly, by accepting the benefits he received from his society.

Perhaps the best way to explain how modern contractarians use the idea of the social contract is to exhibit their close affinities with both the Oxford Intuitionists and the rule-utilitarians. Rawls's contract theory retains the intrinsicalism common to intuitionists and rule-utilitarians but, in answer to the question of how we know what are these principles or rules to which right acts must conform, offers an answer different from either of these, and closer to those in the contractarian tradition, especially Kant. In Rawls's view, these principles are those universal ones which would be chosen, for adoption in a society of which the chooser is himself a member, by any rational person with a certain, somewhat idealized, psychology (e.g., purely self-interested, nonenvious) and placed in a certain favored position (behind "a veil of ignorance," which precludes his having any advantage or disadvantage relative to others making a similar choice). Rawls conceives of the ideal life for man as necessarily lived in cooperation as well as in competition with others. Hence, though fully recognizing the importance of maximizing those "primary" good things in life whose value does not depend on the manner in which their cooperative production is organized, he places especially heavy emphasis on the values arising out of the satisfaction of the proper conditions of association, such as freedom, autonomy, human rights, dignity, self-respect, and just distribution of the jointly produced primary goods.

Since Rawls regards the emphasis on these values as the essence of the tradition in which he is writing, and since he finds these values overlooked or disparaged in the utilitarian and, more generally, the teleological tradition, he readily adopts the account of "teleology/deontology" first offered by William K. Frankena. Like him, Rawls takes teleology as the basic term; defines as teleological any theory that holds: (1) that the good can be defined independently of the right, and (2) that the right is defined as what maximizes the good thus independently determined; and then defines as deontological any theory that is not teleological. Although this definition has several weaknesses—for example, it turns into a deontological theory Moore's later ideal utilitarianism because it does not satisfy (1), and Christian salvationism because it does not satisfy (2)—it is considered by many moral philosophers in the United States and Great Britain the best now available.

KURT BAIER

[*Directly related are the other articles in this entry:* TELEOLOGICAL THEORIES, UTILITARIANISM, THEOLOGICAL ETHICS, *and* OBJECTIVISM IN ETHICS. *See also:* ABORTION, *article on* CONTEMPORARY DEBATE IN PHILOSOPHICAL AND RELIGIOUS ETHICS; DEATH AND DYING: EUTHANASIA AND SUSTAINING LIFE, *article on* ETHICAL VIEWS; INFANTS, *article on* ETHICAL PERSPECTIVES ON THE CARE OF INFANTS; *and* OBLIGATION AND SUPEREROGATION.]

BIBLIOGRAPHY

ANSCOMBE, G. E. M. "Modern Moral Philosophy." *Philosophy* 33 (1958): 1–19.

BENNETT, JONATHAN. "Whatever the Consequences." *Analysis* 26 (1966): 83–102.

BENTHAM, JEREMY. *Deontology.* London: Longman & Co.; Edinburgh: William Tait, 1834.

BRANDT, RICHARD B. *Ethical Theory.* Englewood Cliffs, N.J.: Prentice-Hall, 1959.

BROAD, CHARLES DUNBAR. *Five Types of Ethical Theory.* London: Kegan Paul, Trench, Trubner & Co.; New York: Harcourt, Brace & Co., 1930.

FOOT, PHILIPPA. "Morality as a System of Hypothetical Imperatives." *Philosophical Review* 81 (1972): 305–316.

FRANKENA, WILLIAM K. *Ethics.* 2d ed. Englewood Cliffs, N.J.: Prentice-Hall, 1963.

PRICHARD, HAROLD ARTHUR. *Moral Obligation.* Oxford: Clarendon Press, 1949, 1968.

RAWLS, JOHN. *A Theory of Justice.* Cambridge: Belknap Press of Harvard University Press, 1971.

ROSS, W. DAVID. *The Foundations of Ethics.* Oxford: Clarendon Press, 1939.

SMART, J. J. C., and WILLIAMS, BERNARD. *Utilitarianism: For and Against.* Cambridge: University Press, 1973.

IV
TELEOLOGICAL THEORIES

Teleological ethics (from Greek *telos*, end, and *logos*, discourse) is a term currently used mainly to refer to a group of ethical theories that are thought to share certain characteristics on account of which they are importantly different from those of another group, called "deontological." Theorists of both types agree that it is their task to provide us with guidelines for the good, or even the best possible, life for man, and they agree further that this can be done only by finding answers to the two fundamental ethical questions, "What is good?" and "What is to be done?" Teleologists then part company with deontologists on the issue of the role of the good in ethical theory. Teleologists regard "What is good?" not only as the logically prior of the two questions, which must therefore be answered first, but also attempt to ascertain what should be done by discovering the best way of attaining the good. Different teleologists then disagree with one another on three main problematic issues: (1) exactly what is good; (2) whose good is to be taken into account; and (3) exactly what sorts of guidance can ethical theory provide for the individual in his deliberations about what is to be done.

What is good?   Teleologists give a great variety of answers to their primary question, "What is good?" We can distinguish between *monistic* answers, which contend that there is only one good, e.g., happiness, satisfaction of desire, self-realization, or perfection, and *pluralistic* answers, which include all or most of the goods embraced by monists and more, e.g., knowledge, friendship, self-respect, freedom, etc., and which maintain that life is the better the more of these goods it holds or the more nearly it holds them in the proper proportion.

We can also distinguish between *objective* (or intersubjective) answers, which claim that the good is the same for all (e.g., Aristotle's happiness in accordance with virtue) so that those who pursue other ends must be considered misguided, and *subjective* answers, which say that two people's conceptions of the good life *for them* may differ, one seeking, say, power, the other contentment, yet neither of them being mistaken.

We can further distinguish between those answers that construe the good as *nonquantifiable*, e.g., salvation, which one must either win completely or lose altogether, and those that make the good *quantifiable*; in some such answers, e.g., when the good is conceived as pleasure, happiness, or power, the good is with no ideal limit other than maximization; in other answers of this type, e.g., when the good is conceived as self-realization, the good has a limit, and then one can approximate and perhaps even reach it, but one cannot have indefinitely more of it.

The last difference to be noted among teleological answers to this question is that between versions of the good that are *forward-looking* or *consequentialist*, such as future happiness, and *nonconsequentialist* versions of the good, which give the future no greater weight than the past and allow consideration of the future in relation to the past. Such *nonconsequentialist* views could consider retribution a good, whereas a *consequentialist* view would tend to stress reform or deterrence as an objective of punishment. It would seem that *nonconsequentialist* teleological theories, especially if pluralistic and objective, could with equal justification be called deontological.

Whose good?   Concerning the second main question, whose good is to be considered in determining what is the right thing for someone to do, we can distinguish two main types of answers, *person-relative* and *person-neutral*.

Person-relative answers conceive of the good as what is welcome from a given point of view, e.g., rain from the farmer's but not the vacationer's. One's own good is what is welcome from one's own point of view. How good one's own life is depends on how much in it is welcome, how much unwelcome from one's own point of view. We can distinguish four major classes of such answers, depending on whose good it is that is taken into account in determining what is the right thing to do.

The first, ethical egoism, says that only the agent's own good should be considered. In this class belong hedonistic and eudaimonistic egoism (in which the good is conceived as quantifiable and without ideal limit other than maximization), personal perfectionism (in which the good is conceived as quantifiable but with an ideal limit), and salvationism (in which the good is conceived as nonquantifiable).

The second type of such answers, which might be called "ethical elitism," says that only the good of the elite is to be considered. In another of its forms, perfectionism would be an instance of this type. Thus, in Nietzsche's view, the right thing to do is what maximizes human excellences. He argues that any individual's life can retain the deepest significance only if he lives for the good of the rarest and most valuable human specimens, that mankind must therefore strive continually to produce great men and make possible the realization of their excellences. Society must therefore set aside the claims of the less gifted to have their good taken care of.

The third, which might be called "ethical parochialism," says that only the good of the agent's appropriate in-group (e.g., class, sex, party, church, race, country) should be taken into consideration. This view can, of course, be combined with any type of answer to the teleologist's primary question, "What is good?"

The fourth, "ethical universalism," insists that the good of mankind as such must be taken into account. To this fourth type belongs utilitarianism, whose most popular versions combine an answer of this fourth type to the second main question ("Whose good?") with some version of a quantifiable conception of the good in answer to the first question ("What is good?").

It should be noted that though all these answers are *person-dependent*, ethical elitism and utilitarianism are *agent-neutral*, while ethical egoism and parochialism are *agent-relative* theories. That is to say, in the case of the former two, the class of persons whose good is to be taken into consideration is not, as with the latter two it is, defined by reference to the agent, i.e., the person for whom the morally right action is to be ascertained. Thus, in dealing with the problem of triage, a utilitarian physician must ignore questions of how his allocation of scarce lifesaving drugs will affect the physician's own or his in-group's good, but must allocate them so as to promote the greatest good of the greatest number of persons (whether they are valuable or not); an ethical elitist must promote the greatest good of the most valuable persons (however many or few they may be); an ethical parochialist must promote the greatest good of members of his in-group (whatever their number or merit); and an ethical egoist must promote his own greatest good. And all of them must do so regardless of the way in which this will affect the good of those who fall outside the purview of the definition.

Person-neutral answers, by contrast, conceive of the good as that whose existence, occurrence, or prevalence is an absolutely, i.e., *person-neutrally,* good thing. In this view, the question of *whose* good is the existence, occurrence, or prevalence of something is at best a secondary, at worst an illegitimate question. Such views can admit that developments favorable from a given point of view will tend to appear (absolutely) good to those who have adopted that point of view, but when the bias caused by the special perspective of that point of view is corrected, the appearance of good may then be revealed as deceptive. Writers such as Hegel and Marx, but oddly enough also G. E. Moore, belong in this category.

For illustration let us consider the case of A, a surgeon, who is a sadistic hedonist. He believes that pleasure and pleasure alone is good in itself, and he derives pleasure from, among other things, watching people suffer. In the person-relative answer, the amount of pleasure A would derive from watching B's pain during and after surgery would necessarily count in determining whether it is right for A to perform such surgery on B. If A derives very great pleasure, that could outweigh, in the calculation of whether A ought to operate on B, the misery inflicted on B by the surgery. By contrast, in the person-neutral view, the fact that A's pleasure is derived from watching B's pain may disqualify A's pleasure from being taken into account at all. It may even make it the case that the occurrence of the operation, if A enjoys it, is (absolutely) worse than if A were to suffer in sympathy with his patient.

The most widely discussed of these theories is undoubtedly utilitarianism. Utilitarians typically conceive of the good as some kind of (positive or negative) "payoff" attaching to things that one brings about or that befall one. These payoffs, sometimes called "utiles," are thought of as a common unit of measure, permitting an evaluative (hedonic, felicific, satisfaction, etc.) calculus, which would enable one to conduct one's moral life in a rational manner comparable to that of the efficient businessman. As the good businessman maximizes profits, so the moral person maximizes the net balance of good over bad (pleasure over pain, happiness over unhappiness). One of the major difficulties with this attractively simple idea has been to reduce the payoffs yielded by different courses of action to an empirically verifiable common denominator, both in the case of a single person and, even more so, in the case of a whole society. The main disagreements about how the good of mankind as a whole is to be conceived revolve around what is meant by the greatest happiness or pleasure of the greatest number.

One issue here is whether what is to be compared is the *sum total* of happiness or the *average* happiness resulting from alternative policies. The "sum-total" view would, for example, advocate an increase in population if that increased the total of the balance of pleasure over pain, even if that balance was decreased in every individual life, while the "average" view would advocate it only if it raised the average amount of pleasure or happiness. A second disagreement is about whether the principle of utility is a test of the moral acceptability of the acts of individual agents or of the institutions of a society. The classical utilitarians (Bentham, Mill, Sidgwick) were more concerned with improving the social order than with improving the morals of private individuals. Bentham, for example, divides ethics into private ethics and legislation, the former concerned with providing principles and rules for use by private individuals, the latter with providing those to be used by legislators. In one plausible interpretation of Bentham, both were to use the same principle (which Bentham calls the principle of utility), namely, of acting so as to maximize the happiness of those "under their direction." In other words, private individuals were to use the principle of maximizing the agent's happiness, legislators that of maximizing the happiness of those subject to the law. Bentham therefore was, as far as private ethics is concerned, an egoist rather than a utilitarian, as these terms are usually defined. The individual citizen is bound by the law only in the sense that the sanctions attached to it make it prudent but not morally obligatory for him to follow it. If the legislator follows the principle of maximizing the happiness of those subject to the law, then the law so weights the subject's choice that if they follow the principle of maximizing their own happiness, they will be maximizing the sum total of society's happiness. Sidgwick by contrast appears to have accepted the moral obligatoriness of the law, at least to the extent to which the laws themselves satisfied the principle of utility, i.e., if they were designed so as to achieve the greatest net balance of good over evil in the society they govern. Later utilitarians (e.g., G. E. Moore) concentrate on what Bentham called private ethics, and devote little attention to the problem of whether or not such social institutions as marriage, private property, and the criminal law impose a moral obligation to do what the rules of these institutions require.

Guidance for individual deliberation. Our third question concerns the extent to which ethical theory can provide guidance to the individual in his deliberation about what to do. This institutional or social problem of ethics arises in the recent controversy between so-called act-utilitarians and rule-utilitarians. Act-utilitarians maintain that the only right-making property is "optimificity," having consequences at least as good as those of any alternative acts open to the agent, and the only wrong-making property is "nonoptimificity." Utilitarians typically interpret optimificity in terms of the hedonic (pleasure) or felicific (happiness) calculus. They do not for instance admit that an act's being, say, an act of craniotomy (the cutting or crushing of the fetal skull to reduce its size for removal when normal delivery is not possible) makes it necessarily a wrong act, or its being required by the law necessarily makes it right. Thus, although Bentham recognized the importance of the function of compulsory social rules and of the difference between acts of legislators and of private individuals, he was nevertheless an act-utilitarian. That is, he held that the rightness of a particular act, whether of a legislator or of a private individual, was determined solely by its optimificity, and not at all by its conformity with certain moral rules.

A related issue concerns the kinds of rules a teleologist can admit in his system. The act-utilitarian can, like Bentham, allow that a society should have compulsory rules, such as laws, but he must insist that, as far as determining the rightness of particular acts is concerned, such compulsory rules are no more than rules of thumb, i.e., rough indicators of what it would be right for an individual to do. On this view, private individuals admittedly will, by and large, do better by following these rules than by working out the optimific act on their own. But it is conceivable, perhaps likely, that an individual will occasionally have adequate reason to think that the optimific act will involve breaking the law. If a physician has information that a particular act of euthanasia (or suicide, etc.) would have the best consequences, then he must regard these particular acts as right, even if they constitute a breach of a compulsory social rule or law whose existence is desirable from the point of view of utility. On this, contemporary act-utilitarians thus agree with Bentham. But they differ from him in insisting that the optimificity of a particular act is to be construed, not in Bentham's way as the greatest happiness of the agent, but that of the greatest number of persons.

Rule-utilitarians, by contrast, contend that the rightness of an act is determined by its conformity with all the compulsory social rules that pass the test of utility. Different rule-utilitarians differ from one another on precisely how this is to be interpreted; whether the rules are actual or ideal rules, whether their utility is the utility of everyone actually following them, or the utility of their being accepted as binding in the community. The debate is still in full swing, and no generally agreed results have so far emerged. It is not even generally agreed whether there is any plausible form of rule-utilitarianism that does not collapse into, that is, does not yield exactly the same moral precepts as, act-utilitarianism.

Among the many objections to teleological theories, one deserves special attention, namely, that they imply that the end justifies the means. It is hard to formulate this general objection clearly, but it appears to make at least two distinguishable accusations. One is that teleological ethics, by setting up one end as the good and therefore as so important that its attainment has an overriding claim on us, and by defining the right as whatever brings about the good, encourages us to ignore the rights of those who stand in the way of our attaining that end. If our end is the Nietzschean maximization of human greatness or the conversion of the whole world to our favorite ideology or the control of fertility, the means needed to accomplish such an aim may well run roughshod over many rights and needs whose recognition and satisfaction would stand in the way of that end. Plainly even the more modest end of maximizing pleasure or happiness is open to this objection, if that maximization is interpreted, in the manner of classical utilitarianism, as bringing about the greatest total balance of happiness or pleasure over unhappiness or pain. For that end may actually require the violation of the rights and the neglect of the needs of some members of a community. In the field of population policy, for instance, the maximization of happiness requires an increase in the number of people whose happiness is summed, even if the happiness of every member is thereby decreased, as long as the total is increased. Similarly, in the area of allocation of scarce resources, it may require (to maximize the sum total of happiness) that more of the available resources be allocated to those who already have plenty in order to eliminate the sufferers living at the minimal level of subsistence. This would hold equally in the international and the national sphere. On this point, too, the debate continues.

The second accusation against teleological theories is that they espouse "consequentialism," the principle that consequences alone determine the rightness of an act, i.e., that the only right-making property of an act is its optimificity. This involves the denial that any acts other than optimific ones are intrinsically right, and in particular the denial of absolutism, the contention that there are acts of certain types that are wrong whatever the consequences. Here we must distinguish between the weaker view, that the consequences of a particular act are never irrelevant to its rightness, and the stronger view that certain types of acts are absolutely wrong, i.e., wrong whatever the consequences. If rule-utilitarians can be classified as teleologists, then there are some teleologists who are not open to the milder version of this accusation, for rule-utilitarians do of course allow that acts other than optimific ones can be right. However, they are open to the stronger accusation, for they reject absolutism.

KURT BAIER

[*While all the articles in this entry are relevant, see especially* UTILITARIANISM, *which builds on this article,* DEONTOLOGICAL THEORIES, *and* NATURALISM. *Also directly related is* OBLIGATION AND SUPEREROGATION.]

BIBLIOGRAPHY

BENTHAM, JEREMY. *An Introduction to the Principles of Morals and Legislation.* Oxford: Clarendon Press, 1907.
BRANDT, RICHARD B. *Ethical Theory.* Englewood Cliffs, N.J.: Prentice-Hall, 1959.
LYONS, DAVID. *Forms and Limits of Utilitarianism.* Oxford: Clarendon Press, 1965.
MILL, JOHN STUART. *Utilitarianism, Liberty, and Representative Government.* New York: E. P. Dutton & Co., 1910.
MOORE, G. E. *Principia Ethica.* Cambridge: University Press, 1903.
SIDGWICK, HENRY. *The Methods of Ethics.* 7th ed. London: Macmillan & Co., 1907.

V
SITUATION ETHICS

This article offers a very brief account of situation ethics as a morality without rules and how it would apply to moral questions about biological and medical choices.

Situation (or "contextual") ethics is best classified as act-utilitarianism. Recent philosophical exponents include J. J. C. Smart in *Outline of a System of Utilitarian Ethics,* Kai Nielsen in *Ethics Without God,* E. F. Carritt in *A Theory of Morals,* and A. C. Garnett in *Ethics: A Critical Introduction.*

Act-utilitarians determine what is right by electing that course of action which offers the most beneficent consequences or greatest utility in each act, each particular situation. On the other hand, rule-utilitarians decide what is right by following preconceived rules (as advocated by R. B. Brandt, A. C. Ewing, Kurt Baier, and, in an earlier day, by Bishops Butler and Berkeley). It should be noted, however, that some rule-utilitarians adumbrate only the most general norms, such as "do good and avoid evil" and the Golden Rule, which are not rules of specified conduct. This was the case, for example, with Hastings Rashdall (*A Theory of Right and Wrong*) and Henry Sidgwick (*Methods of Ethics*).

Most religious ethicists elaborate a divine-command theory of morality, combined with a special or "general" revelation of the rules of God's imperative will. It should not be surprising, therefore, that situation ethics finds little favor in religious circles. Nevertheless, there are a few theological advocates in modern times, including Eberhard Griesbach, Paul Tillich, Dietrich Bonhoeffer, Joseph Fletcher, Paul Lehmann, J. A. T. Robinson, James Pike, and Helmut Thielecke.

Frankena ventured to call situation ethics "modified act agapism," because one exponent (the present writer) has chosen to set it within the framework of *agape*, the Greek word meaning "love" or concern for persons (Frankena, p. 3). By "modified" Frankena means (quite correctly) that although situationism is act rather than rule ethics it still has a place for rules of thumb, as long as they are not treated as always-obliging rules. Thus it is possible to say that ordinarily it is right to tell the truth, yet in some situations it would be wrong if telling the truth, on balance, had "unloving" (i.e., bad) consequences.

When norms are either universalized or absolutized they are perverted into what logicians call the material fallacy of faulty generalization. Cognitively, act ethicists take note of what is most frequently the right action in similar situations, as judged by the benefits gained, and this offers a meaningful rule of thumb. They might say, for instance, "We ought to get the patient's consent to do surgery, especially amputations," but this would be a guideline only—not a moral law or rule. If the patient lay in coma or was psychotic or a small child, they might act without consent.

Love being understood as good will or beneficence, the ethics of love is equivalent to utilitarian ethics. Philosophers commonly identify the two. Mill expounded this equivalence in his *Utilitarianism*: "To do as you would be done by, and to love your neighbour as yourself, constitute the ideal perfection of utilitarian morality" (p. 204). Fletcher has contended that love and justice are the same (1966, pp. 87–102). Mill showed that utility and justice are the same (pp. 226 ff.). In this way love and utility are commensurate. Utility, expressed in nonagapistic language, means the greatest possible preponderance of good over evil, calculated as to remote as well as immediate consequences; i.e., it aims at a net gain of *nonmoral* good. Human happiness is thus the ethical measure of right actions, not moralistic or legalistic rectitude. Agapistic modes of exposition, as in Christian ethics, are complementary but not necessary to situation ethics.

"Net gain" is a key concept here. Act ethics is relativistic; it appreciates the importance of coming to terms with the finite human condition—the need, that is, in all decision making to weigh and choose between competing values. Rarely if ever do we have a chance to select between purely good and evil alternatives. This "gray area" is an elementary parameter in ethical investigation.

Moral agents are in effect choosers in significant situations, trying to choose a course between conflicting values that yields a balance of benefit or, in a classical phrase, the "proportionate good" (Fletcher, 1970). This particular good is conceived qualitatively, not just quantitatively; some moral choices may favor the quality of a nonmoral good over its quantity; sometimes quantity can actually subvert quality—as in the case of resuscitating a patient whose cerebral function is lost irretrievably. So-called cost-benefit judgments are for this reason the main substance of moral decisions. This is the relativity of ethics.

The weight of tradition is on the side of making moral decisions or "forming conscience" according to rules. The conventional wisdom of the past, which is still at work in some parts of the world today, has just assumed that righteousness or rightness means being faithful to set norms. This is ethical legalism, basing good conduct on obedience to moral laws. Some of its exponents have actually held that many acts are morally wrong even though their consequences are good (Ramsey, p. 40).

Conventional rule ethics or legalism was sometimes linked with divine commands as an ultimate sanction for the rules. This is not, however, the case with rule-utilitarianism; its norms are formulated empirically and without dogmatic or revelational claims. We should all be prompt to acknowledge the great debt we owe to the idealism and ethical concern that have gone with the traditional morality, even though some hideous things were done in its name—and still are. Its defenders give ground reluctantly and painfully but meanwhile the maturing debate throws valuable light on the nature and function of ethics.

The deontological–teleological typology of ethical theories in the traditional literature is increasingly unacceptable. Conventional discourse in an earlier era understood "duty" (Greek *deontais*) as obedience to rules. But doing one's duty in some situations might require a moral agent to depart from rules sometimes, in order to realize the greatest good possible. In short, act ethics can be quite as dutiful, as responsive to obligation, as rule ethics. In act ethics one's duty is pragmatically to get the best possible results, and one's goal (*telos*) is to fulfill one's duty to realize beneficial results.

Thus duty means to do what is best in the

situation, which may mean either obeying or flouting any given rule. It is this flexibility that invites the rule-committed to charge act ethics with holding that "the end justifies the means." The only adequate retort is to bow to the charge, for nothing we do (no means) is morally justifiable except by the good end it seeks. (Random behavior is "meaningless.") Ethically, actions as such are not self-validating. What gives a "means" its *meaning* is the end to which it is directed. On this reasoning one could rightly engage in civil disobedience, could not be an absolute pacifist, might violate one or the other of the Ten Commandments, could fail to keep a promise or fulfill a contract, and so on.

Except for those who persist in thinking of duty as faithfully following rules, the traditional division between duty and goal ethics (deontology and teleology) is empty, because each kind of these systems presupposes the other. This makes it a distinction without a difference. All ethics of whatever kind predicates obligation or duty. The act–rule distinction, on the other hand, holds up much more adequately.

In sum, situation ethics is a utilitarian or consequentialist ethics, motivated by concern for human well-being, decisionally flexible in method, and guided in its judgments by the greatest good realizable rather than by adhering to prefabricated norms or moral rules.

How, then, does this mode of ethical analysis work out in bioethics, in biological and medical policy and decision making?

It should be obvious that situationists would not either approve or disapprove things like abortion or artificial insemination *in toto,* as a class or category of human acts. They would not deny patients their freedom to be choosers (to be moral agents) nor condemn them when they exercise it, although realistic counsel, including medical advice, might sometimes cut across a patient's wishes. Each case would be weighed on its own merits, clinically and consequentially. Situationists could not lay down such blanket opinions as "Sterilization is wrong." The closest they could come might be, "In this case sterilization would be wrong." Their judgments would hang on the foreseeable results medically, psychologically, and socially.

Some moralists believe that fetal life possesses human rights (e.g., a right to be born) but such a belief is not an ethical proposition; it is a religious teaching or metaphysical speculation with a moral entailment logically, viz., a taboo on abortion. No situationist could adopt universal negatives of this sort. (A few antiabortion moralists, however, have been consequential enough to use the principle of proportionate good to justify therapeutic abortion, to save patients' lives in certain kinds of cases—for example, tubal pregnancies and uterine cancers.)

Of the many ethical issues posed by the "life sciences" (bioethics) those having to do with life itself, as distinguished from health, are perhaps especially searching. Questions as to whether we may let a patient die in terminal illnesses without further medical intervention ("indirect euthanasia") and even "direct euthanasia" and suicide are appropriate to act ethics. Such solemn decisions might be made where the good to be gained outweighed counter considerations. Life itself in act ethics is a relative rather than absolute value—a value to be seen in relation to other values, at most only *primum inter pares* (first among equals)—and therefore it could be decided occasionally that the benefit balance appraisal favors termination. Situation ethics fits quality-of-life appraisals of human initiatives in death and dying, but not sanctity-of-life prohibitions (Fletcher, 1974, pp. 156–160).

This same situational decision making would be applied to fetal research and experimentation, *in utero* and *ex utero*. Even if it was believed that fetuses have human rights (which would be established by nonethical reasoning), it could still be decided that risk of damage or death in some circumstances is justified by proportionate good. Only if fetal life was declared categorically "untouchable" would fetal research be condemned. The same relativity applies to decisions about abortion and terminating defective newborns who are afflicted, for example, with a severe cerebrospinal defect (such as spina bifida with a myelomeningocele and hydrocephaly).

A wide spectrum of bioethical issues invites analysis. Transplant medicine poses some issues, as do proposals to devise chimeras (man–animal fusions) and cyborgs (man–machine prostheses)—each of which could have medical and social utility. Situation ethics asks what is beneficial rather than what is "natural" or any other criterion. In matters of experimentation, for example, any act ethicist would be open to the possibility of approval for such steps as fetal thymus for production of homologous antibodies (in cancer therapy or control of transplant rejection), or the maintenance of brain-dead cadavers as a source of rare hormones or viable organs for treatment of chronic diseases such as renal failure. But a case of *preponderant nonmoral benefit* would have to be made for each such procedure. Many other illustrative problems could be cited.

Physicians sometimes speak of situation ethics as "clinical" in the sense of looking at each case on its own merits. Through training and practice they are familiar with the importance of diagnosis and prognosis case by case. They know that the "laws" of medical science do not apply categorically to all patients with a given complaint; they are accustomed to judge what is best not so much by general principles as in their light. Being case-centered, they reject any notion that medicine should be practiced according to moral rules. Guidelines they welcome, yes, but not categorical moral rules.

Many emerging bioethical questions take shape in fields such as behavior and genetic control, but in all instances situation ethics would put aside moralistic–legalistic generalities and "class action" rules, asking instead the only serious ethical question, namely, "What is the best thing to do in *this* case, for this particular person or problem?" Bioethics directed to acts rather than rules makes good sense to biologists and physicians.

JOSEPH FLETCHER

[*While all the articles in this entry are relevant, see especially the articles* RULES AND PRINCIPLES, DEONTOLOGICAL THEORIES, TELEOLOGICAL THEORIES, *and* UTILITARIANISM. *For further discussion of topics mentioned in this article, see the entries:* ACTING AND REFRAINING; FREE WILL AND DETERMINISM; JUSTICE; LAW AND MORALITY; NATURAL LAW; OBLIGATION AND SUPEREROGATION; PRAGMATISM; *and* RIGHTS. *This article will find application in the entries* ABORTION; BIOETHICS; CARE; CIVIL DISOBEDIENCE IN HEALTH SERVICES; DECISION MAKING, MEDICAL; FETAL RESEARCH; HUMAN EXPERIMENTATION; LIFE; *and* TRUTH-TELLING.]

BIBLIOGRAPHY

COX, HARVEY. *The Situation Ethics Debate.* Philadelphia: Westminster Press, 1968.

FLETCHER, JOSEPH. *The Ethics of Genetic Control.* Garden City, N.Y.: Anchor Press, 1974.

———. *Situation Ethics.* Philadelphia: Westminster Press, 1966.

———. "Virtue Is a Predicate." *Monist* 54 (1970): 66–85.

FRANKENA, WILLIAM K. *Ethics.* 2d ed. Englewood Cliffs, N.J.: Prentice-Hall, 1973.

MILL, JOHN STUART. *Essential Works.* Edited by Max Lerner. New York: Bantam Books, 1961.

RAMSEY, PAUL. *Fabricated Man.* New Haven: Yale University Press, 1970.

VI
UTILITARIANISM

We have to distinguish between utilitarianism as (1) a *metaethical* view about the *meanings* of the moral words (e.g. that 'right' means 'utility-maximizing'), and (2) a *normative* view about what it is right to do (e.g. that it is always right to do what will maximize utility). Most of the famous utilitarians such as Bentham and J. S. Mill, though they did not always sufficiently distinguish the two questions, were more interested in the second. If interpreted in the first way, utilitarianism is a kind of Ethical Naturalism (provided that we make the somewhat questionable assumption that 'utility' itself is a descriptive, not a normative concept); if in the second, however, it may be embraced by thinkers holding widely differing views about the meanings of the moral words. G. E. Moore, the anti-naturalist, was a utilitarian of a sort, and it is also possible for an adherent of Non-Descriptivist Ethics to be a utilitarian.

As a theory about what it is right to do, utilitarianism is a type of *consequentialism*, holding that the morality of actions is to be judged by examining their consequences. But it is important to understand that the word "consequences" here is to be taken in a broader sense than usual: the consequences of an act, in this sense, include all the differences made to the history of the world by the fact that the act is performed. They thus include the performance itself of the act; any attempt to draw a line between the act and its consequences, and to say that in judging morally we have to pay attention to the act in itself and ignore the consequences, is bound to confuse the issue by taking "consequences" in a narrower sense than a careful consequentialist would. If I give a patient an overdose of some barbiturate, a strict division between act and consequences might lead us to say that my giving him the dose is the act, and his death the consequence. A careful consequentialist, however, would include both under "the consequences". If it be objected that this is a misuse of the word, the consequentialists do not need to wince, because it was their opponents who invented the term "consequentialist" and thus caused the confusion.

It should be noted that it is not possible to draw a line between act and consequences in such a way as to separate what is morally relevant from what is not. In the example just given it is relevant that the patient dies, which is a consequence, even in the narrowest sense, of the giving of the dose. The fact that we commonly say, not "He gave him the dose, with the consequence that he died", but "He killed him by giving him the dose", shows that what on one description appears as a consequence of an act can on another description appear as an act.

There are, however, two other distinctions which *are* morally relevant, and which are often confused with that between act and consequences. The first is between different sorts of consequences, in the wide sense. It is usually thought that certain sorts of consequences are morally relevant, others not. In the above example, some have held that to bring about the patient's death (a consequence of giving him the dose) was morally wrong, and a thing that ought not to have been done, but that a further consequence, that the patient suffered no more pain thereafter, ought not to be considered relevant when judging the morality of the act. Whether it ought can be debated; but it is confusing to represent the debate as one between consequentialists and anti-consequentialists, since for both parties it is the relevance or irrelevance of these respective *consequences* that is in question. In general, nearly everything that anti-consequentialists put in terms of a distinction between act and consequences can be put more clearly in terms of one between different consequences (in the wide sense) of an act.

The second morally relevant distinction is that between (1) the narrower class of consequences intentionally brought about and (2) the more comprehensive class (which includes [1]), of all the consequences which flow from an act, whether they are intended or not. It is usually held that, in judging the morality of the agent, it is the intended consequences of his act that have to be considered, and that unintended consequences do not justify blame. The fact that we blame people for the unintended consequences of their acts when they were negligent is no real exception to this rule: what is blameworthy is the omission to take care to inform themselves of the probable consequences. It is necessary also to distinguish between *direct intention*, of which desire that the intended thing should happen is a necessary condition, and *oblique intention*, where we directly intend A, and in pursuit of this intention knowingly cause B, obliquely intending it, though not desiring it. The surgeon who terminates a pregnancy may directly intend to save the mother's life but only obliquely intend the death of the fetus. Both kinds of intention are relevant to the morality of the agent, and discussions of the principle of double effect become clearer if the distinction is observed.

In this connection it is important to distinguish, also, between judgments about the moral rightness of the act and those about the moral worth of the agent. The use, in theological discussions about the morality of acts, of expressions such as "sinful" obscures this distinction. This word applies most naturally to the agent. If so applied, the agent's intentions and motives will be highly relevant; the same act done with one intention or one motive may justify the imputation of sin to the agent, but done with another, not. Theologians are commonly interested in what will happen on Judgment Day; and for deciding the final disposal of souls it is important to know what state they are in.

Utilitarianism, however, has seldom been advocated primarily as a way of judging agents. If it is so used, it will have to pay as much attention to motives and intentions as any other theory. Good motives and intentions will be benevolent ones, arising from the desire to do what is best for the people affected by our acts. As we shall see (and contrary to what many anti-utilitarians think) this may engender a respect (because of the good which comes therefrom) for the moral principles which anti-utilitarians too revere. But utilitarians have generally been less interested in the question "Will this act put me in the category of good or of sinful men?" than in the question "Ought I now to do this act? Would it be the right thing to do?" and they have said that we must answer this question by examining the consequences.

Here, however, the further difficulty arises that we can never know for sure what the consequences of an act will be. We have to rely on merely probable predictions even for those consequences which we have time to consider; and we never have time even to consider the great majority of the consequences, stretching out to the end of history. To meet this difficulty, we have to make another distinction, different from but related to one already made, namely between a *post eventum* judgment which might be made, say, by the Archangel Gabriel at the end of history, in possession of all the facts, and that made by an agent when he is wondering, in a state of fairly deep ignorance of the future, whether he ought to do a certain act. One of these judgments is made in full knowledge of the act's consequences; the other is made in ignorance of them, and often in circumstances in which it is only too easy, by self-deception, to conclude that the consequences of a certain act would be for the best for all those affected taken as a whole, when what really moves us (only we do not realize it) is that they would be for the best for *ourselves*, never mind about the others.

A utilitarian who does not allow for this source of error may find himself thinking, on what seem to him good utilitarian grounds, that he morally ought to do something, which in the event proves not to have been for the best; or a non-utilitarian may do the opposite, sticking to some well-established moral principle without calculating the consequences, and it may turn out to have been for the best. Thus a utilitarian may give a lethal dose to a suffering terminal patient, convinced that he is acting for the patient's and for everybody else's good, when really it is his own convenience that moves him; and a non-utilitarian may refrain from a similar act because he does not think that innocent life ought to be taken; and it may turn out that the patient, in what life remains to him, gets (say through the extra time that he has with his wife and children, to reconcile them all to the loss of parting) some good that outweighs the pain which he suffers, and which in any case can be controlled by careful medication. Anti-utilitarians have argued, on these grounds, that there are utilitarian reasons for not being a utilitarian; but this is too hasty. It follows only that utilitarian reasoning ought not to be too briskly applied, and that a more careful utilitarian, recognizing the pitfalls mentioned above, may think it safest, even on utilitarian grounds, to stick to a well-tried moral principle, as being most likely to be for the best.

This line of thought enables us to bypass the well-canvassed distinction between act- and rule-utilitarianism. Rule-utilitarianism, of which there are many varieties, was invented in order to defend utilitarianism against the objection that it leads to conclusions which to ordinary moral opinion seem outrageous. *Act-utilitarianism* is the view that it is individual acts which are to be judged according to their utility: i.e., the act which ought to be done is that which will yield the most utility (ignoring cases where there are two acts which tie for this prize). *Rule-utilitarianism* (in one of its forms) is the view that the act which ought to be done is that which is prescribed by the set of principles which has the highest acceptance-utility (i.e., whose general acceptance in society will yield more utility than the general acceptance of any other set). Since, it is assumed, the general acceptance of a set of moral principles which includes most of the well-established ones would have better con-

sequences than the acceptance of the principle that each individual act should be judged on grounds of its own utility without bringing in any other principles, this would be a way of giving a rule-utilitarian justification for conforming to the well-established principles, and thus reconciling utilitarianism (of this rule-utilitarian sort) with received opinion.

The maneuver depends on the assumption that the principles which are well-established in a given society are actually the ones with the highest acceptance-utility; otherwise dilemmas will arise with which there is no time to deal here. But the move to rule-utilitarianism is strictly speaking unnecessary. Given the uncertainties and pitfalls involved in moral decision, a careful *act*-utilitarian can argue, as G. E. Moore did, that the probability of acting for the best is maximized by sticking to the well-established principles (Moore, p. 162). Such a person will be both an act- and a rule-utilitarian, and the two positions will have coalesced. If, unlike Moore, we allow that there may be rare and unusual cases in which it is perfectly plain that it would be for the best to break one of these principles, and that in those cases we ought to do so, we can remain act-utilitarians for those cases, while agreeing that in the vast majority of cases it is rational, even for a consistent act-utilitarian, to stick to the rules.

The cleft between act- and rule-utilitarians can be made to seem wider by concentrating on unusual cases—which is why anti-utilitarians not only harp on them, but invent others more fantastic. Suppose, it is said, you were faced with a situation in which, by deliberately killing one innocent man, you could save many other innocent men from violent deaths at the hands of others: ought you not, as a utilitarian, to kill the one, and is not this at variance with received opinion? Such cases arose when the Nazis ordered the directors of mental institutions to kill off incurables, threatening, if not, to kill many more themselves. The utilitarian should reply that such unusual cases are a bad guide when selecting principles to regulate our lives in general. It is easy to cook up cases in which an act-utilitarian would have to say that some well-established principle ought to be departed from; and he should not be afraid to say this. But he should go on to say that in real as opposed to cooked-up cases there would nearly always be other considerations which would make it for the best to stick to the well-established principle (witness the actual history under the Nazis of the Bethel institution whose director, by a marvellously courageous stand on principle, coupled with brilliant diplomacy, got the authorities to change their policy).

Therefore, in selecting principles (necessarily fairly simple and general) to guide our lives by, to teach to our children, to encourage others to follow, etc., we ought to forget about these unusual cases and concentrate on those which are more likely to occur; for then we shall get a set of principles which will give the right answer in the great majority of cases. If we do get such a set of principles established in society, then we shall be not merely intellectually but emotionally committed to them; breaches of them by us will excite compunction; by others, indignation; and thus a particular morality will have got firmly and generally accepted in our society. The union of rule- with act-utilitarianism thus brought about will have engendered what has been called "motive-utilitarianism": the view that we ought to cultivate and be guided by those motives, traits of character, etc., whose general adoption would be for the best. Our moral intuitions will be in accord with these motives, and will prescribe acts which (given that the principles have been well chosen) are in nearly all cases the right ones. But intuitions are a reliable guide only when they have been schooled in accordance with a good set of moral principles; the intuitions of those who have had a poor moral education can be bad counselors (which is why intuitionism as a theory in moral epistemology has to be rejected).

There is also a theoretical reason why rule- and act-utilitarianism coalesce. To understand this, we have to distinguish between the expressions "general" and "universal" as applied to principles. "General" is the opposite of "specific": a principle has a high degree of generality if it places few and simple conditions on its own application. For example, the principle that the innocent ought never to be killed is more general than the principle that they ought not to be killed except when to kill them would save them from needless suffering, and then only at their own request. Both these principles are, however, equally universal, which means that neither contains a reference to individuals, but only to kinds of individuals. By contrast, the statement that *John* ought to be painlessly killed is not universal, because it contains a reference to the individual, John. It may be "universalizable", if its author is prepared to substitute for it the universal principle that in all cases of a certain sort

(perhaps minutely specified) patients in a certain condition (likewise minutely specified) ought to be painlessly killed. The doctrine of the universalizability of moral judgments holds that all moral judgments have to be so universalizable.

The rule-utilitarian has to choose whether the rules whose acceptance-utility he is to judge are allowed to be highly specific, or whether they must be of above some stated degree of generality. In either case, if they are moral principles, and if the thesis of universalizability is accepted, they will have to be universal. If he allows them to be highly specific, then his view collapses into act-utilitarianism; for if the moral judgments of an act-utilitarian are universalizable, he will be able to substitute for them universal principles (albeit highly specific ones) which give the reasons for the judgments. But in that case the rule-utilitarian, too, can adopt the same universal principles as his rules, which will then also be highly specific. If this can be done in all cases, the two positions become for practical purposes equivalent.

It has been objected to utilitarianism that there are cases where the breach of some well-established principle by one person will be for the best, provided that others observe it, because he will get some advantage, and not enough people will be breaking the principle to do any harm. Suppose that a few people can without detection, and with some financial advantage to themselves, break the laws about exhaust emissions from cars, and that the resulting air pollution is not sufficient to endanger public health. It is said that in such cases a utilitarian should prescribe the breaking of the principle that beneficial laws should be observed, and that this is contrary to received opinion. Rule-utilitarians try to meet this case by saying that although the *act* would be for the best, the *rule* forbidding such acts (i.e., the well-established principle that is being broken) has a high acceptance-utility; and that thus on their view the act would be wrong, because it would be a breach of a principle having a high acceptance-utility. But to this it is objected that there is a principle with an even higher acceptance-utility, namely, the more specific principle that one should observe the general well-established principle except in cases where it is clear that everyone else will observe it, but that then one should break it (Lyons, ch. 3).

Such a move puts the rule-utilitarian and the act-utilitarian (whose views have again coalesced) back at variance with received opinion. But they can escape the ill consequences of this (1) by pointing out that cases in which one can know that all the others are going to observe the principle are very rare; and that (for reasons given above) one should not base one's selection of moral principles on such rare cases, and received opinion has not: it is therefore easy to explain why received opinion condemns the act, and why it is (in general) right to do so. (2) They can point out, also, that there is a hidden disutility involved, namely the fact that all the others are having something done to them (namely, to be taken advantage of) which they do not want to have done to them. They do not know that it is being done; but it is a disutility to me to have things done to me that I very much want not to be done, even if I do not know about it (suppose, for example, that my wife's analyst uses his position in order to seduce her without my discovering). This hidden disutility to so many others might outweigh the advantage gained by the offender.

There has not been space to deal with these difficulties adequately, nor to list all the distinctions between types of utilitarianism, nor all the objections that have been made to them; those that seem the most important have been selected. Four more difficulties should be mentioned briefly. First, utilitarian calculations involve judgments comparing the utility accruing to one person with that accruing to another; this presents theoretical difficulties, although we all do it in practice.

Secondly, in the important issue of population policy, and in other issues (e.g., abortion, contraception) where what is in question is the morality of bringing or not bringing a person into existence, a distinction has to be made between classical or total utilitarianism and average utilitarianism. According to *total utilitarianism*, the utility which has to be maximized is the total utility accruing to all existing beings: this would be increased by the addition of an extra member to the population, if the positive utility accruing to him, however small, was greater than that lost by the others owing to his advent. This view, therefore, requires a more liberal population policy than *average utilitarianism*, which requires us to maximize average utility; on this view, we are not required to increase the population beyond the point at which the average utility accruing to existing beings begins to fall.

Thirdly, it has been debated whether the beings whose utility is to be considered include all beings, including dumb animals, which are capable of suffering and enjoyment, or only humans; Jeremy Bentham took the former view, which seems most defensible.

Fourthly, the merits of *positive utilitarianism* and its rival *negative utilitarianism* have been canvassed. The first, in its calculation of utilities, reckons both benefits and harms and balances them against each other; the second reckons only harms. Since the deprivation of a benefit is a harm, it is difficult to sustain the distinction.

Lastly, it has often been disputed what is meant by "utility", and by such phrases as "for the best" which have been used above. Answers put in terms of pleasure and the absence of pain, as given by Bentham and Mill, are now generally thought to be too restrictive. The easiest short answer is to say that that act is for the best which is in the greatest interest of those affected, taken in sum; and that what is in a person's greatest interest (what maximizes *his* utility) is what he would choose to happen if he were fully informed and completely prudent. Morality, then, on the utilitarian view, emerges as a kind of universalized prudence (utilitarians should not be accused, as they sometimes are, of equating it with *selfish* prudence or expediency). We are to give as much weight to the interests of all as the prudent man gives to his own. The affinity between this maxim and the Christian Golden Rule is obvious.

R. M. Hare

[*For the background and varieties of utilitarianism, see the fourth article in this entry,* TELEOLOGICAL THEORIES. *On act-utilitarianism and the use of rules, see the articles above on* RULES AND PRINCIPLES *and* SITUATION ETHICS. *On the universalizability of moral judgments, see the tenth article in this entry,* NON-DESCRIPTIVISM. *For an extensive discussion of G. E. Moore, see the ninth article in this entry,* NATURALISM. *For discussion of related ideas, see the entries:* ANIMAL EXPERIMENTATION, *article on* PHILOSOPHICAL PERSPECTIVES; DOUBLE EFFECT; *and* RISK.]

BIBLIOGRAPHY

BAYLES, MICHAEL D., ed. *Contemporary Utilitarianism.* Garden City, N.Y.: Doubleday & Co., Anchor Books, 1968. Bibliography.

DIGGS, B. J. "Rules and Utilitarianism." *American Philosophical Quarterly* 1 (1964): 32–44.

HARE, R. M. "Medical Ethics: Can the Moral Philosopher Help?" *Philosophical Medical Ethics: Its Nature and*

Significance: Proceedings of the Third Trans-disciplinary Symposium on Philosophy and Medicine, Held at Farmington, Connecticut, December 11–13, 1975. Edited by Stuart F. Spicker and H. Tristram Engelhardt, Jr. Philosophy and Medicine, vol. 3. Edited by H. Tristram Engelhardt, Jr. and Stuart F. Spicker. Boston: D. Reidel Publishing Co., 1977, pp. 49–61.

HASLETT, D. W. *Moral Rightness.* The Hague: Martinus Nijhoff, 1974.

LYONS, DAVID. *Forms and Limits of Utilitarianism.* Oxford: Clarendon Press, 1965. Bibliography.

MOORE, G. E. *Principia Ethica.* Cambridge: At the University Press, 1903. Especially chapter 5.

QUINTON, ANTHONY. *Utilitarian Ethics.* New Studies in Ethics. Edited by W. D. Hudson. London: Macmillan & Co., New York: St. Martin's Press, 1973. Bibliography.

RESCHER, NICHOLAS. *Distributive Justice: A Constructive Critique of the Utilitarian Theory of Distribution.* Indianapolis: Bobbs-Merrill, 1966. Bibliography.

SMART, J. J. C., and WILLIAMS, B. A. O. *Utilitarianism: For and Against.* Cambridge: At the University Press, 1973. Bibliography.

VII

THEOLOGICAL ETHICS

Meaning of theological ethics

The term "theological ethics" (or "moral theology") in its inclusive sense is employed to designate the activity of critical reflection about the bearing of beliefs in God or gods on the understanding of the moral life. As such, it embraces, at least in principle, analysis of the moralities of Christianity, Islam, Buddhism, Hinduism, Judaism, and other religions, including what are sometimes called "primitive religions." In its restricted sense, however, theological ethics refers to discourse about a particular theistic morality embraced by the writer or by a significant part of the society to which the writer belongs. Thus in European-American society the most common expressions of theological ethics are Christian and/or Jewish.

This understanding of theological ethics may be employed even when the meaning of religion is extended to include such belief systems as Marxism and secular humanism, as has recently become fashionable in some circles. If such belief systems are to be considered "theologies" by virtue of their exhibiting the phenomena of faith (that is, trust and commitment) in valued objects or states of affairs (that is, "gods"), then theological ethics may also take the form either of examining the general bearing of such faiths on morality or of analyzing the particular relation of, for example, secular humanism to morality. Nevertheless, such an extension of the meaning of religion is both problematic and marginal to the enterprise of theological ethics as ordinarily conducted. Therefore, and because of limits of space, no further reference will be made to it in this article.

Three types of normative judgments are basic to theological ethics: judgments of obligation, virtue, and value. Judgments of obligation (or duty) respond to the question, "What morally ought to be done?" Thus a particular action, norm, or policy may be probed as to whether it is morally right, wrong, or permissible, such as whether a physician ought to lie to, or withhold information from, a dying patient, or what kind of policy a hospital morally ought to have in such matters. Judgments of virtue (or moral character) respond to the question, "What qualities or dispositions of a person, for which the person can be said to be accountable, are commendable or reprehensible?" Thus a physician may be considered worthy of praise for conscientiousness or of blame for uncharitableness, and a patient worthy of praise for courage or of blame for incivility. Judgments of value respond to the question, "What objects or states of affairs are good or bad?" or "In what sense and to what degree are particular objects or states of affairs good or bad?" Thus the health of a patient may be judged to be a good in itself, a particular national health program to be not as good as another, and the use of intensive care units to be bad as a means to accomplish certain ends. It is noteworthy that in medical and public policy circles these three types of ethical judgments (obligation, virtue, and value) are occasionally collapsed into one category and simply called "values" or "value judgments," with a resulting tendency to confusion in the identification and assessment of specific moral problems.

Theological ethics shares these three types of normative judgment with philosophical ethics (or moral philosophy). What distinguishes the two enterprises from each other, therefore, is not a difference about the need to employ judgments of obligation, virtue, and value, but rather the orientation that is brought to their employment. Philosophical ethics may, but need not, assess the bearing of theistic beliefs and attitudes on the moral life, and to a very considerable degree proceeds today without doing so in European-American society. It more characteristically finds its orientation, to the extent it acknowledges a need to set forth its general bearings or background beliefs, in secular views of human nature, human worth, or human good, sometimes accompanied by logical, epistemological, and/or cosmological doctrines. Theological ethics, on the other hand, is committed by its very nature to the examination of the moral life from the viewpoint of theistic beliefs and attitudes. It characteristically seeks its orientation in inquiries about the appropriate human response to whatever is held to be God's nature, will, or activity, and examines and advocates theories of obligation, virtue, and value associated with that response.

Sharing the same type of orientation with theological ethics are everyday religious moralities of one sort or another. Such moralities involve beliefs and attitudes about God or gods, and their judgments about obligation, virtue, and value are related in some manner to their theistic beliefs and attitudes. How then are they to be distinguished from theological ethics? The answer is that such moralities are a kind of routine practice that can be participated in with only a minimum of theoretical reflection and criticism, while theological ethics is essentially a theoretical activity. It is a highly developed science that examines theistic orientations, the moralities that are associated with such orientations, and the relations between theistic orientation and morality. This is not to say that two mutually exclusive sets of persons are implied by the distinction, those who practice a religious morality and those who engage in theological ethics. This is no more true than to say that the set of persons who engage in health-enhancing actions and the set of persons who are medical scientists are mutually exclusive. Most (but not all) theological ethicists are participants in one or another religious community, adhering to many (if not all) of its tenets on morality. On the other hand, the overwhelming majority of participants in religious moralities are not also involved in theological ethics, properly speaking.

Theistic orientation

A theistic orientation is one that contains two specifiable characteristics. First, there is a belief in one or more religious objects (that is, God or gods). These objects (or states of affairs) can take various forms in different belief systems, but common to all belief systems of this kind is the understanding that such objects transcend ordinary human experience of the sort natural science can describe (actually or potentially), and that the nature and/or activity of such objects is of very considerable, if not overriding,

importance to human experience. A plurality of such objects in a belief system is an indication of polytheism. A single such object that is also held to be relevant to the experience of all persons and groups of persons points to monotheism. And a single such object whose relevance is affirmed only to a particular group of persons suggests henotheism (Niebuhr, pp. 24–31). The principal focus of this article will be on monotheism, the belief in one such object that is ordinarily referred to as God and considered to be universally relevant.

The second characteristic of a theistic orientation is the response that human beings are called upon to make to God. This response, or attitude of the believer, is dependent for its appropriateness upon how God is conceived. Emphasis may be placed on his being holy, gracious, powerful, loving, compassionate, just, fearsome, merciful, forgiving, etc.; his bringing persons out of bondage, revealing his will through a prophet, suffering for his people, etc.; his ordaining of general norms or duties that human beings should follow, establishing a way of life that if pursued will lead eventually to happiness, etc. Among the types of human response that may be considered appropriate to the believer are penitence, sorrow, joy, trust, hope, commitment, imitation, submission, acceptance of a new relationship, undertaking a pilgrimage, obedience to his law, or embarking on a way of life in pursuit of human excellence (Little and Twiss, p. 61).

There is obviously a wide variety of theistic orientations, not only among the different religions of the world, but even to a considerable degree within the same religion. The effect of this rich plurality of orientations is to make theological ethics, at least in its inclusive sense, a highly complex enterprise. For it must examine and clarify the bearing not only of one but of many theistic orientations on the moral notions of obligation, virtue, and value. This task is made even more intricate by the recognition that these moral notions are themselves subject to varying interpretations.

In order to reduce the variables in this article, most of the theistic orientations will be viewed as sundry expressions of one or more of the three basic orientations, and the remainder left to other writings for those readers wishing to pursue them. It is sufficient here to acknowledge that the three basic orientations do not exhaust the full range of possibilities. The first of these basic types of theistic orientation (TO_1) holds that God is the author of a universal ordering which has always been normative for human persons everywhere. Furthermore, the appropriate response to God is to perceive this normative ordering, by reason and/or by revelation, and freely to abide by it. To do so ordinarily implies the acceptance of a way of life that progressively leads to the fulfillment and happiness of the wayfarers. An example of TO_1 is the traditional Catholic teaching on natural law, in which God is perceived to have created human beings with certain ends discoverable by reason. The pursuit of these ends progressively leads, when aided by grace, to human excellence coupled with supreme happiness in fellowship with God (Thomas Aquinas I-II, 1–5; 94). Another example is the Hindu doctrine of karma, in which a person is and gets today what he deserves from his past. Moreover, he becomes and receives in the future what is fitting to his thoughts, attitudes, and actions today (Sarma, pp. 53–59).

The second type of theistic orientation (TO_2) assumes that God has intervened in history to establish a new relationship with humanity, and that a certain event associated with that intervention becomes revelatory or illuminative for the interpretation of other events in history. The appropriate response of one who is a believer is to make this event central to the understanding of one's own existence, assigning meaning to one's life in accord with the accepted meaning of the event and taking upon oneself the commitments associated with the event. Sometimes the event is seen not so much as establishing an entirely new divine–human relationship, but as renewing a relationship that has always existed though (because of human sin or finitude) has not previously been sufficiently perceived or honored. An example of TO_2 is the Exodus experience of Judaism in which God is understood to have delivered his people out of bondage in Egypt and to have established a covenant with them, specifying the kind of monotheism they are to embrace and the duties they are to perform. The appropriate Jewish response today to this event is to acknowledge it as constitutive of one's own history and to conduct one's life in keeping with the divine–human covenant that is understood to have come about through it (Kadushin, pp. 93–95; Hillers, pp. 46–71). Another example is the event in which God is understood by Muslims to have revealed his will to his prophet Muhammad, as is recorded in the Koran. The appropriate response of the believer is to submit to this will, and in so doing diligently to fulfill the five specified duties of profession of faith, prayer facing Mecca five times daily, almsgiving, fasting in the Arabic month of Ramadan, and pilgrimage to Mecca once in a lifetime (Donaldson, pp. 40, 111).

Theistic orientation of the third type (TO_3) places emphasis on characteristic attributes or qualities of God rather than on a normative order he has established in the world (TO_1) or an intervention he has made into history (TO_2). In some instances these attributes are to be imitated, as when believers affirm that they ought to be loving because God is loving. In other instances the response is not imitation (which may be held to be presumptuous), but the expression of attitudes or emotions that are considered fitting responses to a designated quality of God, as when believers respond with an overwhelming sense of awe to God's majesty and holiness. The ascetic response to Allah's (God's) mercy and providence in Sufism (a Muslim mystical religion) and the Christian response of faith, hope, and love to God's grace are further examples of TO_3 (Donaldson, pp. 194–212; Augustine, pp. 36–38, 132, 135–136). However, Gods' grace in the Christian religion can also be understood as decisively expressed in a particular event such as the life and death of Jesus, in which case the orientation may actually be a combination of TO_2 and TO_3. And when al-Ghazzālī reasserted in Sufi mysticism a strong belief in special revelation by Allah to Muhammad, a similar combination resulted (Ghazzālī, pp. 54–68).

Relation of theistic orientations to moral notions

How do theistic orientations bear on moral notions of obligation, virtue, and value? Most simple answers to this question are quite misleading, such as claims that morality generally depends on religion or, alternatively, has no important connection with it. Actually, a number of possible relations between theistic orientation and moral notions do exist and need to be considered, as recent writers on theological ethics have pointed out (Frankena, pp. 295–296; Graber, p. 54). Among these relations, the chief ones seem to be (1) historical, (2) logical, (3) psychological, (4) epistemological, (5) linguistic, and (6) ontological.

Historical relation. A historical relation is one pointing to the genesis of a moral notion in a particular orientation, as for example agapic love had its origin (or at least played its first major role) in early Christian religion from which it later achieved prominence in Western moral consciousness. However, to identify a moral notion with a particular orientation as its historical source is not to claim that without this orientation the notion would not have developed elsewhere, or that having developed historically in one orientation it cannot be adopted into another one (either religious or secular). Sometimes theistic orientations are recipients, not just generators, of moral notions. For example, the notions of generosity and vengeance in the Koran may have got there in part because of the influence of pre-Islamic nomadic morality on Muhammad. And some Aristotelian and Stoic virtues were adopted by the early Christian community, although considerably transformed by their function in that new orientation.

Logical relation. A logical relation pertains (1) to the explication of moral judgments entailed by theistic (and other) orientations. Thus Jewish belief and worship lead implicitly to the moral obligation to seek justice for those who are deprived of it. And Protestant claims about the acceptance of the grace of God through faith entail claims about love and service to the neighbor. A logical relation may also pertain (2) to the justification of moral judgments by theistic (and other) orientations, a role that historical relations, however important, cannot perform. Such justification can aim at showing that a certain theistic orientation is necessary (whether sufficient or not) to establish that one or more moral judgments are valid. For example, it may be suggested that only if there is a God who has commanded that we provide medical care for the indigent are we morally obligated to do so. If successful, this procedure would make at least one judgment in morality logically dependent on religion, and the idea of a secular morality that is fully autonomous would be, to this extent, invalid (or at least in need of qualification). On the other hand, justification may take the form of showing that a certain theistic orientation is sufficient (although not necessary) to establish the validity of a moral judgment. For example, it may be claimed that if there is a God who has commanded that we provide medical care for the indigent we are morally obligated to do so. But this procedure, if successful, would leave open the possibility that the justification for this moral judgment may also be provided by appeal to some other consideration, and to this extent a secular (or other theistic) orientation fully autonomous from this one would be possible. For the most part, justification in theological ethics in the modern world has concentrated on those

logical relations between theism and morality that involve judgments of their sufficiency and not of their necessity, although passages in some important writings do point more in the direction of logically necessary relations (Barth, 1957, pp. 540–542).

Psychological relation. A psychological relation centers on the motivation that theistic orientation may provide for doing one's duty, for improving one's character, or for developing one's values in a more worthwhile direction. For example, there is obviously a significant incentive for right moral action for those who accept the Hindu doctrine of karma, since one's status in one's next existence is understood to be determined largely by one's moral performance and development in this existence. And the Christian notion that Christ died for the world has provided some persons with a strong motivation to open their lives to philanthropic service of others. The psychological function of theistic orientation, however, cannot also provide justification for particular judgments of morality. Nevertheless, it has often been sufficiently impressive in advancing the level of adherence to morality that some nontheistic philosophers (such as John Stuart Mill) have pondered at length the nature and possibility of a secular alternative to the motivational function of theism in improving moral performance.

Epistemological relation. An epistemological relation pertains to claims of knowledge that theistic orientation is held to contribute to morality. Appeals to this kind of relation generally take the form that there are basic truths of morality not generally (or sufficiently) known except through theistic orientation. An example is the claim that only if one truly loves God does one know what it really means to love one's fellow human beings, a claim made by a number of major religions. Another example is the position of early Calvinism that human sinfulness has so weakened the natural human knowledge of morality that there is need through theistic orientation to accept an extraordinary republication of basic morality, such as the Ten Commandments. Still again, it may be claimed that while some people may have a natural knowledge of morality, others (usually less informed) need the special help that theistic orientation provides. Or it may be believed that while all persons have a rational knowledge of basic duties of morality, none has knowledge of morality's higher duties (such as those practiced by the saint or hero—consider orders of nuns devoted to the medical care of the indigent) except by means of some theistic orientation, a belief that was widely current in medieval Catholicism. Finally, it should be acknowledged that the flow of ideas in the epistemological relation may also move in the opposite direction, such as when it is claimed that the knowledge or practice of morality contributes in some important manner to our knowledge of God.

Linguistic relation. The linguistic relation between theistic orientation and morality usually takes the form of asserting that the meaning of some (or all) moral terms requires appeal to religious terms. Of course, this can be declared true by definition or stipulation, as when all moral terms are held to be religious terms in some quite extended sense of religion. But this is not what advocates of the linguistic relation usually have in mind. Rather they argue for such a position as "good" means "valued by God," or "right" means "ordained by God." The linguistic relation may also take the form of affirming that understanding the meaning of God makes reference to moral terms necessary. It may be held, for example, both that one does not know the meaning of the term "God" except by relating it to the terms "good" and "just," and that "good" and "just" are moral terms.

Ontological relation. The last of these relations between theistic orientation and morality is ontological. Simply put, this holds that the existence of moral obligations, virtues, and values (or some part of them) is vitally connected with the existence or sustaining activity of God. This may take the form of saying that, since everything existing depends on the existence of God, morality could not exist without God. The thrust of this relation may also move in the opposite direction, such as when it is claimed that God's existence is enhanced by the moral lives of his human creatures, a claim especially espoused in the ethics of process theology.

All three types of theistic orientation (TO_1, TO_2, and TO_3) have employed in one or another of their expressions each of these six kinds of relations to morality. Nevertheless, some theistic orientations tend to stress certain relations with morality. Thus when God is conceived as the author of a universal ordering (TO_1), the ontological, psychological, and linguistic relations seem to be especially prevalent. When God is understood to have intervened in history through one or more decisive events (TO_2), historical, epistemological, logical, and psychological rela-

tions are often prominent. And when God is perceived as possessing attributes that appropriately lead to certain human responses (TO_3), logical, linguistic, and psychological relations to morality come to be emphasized.

Moral notions

The notion of obligation has played a more important role in theological ethics in the twentieth century, especially in Western Christianity and Judaism, than have the notions of virtue and value. This also seems to be true of the applied field of bioethics. For here such moral problems as those associated with death and dying, experiments on human persons, and distribution of health care have been formulated more often in terms of what morally ought to be done rather than what human characteristics are morally commendable or what states of affairs are morally to be preferred to others. Nevertheless, in theological ethics an increasing interest in considerations of virtue is now becoming evident (Hauerwas, pp. 48–89; Carney, "Virtue–Obligation"). Whether the notion of virtue will also come to play a larger role in the applied field of bioethics or not will have to await further developments.

Obligation theory. Within obligation theory a controversy about the role of moral rules in religious morality—sometimes called the "rule-situation" debate, at other times the dispute over "situation ethics"—has been especially prominent in recent years. To understand the issue at stake it is necessary to distinguish between two types of moral norms. First, there are those norms that are of very wide generality and do not specify some particular action that is required, forbidden, or permitted. Examples are that "we should love our fellow human beings" and that "we should obey the will of God." Norms of this sort will here be called "principles," although this term bears a different connotation in some other writings. It is distinctive of principles that actions on the basis thereof may be enormously diverse, since no concrete action pattern is included in the statement of these norms. Second, there are norms that do specify some particular action, such as "we should refrain from telling lies to patients" and "we should not use persons in experiments without their consent." Such norms will here be called "rules," although the meaning of this term also varies in some other writings. It is distinctive of rules that actions on the basis thereof center on some concrete action pattern (such as lying, or consent in experimentation), although it is not always clear how to relate such a pattern to a specific situation.

Both situationalists and nonsituationalists agree on the need for ethical principles in moral action. But situationalists hold that rules are advisory and not obligatory for human action, since they are only recommendations that arise out of accumulated human experience. The correct moral procedure is to apply the cherished principle (or principles) directly to the situation encountered and, after perhaps considering the counsel given by relevant rules, to do whatever seems indicated by the principle in the situation, whether or not this conforms with what such rules advise (e.g., is informing a particular dying patient of his situation the most loving thing to do in that situation?). Nonsituationalists, on the other hand, hold that moral rules, if valid, do have a binding force in what they require, prohibit, or permit, and that there are some moral rules which are valid. Decisions about validity come about by inquiring whether a rule under review is the best action-pattern expression of the cherished principle (or principles) for a given class of situations (e.g., would informing the dying of their state be the rule most in keeping with love?). Thus the correct moral procedure for nonsituationalists is to accept valid moral rules as obligatory for the classes of situations for which they are intended, and to review from time to time the validity of the moral rules they follow, especially when events or persons raise challenges about them.

The rule–situation controversy would be misleadingly characterized by claiming that one side in the dispute is not interested in obligatory norms and the other not interested in actual situations. For situationalists do hold to obligatory norms, although only principles and not rules. And nonsituationalists do address themselves to actual situations, both in applying rules and in validating them.

Among situationalists there are differences about the nature of the appropriate principle. Some hold that love is the highest principle or criterion of human action, e.g., Joseph Fletcher, others that the command of God is, e.g., Karl Barth. Among the former the criterion is often interchangeably expressed either as doing for the neighbor what love requires or as promoting the good of the neighbor. In either case the procedure is a teleological one requiring a full-fledged value theory about what is truly good or

loving. Unfortunately such a theory is seldom supplied. Situationalists of the other sort employ a deontological procedure in their obligation theory by emphasizing a formal characteristic of human action (i.e., conformity with God's command) rather than the good to be promoted by human action. This kind of situationalism requires an epistemological theory that clarifies how we are to know God's particular commands, which involves an elaborate doctrine of revelation that is difficult to provide. Of course, one can combine these two types of situationalism in various ways. For example, one can claim that our ultimate principle is to love our neighbor or to promote his good, but the best way of doing this is simply to follow God's commands. Or it can be claimed that the ultimate principle is to obey God's commands and that what he repeatedly commands is that we love our neighbor or promote his good.

Among nonsituationalists there are also both teleologists and deontologists, but of course they also (unlike situationalists) employ obligatory rules as expressions of principles in specified classes of situations. In addition, another kind of difference can be observed among them regarding exceptions or qualifications to moral rules. Augustine of Hippo, for example, held that it is always wrong to tell a lie, whatever the circumstances or consequences thereof, even though the blameworthiness of some lies (e.g., benevolent ones) is not as great as others (e.g., malevolent ones). Thus for him and others who have followed in his footsteps there are no exceptions or qualifications to valid moral rules. Muhammad, on the other hand, claimed that one should refrain from telling lies when one is not involved in any of three types of circumstances, namely, in war, in love, and in attempting to reconcile friends who have become alienated. There are two ways of conceiving of such limits to a rule about lies or other practices in religious ethics, and both have been employed at one time or another by theological ethicists. On the one hand, one can say that there are exceptional circumstances or consequences that make the breaking of a rule morally permissible. On the other hand, it can be claimed that a valid rule contains certain qualifying conditions that, if present in a particular situation, make the rule inapplicable, and thus not to follow it is not to break it. Presumably the latter procedure was the recourse of Muhammad. It is also the recourse most often employed today in life-and-death matters by nonsituationalists in theological ethics who believe, as almost all do, that there are some limited circumstances in which it is morally right to let someone die.

Another issue in the obligation theory of theological ethics is whether there are two levels of duty in religious morality, one level that pertains to all persons and another level that is proper only to some. It is said that some obligations are such that it is justifiable to impose them on everyone whether or not they give their consent, such as telling the truth, keeping promises, and refraining from unprovoked assaults on human persons. Special obligations associated with different occupational roles are also usually included as first-level duties (e.g., the duty of physicians not to abandon patients in their care). On the other hand, it is said that there are some obligations that should not be imposed upon persons without their consent but may be freely adopted by those who covenant themselves to a religious–moral way of life requiring them. Such obligations may include assuming accountability for an act one could not have avoided, accepting responsibility for an act of someone else, and engaging under special circumstances in inordinate self-sacrifice (Carney, "Accountability," pp. 320–327). The performance of such "second-mile duties" is most often referred to as works of supererogation. Sometimes, however, they are called the deeds of "saints and heroes" and are considered to be motivated by personal and group "ideals" (in which case they are often treated more as expressions of virtue than as second-level obligations). They have been especially prominent throughout the history of Roman Catholic ethics but are receiving increased attention in Protestant and philosophical circles.

Nevertheless, there is controversy over the moral validity of dividing duties into first-level and second-level ones. For some theologians, such as Luther, see the employment of this distinction as a means by which some persons avoid the full demands of faith in God and others pervert their works of supererogation into vain claims to moral superiority over their fellow human beings. However one assesses the religious and ethical aspects of this controversy, it seems undeniable that the theory and practice of second-level duties have had a profound influence in history on the establishment of health-care facilities and the enlistment of health-care personnel.

Virtue theory. The moral notion of virtue performs two fundamental functions in theological ethics. First, it indicates the kind of person who is to be rightly considered good, just, faithful, loving, holy, and so forth. As such, it provides both a normative complement to a merely descriptive account of human nature and an ideal of human personhood at which to aim. Second, the notion of virtue offers an alternative to notions of obligation for the discernment of the morality of human acts. It does this not by asking what is required by some principle or rule of obligation, but by inquiring what characteristics or qualities (such as faithfulness, fairness, a loving disposition, and so forth) constitute the goodness of a person, and by designating those acts to be good (or bad) to the extent that they are appropriate to the model of a good (or bad) person.

In addition, the notion of virtue may also perform an important derivative function to that of obligation. This may occur in the following manner. If we first know what acts are right or wrong by appeal to one or another principle or rule of obligation, we may be concerned to develop the personal dispositions or traits of character that provide habituation and motivation to perform or resist those acts. In this derivative employment of virtue theory, we try to develop those virtues that support the general types of obligations we already acknowledge (but perhaps do not always fulfill because of moral weaknesses), and those virtues in turn enable us "to put our hearts into our duties," thus increasing the probability that our performance will more closely approximate our profession.

There are two general theories in religious ethics as to how one becomes virtuous or develops a good character. The first is said (somewhat incorrectly) to derive from the influence of Aristotle on Christianity and Islam, and (more correctly) to be exemplified in much of the medieval literature on cases of conscience. This is the theory that a person becomes good by doing good acts, much as surgeons become better surgeons by regular practice. It may be called the "acquiremental theory," inasmuch as it is largely achieved by the repetition of human acts. But it was vigorously repudiated by the Protestant Reformation, because it was believed to lead to a works-righteousness rather than, as Luther and Calvin advocated, a faith-righteousness. They in turn (drawing upon Augustine and others) set forth, as an alternative theory about how one becomes good, the acceptance in the depths of one's heart of the forgiveness and reconciliation offered by God. It was anticipated that this acceptance would lead to new dispositions toward God (trust) and the neighbor (love), much as a physician or patient might be judged to be a different (and better) person following changed dispositions toward those persons with whom he or she is involved. Since this manner of becoming virtuous or righteous focuses on the development of changed attitudinal relations to God and neighbor, it may be called the "relational theory." The dispute over the alternative theories has occasionally flared up with some intensity, although a few theologians, such as Thomas Aquinas and Jonathan Edwards, can be read as advocating a combination of them as closer to the truth (Thomas Aquinas I-II, 58–63; Edwards, pp. 1–41).

One of the topics in theological ethics that appears in both virtue and obligation conceptualities is that of moral default. When considering such default as an obligation notion, the basic category is one of guilt. The offender is considered by himself or others to have engaged in a violation of an important norm and feels (or should feel) guilty for doing so. On the other hand, the acknowledgement of serious default as a virtue consideration ordinarily takes the form of shame. One is judged by himself or others not so much as being in violation of something, but as having fallen short of some ideal and as needing to overcome his humiliation or to "find cover" for some nakedness of his moral personhood. It is of some note that in many religions the concept of sin is related to both guilt and shame. If one is guilty, the violation must be forgiven; if one is ashamed, the person must be restored. Next to the awakening and nurturing of a sense of the holy in human experience, perhaps nothing is as important for religion as its therapies for overcoming guilt and shame.

Another topic common to both virtue and obligation frameworks in theological ethics is that of rewards and punishments. There would seem to be three answers religion has provided to the problem of relating human character and action to good fortune and bad. The first is that persons actually do get what they deserve, if not in this life then in a later life. This answer is especially central in the Hindu doctrine of karma, in early Islam, and in some expressions of Christianity. The second answer is that the doctrine of rewards and punishments is not so much a description of what people actually do receive in relation to the moral quality and actions of their lives as what they deserve to receive. This is to say, rewards and punishments are symbols, not real states of affairs, that bear testimony to the

worthiness or unworthiness of persons. This notion is more commonly found in abstract systems of theological ethics than in everyday religious moralities. The third answer is that rewards and punishments are not extrinsic states of affairs in persons' lives (now or hereafter), but intrinsic conditions of their characters. According to this doctrine, persons become what they truly worship, honor, and do. It is noteworthy that the first answer (i.e., that persons actually get what they deserve) can function within a pure obligation framework, but that the second answer (i.e., rewards and punishments are simply symbols of worthiness or unworthiness) and the third (i.e., rewards and punishments are intrinsic to one's character) require either a pure virtue framework or an obligation framework that is combined with a virtue one.

Natural law theory has also played a major role in some expressions of theological ethics. This too can be interpreted with primary emphasis either on obligation notions or virtue ones. Most commonly it has been given an obligation focus. Those who employ it in this manner seek an understanding of what constitutes the fullness or perfection of the functioning of human nature in order to discover and declare obligatory those norms of human action that seem most commensurate to human nature so conceived. When this endeavor presupposes that the ordering of human life is part of an ordering by God of his entire creation, and allows its determinations to be guided in part by this presupposition, then the natural law doctrine is a part of theological ethics. Natural law with an obligation focus has also been of interest to some secular thinkers, though of course with little or no theistic orientation to their inquiries and advocacies. On the other hand, there are theists (and nontheists) who have placed the emphasis in natural law doctrine on virtue considerations. They do this by focusing on the normative nature of human persons, and simply set forth an understanding of traits of character and actions appropriate thereto. They are less interested in the law of human nature as something external and obligatory to human nature (though derived therefrom) than they are in human nature itself and its appropriate functioning.

Value theory. The notion of value in theological ethics focuses on the question of what things or states of affairs are worth pursuing in life, or what things or states of affairs are more worth pursuing than others. The most usual answer to this question is that goods of the soul are more important than goods of the body (Augustine referred to them respectively as "eternal goods" and "temporal goods"), and that the primary goods of the soul pertain to the cherishing of God and the neighbor. To these primary goods one's own personal qualities (also goods of the soul) are usually considered to be secondary, chiefly in an instrumental sense. Furthermore, goods of the body are ordinarily to be seen as also worthwhile, and most especially if they are needed by the neighbor for his basic sustenance. It should also be observed that a teleological theory of obligation in theological ethics ideally requires a well-developed and hierarchically ordered theory of value.

The concept of love would seem to be the most central one in theological ethics, especially in the Western world (Outka; Ramsey, 1950, pp. 1–45, 92–132, 234–248). Sometimes this functions as a value notion, as when it is employed to specify the objects or states of affairs that are held to be important. At other times, it is a virtue notion, especially when it is acclaimed as "the form of all virtue" or the inclusive motive of good human action. Still again it is considered to be a general principle of obligation, not only teleologically ("do what love requires") but also deontologically ("conform your actions to the covenant-love of God"). This central relevance of love to so much of the territory that theological ethics covers may be a reason for claiming, as one of the major religions has, that "the greatest of these is love."

FREDERICK S. CARNEY

[Directly related are the entries BUDDHISM; CONFUCIANISM; HINDUISM; ISLAM; JUDAISM; PROTESTANTISM; and ROMAN CATHOLICISM. While all the articles in this entry are relevant, see especially the articles THE TASK OF ETHICS, RULES AND PRINCIPLES, DEONTOLOGICAL THEORIES, TELEOLOGICAL THEORIES, and SITUATION ETHICS.]

BIBLIOGRAPHY

AUGUSTINE. The Enchiridion on Faith, Hope and Love. Translated by J. F. Shaw. Edited by Henry Paolucci. Analysis by Adolph von Harnack. Chicago: Henry Regnery, 1961.

BARTH, KARL. "The Command of God." Church Dogmatics. 4 vols. Vol. 2: The Doctrine of God. 2 pts. Edited by G. W. Bromiley and T. F. Torrance. Edinburgh: T. & T. Clark, 1957, pt. 2, chap. 8, pp. 509–781.

———. "Freedom for Life." Church Dogmatics. 4 vols. Vol. 3: The Doctrine of Creation. 4 pts. Edited by G. W. Bromiley and T. F. Torrance. Edinburgh: T. & T. Clark, 1961, pt. 4, sec. 54, pp. 324–564.

CARNEY, FREDERICK S. "Accountability in Christian Morality." Journal of Religion 53 (1973): 309–329.

———. "The Virtue-Obligation Controversy." Journal of Religious Ethics 1, no. 1 (1973): pp. 5–19.

DONALDSON, DWIGHT M. Studies in Muslim Ethics. London: S.P.C.K., 1953.

EDWARDS, JONATHAN. The Nature of True Virtue. Foreword by William K. Frankena. Ann Arbor Paperbacks, AA37. Ann Arbor: University of Michigan Press, 1960, 1969.

FRANKENA, WILLIAM K. "Is Morality Logically Dependent on Religion?" Religion and Morality: A Collection of Essays. Edited by Gene Outka and John P. Reeder, Jr. Garden City, N.Y.: Anchor Press/Doubleday, 1973, pp. 295–317.

GHAZZĀLĪ, AL- [AL-GHAZĀLĪ]. The Faith and Practice of al-Ghazālī. Translated by W. Montgomery Watt. Ethical and Religious Classics of East and West, no. 8. London: George Allen & Unwin, 1953.

GRABER, GLENN C. "A Critical Bibliography of Recent Discussions of Religious Ethics by Philosophers." Journal of Religious Ethics 2, no. 2 (1974), pp. 53–80.

HAUERWAS, STANLEY. Vision and Virtue: Essays in Christian Ethical Reflection. Notre Dame, Ind.: Fides Publishers, 1974.

HILLERS, DELBERT R. Covenant: The History of a Biblical Idea. Seminars in the History of Ideas. Baltimore: Johns Hopkins Press, 1969.

KADUSHIN, MAX. Worship and Ethics: A Study in Rabbinic Judaism. Evanston: Northwestern University Press, 1964.

LITTLE, DAVID, and TWISS, SUMNER B., JR. "Basic Terms in the Study of Religious Ethics." Religion and Morality: A Collection of Essays. Edited by Gene Outka and John P. Reeder, Jr. Garden City, N.Y.: Anchor Press/Doubleday, 1973, pp. 35–77.

NIEBUHR, HELMUT RICHARD. Radical Monotheism and Western Culture: With Supplementary Essays. New York: Harper & Brothers, 1960.

OUTKA, GENE. Agape: An Ethical Analysis. Yale Publications in Religion, no. 17. New Haven: Yale University Press, 1972.

RAMSEY, PAUL. Basic Christian Ethics. New York: Charles Scribner's Sons, 1950.

———. Deeds and Rules in Christian Ethics. New York: Charles Scribner's Sons, 1967.

———. The Patient as Person: Explorations in Medical Ethics. The Lyman Beecher Lectures at Yale University. New Haven: Yale University Press, 1970.

SARMA, DITTAKAVI SUBRAHMANYA. "Hindu Ethics." Essence of Hinduism. Bhavan's Book University, no. 171. Bombay: Bharatiya Vidya Bhavan, 1971, chap. 4, pp. 37–59.

SATHAYE, SHRINIWAS G. Moral Choice and Early Hindu Thought. Jaico Books, no. J-353. Bombay: Jaico Publishing House, 1970.

THOMAS AQUINAS. Summa Theologiae I-II 1–5; 55–67; 90–108; II-II 64, 7. Translated by the Fathers of the English Dominican Province as "Treatise on the Last End," "Virtues," "Treatise on Law," and "Whether It Is Lawful to Kill a Man in Self-defense?" Summa Theologica: First Complete American Edition. 3 vols. Vol. 1: First Part, QQ. 1–119 and First Part of the Second Part, QQ. 1–114, with Synoptical Charts. New York: Benziger Brothers, 1947, questions 1–5, pp. 583–615; questions 55–67, pp. 819–877; questions 90–108, pp. 993–1119; vol. 2: Containing Second Part of the Second Part, QQ. 1–189 and Third Part, QQ. 1–90, with Synoptical Charts, question 64, art. 7, pp. 1471–1472.

VIII
OBJECTIVISM IN ETHICS

For those interested in bioethics, an ethical theory is primarily of value insofar as it provides some help in solving the perplexing moral problems that arise in the practice of medicine and related fields. Ethical theories that attempt to provide such help are called normative ethical theories.

In some sense all normative ethical theories should be regarded as objectivist theories, for a normative ethical theory is an attempt to provide a systematic account of morality such that one will be able, at least in principle, to determine correct answers to at least some moral problems. Most objectivist theories claim that there is a correct answer to every moral problem, and it is this more extreme claim that has given rise to the various forms of ethical skepticism, e.g., emotivism, relativism, and subjectivism, which deny that there is one and only one right answer to any moral problem. Some objectivist theories amount to little more than the claim that there is, at least in principle, a correct answer to all moral problems, their main claim to philosophical interest being that they are stated in philosophical terminology, e.g., the moral sense theory and intuitionism.

As a guide to conduct

The unique feature of the moral sense theory is its claim that the object of moral perception is the actual particular situation just as the object of our sense of beauty is the actual particular painting, etc. It is the real situation with all of its detail that each person is to perceive morally. This theory has the virtue of noting that moral agreement is, in fact, fairly widespread. It also makes clear that disagreement in moral judgments counts against the objectivity of morality no more than disagreement in perception counts against the objectivity of colors or sounds. However, it does not account for the many differences between moral perception and seeing and hearing, e.g., the absence of any specific sense organ and the absence of any scientifically determined objective correlation, such as with light waves and sound waves. This theory really is little more than an extended metaphor; it amounts simply to the claim that we often do know what the morally correct answer to a moral problem is, but it does not explain in any way how we know this.

Intuitionism is a slightly more sophisticated theory. The object of intuition is not a particular situation, but something more general. The different versions of intuitionism differ from one another in what they claim to be the object of intuition. In the most common form of intuitionism, we are said to intuit certain prima facie duties, or moral rules, and we then look at particular situations and apply the relevant rule. This form of intuitionism takes mathematics rather than sense perception as its model. Just as people see that five plus five is ten, or that twenty-eight divided by four is seven, so everyone sees that one morally ought not to kill or steal or lie. Moral disagreements are explained away in the following ways: (1) Just as some people are so mentally defective that they do not see the obvious mathematical truths, so some people are so morally defective that they do not see the obvious moral truths; (2) the situation may be unclear so that people disagree about what rules are applicable; and (3) emotional factors are sometimes distorting.

Intuitionism allows for a slightly more articulate account of moral thinking than the moral sense theory. An intuitionist who observes a doctor performing some medical experimentation on his patients by leading them to think it is part of their treatment says the doctor is doing wrong because he sees the situation as one involving deception and intuits that deception is morally wrong. Thus the intuitionist can say why what the doctor is doing is wrong, viz., because it involves deception, whereas the moral sense theorist is limited to saying that he simply sees that it is wrong. This makes it seem as if all the advantage is with the intuitionist. However, he has a problem that the moral sense theorist does not have. The intuitionist, because he gives deception as a reason for saying that what the doctor did was morally wrong, seems to be committed to holding that all deception is wrong. This does not seem to accord with the ordinary view, for almost all agree that deception may sometimes be morally justified, e.g., when its intent is to prevent significant suffering. It turns out that the various duties or rules of the intuitionist may conflict. Thus he needs a second intuition to tell what is morally right in a situation involving a conflict between two or more rules. The moral sense theorist deals with each situation on its own and so never runs into this kind of problem.

This problem has led some intuitionists, e.g., Sidgwick and Moore, to the view that we intuit not rules of conduct but good consequences. Rules of conduct or moral rules (the two are generally, though mistakenly, taken to be equivalent; Baier, chaps. 4 and 5; Gert, chaps. 1 and 4) are then treated as those rules which if acted upon result in more of the intuited good being produced than any other rules. There are many variations of this teleological form of intuitionism. The most common form is a version of utilitarianism in which pleasure or happiness is taken as good and moral rules are taken as those which result in the greatest amount of happiness for the greatest number. The problem with such a form of intuitionism is that it not only seems to allow any kind of deception practiced by a doctor as long as no harm comes to the patients but also allows involuntary experimentation on patients if such experimentation results in benefits to others that are greater than the harm caused the patient. And though some doctors seem to agree with this conclusion, it is not universally accepted (Gert, p. 99).

Teleological intuitionism differs, only in a technical sense, from another group of theories, which we can call "naturalist" theories. The naturalists are suspicious of the faculty of intuition required by intuitionism and thus, instead of saying that we intuit what things are good, make it a matter of meaning rather than intuition that such things are good (Bentham, chaps. 1 and 2). So they not only deny that we have any special faculty of intuition which enables us to say that pleasure is good but also deny that any such faculty is needed; for they claim that good simply means pleasure—or whatever else it is that they want to substitute for what the intuitionist intuits as good. But besides facing most of the objections that teleological intuitionists face, the naturalists have the additional problem that their proposed definitions of good do not seem very plausible (Moore, chap. 1).

All of the theories discussed so far may seem to be simply academic discussions of moral matters, that is, they may seem to be discussing moral problems as if they were merely problems in some academic subject. But it is generally recognized that the primary function of moral judgments is not to provide information; it is to guide conduct. Thus theories were developed in which correct moral judgments were explicitly put forward as the advice that would be given by an ideal observer about how to act in a moral situation. These "ideal observer theories" can be viewed as variants of moral sense theories, with the ideal observer looking at the actual situation in all of its detail, or as an intuitionist applying all of the relevant moral rules and ideals and balancing them in the appropriate fashion. The focus of attention shifted from determining how the ideal observer came to his moral judgments, e.g., by a moral sense, intuition, or by definition of terms, and to a consideration of the characteristics of the ideal observer. Among the characteristics discussed, three seemed most important: that the observer be informed, impartial, and sympathetic. Thus the correct moral answer to any moral problem was that which would be arrived at by the ideal observer. The very close connection between the ideal observer and God seems obvious.

All of the objectivist theories discussed so far assume that all rational men, if impartial and fully informed, would arrive at the same moral answers. It is this assumption—that there are unique moral answers to every moral question —that has been primarily responsible for the various skeptical theories that are currently so popular. For none of the standard objectivist theories is able to deal adequately with the fact of moral disagreement. The strength of objectivist theories is that they account for those clear cases in which there is complete moral agreement. Everyone agrees that a doctor should not perform an unnecessary operation simply in order to increase his income. But there is not complete agreement on whether or not to allow a terminally ill patient in severe pain to die. Most objectivists are committed to the view that, given all of the facts of the particular case, there is one and only one morally right course of action. But an objectivist need not hold with this. All that he needs to accept is that it is an objective matter as to what are the morally relevant considerations. Thus everyone agrees that in the absence of countervailing reasons doctors ought to try to keep their patients from dying. Everyone also agrees that the facts that the patient is terminally ill and that he is suffering great pain count as reasons for allowing the patient to die. The disagreement arises in determining when, if ever, these reasons outweigh the obligation to keep the patient alive.

Rationality and impartiality

Most contemporary ethical theorists agree that correct moral judgments are those that would be arrived at by impartial rational persons (sympathy is no longer regarded as necessary). Thus attention has focused on clarifying the concepts of rationality and impartiality. Of course, it is recognized that such persons must be as fully informed about the particular situation as possible, and that many, if not most, moral disagreements arise from a disagreement over facts or estimates of probability, but these problems are considered to be practical rather than philosophical. An objectivist theory is required only to account for moral agreement and disagreement in those (rare) situations where the facts are not in dispute.

For almost all theorists, the account of impartiality is such that it follows analytically that, if one rational person makes an impartial judgment, then other rational persons with the same information will make exactly the same judgment. It is easy to see that, with this account of impartiality, any moral question can have only one answer. But it does not seem to be an essential feature of impartiality that all impartial persons will agree. Judges on various courts, all of whom are considered impartial, often reach different decisions, even though they are all presented with the same set of facts, because they weigh the facts differently.

What is required by impartiality is that one base one's decision in a situation only on the relevant features of the case. In a moral decision that means that one uses only morally relevant considerations in making that decision. Objectivist ethics is distinguished from the various skeptical positions (i.e., subjectivism, relativism, emotivism, and prescriptivism) by its claim that what are the morally relevant considerations is an objective matter. Objectivists would hold that any moral judgment incompatible with the one favored by all of the morally relevant considerations is incorrect. And it is incorrect even if the judgment (1) accurately *describes* my feelings or attitudes (subjectivism), or (2) is accepted by my society (relativism), or (3) genuinely *expresses* my feelings or attitude (emotivism), or (4) is one that I would prescribe, even universally (prescriptivism). However, objectivism need not hold (though almost all objectivists have held) that all rational impartial observers will give the same weight to all of the morally relevant considerations.

What are the morally relevant facts? Here again most objectivists are in substantial agreement. The fact that someone will be harmed— e.g., killed; made to suffer pain, anxiety, sadness, or displeasure; disabled; or deprived of freedom, opportunity, or pleasure—is a morally relevant fact. Similarly, the fact that someone will be prevented from suffering one or more of these harms is morally relevant. Also morally relevant are facts concerning deception, the breaking of a promise, cheating, the breaking of a law, or the neglect of one's duty, e.g., as a doctor. What is in dispute is whether facts about a person's gaining greater abilities, opportunities, pleasure, or even the mere satisfaction of a desire are also morally relevant. An impartial person making a moral decision must take into account only these morally relevant facts; he cannot take into account any other facts, such as that it is he and his friends rather than people for whom he does not care who will suffer if this decision is taken rather than that one. One way of guaranteeing impartiality of this kind is to say that the person cannot use any fact about himself that distinguishes him from any other person (Gert, pp. 89 ff.; Rawls, pp. 136–142). He must make his moral decision as if he knew nothing about the identity of the various parties involved.

It may seem that, following this procedure, all impartial persons would always reach the same decision, but that is not the case. Two persons, completely impartial, may reach different decisions in a particular case because they may give different weights to the different harms involved. For example, one doctor may recommend compulsory genetic screening of all married couples because he holds that the harm preventable by such screening outweighs the deprivation of freedom that it involves, while another who believes that exactly the same amount of harm will be prevented by the screening does not think that it justifies the deprivation of freedom involved. An objectivist need not be dismayed by this conclusion, for he can hold that this disagreement occurs only within a very limited area and that both parties agree on the morally relevant facts. Thus, he knows that both doctors would hold it immoral to prevent genetic screening of those couples who desire it, and both would hold that such screening should be made available to all who want it. For in these cases harm can be prevented, and there is no countervailing deprivation of freedom.

Rationality and desire

The final issue that needs to be discussed is an explanation of agreement concerning the morally relevant considerations. This is where the concept of rationality becomes central, for it is the agreement of all impartial rational persons that determines the morally relevant considerations. Unfortunately the standard account of rationality (Rawls, p. 142 f.) in philosophy and in the social sciences, especially economics, puts no limit on the content of rational desires. On this account, to act rationally is simply to act in such a way as most efficiently to bring about the maximum satisfaction of one's desires, taking into account only their intensity, probability, etc. Since there is no limit to the content of rational desires, there is no limit to what counts as a morally relevant consideration. It may seem that this account of rationality is therefore incompatible with objectivity in ethics, but in fact it results in the most extreme form of objectivism. For objectivity can be obtained with this account of rationality only by having each desire count the same as every other desire of equal intensity and probability. Thus the standard account of rationality requires that impartiality, by ruling out all consideration of content, rule out all disagreement.

But there does seem to be a limit to the content of rational desires. Certain desires, viz., for death, pain, disability, or loss of freedom, opportunity, or pleasure, are taken by laymen as well as by psychiatrists as irrational, if one has no reason for so wanting. It is an essential feature of rationality to desire to avoid these harms or evils for oneself, unless one has some reason not to. This explains why there is universal agreement on the morally relevant considerations. All rational persons, if impartial, agree that these evils are to be avoided or prevented for everyone, unless there is an adequate reason for not doing so.

Once we have given this content to the concept of rationality, we are not threatened by anarchy if we allow impartial rational persons to disagree. The content we have given to reason limits the possible disagreement to the ranking of the various evils. This is not only a disagreement that an objectivist can accept, but one that he must accept if he is to provide an acceptable account of our actual moral experience. Moral discussions can then be explicitly focused on the relevant matters. When we have a moral disagreement due to a different ranking of the evils, then we see if we can come up with an alternative that lessens the evils on one side or the other. In this way, moral disputes need not result in each party's regarding the other as ill-informed, irrational, or partial, whereas if one accepts most objectivist theories one must regard all moral disagreement as due to ignorance, irrationality, or partiality. Nor, in reaction to

these extreme objectivist theories, are we tempted to fall into skepticism and regard no moral problems as capable of a correct solution. Rather we can acknowledge the common ground, and thus have the opportunity to work together to see if we can lessen what all of us regard as evils, even though we may disagree on whether one evil is more or less important than some other evil.

Thus an objectivist theory that does not insist on unique answers to every moral problem, while it does not provide the kind of mechanical decision procedure that some doctors may have hoped for, does provide some help in solving the perplexing moral problems that arise in medicine and related fields. For it makes clear what factors are morally relevant, and thus guides the decision maker (physician, scientist, patient, subject, policymaker, etc.) toward that alternative that seems to be favored by most of the morally relevant considerations. But it also makes clear what these parties already knew: that there are some cases in which no single alternative is favored by most of the morally relevant considerations. But even in these cases, where each must decide which alternative he will adopt, the objectivist theory can be useful in helping him to rule out all of the morally unacceptable alternatives.

BERNARD GERT

[*For further discussion of topics mentioned in this article, see the entries:* NATURAL LAW; *and* OBLIGATION AND SUPEREROGATION. *While all the articles in this entry are relevant, see especially the articles* RULES AND PRINCIPLES, MORAL REASONING, *and* RELATIVISM. *See also:* DECISION MAKING, MEDICAL; DOUBLE EFFECT; JUSTICE; LAW AND MORALITY; *and* PRAGMATISM. *This article will find application in the entries* DEATH AND DYING: EUTHANASIA AND SUSTAINING LIFE, *article on* ETHICAL VIEWS; ENVIRONMENTAL ETHICS; HEALTH CARE, *articles on* RIGHT TO HEALTH-CARE SERVICES *and* THEORIES OF JUSTICE AND HEALTH CARE; INFORMED CONSENT IN THE THERAPEUTIC RELATIONSHIP, *article on* LEGAL AND ETHICAL ASPECTS; *and* TRUTH-TELLING, *article on* ETHICAL ASPECTS.]

BIBLIOGRAPHY

MORAL SENSE THEORIES

SHAFTESBURY, ANTHONY ASHLEY COOPER. *Characteristicks of Men, Manners, Opinions, Times . . .* London: 1711.

HUTCHESON, FRANCIS. *A System of Moral Philosophy.* London: 1755.

BONAR, JAMES. *Moral Sense.* Library of Philosophy.

Edited by J. H. Muirhead. New York: Macmillan Co., 1930.

DEONTOLOGICAL INTUITIONISM

REID, THOMAS. *Essays on the Active Powers of Man.* Edinburgh: 1788.

PRICHARD, HAROLD ARTHUR. *Moral Obligation: Essays and Lectures.* Oxford: Clarendon Press, 1949.

ROSS, WILLIAM DAVID. *The Right and the Good.* Oxford: Clarendon Press, 1930.

TELEOLOGICAL INTUITIONISM

SIDGWICK, HENRY. *The Methods of Ethics.* London: Macmillan & Co., 1874.

MOORE, GEORGE EDWARD. *Principia Ethica.* Cambridge: University Press, 1903.

NATURALISM

BENTHAM, JEREMY. *An Introduction to the Principles of Morals and Legislation.* London: 1789.

MILL, JOHN STUART. *Utilitarianism.* London: 1861.

PERRY, RALPH BARTON. *General Theory of Value.* New York: Longmans, Green & Co., 1926.

IDEAL OBSERVER THEORIES

SMITH, ADAM. *The Theory of Moral Sentiments.* London: 1759.

FIRTH, RODERICK. "Ethical Absolutism and the Ideal Observer." *Philosophy and Phenomenological Research* 12 (1952): 317–345.

THEOLOGICAL VIEWS

THOMAS AQUINAS. *Summa Theologiae,* I–II (1266–1274). Especially questions 90–97.

NIEBUHR, REINHOLD. *An Interpretation of Christian Ethics. Living Age Books,* no. 1. New York: Meridian Books, 1956.

RAMSEY, PAUL. *Deeds and Rules in Christian Ethics.* New York: Charles Scribner's Sons, 1967.

IMPARTIAL RATIONALITY

HOBBES, THOMAS. *Man and Citizen.* Edited with an introduction by Bernard Gert. Garden City, N.Y.: Anchor Books, 1972. Contains *De Cive* (1651), translated by Thomas Hobbes; and *De Homine* (1658), translated by Charles T. Wood, T. S. K. Scott-Craig, and Bernard Gert.

KANT, IMMANUEL. *Grundlegung zur Metaphysik der Sitten.* Riga: 1785.

BAIER, KURT. *The Moral Point of View: A Rational Basis of Ethics.* Ithaca: Cornell University Press, 1958.

GERT, BERNARD. *The Moral Rules: A New Rational Foundation for Morality.* New York: Harper & Row, 1970. Revised paperback. Torchbook, 1973.

RAWLS, JOHN. *A Theory of Justice.* Cambridge: Harvard University Press, Belknap Press, 1971.

IX
NATURALISM

The expression "ethical naturalism" is a common noun rather than a proper name. It is used as a label to classify ethical theories rather than as a name to refer to any single ethical thesis. It is commonly and properly used in at least three senses. Ethical naturalism is any ethical theory that (1) holds that the standard of value or obligation is provided only by nature or the natural; (2) explains the nature of value and obligation entirely within a naturalistic metaphysics; or (3) defines ethical words in terms of natural characteristics. The first definition provides a foundation for the moral rules and human rights so crucial to issues in medical ethics. The second claims to be the ideal philosophical basis for bioethics. The third explains how the life sciences can be logically relevant to judgments of value or obligation.

Main types of ethical naturalism

In the first sense, an ethical naturalism is any theory that takes nature or the natural as its standard of value or obligation. It stands opposed to any act or way of life that is artificial, unnatural, or a perversion of nature. One version takes natural purposes as its standard. Aristotle, for example, believed that each kind of thing has its specific end or goal determined for it by its very nature. The good of each individual is to realize its natural end. Another version takes natural law as determining right and wrong. Thus, Cicero claims that specific rules commanding certain kinds of conduct and forbidding others exist in the laws of nature independent of society and its laws. This moral law of nature dictates what humans ought or ought not to do. An important offshoot of the natural law theory is the view that all men possess certain natural rights. Locke defended the inalienable rights to life, liberty, and property. Still another version of ethical naturalism in the first sense takes presocial, primitive human nature as its standard. Rousseau claimed that innate human nature is fundamentally good but that it becomes corrupted and perverted by society with its artificial institutions. His ethical ideal was to live naturally, spontaneously acting upon innate human feelings and impulses. All versions of ethical naturalism in the first sense agree that the moral ideal is the natural life; they disagree as to the precise definition of "nature" and "the natural" (Lovejoy, Chinard, Boas, and Crane).

Ethical naturalism in the second sense is any theory that interprets value and obligation within the framework of a purely naturalistic metaphysics. It refuses to appeal to any supernatural entities like God, an immortal soul, or Platonic forms in explaining the good for man and the grounds of obligation. It may well be that Aristotle was an ethical naturalist in this sense as well as the first, but Cicero certainly was not, because he thought of the natural law as expressing the will of God and morally binding for just that reason. Some philosophers seem to be metaphysical naturalists first, in order to avoid any ontological commitment to supernatural entities, and then become ethical naturalists in order that their ethical theory may be consistent with their ontology. Thus, Samuel Alexander tries to show how he can extend his analysis of spatio-temporal nature to include an explanation of value, and John Dewey argues at length that both the existence of values and our knowledge of them can be understood purely in terms of the interests and intelligence of natural organisms. Others seem to reject all supernatural religion and morality and become ethical naturalists because they wish to place human life and human well-being at the center of ethics. Humanists, both non-Marxist and Marxist, are less concerned with ontological commitment than with the import of their ethical theories for individual self-realization and social reform.

Ethical naturalism in the third sense is any theory that defines ethical words in terms of natural characteristics. It rejects both ethical intuitionism, which holds that ethical words stand for nonnatural characteristics, and nondescriptive ethics, which maintains that ethical words do not refer to any kind of quality or relation. No very satisfactory definition of what counts as an ethical word has been given, but examples are "good," "bad," "right," "wrong," and "ought." Nor is it at all clear just what makes any characteristic "natural." The two most plausible suggestions are that natural characteristics are qualities or relations that exist in the spatio-temporal realm of nature *or* that they are qualities or relations that are given in experience or analyzable into such empirically observable characteristics. In any event, it is helpful to classify each version of ethical naturalism in the third sense according to the natural science from which it borrows its defining terms. To hold that "good" means either pleasant or desired is to hold a psychological version of ethical naturalism. To define "good" as that which serves physiological needs, or "right" as that which is conducive to the survival of the species, is to adopt a biological form of ethical naturalism. Finally, an anthropological or sociological version would be the proposition that "right" means to be in conformity with the mores of the agent's society. Diverse as these

ethical theories are, they share a fundamental allegiance to empiricism, the view that experience is the source of all concepts and the ground of all knowledge.

Naturalistic fallacy

George Edward Moore charged all versions of ethical naturalism in the third sense with committing "the naturalistic fallacy." Although he repeated this charge frequently throughout the first three chapters of *Principia Ethica*, he never did make it clear which of several alleged errors he had in mind. Since the nature and fallaciousness of "the naturalistic fallacy" have been much debated for decades, the interpretation and evaluation of Moore's critical arguments are of considerable philosophical importance.

Moore often suggests that the fundamental error of ethical naturalism lies in defining, or trying to define, what is incapable of definition (Moore, p. 7). He argues that goodness, the primary ethical characteristic, is simple rather than complex and claims that the only philosophically illuminating sort of definition is one that analyzes some complex object into its parts. It follows, of course, that the word "good" cannot be defined in any philosophically relevant way. Since the fundamentally irreducible quality of goodness cannot be defined at all, it obviously cannot be defined in terms of natural characteristics. Ethical naturalists have typically tried to rebut this charge by arguing either that goodness is a complex property or that definitions that do not analyze a complex object are philosophically legitimate.

In other passages, Moore says (p. 13) that the error of ethical naturalism is in mistaking the proper subject matter of ethics. The crux of this charge is that the naturalists assign the wrong ontological status to values and obligations. By defining the vocabulary of ethics in terms of the concepts of the natural sciences, they locate the subject matter of ethics within the realm of nature. Actually, the ethical characteristics of goodness and oughtness are *non*natural properties that have a kind of being quite different from that of natural properties like yellowness, sweetness, or pleasantness. Moore agrees with the naturalists that values and obligations are facts, but he insists that they are nonnatural facts known only by intuition. Other critics of naturalism give a more radical interpretation of the ontological error by denying that values and obligations are facts of any kind. They maintain that values are ontologically different from facts and that what *ought to be* the case has a different metaphysical status from what *is* the case. Since the subject matter of ethics is values and oughts, it is a metaphysical muddle to define ethical words in terms of any kind of facts, either natural or nonnatural. Ethical naturalists have argued vigorously, on both metaphysical and epistemological grounds, against any ontological commitment to a nonnatural realm or to the being of "oughts." Even if their arguments are granted, however, it need not follow that the subject matter of ethics is the facts of nature. If either emotivism or prescriptivism is on the right track, ethical sentences do not describe any facts at all.

In still other places (e.g., p. 11), Moore says that the error of ethical naturalism consists in misrepresenting our ethical knowledge. This epistemological error treats our rational insight into values and obligations as though it were a species of empirical knowledge essentially like the knowledge provided by the natural sciences. Since the goodness of something is not a property that can be observed by external perception or felt by inner sensation, our knowledge of values must come from reason rather than experience. And since how people ought to act, as contrasted with how they do act, cannot be established by observation or experiment, our knowledge of obligations must also be a priori. Ethical naturalists have replied that, if values and obligations are properly interpreted through their naturalistic definitions, it is clear how scientific information can answer ethical questions. Much of the debate between the intuitionists and the naturalists from 1903 until about 1944 centered upon just this epistemological issue. The ethical naturalists were trying to show how empiricism can explain our knowledge in ethics just as it explains our scientific knowledge; the ethical intuitionists were insisting that only rationalism can give an adequate account of our ethical insight.

A fourth set of passages implies that Moore intended to charge the ethical naturalists with making a logical error. His complaint is that they try to establish their conclusions by using logically invalid arguments. One of his prime targets is Mill's notorious proof of utilitarianism. Mill argues that happiness is the one and only thing that is intrinsically desirable on the ground that it is the one and only thing desired for itself. Moore insists that from the psychological fact that happiness is desired it does not follow that it is desirable, worthy of being desired (p.

67). He also objects, on logical grounds, to Rousseau's argument that the simple life is best *because* it is natural (p. 42). From the fact that something is natural it does not follow that it is good, much less that it is the best. More contemporary examples of arguments that might be charged with this sort of logical fallacy are that genetic engineering is wrong because it is artificial and the argument that all men have a human right to medical care because all human beings need medical care. Roughly, the logical error can be said to consist in deducing an ethical conclusion from purely factual premises or, to use a slogan modeled on a passage in Hume, deducing an "ought" from an "is."

In spite of considerable disagreement about the precise nature of "the naturalistic fallacy," it used to be widely agreed that any argument from facts to values or from "is" to "ought" does commit some sort of logical error. More recently, however, serious attempts have been made to show that some such arguments are logically valid. Logicians, such as Prior, have constructed arguments that meet all the requirements of formal logic and by which one can infer an allegedly ethical conclusion from apparently factual premises (1960, pp. 201–202, 204). Cautious language is imperative here because it remains undecided whether such arguments show that ethical conclusions can be inferred from factual premises or merely that the distinction between factual and ethical sentences is vague. Other philosophers have advanced arguments that, they claim, move from purely factual premises to ethical conclusions and are valid not by virtue of their logical form, but by virtue of their content. Searle, for example, has defended the validity of an argument from the fact that someone has promised to do something to the conclusion that he ought to do it (p. 44). Although such arguments have been widely criticized, their plausibility leaves it an open question whether "the naturalistic fallacy" is genuinely a logical error at all.

Science and ethics

What is primarily at stake throughout the debate about the alleged fallaciousness of "the naturalistic fallacy" is the relevance of science to ethics. What bearing, if any, do the findings of the life sciences have upon bioethics? Suppose that medical science should establish the fact that in some cases of terminal cancer there is no way to relieve the intense pain while sparing the life of the patient. This factual premise might seem to some to support the ethical conclusion that in some cases euthanasia is right. Or suppose, to take a different sort of example, medical sociology should find that the medical resources required to save one life by organ transplant would, if allocated to chemotherapy, save two or even three lives. Many would conclude, in this instance, that the use of medical resources for organ transplantation is not the best allocation. The philosophical problem is to explain just how scientific facts like these can be relevant to ethical conclusions about what is right or good. Leaving aside the possible, but implausible, view that factual information has no bearing whatsoever upon bioethics, there are four solutions proposed to this problem.

1. The traditional solution is that factual information is relevant to ethical conclusions insofar, and only insofar, as it can be subsumed under some universal ethical principle. Thus, granted that the right act is always the act that is most conducive to pleasure or the absence of pain, the fact that in some cases euthanasia is the only effective way to remove great pain implies that euthanasia is sometimes right. Again, the factual minor premise that the use of medical resources for organ transplant does not save the largest number of lives implies that it is not the best allocation of medical resources only when coupled with the ethical major premise that the best allocation of medical resources is the one that saves the most lives. On this view, the findings of the life sciences are reasons for ethical conclusions only when combined with universal principles provided by a very different discipline, ethics.

2. The solution proposed by ethical naturalism in the third sense is that factual premises imply ethical conclusions by virtue of the defined meaning of ethical concepts. There is no need to add any moral principle to the factual premise because the naturalistic definition of the ethical word used in the conclusion shows that the conclusion merely reaffirms what has already been asserted in the premise. If the word "right" really does mean "most conducive to pleasure or the absence of pain," then to conclude that in some cases euthanasia is right is merely to reassert in other words what is asserted by the premise that in some cases euthanasia is the only means to the absence of pain. Again, the fact that the use of medical resources for organ

transplant does not save as many lives as some alternative allocation clearly implies that it is not the best allocation if "the best allocation" is defined, at least for medical contexts, as "the allocation that saves the most lives."

3. A more recent suggestion is that factual information supports ethical conclusions by some special sort of nondeductive inference (Toulmin, pp. 160–161). Just as the scientific method reasons in terms of an inductive logic that cannot be reduced to any form of deduction, so ethical reasoning is governed by a special logic of ethics. What links the factual premise to the ethical conclusion is neither a tacit ethical principle nor a naturalistic definition, but a rule of ethical inference. Since these arguments do not follow the rules of standard deductive logic, they are not deductively valid; since they do claim to follow a different set of logical rules appropriate to ethics, they are still valid in some logical sense. Although this sort of solution has been advocated by several philosophers, they have not been able to agree on the rules for this special sort of logic or on what gives logical validity to it.

4. Finally, some emotivists argue that factual information is not *logically* relevant to ethical conclusions at all, but that it is relevant in some *psychological* sense. The fact that in some cases euthanasia is the only way of terminating intense pain does not logically imply that in some cases euthanasia is right; but since most people dislike pain and approve of whatever removes pain, the factual information does psychologically support the conclusion that euthanasia is sometimes right just because the belief in this factual premise tends to cause one to have a favorable attitude toward euthanasia. Similarly, the fact that the medical resources used to save one life by organ transplantation could be used in some other way to save two or more lives is psychologically relevant to the conclusion that it is not the best allocation of medical resources because, given our human desire to save as many lives as possible, belief in this fact tends to cause a less favorable attitude toward this allocation than to some alternative one.

Debate continues among philosophers as to just how factual statements can serve as reasons for or against ethical conclusions. Ethical naturalism remains one of the more plausible ways of explaining how the life sciences can make their contribution to the solution of the problems of bioethics.

Further implications

Ethical naturalism, in one or another of its various senses, is of considerable importance to bioethics in a number of additional ways. First, conclusions in medical ethics are frequently defended by an appeal to moral rules. The practice of taking organs for transplant from live donors is often criticized as a violation of the no harm rule, i.e., the general rule that the physician or surgeon ought never intentionally to injure a patient except for the greater medical benefit of that patient. Euthanasia and abortion pose moral problems for bioethics just because most people accept the rule that it is generally wrong to kill a human being. What status are we to ascribe to such moral rules? Unless one is willing to admit that moral rules are mere conventions—artificial and arbitrary—one is committed to the view that they are in some sense natural. And this, of course, is the view that the standard of right and wrong is the natural, where the natural is conceived in terms of the law of nature. Although the traditional language of natural law theory is generally rejected in contemporary bioethics, the substance of this version of ethical naturalism in the first sense remains in any view that takes moral rules seriously.

Second, many issues in bioethics hinge on the existence and content of certain human rights. Whether the routine harvesting of organs from cadavers without express consent is morally justified depends in part upon whether the human right to property implies that either the deceased individual or the next of kin "owns" the cadaver. It is widely taken for granted that certain types of experimentation with human subjects are morally right only if the subjects have given their free informed consent. But this presupposes the existence of some human right to privacy or personal security that such experimentation would violate were it not waived by consent. These human rights, implicitly affirmed or denied in medical ethics today, are simply the traditional natural rights under a new name. Once more ethical naturalism in the first sense, viz., the offshoot of natural law theory that upholds the existence of natural rights, turns out to be of unsuspected importance for bioethics.

Third, if bioethics is to reach any conclusions whatsoever about what is good or bad, desirable or undesirable, it must have some theory of value. While philosophy offers a wide array of value theories, not all of these are equally suitable for the purposes of bioethics. A supernatural or nonnatural theory of value will at least place ethics at a considerable distance from the life sciences and may sever the connection between them entirely. A naturalistic ethics, even in the second sense, will interpret values and disvalues in terms of categories such as pleasure, desire, human needs, life, or species survival. Ethical naturalism, therefore, claims to be the ideal philosophical basis for bioethics, since it offers an ethical theory that makes the life sciences directly and decisively relevant to the solution of ethical problems. This does not, however, prove that any version of ethical naturalism is true, but it does indicate both its theoretical and practical importance for bioethics.

CARL WELLMAN

[*Directly related are the entries* BIOLOGY, PHILOSOPHY OF; MEDICINE, ANTHROPOLOGY OF; NATURAL LAW; RIGHTS; *and* SCIENCE: ETHICAL IMPLICATIONS.]

BIBLIOGRAPHY

ADAMS, ELIE MAYNARD. *Ethical Naturalism and the Modern World-View.* Chapel Hill: University of North Carolina Press, 1960.

ALEXANDER, SAMUEL. *Space, Time and Deity.* London: Macmillan, 1920, vol. 2, pp. 236–314.

ARISTOTLE. *Nicomachean Ethics.* William David Ross, trans. *The Basic Works of Aristotle.* Edited by Richard McKeon. New York: Random House, 1941, pp. 927–1112. See pp. 935–952, bk. 1.

BRANDT, RICHARD B. *Ethical Theory.* Englewood Cliffs, N.J.: Prentice-Hall, 1959, pp. 151–182.

CICERO. *De Legibus.* Clinton Walker Keys, trans. *De Re Publica, De Legibus.* Loeb Classical Library. London: William Heinemann; New York: G. P. Putnam's Sons, 1928, pp. 287–519. See especially pp. 317–331.

DEWEY, JOHN. *Theory of Valuation.* Chicago: University of Chicago Press, 1939.

HUDSON, WILLIAM DONALD, ed. *The Is–Ought Question.* London: Macmillan, 1969.

HUME, DAVID. *Treatise of Human Nature* (1738). Edited by L. A. Selby-Bigge. Oxford: Clarendon Press, 1888, pp. 455–476.

LOCKE, JOHN. "An Essay Concerning the True Original Extent and End of Civil Government" (1690). *Treatise of Civil Government and A Letter Concerning Toleration.* Edited by Charles L. Sherman. New York: Appleton-Century Co., 1937, pp. 3–162.

LOVEJOY, ARTHUR ONCKEN; CHINARD, GILBERT; BOAS, GEORGE; and CRANE, RONALD S., eds. *A Documentary History of Primitivism and Related Ideas.* Contributions to the History of Primitivism. Baltimore: Johns Hopkins Press, 1935. Contains fifty-seven meanings of "Nature."

MILL, JOHN STUART. *Utilitarianism* (1863). *Utilitarianism, Liberty and Representative Government.* Edited by A. D. Lindsay. New York: E. P. Dutton & Co., 1950, pp. 1–80.

MOORE, GEORGE EDWARD. *Principia Ethica.* Cambridge: Cambridge University Press, 1903.

PRIOR, ARTHUR N. "The Autonomy of Ethics." *Australasian Journal of Philosophy* 38 (1960): 199–206.

———. *Logic and the Basis of Ethics.* Oxford: Clarendon Press, 1949.

ROUSSEAU, JEAN JACQUES. *A Discourse on the Origin of Inequality* (1755). G. D. H. Cole, trans. *The Social Contract and Discourses.* London: J. M. Dent & Sons, New York: E. P. Dutton & Co., 1913, pp. 155–246.

SEARLE, JOHN R. "How to Derive 'Ought' from 'Is'." *Philosophical Review* 73 (1964): 43–58.

STEVENSON, CHARLES LESLIE. *Ethics and Language.* New Haven: Yale University Press, 1944, pp. 152–173.

TOULMIN, STEPHEN EDELSTON. *An Examination of the Place of Reason in Ethics.* Cambridge: Cambridge University Press, 1950, pp. 130–165.

X

NON-DESCRIPTIVISM

When classifying ethical theories, it is essential to make clear the questions to which they are answers; for if different theories are answers to different questions, they do not necessarily conflict. The main division is between theories about the meanings of the moral words or the analyses of the moral concepts, and theories about the rules of valid reasoning on moral questions of substance. Non-descriptivism belongs to the former class, whereas utilitarianism, for example, belongs to the latter. Thus utilitarianism, which answers the question "How ought we to decide what we ought to do?" is not necessarily in conflict with non-descriptivism, which is an answer to the question "What does 'ought' mean?" The relation between the two types of question is that the rules of valid reasoning in any field depend upon the rules governing the uses of words (that is, upon the conceptual framework) in that field. Thus the fact that "all" and "some" have the meanings that they have makes the following an invalid inference: "Some abortions are wrong; therefore all abortions are wrong." We shall see that, so far from utilitarianism and non-descriptivism being incompatible, a certain form of the first is a consequence of a certain form of the second.

Within theories about the meanings of the moral words the main division is between descriptivist and non-descriptivist theories. A crude and unilluminating first attempt at stating the difference between them is to say that descriptivism regards moral judgments as factual statements *describing* people, acts, etc., or attributing properties to them, whereas non-descriptivism treats them as having an altogether different role in our language (see below). But the difference is best illustrated by examples. Examples of descriptivist theories are various forms of ethical naturalism according to which moral judgments are equivalent to certain statements of empirical, or at least not specifically moral, fact; when their analysis is understood, they can be verified or falsified by observation of these non-moral facts. For example, if it were true (as it would be on a very crude type of naturalistic theory) that "wrong" meant "forbidden by the Church", then we could determine that euthanasia was wrong simply by observing the verbal behavior of those in ecclesiastical authority (e.g., by reading papal encyclicals). This assumes that the word "authority" is a purely descriptive word, which in many uses it is not.

An important sub-class of naturalism is subjectivism (a view which goes back to the ancient Greek philosopher Protagoras). This is a descriptivist theory, in that it holds that moral judgments state facts of a sort. But whereas on some descriptivist theories (the objectivist ones) the facts in question will be facts about the external world, independent of the thoughts, dispositions, etc., of people, on others (the subjectivist ones) they will be facts about these latter. It is an interesting exercise to determine to which of these classes the "ecclesiastical" type of naturalism just mentioned belongs. Subjectivism is a type of naturalism because it equates moral facts with a certain kind of non-moral facts, namely, facts about people's thoughts, etc.

Another example of a descriptivist theory is ethical intuitionism. This rejects naturalism, but maintains that moral judgments are statements of a different sort: they attribute certain specifically moral (sometimes called non-natural) properties of rightness, wrongness, goodness, badness, etc., which are not the same as, nor analyzable in terms of, non-moral properties of any kind. Moral properties are, as was said, *sui generis* (of a sort all their own). The way we ascertain whether something has or lacks these properties is by intuition, i.e., by exercising a special moral faculty whereby we apprehend their presence or absence. The distinguishing mark of intuitionist theories, among descriptivist theories, is their irrationalism; that is to say, at certain crucial points in the process which is supposed to end with an answer to a moral question, they appeal, not to argument, but to our alleged ability to know, without argument, the truth of certain moral facts. Although intuitionism was generally thought to have been discredited by its essential irrationalism, and now has few overt defenders, a great number of present-day philosophers (perhaps the majority) become crypto-intuitionists when they descend to discuss practical issues; i.e., they think that the way to do this is to look for moral judgments which they and their readers can accept without argument. This often amounts to a mere appeal to received opinion (to what people, including the philosopher in question, think), and thus comes close to a form of ethical relativism or subjectivism, the dividing line between which and intuitionism is often invisibly narrow.

The terms "cognitivism" and "non-cognitivism" are commonly used to distinguish the same types of theory as are "descriptivism" and "non-descriptivism". The former pair make the division according to whether a theory does or does not allow of the existence of *knowledge* of some moral facts. Other ways of making the distinction are by asking whether or not a theory allows that moral judgments may be *true* or *false,* or whether or not it allows that moral adjectives may be the *"names"* of *properties.* All these alternative ways of marking the distinction are unreliable, because of the obscurity of the words "knowledge", "true", and "property". Some non-descriptivist theories may well be able to give a sense to the claim that we can know that a moral judgment is true, or that an act has the property of being wrong. But we may perhaps define descriptivism and non-descriptivism by saying that the former, unlike the latter, claims that the meanings of the moral words are a function solely of the truth-conditions of propositions containing them; that is to say, there is no further element in their meaning which could leave us the choice of asserting or denying them, once the facts of the case are given. Thus descriptivism, unlike non-descriptivism, is committed to a "verificationist" account of the meanings of the moral words.

Non-descriptivism arose because of dissatisfaction with all these kinds of descriptivism. It was thought that G. E. Moore had produced conclusive arguments against all forms of naturalism, including subjectivism; but his own and other attempts to produce a viable intuitionist theory had encountered insuperable difficulties over the nature of the *sui generis* moral properties and our means of discerning them. The first

non-descriptivist theory to hold the field was of an irrationalist type, called "emotivism" (although non-descriptivism does not *have* to be irrationalist). Leaving aside certain premonitory remarks of Berkeley and Hume, and a longer and very Humean passage of J. S. Mill, the first full-scale exposition of non-descriptivism was by the Swedish philosopher Hägerström; this was succeeded by Ogden and Richards' work. Emotivism was embraced by some, though not all, of the Logical Positivists (the "Vienna Circle") and their followers. Its most trenchant expositions were by Carnap and Ayer; and its fullest and most considered defense by Stevenson.

Emotivists are non-descriptivists because they hold that there is a central element in the meaning of moral judgments in their typical uses which goes beyond the describing of the acts, people, etc., judged, or the ascribing to them of properties, whether objective or subjective. This element, called by Stevenson the emotive meaning, does not necessarily exhaust the meaning (there may be descriptive elements as well), but it prevents any analysis in wholly descriptive terms. The emotive meaning of a moral term consists in its tendency to express or evince feelings or attitudes (e.g., of approval) that the speaker has, or to produce or evoke such attitudes in a hearer. One of the commonest and most time-wasting confusions in moral philosophy is to equate these non-descriptivist views with the subjectivist view (a form of naturalism; see above) that moral judgments are *statements that* the speaker as a matter of psychological or behavioral fact has such feelings or attitudes. Though both views are opposed to the objectivist kind of descriptivism, and are therefore sometimes loosely grouped together under the name "subjectivism", this wide use of the term is highly misleading, because it obscures the main division of ethical theories into descriptivist and non-descriptivist, and because it suggests that all types of non-descriptivist theory are open to the same objections as are subjectivist descriptivist theories; this is not so.

The mistake becomes even more serious when made about the form of non-descriptivism which has largely superseded emotivism. This is sometimes called prescriptivism. It holds that the peculiar element in value-judgments (of which moral judgments are a sub-class) which prevents their being wholly descriptive, is their prescriptivity, i.e., their action-guiding function. There are prescriptivist elements clearly detectable in the moral philosophies of Socrates, Plato,

Aristotle, and Kant, though overlaid by their predominant descriptivism. Some of the earlier emotivists, by comparing moral judgments with imperatives, adopted a form of prescriptivism (Carnap; Ayer, p. 160; Stevenson, p. 21). More recent writers, however (e.g., Hare, 1952, 1963) have departed in two important respects from emotivist views. First, they have insisted that prescriptive judgments (including imperatives) can function as premises or as conclusions in logical inferences; the term "emotive", which suggests irrationalism, is therefore inappropriate in characterizing the meaning of moral judgments, even if it has a prescriptive element. Secondly, they have claimed, in agreement with many other ethical writers who are not prescriptivists, that moral judgments are universal or at least universalizable. This feature, which they share with descriptive judgments, can be explained as follows: it is self-contradictory to make dissimilar moral judgments about two cases which one admits to be similar in all non-moral respects.

On these two features of prescriptivity and universalizability, it has been the hope of recent writers to found a theory of moral reasoning which would enable moral questions, such as those in bioethics, to be rationally discussed, and thus escape the imputation of irrationalism which attached to the earlier emotivists. Such a theory owes a great deal to Kant: we are to seek prescriptions which we can universalize; i.e., the "maxims of our actions" (Kant's phrase) are to be such as we are prepared to accept for identical cases in which we are at the receiving end. Such cases can be hypothetical ones (it is not necessary for there to be any likelihood that we shall actually find ourselves in the situations of our victims); all that is necessary is that we should prescribe as if we were to be the sufferers from the consequences of the actions prescribed. In the hypothetical case, the sufferer is to be supposed to have the same desires as the present victim has, not as the present agent has; therefore objections of the sort "If it were done to me I would not mind" are ill-taken.

Such a theory of moral reasoning leads naturally to the requirement of impartiality in moral judgment, i.e., the requirement to treat the equal interests of every affected party as of equal weight. It thus leads, in spite of its Kantian connections, to a form of utilitarianism; for if one gives equal weight to the equal interests of each party, one will be led to maximize the satisfaction of those interests, taken as a whole. The theory also has affinities with the Christian (and indeed pre-Christian) Golden Rule that we should do to others as we wish them to do to us sc. in precisely similar situations (Hillel, Babylonian Talmud, *Sabbath*, 31a; Matthew 7:12; see also Tobias 4:16).

It also has links with the so-called rational-contractor theory, which holds that we should adopt those principles which would be agreed to by a set of self-interested parties who were without knowledge of their roles in the society to be governed by the principles (Rawls; Richards; both, however, attempt to draw non-utilitarian conclusions from their theories). It also has affinities with the so-called ideal-observer theory, which holds that we should adopt those principles which would be prescribed by an impartially benevolent spectator who knew all the facts (Haslett). In Christian morality God often serves as this ideal prescriber. Most of these theories are, however, propounded by descriptivists (for an interesting reference to the possibility of formal analogies between descriptivist and non-descriptivist theories in their approaches to actual moral issues, see Richards, p. 85).

All these theories have considerable bite when discussing questions in bioethics. For example, questions about the legitimacy of euthanasia can be handled as follows: if, in a particular case, we can determine that to kill the patient would be, in sum, most in the interests of all affected parties, including his own, then it is legitimate. However, if it could be shown that a law, or even a rule of medical ethics, permitting this would (as it well might) lead in practice to abuses (i.e., to the use of euthanasia in many cases where the conditions for its legitimacy were not in fact realized), then the law or rule ought not to be adopted. This would be especially important if cases in which euthanasia would be justified (i.e., in which there was no way of doing better for the interests of the parties) are rare, as is plausibly claimed. These two arguments (which, though contrary in tendency, are not actually inconsistent) lead together to the conclusion that euthanasia is sometimes morally right but that it would be morally wrong to make it legal (a combination of views actually held by many medical men). If such a conclusion can be shown to be in accord with the Golden Rule (as it probably can), it should be of interest to Christian moralists (Hare, 1975).

R. M. HARE

[*While all the articles in this entry are relevant, see especially the articles* UTILITARIANISM *and* NATURALISM.]

BIBLIOGRAPHY

AYER, A. J. *Language, Truth and Logic.* London: V. Gollancz, 1936, chap. 6.

BERKELEY, GEORGE. *A Treatise Concerning the Principles of Human Knowledge* (1710). Introduction, sec. 20.

CARNAP, RUDOLPH. *Philosophy and Logical Syntax.* London: Kegan Paul, Trench, Trubner & Co., Psyche Miniatures, 1935. Partial reprint. *The Age of Analysis.* The Great Ages of Western Philosophy, no. 6. Edited by M. White. Boston: Houghton Mifflin, 1955, pp. 209–225.

HÄGERSTRÖM, AXEL, "Kritiska Punkter i Värdepsykologien." [Critical Points in the Psychology of Value] *Festskrift tillägnad E. O. Burman.* Uppsala: K. W. Appelbergs Boktryckeri, 1910, pp. 16–75. For references and summary, see his *Philosophy and Religion.* Translated by Robert T. Sandin. London: G. Allen & Unwin, 1964, p. 315.

HARE, R. M. "Ethical Theory and Utilitarianism." *Contemporary British Philosophy.* 4th sers. Edited by H. D. Lewis. The Muirhead Library of Philosophy. London: George Allen & Unwin, 1976.

————. "Euthanasia: A Christian View." *Philosophic Exchange* 2, no. 1 (1975), pp. 43–52.

————. *Freedom and Reason.* Oxford: Clarendon Press, 1963.

————. *The Language of Morals.* Oxford: Clarendon Press, 1952.

————. *Practical Inferences.* London: Macmillan & Co., 1971. Bibliography.

HASLETT, D. W. *Moral Rightness.* The Hague: Martinus Nijhoff, 1974.

HUME, DAVID. *Treatise of Human Nature* (1738). Bk. 3 pt. 1, sec. 1.

KANT, IMMANUEL. *Grundlegung zur Metaphysik der Sitten* (1785). Translated by Lewis White Beck as *Foundations of the Metaphysics of Morals.* Indianapolis, Ind.: Bobbs-Merrill, 1956.

MILL, J. S. *A System of Logic* (1843). Bk. 6, chap. 12.

MOORE, G. E. *Principia Ethica.* Cambridge: At the University Press, 1903.

OGDEN, C. K., and RICHARDS, I. A. *The Meaning of Meaning.* London: Kegan Paul, Trench, Trubner & Co.; New York: Harcourt, Brace & Co., 1923, chap. 6, p. 125.

PROTAGORAS. "Protagoras." *Die Fragmente der Vorsokratiker, griechisch und deutsch.* Edited by Hermann Diels. Berlin: Weidmannsche Verlagsbuchhandlung, 1951–1952, vol. 2, pp. 253–271. Also in Philip Wheelwright. *The Presocratics.* New York: Odyssey Press, 1966, pp. 239–248.

RAWLS, JOHN. *A Theory of Justice.* Cambridge: Harvard University Press, 1971.

REICHENBACH, HANS. *The Rise of Scientific Philosophy.* Berkeley: University of California Press, 1951.

RICHARDS, D. A. J. *A Theory of Reasons for Action.* Oxford: Clarendon Press, 1971.

STEVENSON, CHARLES L. *Ethics and Language.* New Haven: Yale University Press, 1944.

URMSON, J. O. *The Emotive Theory of Ethics.* London: Hutchinson, 1968. Bibliography.

XI
MORAL REASONING

What is moral reasoning? Reasoning is the process by which one arrives at a conclusion from premises, and in moral reasoning one arrives at a moral conclusion. It may contain the word "moral" or its cognates, or an expression such as "virtue" or "good action" that is normally understood in a moral sense. But no vocabulary peculiar to ethics is required; one may merely say that something should be, or ought to be done, implying that it is for moral reasons that this is so. A moral conclusion is a moral judgment, however expressed.

To describe moral reasoning we must find the premises from which moral conclusions can be derived, and one way of seeing the task is as that of finding criteria for the application of the concepts used in moral judgment. In moral reasoning we use the criteria; in moral philosophy we search them out. Thus, when Plato asked about the nature of justice, or courage, or temperance, he insisted that we needed this knowledge if we were to argue correctly about the morality of something that was done, and much of the history of ethics is about discussions of this kind. Kant, for instance, proposed that we test the moral permissibility of an action by considering whether the principle under which it fell could be willed as a universal law. And Bentham and his Utilitarian followers thought that an action could be shown to be right by showing that it tended to produce the greatest happiness of the greatest number. For reasons that will be mentioned later many philosophers of the present century have abandoned the search for such criteria of morality; nevertheless John Rawls's *Theory of Justice*, one of the most important and interesting of contemporary books on ethics, is precisely concerned with the criteria by which institutions and actions may be judged to be just.

So far nothing has been said to show why there should be any special difficulty about describing moral reasoning or why, indeed, moral reasoning should be any different from reasoning about any other subject. Obviously there are difficult concepts involved, but there are many elusive concepts outside of ethics, as, for instance, that of *metaphor* or *tragedy* or *intelligence* or *genius*. Why is the problem of moral reasoning different from the problem of reasoning elsewhere?

Undoubtedly there is a special difficulty about

moral reasoning, and it comes from the fact that in some sense or other (and the interpretation is a matter of controversy) moral reasoning is practical reasoning: it is reasoning about what to do. David Hume made the minimal claim when he said that morals excite passions and produce or prevent actions, and insisted that our theory of moral reasoning must take this into account. He himself went farther, demanding a quite general connection between moral judgment and the will; but the mere fact that men ever do something because they think it right to do so is enough to create problems for certain philosophers. For some have had theories of the psychology of human action by which the search for pleasure and the avoidance of pain is the only motive on which anyone can act. Bentham, for instance, believed this and had to reconcile it with the fact that moral action is possible. It was public interest that determined morality but private interest that determined what was done. Reasoning about what was right and good was reasoning about the general happiness; reasoning about what to do was about one's own pleasure and pain. No one could be influenced by moral considerations unless public and private interest seemed to coincide, and no one ever acted morally except for the sake of gaining pleasure or avoiding pain. Bentham accepted both conclusions. For Kant, however, the problem was more acute. He insisted that only action done for the sake of duty had true moral worth, while no action was done for the sake of duty if done purely to satisfy the agent's desire. How could there be actions not determined by the usual causality of desire? This is not the place to discuss Kant's solution; his problem is mentioned to show that even on the minimal interpretation of the dictum that moral reasoning is practical some philosophers find themselves in trouble. They ask, "How is moral action possible at all?"

For most, however, the problem arises only upon a different understanding of the practical nature of moral judgment and hence of moral reasoning; it is not just that men sometimes do what they think they ought to do, but that there is a general, or even universal, connection between moral judgment and conduct. How close a connection should we see? Some, following Plato, go so far as to deny that anyone ever sees that he ought to do one thing and then deliberately does something else. No one, they say, ever really sees the better and chooses the worse.

So if, in what looks like moral reasoning, he seems to draw the conclusion that he should do a thing, but does not choose to do it, the conclusion has not really been drawn. One may, however, insist that the phenomenon called (somewhat misleadingly) "weakness of will" does exist, that people may be fully aware that they should do a thing but have no intention of doing it. Taking this line, one will say that moral judgment and action are not quite as closely tied together as some have thought and will allow the possibility of reasoning to a moral conclusion without the accompanying action or intention.

Whether or not this is to be called "practical reasoning" is another matter. There is a tradition that follows Aristotle in insisting that the conclusion of a piece of practical reasoning is an action, and it would be possible to adopt this terminology whatever one said about the problem of "weakness of will." It will be more natural, however, to say that moral reasoning may be to a conclusion not accompanied by action (or intention) if one is satisfied that a moral judgment may on occasion be like this.

In what sense then is moral reasoning practical reasoning, if not in the sense that it leads to a conclusion that is necessarily accompanied by a choice? The answer seems to lie in the idea that certain considerations give reasons for acting, and that the premises from which a moral conclusion follows must be premises of this kind. In moral reasoning we argue that something should or should not be done, and if it should be done this implies that there are reasons for doing it. This account has the advantage of applying directly to reasoning about other people's action as well as one's own.

Practical reasoning that meets these conditions is something extremely familiar in everyday life. A doctor starts, for instance, with the objective of curing his patient and reasons that it will be necessary to get his blood pressure down. Further he calculates that the administration of a certain drug will have this effect. He reasons, in other words, about the necessary conditions and the sufficient conditions (the lowering of the blood pressure necessary for the cure; the taking of the drug sufficient for the lowering of the blood pressure) until he comes to something that is within his power, such as the administration of the drug. This is something he can do, and it is seen as the first link in a chain leading to the desired end. The starting point is, as Aristotle says, "*to orekton*," something wanted, and the reasoning is with a view to achieving the desired thing, which may be, but is not necessarily, external to what is to be done. So the doctor might reason about how to cure the patient or about how to act in accordance with his wishes.

Similarly, it might be supposed, moral reasoning has as its starting point something wanted; either an end stated in terms that are already moral, such as to be just, to do morally good actions, or perhaps an end such as the relief of suffering or the preservation of the dignity of human life. The problem about moral reasoning, seen as a form of practical reasoning, lies in the status of these ends. For suppose that a certain individual does not have them? How, then, shall we be able to proceed by practical reasoning to the conclusion that he should, for example, refrain from killing or injuring others, or should help those in need? We have a very strong desire to say that we can always draw this conclusion, if only because "should" and "should not" are instruments of social pressure, and we want to bring pressure against *anyone* who acts in an antisocial way. What is more, we should like to be able to say that each and every man *has reason* to be moral whatever his particular ends may be.

It is not surprising, therefore, that there should have been many attempts to show that there are ends which everyone must have and to use these as the starting point for practical moral reasoning. Can it not be said, for instance, that we necessarily desire our own happiness, and may it not be possible to show that therefore we should live a virtuous life? Plato's *Republic* contains one of the most famous examples of a theory of this type. It is argued that, although just actions apparently benefit others and are to the disadvantage of the just man, nevertheless the way to be happy is to be just. Some have elaborated such theories, but others have rejected them out of hand. For one thing it is really very difficult to show that an unjust action could never be advantageous. And in any case it has seemed to many that no one who wants to be just in order to be happy is truly moral.

Kant put forward this latter point of view in an extreme form, insisting that a moral judgment is a categorical imperative, not one telling us how to achieve the end of happiness, or any other that we might happen to have. Kant's own

solution was complex, and it is hard to interpret at certain points. But it consisted essentially in equating moral action with rational action, not because in acting morally a man did what was likely to get him what he wanted, but because moral action was action determined merely by the principle of universalizability and therefore (Kant said) by the faculty of reason.

Most philosophers agree that neither Plato nor Kant was successful in solving the problem. How can we represent moral reasoning as practical and also universally applicable?

At present the answer most often given is one that derives from Hume's moral philosophy. Hume's answer to his own question about how we can guarantee a connection between moral judgment and the will lay in his theory of moral sentiment. He distinguished, on the one hand, judgments of fact (which he called conclusions of reason) and, on the other, sentiments or feelings (which he called passions). Conclusions of reason were, in themselves, inert; only in conjunction with a passion could they produce or prevent action. Moral judgments were expressions corresponding to sentiments; to judge an action virtuous was (at least in one rather simple version of Hume's theory) to say that one felt a pleasing sentiment of approbation when it was contemplated; and there seemed to be no difficulty in seeing why we should do the actions that pleased us thus. The connection between moral judgment and the will had, let us suppose, been taken care of. What had become of reasoning to a conclusion about what was right and wrong?

The answer is that a gap had appeared between the facts from which moral reasoning may be supposed to proceed and the conclusion to which it led. On the one hand, there is the contemplation of the facts and reasoning about them, on the other, a moral sentiment, and between the two there is a gap: Hume's famous gap between "is" and "ought." There is some disagreement about the interpretation of Hume's theory at this point; some say that the gap only consists in this: that *deductive* reasoning cannot join the two. (In other words, one will never be forced on pain of contradiction to move from premises to conclusion.) But one may doubt whether any form of reasoning is possible from "is" to "ought" if there are not even rules of evidence linking the two. And Hume does not suggest that there are; he thought that as a matter of fact sentiments of approbation were felt toward what was "useful or agreeable to ourselves or others," but he did not suggest that any other connection linked the two.

An even more thoroughgoing version of this theory was worked out in the thirties and forties of the present century, under the influence of logical positivism, but having as its adherents many who would not count themselves as logical positivists. C. L. Stevenson, who did more work on this than anyone else, argued in *Ethics and Language* that moral language expresses attitudes and that there is no logical connection between a man's attitudes and his beliefs. The connection between beliefs and attitudes is merely causal, and there is no reason why a given set of "premises" may not bring one individual to one "conclusion" and another to another conclusion. In fact there is no limit—except that imposed by the requirement that attitudes be consistent—to the moral judgments that may be "derived" from a given set of facts. Stevenson talks about moral "arguments" and "rational methods" of trying to resolve moral disputes, but it is not clear that such descriptions are warranted. When A. J. Ayer, who had put forward a similar view, said that in his opinion there was argument about facts but not about moral values, he was perhaps representing the position more accurately.

A similar doubt as to whether argument from fact to value is left standing can be raised about the imperativist theory of R. M. Hare. He too denies that there are rules of evidence linking facts to moral judgment, except those requiring not only consistency but also that moral judgments shall ultimately concern kinds of facts, not individuals or individual occasions. Within these limits one may make any moral valuations one chooses, and in fact Hare stresses the element of decision in adopting principles after rehearsing the facts. He speaks of the decisions as being "based on" the facts, but again the description may be challenged. On this theory it does not seem to be here that one finds something properly called moral reasoning, but rather in the reasoning from one moral imperative to another. The latter is of course an important kind of reasoning, whose rules have been developed by Hare himself. But so far as the original problem of practical reasoning is concerned one may say that it has been banished rather than solved.

The correct theory of moral reasoning is thus a matter of current controversy. Will our actual moral reasoning necessarily be affected by these uncertainties? The answer seems to be that sometimes it will not be affected. So long as certain ends are taken for granted, we can proceed as if the theoretical difficulties about the foundations of moral reasoning did not exist. Aristotle points to this kind of case when he says that a doctor does not deliberate about whether to cure his patient; he takes the end for granted and asks how it may be achieved. But Aristotle's example raises for us the difficulties that can so often be put aside. Debating the moral issues of euthanasia we ask whether a doctor must always try to cure his patient and, if not, when he should give up this end, and whether he should ever actually seek the patient's death. Can the philosophers help us here? Obviously they can so far as what is wanted is a clarification of ideas such as that of passive and active euthanasia; but when the question touches problems about the ultimate starting point of moral reasoning the area of uncertainty and controversy is reached.

PHILIPPA FOOT

[*While all the articles in this entry are relevant, see especially the articles* THE TASK OF ETHICS, RULES AND PRINCIPLES, NON-DESCRIPTIVISM, *and* RELATIVISM. *See also:* DEATH AND DYING: EUTHANASIA AND SUSTAINING LIFE, *article on* ETHICAL VIEWS.]

BIBLIOGRAPHY

ANSCOMBE, G. E. M. *Intention.* 2d ed., Oxford: Basil Blackwell, 1963. See sections 33–44.

———. "Thought and Action in Aristotle." *New Essays on Plato and Aristotle.* Edited by R. Bambrough. London: Routledge & Kegal Paul, 1965.

ARISTOTLE. *Nicomachean Ethics.* Translated by Martin Ostwald. Indianapolis: Bobbs-Merrill Co., 1962.

AYER, A. J. *Language, Truth and Logic.* 2d ed. London: Victor Gollancz, 1947. See Chapter VI, pp. 102–120.

BENTHAM, JEREMY. *An Introduction to the Principles of Morals and Legislation* (1780). New York: Humanities Press, 1970.

GEACH, P. T. "Dr. Kenny on Practical Inference." *Analysis,* January 1966, pp. 76–79.

HARE, R. M. *Freedom and Reason.* Oxford: Oxford University Press, 1963.

———. *The Language of Morals.* Oxford: Oxford University Press, 1952.

———. *Practical Inferences.* London: Macmillan, 1971. See pp. 69–73.

HUME, DAVID. *A Treatise of Human Nature* (1739). Oxford: Oxford University Press, 1941.

KANT, IMMANUEL. *Critique of Practical Reason* (1788). Translated by Lewis White Beck. Indianapolis: Bobbs-Merrill, 1956.

————. *Foundations of the Metaphysic of Morals* (1785). Translated by Lewis White Beck. Indianapolis: Bobbs-Merrill, 1959.

KENNY, A. J. "Practical Inference." *Analysis* 26 (1966): 65–75.

MACINTYRE, ALASDAIR C. "Hume on 'Is' and 'Ought'." *Against the Self-Images of the Age.* New York: Schocken Books, 1971, pp. 109–124.

PLATO. *Republic.*

RAWLS, JOHN. *A Theory of Justice.* New York: Oxford University Press, 1972. Cambridge: Belknap Press of Harvard University Press, 1971.

STEVENSON, CHARLES L. *Ethics and Language.* New Haven: Yale University Press, 1944.

THOMSON, JUDITH J. and DWORKIN, GERALD, eds. *Ethics.* New York: Harper & Row, 1968.

WALLACE, G., and WALKER, A. D. *The Definition of Morality.* London: Methuen & Co., 1970.

XII
RELATIVISM

The expression "ethical relativism" refers to a number of diverse theories, each of which asserts that something ethical is relative to something else, for example that what one ought to do is relative to the mores of one's society or that one's values are relative to one's personality. There are many versions of ethical relativism, not all of equal importance for bioethics. Some, such as cultural relativism, threaten the truth of any objective bioethics and the legitimacy of any innovative medical practice. Others, such as situation ethics, maintain ethical absolutism in our changing world. One version differs from another either in what it asserts to be relative or in that to which it takes it to be relative. In all versions, however, to assert that one thing is relative to another is to assert that the former varies with and depends upon the latter.

It is helpful to distinguish between ethical relativism and ethical nihilism. While the relativist asserts that something ethical is relative, the nihilist denies its very existence or reality. Reflecting upon the fact that an act practiced with approval in one society is condemned in another, the relativist concludes that right and wrong are relative to culture, and the nihilist concludes that there really is no difference between right and wrong. Confronted with ethical disagreement among different sorts of individuals, the relativist asserts that the truth of any ethical statement is relative to the personality of the speaker, while the nihilist denies that ethical sentences have any truth-value at all.

Any version of ethical relativism can most fruitfully be classified according to the status of its central thesis. If the thesis is a factual statement, the theory is an instance of descriptive relativism. If the thesis is an ethical statement, a judgment of value or obligation, it is a normative relativism. If the thesis is an epistemological claim, i.e., a statement about our ethical knowledge, pertaining to the meaning of ethical statements or the validity of ethical arguments, it is a metaethical relativism.

Descriptive relativism

Any ethical relativism in which the central thesis simply asserts that as a matter of fact something ethical varies with and depends upon something else is a descriptive relativism. The two most important species of descriptive relativism are cultural and psychological. A cultural relativism asserts that something ethical (such as the mores, the institutions creating rights and duties, the human goals or ends, and the moral concepts or ethical judgments) is relative to culture. Psychological relativism asserts that something ethical (such as goals, evaluations, or conscience) is relative to the psychology of the individual.

In its Statement on Human Rights, the Executive Board of the American Anthropological Association asserted in 1947 that "standards and values are relative to the culture from which they derive" (Executive Board, p. 542). This assertion is far from unambiguous. If it means that one is morally bound only by the standards of one's own society and that what is good in one society may be evil in another, then it is a version of normative relativism. If, on the other hand, it means to assert that in point of fact the moral standards accepted by one society and the goals valued by any people vary with and are causally determined by the culture of that society or people, it is a version of descriptive relativism. Since the Executive Board clearly takes this assertion to be established by the sciences of anthropology and social psychology, the latter interpretation is the more plausible.

The Executive Board argues that this cultural relativism poses an awkward dilemma for any contemporary declaration of human rights (ibid., pp. 542–543). If the declaration affirms the moral standards and human aspirations of Western cultures, it will be inapplicable to the many non-Western societies with their very different standards and values. But given the cultural variation in standards and values, there is no universal code of human rights that could be asserted by all men and applied to all societies. What status, then, is one to assign to article 25 of the United Nations' Universal Declaration of Human Rights, which affirms the right of every human being to medical care, or to the Declaration of Helsinki, which proclaims the right of all persons to be subjected to potentially dangerous clinical research only after free informed consent? Are these declarations morally applicable to medical practice and public health programs throughout our world, or are they merely ethnocentric expressions of our provincial biases?

Another version of descriptive relativism is the theory that the individual's values, in the sense of goals and evaluations, are relative to his or her personality. A timid person will shun danger and consider it a great evil, but a more adventurous individual will discount risk and even value it as a source of excitement. Similarly, the importance an individual attaches to sexual satisfaction will vary with and depend upon the strength of his or her sex drive. Since this version of psychological relativism simply asserts an empirical fact about the individual, it is a descriptive relativism.

This descriptive relativism may, however, have important implications for bioethics, specifically for the moral justification of medical advice. When a physician or surgeon advises a patient, the advice typically does not limit itself to factual information about the available procedures and the probable outcomes of each. Medical advice is most helpful to the patient when it includes some judgment of what would be best for the patient in the light of all this complex technical information. But evaluations, including judgments of which course of action is best, are supposed to be relative to the personality of the individual. Presumably, then, a somewhat timid physician or surgeon will be less inclined to advise risky procedures and a more adventurous doctor will evaluate potentially dangerous treatments more favorably. The patient, however, will probably have a rather different personality and, accordingly, a different set of values from that of the doctor. Since it is the patient's life and health that are at stake, it is the patient's values and not the doctor's that determine the ethical propriety of the advice. How, then, is it morally justifiable for one individual, the physician or surgeon, to give medical advice to another individual, the patient?

Normative relativism

When the central thesis of some version of ethical relativism is an ethical statement, rather than a factual statement, it is a version of normative, rather than descriptive, relativism. Once more, the most important varieties are either cultural or psychological, but some interesting versions fall into neither of those two classes.

It is often claimed that right and wrong are relative to culture, that the very same kind of act is right in one society and wrong in another because of the different mores of the two societies. Since this claim goes beyond describing the facts about what people believe right and wrong in order to take a stand on which acts really are right and wrong, it is a normative relativism. If true, this version of cultural relativism is important for bioethics in at least two ways. First, many medical acts are of the kinds forbidden, permitted, or required by the mores of many societies. Some societies harshly condemn the mutilation of corpses, an act involved in the harvesting of cadaver organs for transplant, while other societies permit such actions. Similar prohibitions and permissions apply to the acts of abortion, infanticide, and euthanasia. It makes all the difference in the world to the moral status of such acts whether their rightness or wrongness is relative to culture or somehow independent of the mores of the agent's society. Second, the explosion of knowledge in the life sciences and the application of this new knowledge to medicine have inevitably led to great innovation in medical practice. But new practices, such as organ transplantation or artificial insemination, often deviate dramatically from traditional culture and established custom. Are we to conclude that new medical procedures are morally justifiable only so long as they remain within the bounds of custom, or is there some moral standard independent of the mores by which medical innovation can be morally justified?

A second version of normative relativism is the theory that values are relative to the desires, preferences, or interests of the individual (Perry, pp. 115–116). Notice that this theory differs from the previous one in two ways. What is declared to be relative is values rather than obligations, and that to which they are held to be relative is the psychology of the individual rather than culture. The word "values" in this theory means "things that have value or disvalue," not "goals or evaluations." This change in the meaning of the word "values" is crucial, for it distinguishes the normative relativism of this section from the descriptive relativism of the previous section. This theory denies that anything can be good or bad in itself and asserts that everything of value is good or bad *for* some individual. It goes on to assert that what makes anything good or bad for someone is that individual's desires, preferences, or interests. Bioethics often presupposes that medical treatment is morally justified only if it is beneficial for the patient. But if this version of ethical relativism is true, there can be no universal rule on such matters; one must ask for whom the treatment is to be beneficial. The act of taking out one kidney for transplant may be beneficial for the altruistic person who cares more deeply about the welfare of a loved one than about his or her own health, but harmful for the individual who prefers his or her own health to the life of another. Similarly, the relative value of length of life as compared with the quality of life may depend upon the desires of the individual patient. If so, there can be nothing like *the* moral solution to the ethical problems of organ transplantation or euthanasia; such problems must be solved anew in the case of each patient.

A third version of normative relativism, and one that is neither cultural nor psychological, is situation ethics. The central thesis of this theory is that obligation is relative to the situation in which the agent is acting, that what one ought to do varies with and depends upon the circumstances (Fletcher, p. 65). Thus the very same kind of act, for example an act of euthanasia, may be right in one situation (where a terminally ill patient is in pain too intense to be allayed and has begged for release) but wrong in another situation (where the pain can be reduced considerably by medication and the patient is psychologically prepared to go on living). Situation ethics stands opposed to ethical legalism, the view that there is a set of moral rules specifying which kinds of action are always right and which kinds are always wrong. Situation ethics tends to emphasize the differences between cases and to make it easier to justify untraditional conduct in changing circumstances; ethical legalism tends to emphasize the similarities between acts and to insist that exceptional circumstances do not justify exceptions to accepted moral standards. That these opposed approaches to bioethics do frequently lead to different conclusions is illustrated by the recent literature dealing with issues such as euthanasia, abortion, organ transplants, and genetic engineering.

Metaethical relativism

Any ethical relativism in which the central thesis is an epistemological claim about (i.e., a statement about our knowledge of) ethical statements or ethical arguments is metaethical. One version of metaethical relativism is the view that the meaning of the expressions "normal" and "abnormal" as used in clinical psychology is relative to culture. This is an ethical relativism because the expressions "normal" and "abnormal" are ethical words used to brand some person or action as socially acceptable or unacceptable; it is a *meta*ethical relativism because its central thesis is an epistemological claim about the meaning of these ethical words. Ruth Benedict has argued that every society has its distinctive pattern of culture in which certain values are selected and emphasized while other possible objects, acts, and personalities are devalued or even excluded. She gives many illustrations of the way in which a personality type or mode of conduct is judged normal or abnormal to the degree that it does or does not fit into the accepted pattern of culture. She concludes that "normality is culturally defined" (Benedict, p. 72). The relevance of this metaethical relativism to medical ethics is obvious. A diagnosis of mental illness is often made on the basis of a judgment of psychological abnormality, and the goal of psychotherapy is typically to restore the patient to normality. But is the diagnosis of mental illness more than an expression of the cultural bias of the psychologist? And what is the moral justification for attempting to get the patient to conform to a cultural pattern that may be alien to him or her? Both the way in which one conceives of mental illness and the stand one takes on the morality of psychotherapy will hinge upon whether one accepts or rejects this version of metaethical relativism.

Conclusion

It is of considerable importance to distinguish carefully among descriptive, normative, and metaethical relativisms, because the evidence for or against each is so very different. Since descriptive relativisms make purely factual assertions, they can presumably be shown to be true or false by scientific investigation. Since normative relativisms assert something about value or obligation, they can be established or refuted only by the very different methods of ethics. Since metaethical relativisms make claims about meaning, truth, or reasoning, they are to be accepted or rejected on the basis of epistemological considerations. Only by sorting out the various kinds of ethical relativism is there any hope of distinguishing the true versions from the false ones.

Although the three kinds of ethical relativism are very different, they are not unrelated. One version of ethical relativism often serves as a premise in an argument to support some other version. For example, the mores of any society vary with and are dependent upon the culture of that society (descriptive relativism); it is the mores of the agent's society that make an act right or wrong; therefore, right and wrong are relative to culture (normative relativism). The logic of the argument is cogent, but the truth of its premises can, and should, be questioned. Some anthropologists and social psychologists have challenged this descriptive relativism by presenting empirical evidence that there are some cultural and psychological universals, e.g., the values of loyalty or love and the taboo against incest. Many philosophers deny that the mores are the standard of right and wrong on the grounds that we condemn some mores as unjust or inhumane. The proper conclusion to draw after critically assessing the many arguments for and against the various kinds of ethical relativism is not The Truth about Ethical Relativism, but many truths about the several versions of ethical relativism.

CARL WELLMAN

[While all the articles in this entry are relevant, see especially the articles RULES AND PRINCIPLES, OBJECTIVISM IN ETHICS, and MORAL REASONING. For further discussion of topics mentioned in this article, see the entries: RIGHTS; and RISK. Also directly related are the entries HUMAN EXPERIMENTATION; MEDICINE, ANTHROPOLOGY OF; MENTAL HEALTH; MENTAL ILLNESS; and THERAPEUTIC RELATIONSHIP. See also: HEALTH CARE, articles on RIGHT TO HEALTH-CARE SERVICES and THEORIES OF JUSTICE AND HEALTH CARE; and LIFE.]

BIBLIOGRAPHY

BENEDICT, RUTH (FULTON). "Anthropology and the Abnormal." *Journal of General Psychology* 10 (1934): 59–82.

BRANDT, RICHARD B. *Ethical Theory.* Englewood Cliffs, N.J.: Prentice-Hall, 1959, pp. 83–150, 271–294.

Executive Board, American Anthropological Association. "Statement on Human Rights: Submitted to the Commission on Human Rights, United Nations." *American Anthropologist* n.s. 49 (1947): 539–543.

FLETCHER, JOSEPH FRANCIS. *Situation Ethics: The New Morality.* Philadelphia: Westminster Press, 1966.

HERSKOVITS, MELVILLE JEAN. *Man and His Works.* New York: Alfred Knopf, 1948, pp. 61–78.

LADD, JOHN. *Ethical Relativism.* Belmont, Calif.: Wadsworth, 1973.

MACBEATH, ALEXANDER. *Experiments in Living.* London: Macmillan, 1952.

MOSER, SHIA. *Absolutism and Relativism in Ethics.* Springfield, Ill.: Charles C. Thomas, 1968.

PERRY, RALPH BARTON. *General Theory of Value.* New York: Longmans, Green & Co., 1926; Cambridge: Harvard University Press, 1954, pp. 115–145.

WELLMAN, CARL. "The Ethical Implications of Cultural Relativity." *Journal of Philosophy* 60 (1963): 169–184.

WESTERMARCK, EDVARD ALEXANDER. *Ethical Relativity.* London: Kegan Paul, Trench, Trubner & Co., 1932.

ETHICS COMMITTEES

See DEATH AND DYING: EUTHANASIA AND SUSTAINING LIFE, *article on* PROFESSIONAL AND PUBLIC POLICIES; INFANTS, *articles on* PUBLIC POLICY AND PROCEDURAL QUESTIONS *and* ETHICAL PERSPECTIVES ON THE CARE OF INFANTS; RESEARCH POLICY, BIOMEDICAL; HUMAN EXPERIMENTATION, *article on* SOCIAL AND PROFESSIONAL CONTROL.

EUGENICS

I. HISTORY   *Kenneth M. Ludmerer*
II. ETHICAL ISSUES   *Marc Lappé*

I
HISTORY

"Eugenics" is a term with several connotations. Literally meaning "well-born," the term at different times has meant different things: a science that investigates methods to ameliorate the genetic composition of the human race; a program to foster such betterment; a social movement; and, in its perverted form, a pseudo-scientific retreat for bigots and racists.

Background and origins

Although the idea of improving the hereditary quality of the race is at least as old as Plato's *Republic*, modern eugenic thought arose only in the nineteenth century. The emergence of interest in eugenics during that century had multiple roots. The most important was the theory of evolution, for Francis Galton's ideas on eugenics—and it was he who created the term "eugenics"—were a direct logical outgrowth of the scientific doctrine elaborated by his cousin Charles Darwin. Galton advanced his ideas, moreover, just when it was becoming current to apply the doctrine of evolution to nonbiological situations. He developed his views during the period when evolutionary theory was exerting its greatest impact upon intellectual thought, having flavored doctrines known as "naturalism" and "Social Darwinism." These doctrines encompassed a group of ideas, the most important of which were the analogy between biological organisms and social systems, the conviction that scientific research represented the most accurate approach to knowledge, and the appeal to scientific method for solutions to social problems. Social Darwinists also tended to equate a person's genetic "fitness" with his social position and popularized the catchwords "survival of the fittest" and "struggle for existence."

However, other factors were also important in the growing interest in eugenics. One in particular was the philosophical belief, inherited from certain eighteenth-century thinkers, in the notion of human perfectibility. Another was the rising fear, which coexisted with this faith in progress, that the quality of the American stock was deteriorating. According to this view, the "unfit" in civilized societies constituted a major menace; they were surviving in increasing numbers because of modern medicine and charity, and they were procreating far more rapidly than the "fit," thereby diluting the concentration of valuable hereditary characteristics in the population.

Despite those factors favoring an interest in eugenics, an organized eugenics movement did not occur in the United States or elsewhere before 1900. The principal reason was ignorance regarding the process of heredity. The physical basis of heredity was still unknown; chromosomes were not found in the nucleus until the 1880s, and only after 1900 were they shown to be carriers of genes. Furthermore, no rule was known to govern the transmission of traits from one generation to the next; the only formula biologists could follow was the broad theory used by breeders that "like produces like" and the assumption that all traits result from a "blend" of parental characteristics. Finally, popular belief in the inheritance of acquired characteristics vitiated the supposed need for eugenic proposals, since this theory contradicted the idea that improvements in the hereditary composition of man could occur only from breeding programs.

The birth of modern genetics in 1900 enabled earlier interest in eugenics to be mobilized into an organized movement. Mendel's law provided an explanatory framework in terms of which the transmission and distribution of traits from one generation to the next could be understood, thereby permitting eugenic proposals to be conceived on a heretofore impossible scale. Eugenic breeding programs now became widely appealing because at last they could be based upon biological theory rather than upon the imprecise rules used by breeders. Other early developments in genetics stimulated further interest in eugenics: the emergence of a belief that most traits are determined by single genes acting independently, and the popularization after 1900 of the work of August Weismann, who disproved the Lamarckian theory that acquired characteristics can be inherited.

The eugenics movement; positive and negative eugenics

The potential applicability of the science of genetics to social problems was recognized almost immediately. Organizations focusing on eugenics were created around the world: in England, the United States, Germany, Scandinavia, Italy, Austria, France, Japan, and South America. The eugenic societies in each country exhibited some national differences, but all were committed to the popularization of genetic science, demanding that social legislation be directed by what they judged to be biological wisdom. The center of this trend was the American eugenics movement, whose national headquarters was at the Eugenics Record Office at Cold Spring Harbor, Long Island, and whose acknowledged leader was the geneticist Charles B. Davenport. Unless otherwise specified, the remainder of this discussion will refer to eugenics in America.

From approximately 1905 to the early 1930s, eugenicists in the United States presented a two-part policy to improve the hereditary level of the American people. One part they called "negative eugenics," the elimination of unwanted characteristics from the nation by discouraging "unworthy" parenthood. Through specific devices—including marriage restriction, sterilization, and permanent custody of defectives—eugenicists hoped to stop the breeding of people whose physical disabilities or behavioral characteristics they thought to be genetically determined. Such hereditary "degenerates" included epileptics, criminals, alcoholics, prostitutes, paupers, the feebleminded, and the insane. The second part of eugenic policy was "positive eugenics," the striving to increase wanted traits in the population by urging "worthy" parenthood. Since eugenicists recognized that the social and technical difficulties facing positive eugenics were enormous, most of them recommended only that the public be educated about the "facts" of heredity to encourage "superior" couples to respond voluntarily to the plea to have more children.

At the turn of the century the movement attracted a diverse group of individuals. Eugenicists came in largest numbers from the native-born, Anglo-Saxon, Protestant, upper middle class and formed part of that generation's educators, scientists, scholars, journalists, physicians, lawyers, and clergy. They lived in all sections of the country and in both urban and rural areas. It is notable that until around 1915 many of the most enthusiastic members of the movement were geneticists. It is also notable that some eugenicists were racists who claimed a scientific sanctuary in eugenics for their bigotry. After the First World War leadership of the movement fell predominantly into the hands of such persons, the most famous of whom was the New York socialite Madison Grant.

Early in the century eugenic programs seemed feasible in light of the scientific knowledge of the day. By the First World War, however, additional developments in genetic science had cast doubts upon the scientific merit of eugenic proposals. A number of investigations showed that environment as well as heredity significantly influences human development; other studies demonstrated that many characteristics are produced by multiple genes interacting rather than by single genes acting independently as previously supposed. Moreover, early studies in statistical genetics showed that the process of reducing the frequency of a gene in a population by breeding programs would require a prohibitively long period, not the short time that eugenicists had assumed. Taken as a whole, these developments demonstrated that the process of inheritance was much more complex than originally had been thought, and they effectively invalidated the genetic assumptions underlying the movement.

In response to this new scientific information, many geneticists during the First World War years lost interest in the eugenics movement. Still, the majority of the eugenicists remained as captivated by the movement as they had been at the beginning. Although they debated the particulars of the programs they advocated, they did not, for the most part, examine the ethical and scientific assumptions underlying their proposals. Few of them ever bothered to examine such fundamental issues as whether their programs made scientific sense in view of the more recent findings in genetics or whether mankind really is wise enough to decide which characteristics are desirable.

In their continuing allegiance to the movement, most eugenicists were sincere and well-intentioned. However, the majority had no scientific training, and their claim that the eugenic program rested firmly upon a valid genetic foundation rested more on faith than on personal acquaintance with the experimental evidence. To most of them, eugenics assumed the proportions not of a science but of a social and moral crusade. Some so venerated science and the scientific method that they came to regard the acceptance of eugenic programs as a religious duty imposed by the theory of evolution. Like many Americans of the time, eugenicists were frightened by what they interpreted as a sharply increasing incidence of physical and mental degeneracy, and they were equally alarmed at civilization's supposed interference with the working of natural selection. Accordingly, they were interested in eugenics because it offered a "scientific" solution to pressing social "problems" compatible with the world view of the naturalistic mind. The intellectually stagnant qualities of the eugenics movement can best be understood in this light.

Impact of the eugenics movement

Ironically, it was at the time that the scientific justification of eugenics was weakening that the movement started to achieve its greatest political triumphs. As the First World War closed, the movement began a decade of intensive and successful campaigning for "eugenic" legislation. Eugenicists were active peripherally in a variety of issues, including prohibition, birth control, custodial care for "defectives," and antimiscegenation bills. More important, however, they made a significant impact in two areas of major social import: sterilization legislation and immigration restriction.

The first American state to pass a sterilization law was Indiana, which in 1907 enacted a bill requiring the compulsory sterilization of inmates of state institutions who were insane, idiotic, imbecilic, or feebleminded, or who were convicted rapists or criminals, upon the recommendation of a board of experts. By 1931 thirty states had passed compulsory sterilization measures, some of which applied to a very wide range of "hereditary defectives" including "sexual perverts," "drug fiends," "drunkards," and "diseased and degenerate persons." The laws were passed primarily in response to the lobbying in the various state legislatures of zealous eugenicists, who viewed the measures as important planks of "negative eugenics." The most influential person was Harry Laughlin, Davenport's assistant at the Eugenics Record Office, who pursued the sterilization campaign with missionary fervor and whose writings on the subject guided interested lawmakers and citizens for more than twenty years.

More important than the sterilization laws was the Immigration Restriction Act of 1924. The controversial feature of this law was not the restriction of immigration per se but the *selective* restriction clause. This provision drastically limited the entry of individuals from Southern and Eastern Europe on the grounds they were "biologically inferior," favoring instead the admission of "Nordics" from the northwest corner of the Continent. Following the First World War, at a time of intense nationalism and isolationism, of deep hostility and animosity toward anything foreign, the social climate was ripe for the enactment of a law restricting immigration. Nevertheless, the racist leaders of the eugenics movement, masking their hatreds under a veneer of scientific objectivity, seized this opportunity to argue that selective immigration restriction was a biological imperative. They stressed the Social Darwinistic supposition that economic and social status indicate hereditary value; they insisted that heredity is far more important than environment; and they claimed that any mixing between "American" and "foreign" blood would produce offspring inferior to both parental types. The leading popularizer of this view in Congress was Laughlin, who had been appointed "expert eugenics agent" of the House Committee on Immigration and Naturalization in 1920, and whose most important congressional testimony, "Analysis of America's Modern Melting Pot," greatly influenced congressmen and the public alike. By this time, as previously mentioned, eugenicists' view of biology had lost its scientific validity, but the public did not appreciate this, in part because few geneticists let their disapproval of the movement be generally known. During the course of the immigration debates, eugenicists' authority was effective and uncontested; their misappropriation of genetic theory gave their view a scientific sanction which opponents could not combat. Eugenicists considered the passage of this law to be their greatest triumph.

In the 1920s the racist side of eugenics was emerging in the German as well as in the American eugenics movement. With the rise to power of Hitler, who himself had long emphasized eugenic strictures for race improvement, the eugenics movement in Germany became irrevocably intertwined with the Nazi regime. Leading eugenicists became Nazi officials, and other government leaders also found eugenic concepts appealing. Eugenic ideas of race and of Aryan superiority were sanctioned by law on 14 July 1933, when Hitler decreed the Hereditary Health Law, or Eugenic Sterilization Law, which was created to make certain that "less worthy" members of the Third Reich did not transmit their genes. This law started the process that resulted in the experimentation with euthanasia in 1939 and ultimately to the mass murder of millions of other "undesirables."

Decline and rebirth of the movement

In the 1930s, in the aftermath of the eugenics movement's greatest political victories, the American people repudiated it. Several factors contributed to the movement's downfall. To a generation frightened by the Nazis' creed of Aryan superiority and alarmed by their morbid fascination with biological fitness and human breeding, the racist ideology of the American eugenics movement no longer carried its earlier appeal. Distrust of eugenics in the United States seemed well-founded, since throughout the 1930s some American eugenicists had publicly applauded the Nazi "eugenic" measures. The eugenics movement lost further ground as other social conditions changed. The Great Depression castigated economically, without distinction, both the Nordic and non-Nordic; people whose incomes had disappeared could no longer maintain with impunity that money and social prestige are indicators of genetic excellence. Finally, in the 1930s the scientific argument against eugenic proposals became fully developed. Increasingly, traits claimed by eugenicists to be the result of single genes acting alone were found to have complex etiologies—some were discovered to be the product of many genes interacting together, some of heredity interacting with environment, and many of environment alone. Research in psychology and anthropology also began to emphasize the influence of culture and environment in the development of an individual, race, or society, thereby providing further evidence against those eugenicists who held the Social Darwinist view that social position measures biological fitness. Perhaps the most devastating argument against eugenic schemes came in the 1920s and 1930s from the culmination of the earlier work in population (statistical) genetics. Research in this field showed that even allowing eugenicists their claim of the omnipotence of heredity and of the Mendelian recessive mode of inheritance of many traits, a eugenic breeding program would not cause the swift elevation of the genetic level of the population that eugenicists had predicted. As a result of all these events, eugenics in the 1930s fell into disrepute.

Though the old eugenics movement underwent an ignominious fall, the period from the 1950s to the 1970s witnessed a rekindling of interest in eugenics. The roots of this renewed interest began in the 1930s, when a new leadership, genuinely concerned with mankind's genetic future, rescued the eugenics movement from its ruins and assumed the task of rebuilding it. The new leaders cast off the class and race biases of the movement's founders, conceded the absurdity of earlier eugenicists' biological claims, and put together a new eugenics creed that was both scientifically and philosophically in keeping with a different America.

Since the Second World War, the revived eugenics program has developed along two main paths. The first and less dramatic is genetic counseling, the instructing of prospective parents about the likelihood that their children will be born with a genetic condition, a service which many medical centers are already offering. The second and more controversial part, sometimes itself called the "new eugenics," is the startling new view of man's future resulting from the postwar advances in molecular biology. With the composition of the gene and the principal molecular mechanisms of inheritance having been clarified, futurists foresee a day when physicians will distribute test-tube babies and do away with hereditary conditions by genetic surgery. The new eugenics is often referred to as "genetic engineering," though in fact it involves more than just genetic surgery as that name implies. In a narrow sense it may require environmental manipulation; nonetheless it utilizes genetic techniques. Although at present genetic engineering is still a branch of experimental biology, not yet ready for application to man, its overtones for eugenics are clear. The "new eugenics," like the old, is highly controversial; but the modern controversies center primarily on ethics rather than science, focusing on issues of means and not of ends.

The future of eugenic applications in the United States is not easy to determine, for American society today provides no clear signs, only ambiguous and contradictory clues. Modern medical research is increasingly interested in utilizing genetic techniques. For example, recent discoveries have made it possible to detect *in utero* fetuses afflicted with certain genetic diseases by examination of amniotic fluid. At the same time, however, contemporary medicine has not lost its traditional determination to conquer disease by utilizing the environmental procedures of surgery, diet, and drugs. If completely successful, the environmental approach theoretically might end the need for any further consideration of eugenics. Of course, there is no reason why the eugenic and environmental approaches cannot be pursued together, but so far there is much disagreement concerning their relative desirability and merit. Moreover, at a time when American society is struggling to determine how to foster individualism without encouraging lawlessness or civil disobedience, and how to contain crime and violence without resorting to repression, the ancient problem of clarifying the responsibility of the individual to the group and of the present generation to the future remains unresolved. On no other issue is it so important to reach a consensus before enacting far-reaching eugenic programs.

KENNETH M. LUDMERER

[*Further discussion of the history of the ethical issues in eugenics is found in the entry* EUGENICS AND RELIGIOUS LAW. *Also directly related are the entries* EVOLUTION; GENETIC ASPECTS OF HUMAN BEHAVIOR; GENETIC CONSTITUTION AND ENVIRONMENTAL CONDITIONING; GENETIC DIAGNOSIS AND COUNSELING, *article on* GENETIC COUNSELING; GENETIC SCREENING; REPRODUCTIVE TECHNOLOGIES; *and* STERILIZATION, *articles on* ETHICAL ASPECTS *and* LEGAL ASPECTS. *Other relevant material may be found under* BIOLOGY, PHILOSOPHY OF; EUPHENICS; GENETICS AND THE LAW; MEDICAL ETHICS UNDER NATIONAL SOCIALISM; POPULATION POLICY PROPOSALS, *article on* GENETIC IMPLICATIONS OF POPULATION CONTROL; PRENATAL DIAGNOSIS, *article on* ETHICAL ISSUES. *See also:* RACISM.]

BIBLIOGRAPHY

DAVENPORT, CHARLES BENEDICT. *Heredity in Relation to Eugenics.* New York: Henry Holt & Co., 1911.
DUNN, L. C. "Cross Currents in the History of Human Genetics." *American Journal of Human Genetics* 14 (1962): 1–13.
GALTON, FRANCIS. *Hereditary Genius: An Inquiry into Its Laws and Consequences.* London: Macmillan &

Co., 1869. Reprint. Gloucester, Mass.: Peter Smith Publisher, 1976.

GRANT, MADISON. *The Passing of the Great Race: Or, the Racial Basis of European History*. New York: Charles Scribner's Sons, 1916.

HALLER, MARK HUGHLIN. *Eugenics: Hereditarian Attitudes in American Thought*. New Brunswick: Rutgers University Press, 1963.

HOFSTADTER, RICHARD. *Social Darwinism in American Thought*. Rev. ed. Beacon Paperbacks, no. 16. Boston: Beacon Press, 1955.

LAUGHLIN, HARRY HAMILTON. *Eugenical Sterilization in the United States*. Chicago: Psychopathic Laboratory, Municipal Court of Chicago, 1922.

LUDMERER, KENNETH M. *Genetics and American Society: A Historical Appraisal*. Baltimore: Johns Hopkins University Press, 1972.

OSBORN, FREDERICK HENRY. *Preface to Eugenics*. Harper's Social Science series. Edited by F. S. Chapin. New York: Harper & Brothers, 1940.

PICKENS, DONALD K. *Eugenics and the Progressives*. Nashville: Vanderbilt University Press, 1968.

II
ETHICAL ISSUES

Objectives and means in eugenic practice

Attaining any eugenic objectives for improving the effective genetic quality of human populations over time will entail policy considerations that challenge contemporary values. The scope of a hypothetical eugenic policy would impinge on virtually every facet of human life. Eugenics, in Sir Francis Galton's words, deals with *"all* the influences that improve the inborn qualities of a race" (emphasis added).

In animal populations, the objectives of eugenics were attained through programs that selectively bred individuals whose gross physical characteristics corresponded to arbitrary ideals. Undesirable stock were prevented from procreation through sterilization or slaughter. In human populations, the early eugenicists sought to decrease the propagation of the physically or mentally handicapped and to encourage the procreation of those they deemed to embody the best features of the "race." A broad range of disabilities was considered to be genetically caused, and effective elimination of the affected individuals was sought by means remarkably similar to those used by animal husbandmen. Such steps were expected to reduce the incidence and ultimately the gene frequency for presumptively deleterious "genetically based" conditions like degeneracy, paraplegia, tuberculosis, promiscuity, and criminality, as well as those conditions which had a bona fide genetic basis, like albinism. Other geneticists, notably Hermann Muller, advocated *positive* eugenic ends through the selective use

of semen from "more desirable" persons to propagate their kind.

The chief stumbling block in attaining any of these early objectives of human eugenics has been the absence of adequate data on which to formulate policies that would be scientifically and ethically sound. More recently, genetic policy has shifted attention from broad eugenic objectives to focus on specific disease entities or physical disabilities with straightforward genetic causes. Most of the objectives of positive eugenics remain unattainable because of fundamental uncertainties regarding the genetic contribution to "positive" attributes like stature and intelligence.

In animal populations the only measurable eugenic successes have been made by extraordinary winnowing of less desirable sires or dams in favor of their more desirable counterparts. Applied to humans, such mechanisms would seem inevitably to violate traditional societal norms and breach virtually all rules of justice. Indeed, extreme forms of genetic intervention such as were practiced in Nazi Germany are stark reminders of the extremes to which pseudoscience can be bent to meet ideological objectives.

Value questions in genetic intervention

Ethical issues arise even when extremely modest eugenic ends are sought or less coercive measures are contemplated to bring about genetic change in human societies than were used by the Nazis. For instance, a decision to embark on a marriage counseling program that includes genetic information raises important questions of the propriety of the state's interest in genetic aspects of the reproductive decision making of couples. Any policy to discourage the marriage or procreation of individuals raises the question of possible infringement of privacy—a concept recently expanded by U.S. Supreme Court decisions to encompass reproductive acts, e.g., in *Griswold* v. *Connecticut* and *Eisenstadt* v. *Baird*.

Whether or not the state should embark on eugenic programs at all hinges on unexamined features of the ethos of the body politic. Some eugenicists have maintained that there is a fundamental obligation to improve the human species, while theologians like Paul Ramsey have maintained that an obligation for improvement is a derivative notion bereft of fundamental justification (Ramsey). Other scholars, like Bentley Glass, maintain that there is an irreducible obligation, in the light of genetic knowledge, not knowingly to produce a child with the prospect of physical or mental defect.

Progress through genetic improvement is part of a natural law ethic held by several major scholars. Sperry maintains that the preeminent place of humans in the order of nature makes manifest the direction of evolution. He argues that being human confers an obligation to continue this pattern of improvement (Sperry). Some evolutionary and molecular biologists (Simpson; Stent) contest this viewpoint and argue that there is nothing in the evolutionary program that would suggest an innate tendency toward evolutionary progress, nor is there any reason to conceive of human destiny as having a divine imperative toward species improvement.

Another viewpoint is that the very fact that humans can be aware of their origins and of the forces that shape their future mandates active use of that knowledge; to be human means to change nature and the human estate, and human consciousness and rationality argue for building on and directing the processes of nature (Fletcher). On the other hand, it is contended that there is nothing in nature or in any doctrine of divine providence that would require that a person succeed in achieving eugenic ends (Ramsey).

Minimal ethical considerations

Recent definitions of eugenics now embrace the concept of a basic obligation to *maintain* as well as to improve the genetic potentialities of the species. According to the theologian James Gustafson, responsibility for preventing deterioration of human genetic systems becomes enlarged because of our increased contemporary knowledge of genetics. We now know that present generations *are* causally linked with the genetic health of future generations, and thus, he argues, we have a moral responsibility to them. He identifies the injunction of not harming others as a minimal guiding principle undergirding any genetic policy (Gustafson). The rabbinical tradition, as well as that of Theravedic Buddhism, emphasizes that obligation by stressing the moral requirement that one not knowingly multiply the individual or collective griefs of mankind through taking even the most "mild" genetic risks (Narot).

Several theologians go farther in arguing that the moral principle of *primum non nocere* (first, do no harm) should be assigned the greatest weight in policymaking, and hence would preclude any attempt at genetic intervention that might generate unintentional harms. In traditional medical ethics, the basic precept of not harming was considered more important than attempting to improve an individual's condition. Medical interventions before the twentieth century often led to more lives lost than saved. Even today, where surgical practice is involved, the physician is under a primary injunction not to *add* to the patient's injuries. Before intervening, the surgeon must establish that reasonable cause exists for breaching the integrity of the body; that the techniques or explorations under consideration are appropriate to the ends being considered; that a reasonable attempt has been made to enlist the cooperation of the patient in consenting to the risks entailed in the intervention; and, finally, that informed consent to proceed has been obtained.

Validating eugenic policy

Analogous arguments can be applied to the propriety of initiating genetic interventions. A minimum ethical requirement for eugenics might include answers to he following: (1) Has the human genetic condition been demonstrated to be sufficiently impoverished or endangered to justify intervention? (2) Are the ends sought desirable, and who makes that judgment? (3) Are the means to be used necessary and sufficient ethically to achieve those ends? (4) Are the individuals whose lives will be affected by the interventions given a voice in the decision making? (5) Can assurances be given that implementing eugenics programs will not generate more harm than good? This approach links policy decisions to both utilitarian (e.g., the greatest genetic good for the greatest number) and deontological (are the inherent moral duties acceptable on their face?) considerations.

Should those requirements be met, second order ethical issues enter. One is the question of the appropriate level at which eugenic policies ought to be applied. For instance, it might be possible to achieve strictly limited eugenic ends for a specific disease entity whose gene frequency *was* in fact endangering individual families, while difficult or impossible to achieve the same ends for a more complex disease. A second problem is the weight to be given to efficacy in reaching eugenic ends. Some policies for achieving eugenic objectives could focus on specific disease entities and embrace intrauterine diagnosis and abortion of carriers of deleterious genes, while others could center on more prevalent manifestations of complex gene–environment interactions, such as hypertension. Programs to minimize the transmission of the responsible genes for hypertension would nevertheless be likely to prove cumbersome and inefficient. But it is a basic ethical tenet that inefficiency or any other index of likely efficacy alone does not invalidate the ends being sought.

Defining the genetic status quo

All objectives of eugenic policy must ultimately be measured against the perceived necessity of change. And any rationale for changing the human gene pool requires an understanding of its present state. What is the genetic status quo? Is the genetic composition of society deteriorating in such a way that remedial actions are mandatory in order to keep the situation from getting worse? Geneticists (e.g., Sang) believe that the apparent increase in human heterozygosity for deleterious genes will inevitably lead to their spread through the population. J. H. Sang sees the present genetic condition as being roughly equivalent to the beginnings of environmental pollution a generation ago. Others challenge this view (Medawar). They argue that, while some genetic dangers confront mankind, most are not of great urgency or gravity.

The truth appears to lie closer to the moderate view. Most contemporary geneticists downgrade the weight to be assigned to presumptive genetic deterioration and focus on the consequences of dynamic trends in populations instead. They are unclear about the ultimate meaning of the vast amount of genetic heterogeneity revealed by study of human genetic polymorphisms (situations in which two or more forms of the same allele or gene pair are present in a frequency greater than that generated by mutation alone). For example, it is uncertain whether selective forces or purely neutral events like genetic drift have generated the degree of genetic diversity observed in human populations. The ethical weight one should give to sustaining, reducing, or increasing the current level of diversity depends basically on an as yet unobtainable understanding of the evolutionary significance of genetic heterogeneity or the complex sources for the load of mutations we carry (Neel).

Ultimately, the genetic status quo of a given population is determined by dynamic factors and its exposure to mutagens like ionizing radiation. The average fertility, differential mortality, and age characteristics of the breeding members of a population can themselves affect the genetic

"load" that the population bears. Geneticists have identified many components that contribute to the load of deleterious genes a population carries, including radiation, mutation rate, and age at reproduction, each of which is an independent variable requiring its own analysis for weighting and policy decisions.

In addition to those factors, the intrinsic rate of increase of the population will have major impacts on genetic load. For example, if the population is growing rapidly it will tend to have a lower mutation rate and lower genetic load than will a stationary or declining population, because spouses will tend to reproduce when younger and hence prior to the accretion of excessive numbers of new mutations. Demographic effects of this sort mean that eugenic policies may conflict with other valued policies, like those for population limitation. In turn, "slow growth" policies in which reproductive age is protracted and/or delayed, will decrease the incidence of deleterious traits that are expressed with increasing probability with age (e.g., Huntington's chorea or multiple polyposis coli), but increase the risk of age-associated reproductive damage (e.g., Down's syndrome).

It is likely to prove crucial for eugenic considerations to recognize that the current population is not in genetic equilibrium and that acting to sustain or change demographic patterns will itself have potentially important effects on the frequency of specific genetic conditions. Slower-growing populations will have progressively less opportunity for sudden fluxes in the numbers of rare or novel genotypes, and the progressive trend toward equalizing family size seen in developing countries will minimize the differential fertility necessary for evolutionary change. While reduction of family size in itself does not mean that changes in gene frequency cannot still occur, in concert with population constraints it will reduce the variance in offspring and the effective number of breeding couples. Such a reduction means that the effective breeding population itself will shrink and that the opportunity for selection, so crucial to eugenic improvement, will also diminish.

Initially, that trend will give the appearance of eugenic effect since under the conditions of fertility limitation the frequency of recessive genes actually declines for the first few generations. But the long-term effect of reduction in population size, coupled with improved hygienic conditions and medical care, is to push frequencies for deleterious genes higher by "saving" affected and carrier individuals for procreation (Imaizumi, Nei, and Furusho). But what constitutes a tolerable load of harmful recessive genes, and how "deleteriousness" is to be defined, are still major value questions to be answered.

Defining "desirable" and "undesirable" genes

Like demographic shifts that affect gene frequencies, all eugenic policies require changes in the relative frequencies of human genes. But intentionally changing gene frequencies means determining which genes are to be assigned "favorable" and which "unfavorable" status. Definitions of "good" and "bad" genes are clouded in the ambiguities inherent in complex genetic causation. The classic example is the gene for hemoglobin S in which carriers of a single gene are afforded protection against the adverse health consequences of malaria, while those with two genes have sickle-cell anemia. Even as straightforwardly "harmful" a gene as that for retinoblastoma, an eye tumor, may be so closely coupled with one or more genes for intelligence as to be inseparable in any attempt at eugenic practice. Indeed, the gene for retinoblastoma itself may be so "pleiotropic" that one of its ancillary effects could affect factors bearing on intelligence.

Thus, significant questions of fact remain for all but the most egregiously lethal or semilethal genetic combinations. Even greater questions of value lie in determining how one should assign ethical weight to such genes when they are known. For instance, the gene involved in hyperbetalipoproteinemia, a familial condition characterized by high cholesterol levels and deficient receptors for low-density lipoproteins, is associated in white male carriers (heterozygotes) with over a fifty percent chance of a first heart attack before the age of fifty. Fully 0.1 to 0.5 percent of the population carry the responsible gene. Yet the policy one should implement in newborns or adults found to have this disorder is far from simple (Erbe). Moreover, for eugenic effects to be of consequence, aggressive genetic counseling must be exerted against procreation *prior* to the manifestation of the gene's full deleterious consequences, a difficult task both in practice and in principle.

In part, the dilemma of eugenic policy is that its effectiveness is conditioned on the long-term scope of its application, while the genetic decisions made by individual couples are most often predicated by more immediate life-style and personal decisions. Should some or most couples confronting the prospects of reproduction where Type II hyperbetalipoproteinemia is at stake be counseled to consider the more future-related, populationwide implications of their decision? By and large, genetic counselors have shied away from the inevitable eugenic "taint" of long-range goals. Emphasis on seeing "good" and "bad" genes in the context of genetic heterogeneity with wide variability in expression has become the rule rather than the exception.

Problems in changing the genetic status quo

It is widely recognized that the *effective* genetic makeup of any individual as expressed in that person's phenotype is the end result of a series of interactions between genes and the environment. Gene expression itself is affected by modifier genes, position effects, and the constellation of other genes in the person's genetic makeup. Most important, several key ethical considerations essential to any scientifically sound eugenics policy would focus on the nongenetic factors that might distort the expression of the genotypes in question.

Socioeconomic factors are strongly associated with increased incidences of birth defects like anencephaly (a lethal congenital condition in which the upper brain case and cerebrum fail to form) or reduced scores on intelligence tests. "Eugenic" policies could conceivably be implemented for these or other socioeconomically associated "defects" on the assumption that their statistical associations with class standing accurately reflect social differentials in gene frequency. This was, of course, the rationale behind extremely oppressive eugenics programs in the past. Class-related genetic policies are not only inappropriate where the conditions of life of the persons involved are in fact the major causative factors of disability, but politically freighted as well. Environmental influences that affect gene expression, such as diet (vitamin B deficiency), trace elements (lead contamination), and intrauterine existence, are known to lead to the appearance of "familial" patterns of defect or disability that are in fact largely or solely environmental rather than genetic in origin. In such instances, policies predicated on genetic models will almost always be socially injurious and unjust. Additionally, defects and tumors might be the result of sporadic somatic mutations rather than germinal ones, and hence not subject to the influence of procreative policies. Hemophilia and retinoblastoma are both examples. Hence, complexity in genetic causation calls for constraint in policy implementation if breaches of individual rights are to be avoided.

The state versus the individual

In addition to adequate consideration of the possible confounding effect of environmental influences, eugenic policymakers would need to consider the ethical issues around the weight to be given to personal autonomy. Theoretically, an operating principle for justifying eugenic policies could be derived form the demonstrated eugenic effect of population policies in which the reproductive behavior of individuals is constrained or otherwise influenced. Incentive programs in the form of tax credits, or disincentives in the form of penalities for those carrying presumptively deleterious genes, have been suggested at different times in the history of the eugenics movement. Such policy considerations place a greater weight on the public good to be obtained by compliance with a politically mandated solution than with autonomously derived decisions about reproduction that place the individual or his or her family above the state. The relative primacy of the state or the individual has traditionally underscored much of the eugenics debate.

Seen in modern terms, increased genetic knowledge and the enhancement of our ability to predict the consequences of reproductive behavior with an unprecedented degree of accuracy bring two ethical traditions into conflict: One assigns a high value to autonomy and self-determination in decision making, while the other imbues individuals with a sense of duty to act for the common good. When faced with these alternative orientations, ethicists have differed on where to place the greatest moral weight. Some ethicists believe that society does not have an unmitigated right to intervene in parenthood and reproductive behavior (Twiss). Others allow that right and accept that the state has the minimal moral obligation to educate and instruct in matters affecting reproduction. Such instruction is appropriate to raise the consciousness of persons with regard to the future, specifically the immediate social consequences of their reproductive behavior (Gustafson). The ethical arguments for the latter position are based on society's implicit obligation to future generations at least not to leave them worse off genetically than we are.

This obligation is reinforced by the recognition that our increasing sophistication in developing predictive techniques allows us to project the genetic consequences of individual human actions with unprecedented statistical accuracy. For instance, we now have a growing awareness of the legacy left by individuals who carried the gene for Huntington's chorea into this country in the eighteenth century, unknowingly spreading the deleterious gene they bore (as well as an indeterminate number of beneficial ones) to thousands of descendants. Under similar circumstances today, some ethicists believe that the range of moral accountability is greatly increased, and the notion of negligence becomes a more dominant reason for assessing moral liability.

Can eugenic policy be just?

Ethicists concur that any eugenic policy should incorporate some of the features of a just system. However, they disagree on what the achievement of "justice" requires. Those who believe that justice requires doing the greatest good for the greatest number might be expected to support those eugenic programs which achieved the "greatest genetic good." Others believe that the violation of one person's rights, especially those that embody basic liberties like procreation, for the benefit of others is only rarely, if ever, justified. Indeed, many follow John Rawls's suggestion that justice requires a fundamental kind of fairness in the allocation of goods, and they propose that justice requires that such goods and opportunities be distributed in a manner that benefits those who are least advantaged. While Rawls does not specifically apply this notion to eugenic policies, many if not most such policies seem to require sacrifices from those who are already (genetically if not otherwise) the less advantaged. Whether a specific program would be "fair" from a Rawlsian viewpoint depends on the priorities assigned to human goods and identification of those goods which are fundamental (Lappé).

Ultimately, we do not know which goods are considered sufficiently fundamental such that they *must* be distributed equally; nor do we know which ones are able to be distributed unequally without compromising the status of those most well off while aiding those who are least advantaged. Rawls does identify one human good, that of liberty, as being irreducible. In his view, liberty may be restricted only for the sake of liberty itself (Rawls).

At face value, the attainment of eugenic aims conflicts strongly with liberty. The implementation of eugenic programs has historically entailed selective, and often arbitrary and coercive, restrictions on some members of society and not others. The problem of justice is exacerbated by the fact that by definition the negative aspects of any eugenic policy on liberties would be directed at the least, rather than the most, fortunate members of society.

Some geneticists believe that any inequalities in social policies that flow from eugenic considerations could be rectified by allotting an individual's genetic contribution to the next generation on the basis of some assessment of his or her social worth. Two prominent geneticists have advocated assigning an Index of Social Value which apportions social value to some traits and not others (Gottesman and Erlenmeyer-Kimling). In practice, it would probably prove difficult to separate those traits that have little or no genetic contribution from those that have much, since ascertainment of the heritability of complex human traits is notoriously difficult. Any such exercise would ultimately require some determination of an individual's "genetic health," a concept that itself is fraught with ambiguities.

One manner of handling the problem is to allow a mechanism to produce a consensus in order to restrict liberty according to certain rules. Those who submit to restrictions, for instance, might then have a claim on those who have benefited from their actions. In the case of the mentally retarded, it might be considered ethically acceptable to have them or their proxies involved in any decisions to restrict childbearing in return for better conditions for their fewer offspring—conditions better than they themselves received.

But Rawls asserts that it is axiomatic for each person to wish to have greater natural assets and hence to wish such assets for one's own or another's children. Would we encourage donor insemination for the mentally retarded if the donor semen from high-IQ persons could be used? Certainly it is problematic to assume that actions should be taken that ensure for every person's descendants the best genetic endowment possible. While it is possible to argue that for a period of time a society should take steps at least to preserve the general level of natural abilities and to prevent the diffusion of serious defects, it is not clear how those aims would now be ethically realized.

Conclusions

The problem of reaching consensus on ethically acceptable approaches to eugenic policy is likely to remain knotty. Encouraging policies that already have public sanction—such as restricting consanguineous marriages or encouraging prospective genetic counseling, with amniocentesis and selective abortion—could effect a reduction in the incidence of rare genetic *diseases* but would not appreciably affect genetic load. Populationwide policies whose fundamental effect is to shift childbearing or other demographic characteristics through provision of public information, counseling, voluntary screening, and other noncoercive public devices would appear to be more consistent with equity and justice than are policies directed at compulsory control of individuals or groups; yet they are the very ones that would be most hampered by lack of compliance or participation.

At present we also lack a sufficient understanding of the critical demographic factors that already affect gene frequency, the incidence of chromosomal aneuploidy, as is found in Down's syndrome, and the opportunity for selection in human populations. Thus, we do not know with reasonable certainty that the current genetic status of the population (as it is affected by shifts in demographic variables) is in fact undergoing a dysgenic trend, or whether it is stabilizing in terms of the genetic load.

We have not systematically studied the socioeconomic factors that interact strongly with environment to produce disparate incidences of congenital malformations, many of which have appreciable genetic components. Furthermore, we have not sufficiently evaluated the desirability of utilizing existing methodologies for genetic intervention—such as population screening for carrier status, or genetic counseling and amniocentesis, which are now of value to *individuals*—as means of effecting populationwide change.

In our current state of ignorance of the benefits and consequences of the options, the consensus of most geneticists (Neel) is that our obligations to improve environmental components are prior to eugenic considerations. Chief among these environmental factors are those which increase the genetic load (mutagens) and those which undermine the expression of human genetic potential (and here poverty would rank highest). Stabilizing the quantity of the population so that equitable distribution of resources remains possible also has priority over eugenic considerations. Many geneticists would also concur that, where eugenic policies are to be put into effect, they should preserve the status quo of the gene pool, particularly by minimizing the contribution of novel mutations.

Ultimately, the fundamental ethical issues broached by eugenics embrace the problem of the relative primacy of the individual or the collective whole. Should the ends of medicine serve the race or individuals? Should any aspect of human procreation be placed under state control? How can desirable eugenic programs best be implemented to enhance individual responsibility, justice, and equity in the distribution of society's resources? These remain among the strongest unanswered ethical questions in eugenics.

MARC LAPPÉ

[*For further discussion of topics mentioned in this article, see the entries:* FUTURE GENERATIONS, OBLIGATIONS TO; JUSTICE; PATERNALISM; PRIVACY; *and* STERILIZATION. *Also directly related are the entries* GENE THERAPY; GENETIC DIAGNOSIS AND COUNSELING; GENETIC SCREENING; *and* GENETICS AND THE LAW. *See also:* POPULATION POLICY PROPOSALS, *article on* GENETIC IMPLICATIONS OF POPULATION CONTROL; *and* REPRODUCTIVE TECHNOLOGIES, *article on* ETHICAL ISSUES. *For discussion of related ideas, see the entry* MEDICAL ETHICS UNDER NATIONAL SOCIALISM.]

BIBLIOGRAPHY

CROW, JAMES F. "The Quality of People: Human Evolutionary Changes." *BioScience* 16 (1966): 863–867.

ERBE, RICHARD W. "Mass Screening and Genetic Counseling in Mendelian Disorders." *Ethical, Social and Legal Dimensions of Screening for Human Genetic Disease.* Edited by Daniel Bergsma. *Birth Defects: Original Article Series* 10, no. 6 (1974), pp. 85–99.

FLETCHER, JOSEPH F. *The Ethics of Genetic Control: Ending Reproductive Roulette.* Garden City, N.Y.: Anchor/Doubleday, 1974.

GOTTESMAN, IRVING I., and ERLENMEYER-KIMLING, L. "Prologue: A Foundation for Informed Eugenics." *Social Biology* 18, suppl. (1971), pp. S1–S8.

GUSTAFSON, JAMES M. "Genetic Engineering and the Normative View of the Human." *Ethical Issues in Biology and Medicine.* Edited by Preston N. Williams. New York: Schenkman Press, 1973, pp. 46–58. Symposium on the Identity and Dignity of Man, Boston University, 1969.

HUXLEY, JULIAN. "Eugenics in Evolutionary Perspective." *Perspectives in Biology and Medicine* 6 (1963): 155–187.

IMAIZUMI, YOKO; NEI, MASATOSHI; and FURUSHO, TOSHIYUKI. "Variability and Heritability of Human Fertility." *Annals of Human Genetics* 33 (1970): 251–259.

INGLE, DWIGHT JOYCE. *Who Should Have Children? An Environmental and Genetic Approach.* Indianapolis: Bobbs-Merrill, 1973.

JONES, ALUN, and BODMER, WALTER F. *Our Future Inheritance: Choice or Chance? A Study.* London: Oxford University Press, 1974.

LAPPÉ, MARC. "Can Eugenic Policy Be Just?" *The Prevention of Genetic Disease and Mental Retardation.* Edited by Aubrey Milunsky. Philadelphia: W. B. Saunders Co., 1975, chap. 21, pp. 456–475.

LIPKIN, MACK, JR., and ROWLEY, PETER T., eds. *Genetic Responsibility: On Choosing Our Children's Genes.* New York: Plenum Press, 1974. Proceedings of the Symposium "Genetics, Man, and Society" held at the American Association for the Advancement of Science meeting, 29 December 1972.

MEDAWAR, PETER. "The Genetical Impact of Medicine." *Annals of Internal Medicine* 67, no. 3, pt. 2 (1967), pp. 28–31.

MULLER, HERMANN J. *Man's Future Birthright: Essays on Science and Humanity.* Edited by Elof Axel Carlson. Albany: State University of New York Press, 1973.

NAROT, JOSEPH R. "The Moral and Ethical Implications of Human Sexuality as They Relate to the Retarded." *Human Sexuality and the Mentally Retarded.* Edited by Felix F. de la Cruz and Gerald D. La Veck. New York: Brunner/Mazel, 1973, chap. 15, pp. 195–205. Conference on Human Sexuality and the Mentally Retarded, Hot Springs, Arkansas, 1971.

NEEL, JAMES V. "Lessons from a 'Primitive' People." *Science* 170 (1970): 815–822.

OSBORN, FREDERICK HENRY. *The Future of Human Heredity: An Introduction to Eugenics in Modern Society.* New York: Weybright & Talley, 1968.

RAMSEY, PAUL. *Fabricated Man: The Ethics of Genetic Control.* A Yale Fastback, no. 6. New Haven: Yale University Press, 1970.

RAWLS, JOHN. *A Theory of Justice.* Cambridge: Harvard University Press, Belknap Press, 1971.

SANG, J. H. "Nature, Nurture, and Eugenics." *Postgraduate Medical Journal* 48 (1972): 227–230.

SIMPSON, GEORGE GAYLORD. "The Concept of Progress in Organic Evolution." *Social Research* 41 (1974): 28–51.

SPERRY, R. W. "Science and the Problem of Values." *Zygon* 9 (1974): 7–21.

STENT, GUNTHER. "Molecular Biology and Metaphysics." *Nature* 248 (1974): 779–781.

TURNER, JOHN R. G. "How Does Treating Congenital Diseases Affect the Genetic Load?" *Eugenics Quarterly* 15 (1968): 191–197.

TWISS, SUMNER B., JR. "Ethical Issues in Priority-Setting for the Utilization of Genetic Technologies." *Ethical and Scientific Issues Posed by Human Uses of Molecular Genetics.* Edited by Marc Lappé and Robert S. Morison. *Annals of the New York Academy of Sciences* 265 (1976): 22–45.

EUGENICS AND RELIGIOUS LAW

I. JEWISH RELIGIOUS LAWS   *David M. Feldman*
II. CHRISTIAN RELIGIOUS LAWS
                                 William W. Bassett

I

JEWISH RELIGIOUS LAWS

The laws of incest and consanguinity in the Old Testament would seem to have a rationale in eugenics, though this is never specified in the biblical text. The traditional commentators, too, advert only to the natural repugnance against incest. In the talmudic discussion as well as in the legal codes, the subject is treated as a sexual offense, involving a breach of morality rather than a eugenic error. (The Talmud is the repository of rabbinic exposition of biblical law and teaching, spanning more than five centuries of discussion in the Academies. The legal codes are, in turn, based on the Talmud and on subsequent development of the law, such as in Responsa, or formal opinions in response to new case-law inquiries.)

Even bastardy is a moral rather than a eugenic category. The *mamzer* (in Jewish law, the product only of an adulterous or incestuous liaison, not of an "out-of-wedlock" relation between unmarried persons) is not physically illborn; his status is compromised only legally and socially, rendered so in punitive (or deterrent) judgment against parents not free to have entered the relationship. But no difference obtains between the *mamzer* born of adultery—even technical adultery, such as when the document of divorce for her previous marriage was impugned—and the *mamzer* born of incest. Hence, no eugenic motive can be assigned here.

Moreover, the one "maimed in his privy parts" bears the same legal disabilities as the *mamzer*. Thus, a man of "crushed testicles or severed member" is excluded from "the congregation of the Lord" (Deut. 23:2); this verse is interpreted to mean only that he may not enter into conjugal union with an Israelite woman. Hence, the castrated male is under the ban *because* the act of castration is forbidden. But one "maimed in his privy parts" as a natural result of birth defect or of disease, as opposed to one castrated by his or another's deliberate assault, is free of this disability. The legal situations were thus analogized: "Just as the *mamzer* is the result of human misdeeds, so only the castrated one who is such as a result of human misdeeds is to be banned." With that distinction made in both cases, and with the further fact that the banned *mamzer* and castrated are permitted to marry, for example, a fellow *mamzer* or proselyte, it must be concluded that moral outrage and punitive judgment rather than eugenic considerations are evidently operative.

Eugenics, in the sense of choosing a marriage partner with the well-being of the progeny in mind, is more clearly present in talmudic counsel and legislation. A person is counseled to choose a wife prudently, and guidance is offered in doing so in accordance with the intellectual and moral virtues of the prospective bride; and since, we are told, a child normally takes after its mother's brothers, one should regard the maternal uncles in making his decision (Bava Batra

110a). A hidden physical blemish in a bride is grounds for invalidating a marriage, unless the husband can be presumed to have known of it in advance.

Actually, heredity as a eugenic principle takes its legal model from rulings with respect to circumcision. An infant whose two brothers died as a possible result of this operation may not be circumcised. He is deemed to have inherited the illness (probably hemophilia) that proved fatal to his two brothers. The Talmud goes on to say that an infant whose two maternal cousins showed that weakness may also not be circumcised. That is, the statistical evidence yielded by two sons from the same mother can also be reflected in two sisters of that mother (Yevamot 64b). This is a remarkably early recognition that hemophilia is transmitted through maternal lineage—in itself a significant eugenic discovery.

The statistical evidence, or the presumption, of adverse hereditary factors in a third family member, when those factors are seen to exist in two of them, thus becomes the basis of talmudic laws of eugenics. With modern laboratory means to determine the presence of these factors, the principle would of course operate even sooner, without waiting for statistical evidence in two members. The Talmud rules that a man may not marry into a family of epileptics or lepers, or—by extension—a similar disease (ibid.). This may be the first eugenic edict in any social or religious system.

True, the pure hereditary nature of this recommendation is not unanimously agreed upon. While one view in the Talmud attributes the "heredity" to physical characteristics of the marriage partner, another view sees the basis as "bad luck." In a recent Responsum, where the questioner considered abortion because the mother was epileptic, the Rabbi responded that the latter of the two views above may be the right one, and that fear of bad luck is an inadequate warrant for abortion (Feldman, p. 292).

In an other than legal context, the Mishnah (the foundation layer of the Talmud), speaks of the faculties that a father bequeaths to his son: "looks, strength, riches, and length of years" (Eduyot II, 9). Here, too, the commentaries align themselves on both sides: one sees the bequeathing of faculties as a natural hereditary process, the other sees them as reward for the father's virtues.

Two other talmudic ideas with eugenic motifs have reflections in current practice. In the interests of fulfilling the injunction to "love one's wife as much as himself and honor her more than himself," a man is advised to seek his sister's daughter as a bride; his care for her will be the more tender due to his affection for his own sister. Yet in the thirteenth century Rabbi Judah the Pious left a testamentary charge to his children and grandchildren, which became a source of guidance to others on the level of precedent for subsequent Jewish law. In this famous testament, he advises against marriage with a niece as having adverse genetic results. Modern rabbinic authorities conclude that, if this be the case, "natures have changed" in this regard since the days of the Talmud; but generally they dismiss the fears as medically unjustified.

A second point is a talmudic notion that eugenic factors operate in the matter of intercourse during pregnancy. Conjugal relations, we are told, should be avoided during the first trimester as "injurious to the embryo"; but encouraged during the final trimester as desirable for both mother and embryo, that the child then comes forth "well-formed and of strong vitality" (Niddah 31a). A medieval Jewish authority makes the matter a point of pride in comparative culture: the Talmud recommends coitus during the final trimester, while the Greek and Arab scholars say it is harmful. Don't listen to them, he says (Responsa Bar Sheshet, No. 447). Nonetheless, the Talmud prohibits the marriage of a pregnant or nursing widow or divorcee; the second husband, it is suggested in Maimonides's formulation, may be less considerate of another man's fetus and may inadvertently damage it through abdominal pressure in intercourse (Yevamot 36a); and in the nursing situation, assuming that a pregnancy weakens the mother's milk, the new father may fail to take the necessary steps to supplement the diet of his stepchild. And a pregnant woman who feels either an urgent physical or psychological need for food during the Yom Kippur Fast is to be fed for the sake of her fetus's welfare as well as her own (Yoma, 82a).

More homiletic than legal is the notion that defective children can be the result of immoral or inconsiderate modes of intercourse—an idea expounded but ultimately rejected by the Talmud (Nedarim 20a). Yet in more modern times the Hasidim ("pietistic" Jewish groups with a mystic orientation) maintain that spiritual consequences of the act are indeed possible; that if a man has pure and lofty thoughts during or preparatory to cohabitation he can succeed in

transmitting to the child an especially lofty soul. Hence dynastic succession of leadership, as opposed to democratic selection, obtains among Hasidic groups.

A study of biblical and talmudic sources written by Max Grunwald in 1930, cited by Jakobovits, discerns a broad eugenic motif. Grunwald writes that Judaism

. . . quite consciously strives for the promotion of the quality as well as quantity of the progeny by the compulsion of matrimony, the insistence on early marriage, the sexual purity of the marital partners and the harmony of their ages and characters, the dissolubility of unhappy unions, the regulation of conjugal intercourse, the high esteem of maternity, the stress on parental responsibility, the protection of the embryo, etc. To be sure, there can be no question here of a compulsory public control over the health conditions of the marriage candidates, but that would positively be in line with the principles of Jewish eugenics: the pursuit after the most numerous and physically, mentally, and morally sound natural increase of the people, without thinking of an exclusive race protection [Jakobovits, p. 154].

Though abortion is warranted primarily for maternal rather than fetal indications, screening of would-be parents for actual or potential defective genes, such as in Tay–Sachs disease, would, like premarital blood tests, be much in keeping with the Jewish traditional eugenic concern.

DAVID M. FELDMAN

[For further discussion of topics mentioned in this article, see the entries: ABORTION, *article on* JEWISH PERSPECTIVES; JUDAISM; *and* RELIGIOUS DIRECTIVES IN MEDICAL ETHICS, *article on* JEWISH CODES AND GUIDELINES. *Also directly related are the entries* FETAL–MATERNAL RELATIONSHIP; GENETIC DIAGNOSIS AND COUNSELING; GENETIC SCREENING; *and* PRENATAL DIAGNOSIS.]

BIBLIOGRAPHY

FELDMAN, DAVID M. *Birth Control in Jewish Law.* New York: New York University Press, 1968. Paperback ed. *Marital Relations, Birth Control, and Abortion in Jewish Law.* New York: Schocken Books, 1974.

JACOBS, LOUIS. *What Does Judaism Say About . . . ?* New York: Quadrangle/New York Times Book Co., 1974, pp. 165–166.

JAKOBOVITS, IMMANUEL. *Jewish Medical Ethics: A Comparative and Historical Study of the Jewish Religious Attitude to Medicine and Its Practice.* New ed. New York: Bloch, 1975.

ZEVIN, SHELOMOH YOSEF. *Le'Or Ha-Halakhah.* 2d ed. Tel Aviv: Abraham Zioni, 1957, pp. 147–158.

II
CHRISTIAN RELIGIOUS LAWS

Christian religious laws historically comprehend a large spectrum of rules to guide individual conduct and social relationships among the baptized. The laws most likely to have eugenic significance are the canons prohibiting the marriage of relatives. These regulations also formed the basis for the civil law prohibitions against the marriage of relatives in both the Continental legal systems and in the common law statutory scheme. Though the principal justification given for such prohibitions in Christian law has been ethical and social, there is substantial evidence that they also may reflect considerations classified as eugenic in contemporary scientific research.

The ecclesiastical regulations that forbid marriage between persons closely related by consanguinity are among the most ancient canons of the Christian tradition. Penalties attached to the violation of religious exogamic laws have varied historically in their severity, as, indeed, have the ways of measuring the degrees of kinship and defining within which degrees the crime of incest shall be punished. But the core of the tradition of canon law remains constant and reflects an extreme reluctance to accept the marriages of close relatives as humanly or religiously feasible.

For Roman Catholics all marriages within the direct line of blood relationship, i.e., between an ancestor and a descendant by parentage, and within the collateral line to the third degree, i.e., to second cousins, are forbidden (*Code of Canon Law*). In the Greek Orthodox tradition, marriage in the direct line and in the collateral line to the sixth or seventh degree by the Roman method of computation is prohibited in canon 54 of the Synod in Trullo, 691/2 (Hefele). All Oriental Christians forbid marriages in the direct line; Armenians, Jacobites, and Copts prohibit it in the collateral line to the fourth degree, Melkites to the sixth degree, Serbs and Chaldeans to the third degree, and Ethiopians without distinction. Among the Protestant reformers the restrictions of the medieval canon law were accepted by some, e.g., Melanchthon, Kemnitz, only the Old Testament regulations of Leviticus 18:6–13 by others, e.g., Bucer and, perhaps, Luther, and only the closest tie of direct parental relationship by still others, e.g., Wycliffe. In the Anglican community, *The Book of Common Prayer* contains the table drawn up by Archbishop Parker based on Leviticus in naming relatives incapable of marriage (Wheatly). Most Protestant churches today follow the prohibitions of civil law regarding incest and kinship marriage (Acte for Kynges Succession; Acte for Succession of Imperyall Crowne; Concerning Precontracte and Degrees).

The sources and commentaries upon the Christian laws record debate about the extent of the prohibition, the possibility of dispensation within certain close degrees of kinship, and about the related question of the divine or natural law origin of the laws. They reveal, however, only the most sketchy discussion of the foundations of the regulations themselves.

The classical reasons given for the prohibition of consanguineous marriages are ethical and social. The first reason was called the *respectus parentelae*, namely, that such marriages would undermine the respect due to parents and consequently to all those who are closely related (Thomas Aquinas, *Summa Theologiae* II-II, 154, 9). Secondly, they constitute a moral danger to family life arising from the possibility of early moral corruption of the young dwelling within the same household in which marriage could be allowed (ibid.; Sanchez, 7.52.12; 53). Thirdly, the prohibition of consanguineous marriages prevents the disruption of the family by sexual competition and forces the multiplication of friendships and the spread of charity (Augustine). These three reasons seem to have been sufficient to justify the laws, so that most scholars did not go beyond them to seek a further justification. Esmein, for example, said the laws arose simply out of an instinctive repulsion for incest and were not reflective of any known adverse physical consequences.

It is only in comparatively modern times that an explicitly eugenic reason for the prohibition has received scientific attention. Writing in 1673, Samuel Dugard noted: "There is a *judgment* which is said often to accompany these Marriages, and that is *Want of Children* and a *Barrennesse*" (p. 53). "The Children are weak, it may be; grow crooked, or, what is worse, do not prove well; presently, Sir, it shall be said what better could be expected? an unlawfull Wedlock must have an unprosperous successe" (p. 51). A. J. Stapf's *Theologia Moralis* in 1827 alluded to this possibility (p. 359). A fuller treatment is found in Le Noir's 1873 edition of St. Alphonsus's Moral Theology. Westermarck in 1889 and Laurent in 1895 spoke at length of a physiological justification of the canons to prevent indiscriminate inbreeding and the risk of a high incidence of deleterious genetic effects. Wernz, in 1911 (n. 416 [72]), writing from a comprehensive knowledge of the canonical tradition, said the ancient writers also knew of the undesirable effects of excessive inbreeding. He noted reasons derived from contemporary medical science in the writings of Gratian (early twelfth century) (c. 35 q. 283, c. 20), Pope Innocent III (1161–1216) (Schroeder), and Thomas Aquinas (*Commentum*). Since the late nineteenth century nearly all commentators on the canonical rules speak of eugenic objections to marriages of blood relatives.

It is possible to find in the ancient ecclesiastical commentators an awareness of a eugenic foundation to the prohibition expressed in primitive and undifferentiated modes of speech. For example, a persistent belief was kept alive among theologians and canonists that children of incestuous relationships will die or will be greatly debilitated, or that the familial line will be cursed with sterility. Benedict the Levite (850?) wrote of these marriages: "From these are usually born the blind, the deaf, hunchbacks, the mentally defective, and others afflicted with loathsome infirmities" (Benedict the Levite). Furthermore, in the explanations of the name of the impediment (i.e., the impediment of consanguinity), if one traces their origins through medieval glossography to the *Etymologies* of Isidore of Seville (560?–636), there appears an awareness of a physiological factor in the blood bond of close relatives that must be weakened before marriage safely can be contracted.

The antecedents of the Christian canons in the Mosaic law (Lev. 18:6–13) and the Roman law were taken as expressions of natural law by the canonists and were continued in the barbarian codes. In his *Ecclesiastical History* (I, 27) where the Venerable Bede (673–735) notes these laws, he records a quotation from a letter of Pope Gregory I to Augustine of Canterbury, written in 601. The reason given by Gregory for forbidding marriages of close relatives is, "We have learned from experience that from such a marriage offspring cannot grow up" (Bede). This letter and this reason not only are later picked up and cited by Gratian (c. 35, q. 5, c. 2) and Thomas Aquinas (*Summa Theologiae Suppl.* 54, 3), but may be found in virtually all the canonical collections of the early Middle Ages. Though comment on this passage is rare, comment was, perhaps, unnecessary. The passage from Gregory seems clearly to say that from forbidden consanguineous marriages experience teaches that children are affected or unable to grow up. There is thought to be a physiological consequence to incest. In the light of this it seems probable that the labored argumentation over the question of how close the relationship must be for marriage to be forbidden by natural law must have been conducted in some awareness of a popular belief in the biological consequences of such unions. The fear of genetic anomalies or biological debilitation from indiscriminate inbreeding may not be perfectly articulated. It is difficult to imagine, however, that some physiological dangers to offspring may not have been intended in the frequent citation of Pope Gregory to sustain the severity of the prohibition.

Thomas Sanchez (1625), who wrote the greatest of the canonical commentaries on marriage, says that the most suasive ground for forbidding incestuous unions is that there is a sharing of the blood among close relatives and that the physical image of a progenitor (*imago, complexio, effigies, mores, virtus paterna*) passes to offspring, so that the blood must be weakened through successive generations before marriage should be contracted (7.50; 7.51.1–2). Thus, preventing marriages of close relatives to protect the offspring by allowing several generations to pass before procreation can be called a measure of eugenic foresight, however simple the scientific awareness to support it may have been.

In summary, a eugenic foundation to Christian religious laws forbidding the marriage of close relatives is clearly articulated and commented upon by modern scholars from the late eighteenth and nineteenth centuries. Evidence of this kind of awareness may be discovered earlier in the canonical sources, however, going back at least to the seventh century. It would seem consistent with the eugenic connotation of those laws rooted in antiquity, together with a Christian sense of responsibility for offspring that partly motivated them, to consider further eugenic restrictions on marriage in Christian communities today, in light of contemporary knowledge of genetics.

WILLIAM W. BASSETT

[For a further discussion of topics mentioned in this article, see: EUGENICS. See also: FUTURE GENERATIONS, OBLIGATIONS TO; GENETICS AND THE LAW; NATURAL LAW; and STERILIZATION. This article

will find application in the entries GENE THER-
APY; GENETIC ASPECTS OF HUMAN BEHAVIOR;
GENETIC CONSTITUTION AND ENVIRONMENTAL
CONDITIONING; GENETIC DIAGNOSIS AND COUN-
SELING; GENETIC SCREENING; PRENATAL DIAG-
NOSIS; *and* REPRODUCTIVE TECHNOLOGIES.]

BIBLIOGRAPHY

An Acte for the Establishement of the Kynges Succession. 25 Hen. VIII, c. 22 (1533–1534). *The Statutes of the Realm,* vol. 3, pp. 471–474, especially pp. 472–473.

An Acte for the Establisshement of the Succession of the Imperyall Crowne of this Realme. 28 Hen. VIII, c. 7 (1536). *The Statutes of the Realm,* vol. 3, pp. 655–662, especially pp. 658–659.

AUGUSTINE. "Of Marriage between Blood-Relations, in Regard to Which the Present Law Could Not Bind the Men of Earliest Ages." *The City of God.* Translated by Marcus Dods. Introduction by Thomas Merton. New York: Modern Library, 1950, bk. 15, chap. 16, pp. 500–502. "De jure conjugiorum, quod dissimile a subsequentibus matrimoniis habuerint prima connubia." *Patrologia Latina,* vol. 41, cols. 457–460. Also. *Writings of Saint Augustine.* Vol. 7: *The City of God, Books VIII–XVI.* Translated by Gerald G. Walsh and Grace Monahan. The Fathers of the Church: A New Translation, vol. 14. Edited by Roy Joseph Deferrari. New York: 1952, pp. 450–454.

BEDE [VENERABLE BEDE]. *Bede's Ecclesiastical History of the English People.* Edited by Bertram Colgrave and R. A. B. Mynors. Oxford: At the Clarendon Press, 1969, bk. 1, chap. 27, pp. 78–102, esp. p. 85. Facing texts in Latin and English.

BENEDICT THE LEVITE [BENEDICTI DIACONI]. "Capitularium collectio: Pertz monitum." *Patrologia Latina,* vol. 97, bk. 3, sec. 179, col. 820.

Code of Canon Law: A Text and Commentary. Edited by Timothy Lincoln Bouscaren and Adam C. Ellis. Milwaukee: Bruce Publishing Co., 1946, canon 1076, secs. 1, 2; pp. 487–489. English with commentary.

Concerning Precontracte and Degrees of Consanguinite. 32 Hen. VIII, c. 38 (1540). *The Statutes of the Realm,* vol. 3, p. 792.

COUSSA, ACACIO. *Epitome Praelectionem de Iure Ecclesiastico Orientali.* 3 vols. Vol. 3: *De Matrimonio.* Rome: Typis Monasterii Exarchici Cryptoferratensis, 1948.

DAUVILLIER, J.-DECLERCQ C. *Le Mariage en droit canonique oriental.* Paris: Recueil Sirey, 1936.

DUGARD, S[AMUEL]. *The Marriages of Cousins German, Vindicated from the Censures of Unlawfullnesse, and Inexpediency, Being a Letter Written to His Much Honour'd T. D.* Oxford: Printed by Hen: Hall for Thomas Bowman, 1673. Work attributed to Dugard although taken largely from Jeremy Taylor's *Ductor Dubitantium.* Attributed to Simon Dugard in the British Museum Catalog.

ESMEIN, ADHÉMAR. *Le Mariage en droit canonique* (1891). 2 vols. 2d ed. Paris: Recueil Sirey, 1929.

FLEURY, J. *Recherches historiques sur les empêchements de parenté dans le mariage canonique des origines aux fausses décrétales.* Paris: Recueil Sirey, 1933.

GRATIAN [GRATIANUS, THE CANONIST]. *Decretum divi Gratiani, universi iuris canonici pontificias constitutiones & canonicas brevi compendio complectens.* Lyons: I. Pideoius, 1554, pt. 2, causa 35, question 2, canon 20, p. 1217; question 5, canon 2, pp. 1218–1221.

GREGORY I. "Gregorius Augustino Episcopo." *Registrum Epistolarum.* 2 vols. 2d ed. Edited by Paulus Ewald and Ludovicus M. Hartman. Monumenta Germaniae Historica, Epistolarum, vols. 1, 2. Berlin: Apud Weidmannos, 1957, vol. 2, pp. 332–343, especially pp. 335–336.

HEFELE, CHARLES JOSEPH. "The Quinisext or Trullan Synod, A.D. 692." *A History of the Councils of the Church: From the Original Documents.* Translated and edited by William R. Clark. Vol. 5: A.D. 626 *to the Close of the Second Council of Nicaea,* A.D. 787. Edinburgh: T. & T. Clark, 1896, sec. 327, pp. 221–239, especially canon 54, p. 231.

ISIDORE OF SEVILLE. "De affinitatibus et gradibus." "De agnatis et cognatis." "De conivgiis." *Etymologiarum sive originum, libri XX.* 2 vols. Edited by W. M. Lindsay. Oxford: E typographeo Clarendoniano, 1911, vol. 1, bk. 9, chaps. 5–7, unpaginated. *Patrologia Latina,* vol. 82, cols. 353–368.

LAURENT, E. *Mariages consanguins et dégénérescences.* Paris: A. Maloine, 1895.

LIGUORI, ALFONSO MARIA DE'. "De matrimonio." *Theologia moralis.* 4 vols. Edited by D. Le Noir. Paris: Ludovicum Vivès, 1872–1874, vol. 3, bk. 5, tractate 6, pp. 661–858, especially pp. 783–784.

MEYVAERT, PAUL. "Bede's Text of the *Libellus Responsionem* of Gregory the Great to Augustine of Canterbury." *England before the Conquest: Studies in Primary Sources Presented to Dorothy Whitelock.* Edited by Peter Clemoes and Kathleen Hughes. Cambridge: Cambridge University Press, 1971, pp. 15–33.

Patrologiae cursus completus: Series Latina [Patrologia Latina]. 221 vols. Paris: Apud Garnier Fratres, editores & J.-P. Migne successores, 1851–1894. *Supplementum.* Paris: Éditions Garnier frères, 1958– .

SANCHEZ, TOMÁS. "De impedimentis." *Disputationum de sancto matrimonio sacramento.* 3 vols. in 4. Vols. 1, 2, Genoa: Iosephum Pavonem, 1602. Vols. 3, 4, Madrid: Ludouici Sanchez, 1605, vol. 3, bk. 7, disputation 50, pp. 332–336; disputation 51, pars. 1–2; pp. 336–337; disputation 52, par. 12, p. 352; disputation 53, pp. 352–354.

SCHROEDER, HENRY JOSEPH. "The Twelfth General Council (1215): Fourth Lateran Council." *Disciplinary Decrees of the General Councils: Text, Translation, and Commentary.* St. Louis: B. Herder Book Co., 1937, pp. 236–296, in particular canon 50, pp. 279–280. Latin text. "Canones Concilii Lateranensis IV (Oecumen. XII): Anno 1215 Habiti." *Disciplinary Decrees,* pp. 560–584, in particular canon 50, p. 578.

STAPF, AMBROSIUS JOSEPH. *Theologiae Moralis.* 2 vols. Innsbruck: Typis & sumptibus Wagnerianis, 1827, vol. 2, sec. 312, p. 359.

The Statutes of the Realm, Printed by Command of His Majesty King George the Third, in Pursuance of an Address of the House of Commons of Great Britain, from the Original Records and Authentic Manuscripts (1810–1833). 11 vols. in 12. Reprint. London: Dawsons of Pall Mall, 1963.

THOMAS AQUINAS. *Opera omnia.* Vol. 30: *Commentum in Libros IV Sententiarum.* Edited by Stanislai Eduardi Fretté. Paris: Ludovicum Vivès, 1878, distinctions 40 & 41, question 1, article 4, pp. 770–771.

———. *Summa theologiae* II–II 154, 9. "Utrum incestus sit species determinata luxuriae." *Summa theologiae*. Vol. 3: *Pars secunda secundae*. Rome: Marietti, 1948, pp. 722–723. Translated by the Fathers of the English Dominican Province as "Whether Incest Is a Determinate Species of Lust?" *Summa Theologica: First Complete American Edition*. 3 vols. Vol. 2: *Second Part of the Second Part, QQ 1–189 and Third Part, QQ 1–90, with Synoptical Charts*. New York: Benziger Brothers, 1947, question 154, article 9, pp. 1823–1824.

————. *Summa theologiae suppl.* 54, 3. "Utrum consanguinitas de iure naturali impediat matrimonium." *Summa theologiae*. Vol. 4: *Pars tertia et supplementum*. Rome: Marietti, 1948, pp. 838–840, especially "Sed contra," p. 839. Translated by the Fathers of the English Dominican Province as "Whether Consanguinity Is an Impediment to Marriages by Virtue of Natural Law." *Summa Theologica: First Complete American Edition*. 3 vols. Vol. 3: *Supplement QQ 1–99, Appendices, Articles, Index*. New York: Benziger Brothers, 1948, question 54, article 3, pp. 2758–2760, especially "On the contrary," p. 2759.

WAHL, FRANCIS X. *The Matrimonial Impediments of Consanguinity and Affinity*. Washington: Catholic University of America Press, 1934.

WERNZ, FRANZ XAVER. *Ius decretalium*. 6 vols. Rev. ed. Vol. 4: *Ius matrimoniale ecclesiae catholicae*. Florence: Libraria Gaichetti, 1911.

WESTERMARCK, EDWARD A. *The History of Human Marriage* (1889). 3 vols. 5th ed. rev. London: Macmillan & Co., 1921; New York: Allerton Book Co., 1922. Reprint. New York: Johnson Reprint Corporation, 1971.

WHEATLY, CHARLES. "Of the Preface and Charge and the Several Impediments to Matrimony." *A Rational Illustration of the Book of Common Prayer of the Church of England*. 8th ed. London: C. Hitch et al., 1759, chap. 10, sec. 3, pp. 376–383. A commentary.

EUPHENICS

Euphenics (Greek *eu* = good or well, plus French or Greek *phen* = to show) was coined by Lederberg in 1963 as a noun to describe the engineering of human development. Currently it refers to the application of medical and surgical treatments to genetic disease (Lederberg, p. 521). Euphenics represents the realization of biological knowledge applied to human hereditary malfunctions, i.e., therapeutic medical genetics. It is an alternative to eugenics that has as its goal the reshaping of the gene pool of an entire population.

Nearly two thousand hereditary diseases are now known to afflict the human species; some such diseases have been medically cured symptomatically, but no genetic cure at the level of the gene itself has yet been effected. To date only about one hundred of these are understood at the level of primary gene products (enzyme or protein). For nongenetic diseases such as invasions by pathogenic microorganisms, a cure rids the afflicted of that which was the cause. However, in the case of hereditary diseases the source of affliction is a malfunctioning or nonfunctional gene, a component of the very biologic core of each individual. Treatment of such diseases relieves or even eliminates their symptoms, but the defective gene or genes persist and can be passed on to offspring.

Even though no effective method of altering or replacing abnormal genes in human patients is yet available, more and more genetic diseases are being treated by alleviating the malfunctions involved. Medical strategies currently in use as therapies for genetic diseases are enumerated with examples in Table 1.

Many genetic diseases, such as phenylketonuria, hemophilia, and cystic fibrosis, reduce the reproductive potential of the afflicted individual to nearly zero when untreated. These individuals are not sterile in the sense of lacking in functional gamete production; their low reproductive potential is a result of physical debilitation, social unacceptability, or prereproductive death caused by the genetic disorder they suffer. In most cases successful treatment of the disease symptoms also removes barriers to reproduction. Thus euphenics commonly raises the reproductive potential (Darwinian fitness in evolutionary terms) of the treated individual. It is a fundamental evolutionary precept and axiom of population genetics that whenever the Darwinian fitness of a particular genotype is raised relative to all others in a population the frequency of the genes characterizing the "selected" or more advantaged type will increase in the gene pool of subsequent generations. Herein lies a principal ethical dilemma of euphenics. As medical science is able to treat more genetic diseases, the frequency of each malfunctioning gene concerned will increase in subsequent generations. Indeed, it has been estimated that, at our current rate of medical advancement in the treatments of genetic defects, within five to ten generations the frequency of serious genetic defects could double from its current one in every twenty live births to one in ten (Augenstein, p. 32; see also Holloway and Smith).

Although each genetic disease may be rare in the populations surveyed, collectively these diseases already pose serious challenges to our medical resources and health-care delivery systems. It is estimated that currently twelve million Americans suffer from genetic diseases; at

TABLE 1

Medical Strategies Currently in Use as Euphenic Measures with Examples

1. Addition of a missing product
   Insulin for diabetes mellitus
   Antihemophilic globulin for hemophilia
   Gamma globulin for gamma globulin deficiency
   Thyroid hormone for familial goiter
   Human growth hormone for pituitary dwarfism

2. Restriction of a substance
   Dietary restriction of phenylalanine for phenylketonuria
   Dietary restriction of galactose for galactosemia
   Dietary restriction of fructose for fructose intolerances
   Dietary restriction of protein for arginosuccinicaciduria, citrullinemia, hyperammonemia, and hyperargininemia
   Avoidance of muscle relaxants for cholinesterase deficiency

3. Drug therapy
   Allopurinol for gout and Lesch-Nyhan syndrome
   Phenobarbital for hyperbilirubinemia and Crigler–Najjar syndrome
   D-penicillamine for Wilson's disease
   Cortisol for adrenogenital syndrome
   Pyridoxine for primary hyperoxaluria

4. Immunologic inhibition
   Rhogam for Rh incompatibility between mother and child

5. Surgery
   Remove lens for inherited cataracts
   Remove eye for retinoblastoma
   Remove spleen for spherocytosis
   Open valve for pyloric stenosis
   Close spinal column for spina bifida
   Transplant kidney for cystinosis, polycystic kidneys, and Fabry's disease
   Transplant bone marrow for Thalassemia and agammaglobulinemia

Source: Adapted from Howell, pp. 278–279, and Omenn, p. 56.

least forty percent of all infant mortality results from genetic factors; and every married couple stands a three percent risk of having a genetically defective child (United States, National Institutes of Health, p. 6). It is the compounding effects of all treatable genetic diseases that lead to concerns about the deterioration of the gene pool in future generations if the reproductive potential of large numbers of individuals is significantly raised by treating a multitude of different genetically defective conditions.

Conversely, it has been argued that genetic deterioration of the human species is a red herring (Lappé, p. 419), that the genetic consequences of the successful treatment of diseases caused by rare recessive genes are slight (Crow, p. 865), and that the rate of genetic deterioration is so slow that future generations will certainly find solutions to cope with any difficulties that arise (Medawar, p. 33). Positions such as these are usually based on single examples of rare genetic diseases, which show that more than a thousand years would be needed to double the frequency of any particular gene in question following successful treatment. It is also common to slip into "eugenic rationales" in discussions of the prevention of genetic deterioration. Thus, the possibility of sterilizing carriers (heterozygotes) becomes an issue, while this has nothing to do with euphenic practices.

The relationship of euphenics to genetic deterioration of the gene pool must be clearly known (1) before considering the collective impact on society of all current and potential genetic ameliorations and (2) in order to clearly separate eugenic goals or objectives from the problems created by euphenics. Euphenics may be an alternative to eugenics, and the two practices can, and we think should, be mutually exclusive. We suggest that this distinction must permeate all discussions of the euphenics–genetic deterioration dilemma. The solution to any such dilemma will eventually have to be an ethical compromise, and we should not unduly complicate our task by superimposing eugenic issues on an already difficult situation.

Several important factors that are generally not included in cursory views of the euphenics–genetic deterioration dilemma must be enumerated before moving on to remaining ethical problems. First, although the incidence of any particular treated genetic defect increases only slightly in a population as a whole, the effects within any family expressing the defect are much more pronounced. For example, pyloric stenosis (constriction of the passageway between the stomach and small intestine) produces obstructions in about 3 per 1,000 newborn infants. Before corrective surgery (to release and open the pyloric sphincter between the stomach and the small intestines) was available most individuals with this polygenic condition (produced by the action of many genes) died as children without making any contribution to the gene pool. When the condition became surgically treatable, afflicted children were then enabled to reach adulthood and reproduce. It was found that among their children 70 out of each 1,000 needed surgical treatment for pyloric stenosis. This is more than a twentyfold increase in one generation within families harboring this genetic defect (Stern, p. 628). Because inherited diseases are familial, the impact of even a slight populational increase becomes localized and hence intensified in particular families. Such situations may result in heavy burdens within certain families, while any effects go virtually unnoticed in the rest of society.

Second, because each genetic disease is rare and is held at low frequency by the low or zero reproductive fitness of those afflicted, the human mating system has not routinely generated recombinants (new genetic combinations) bearing two or more serious conditions within the same genotype. We have never observed the interaction of two or more genetic diseases in one person, e.g., someone with hemophilia and sickle-cell anemia or someone with phenylketonuria (inability to metabolize an essential amino acid) and galactosemia (inability to digest milk sugar). We are totally ignorant of the genetic interactions and phenotypic expressions of any such recombinants. We do know that in other organisms where double and triple mutants can be derived experimentally (they are never found in nature), the interaction of two or more mutations effecting lower viability or fertility typically exceeds the detrimental effects of either mutant alone. This problem is well known to animal and plant breeders and to anyone who has conducted Mendelian transmission exercises with the geneticist's favorite, *Drosophila melanogaster* (fruit fly). The treatment and subsequent reproduction of human beings with viability and/or fertility debilitations not only raise the frequency of each condition separately, but they progressively increase the probability of producing genotypes with multiple disorders. This potential needs to be thoroughly evaluated before the incidences of too many genetic diseases are allowed to increase unchecked.

Third, besides being ignorant about phenotypes due to genetic interactions involving multiple afflictions, we also know nothing of treatment interactions that might result. The array of genetic interactions possible from the collective accumulation of ten, or a hundred, or a thousand treatable genetic diseases makes even speculation on treatment interactions impossible.

Euphenics creates another set of ethical problems with regard to the distribution of medical care and the priorities given to medical services. It has been suggested that, once we accept the premise of equal right and access to medical care along with the present reality that we simply cannot, physically cannot, treat all who are in need, it seems more just to discriminate by virtue of categories of illnesses, for example, rather than between the rich ill and the poor ill (Outka, p. 24). Thus, with our assuredly less-than-optimal conditions for supplying medical services, it can be argued that persons with rare, noncommunicable disease should receive low priority, especially when costs are high and resources are scarce. Acceptance of this stance would place virtually all euphenic measures at a very low priority, because each measure is bound to treat a rare, noncommunicable (in the usual public health sense of the word) disease. Yet collectively, as we have noted, genetic diseases constitute a major medical problem. Again we urge that genetic diseases be considered collectively as a class of medical problems for which we are ethically obligated to provide medical services. It must also be recognized, however, that, if this view served to accelerate medical treatments of numerous genetic diseases, it would at the same time intensify the euphenics–genetic deterioration dilemma.

It has been pointed out that, in cases where normally functioning carriers (individuals with one dose of a detrimental recessive gene and one of the normal functioning gene) actually display "hybrid vigor," i.e., higher reproductive ability than individuals with two doses of the normal gene (homozygotes), public health might be better improved by treating "normals" than by treating sufferers (Turner, p. 196). Thus, for diseases such as sickle-cell anemia, cystic fibrosis, and Tay-Sachs, where carriers may have a higher reproductive potential than normal homozygotes, it may be argued that in the interest of future generations normal homozygotes also need, and are entitled to, some sort of treatment to compensate for their lower fitness. Do normal homozygotes in these situations have any claim to medical care? If so, what kinds of treatment would be appropriate, how would they be distributed, and what priority should they receive?

Yet another set of ethical issues concerning euphenics is that associated with partially treatable genetic defects. The concerns here regard situations where the rescuing of individuals from certain death seriously compromises their quality of life (Motulsky, p. 656). For example, it is now possible to isolate children born with immunodeficiency diseases inside a germ-free bubble to protect their defenseless systems from contracting any infections. They would prove fatal. This rare class of inherited diseases has little treatment other than the artificial bubble environment. Unless or until an efficient treatment is found, some kind of bubble is the only environment afflicted individuals can look forward to. Such partial treatments place "quality of life" and "sanctity of life" in an ethically difficult juxtaposition. Whether or not children might have the right to sue their parents for wrongful life in view of the psychological stresses experienced as a result of parental decisions to produce them and/or sustain them in spite of known genetic malfunctions and prognoses has already been questioned (Stern, p. 627; Ghent).

We must also ask how far any "right to reproduce" extends to such partially treated individuals. For example, suppose a boy with the form of immunodeficiency disease known as X-linked infantile agammaglobulinemia (also known as Bruton agammaglobulinemia) grew up in a germ-free bubble to adulthood, fell in love with a young nurse, and married her. Does this couple have a right to children, possibly by collecting sperm from the young man and using it to artificially inseminate his wife to produce their child? We know that all daughters will be carriers of their father's defective gene and all sons will be normal in this respect. Should there be any restriction on reproduction or on the production of female carriers? Should there be concern about increasing the frequency of a gene that produces a disease that has such a currently restrictive medical prognosis? Should we supply all the bubbles needed in anticipation of a cure? There are many proposed answers to these questions, but no unanimity. The difficulties exist entirely at the euphenic level; none needs to be extended into the realm of eugenics to conjure up ethical dilemmas.

Are we at an impasse—damned if we do and damned if we do not? Golding (p. 463) has said that the tragedy of the euphenic situation may be that we will have to reckon with the fact that the amelioration of short-term evils and the promotion of good (avoidance of gene pool deterioration) for the remote future are mu-

tually exclusive alternatives. Is this so? Is there any way out of this "euphenic fix?" Callahan (p. 7) says that there are only two ways to bridge the middle ground between unlimited individualism (individual rights) and unlimited regard for the community (societal rights): by establishing upper limits to what individuals can demand and by establishing internal restraints on the harm communities may do to individuals. The task is to arrive at an ethical compromise that properly balances the rights of individuals and those of society.

There seems to be a divergence of views regarding the individual–societal rights balance that ranges from abstention from reproduction by persons receiving euphenic aid (Wallace, p. 44) to claims of no responsibility to society's gene pool on the part of families receiving treatment for genetic disorders (Kushnick, p. 624).

As a "working" solution to the myriad problems raised by euphenics we propose the following concept as a humanitarian "stopgap," given the complexities and perplexities inherent in current euphenic implications.

It would seem most efficacious, given all the problems discussed above, that a "holding stance" be taken with regard to any deliberate change whatsoever in the human gene pool for the immediate future. At the same time it seems imperative that we continue to relieve to the best of our abilities the pain and suffering of individuals afflicted with genetic diseases and anomalies. We therefore suggest that the ethical compromises that must accompany euphenic manipulations be formulated about the objective of producing no change in the frequency of any genes whose function is altered by euphenic measures. We term this concept *genetic conservation* and define it as the maintenance of the genetic composition of the human gene pool in its present proportions. This must be understood to include active measures such as various degrees of control over reproductive potentials of individuals in whom euphenic measures would raise fitness and thereby produce future changes in gene frequencies. Genetic conservation includes acceptance of neither dysgenic nor eugenic gene frequency alterations given our current lack of knowledge regarding the compounding and interaction effects of increasing genes involved with genetic diseases and the pleiotropic (multiple, secondary) and evolutionary effects of decreasing or eliminating these same genes. We recommend genetic conservation because we do not currently have the requisite armamentaria with which to interfere either profitably or wisely with the structure of the human gene pool.

Genetic conservation focuses our problems squarely on the balance between individual and societal rights and responsibilities. It is not an answer but a way of approaching an answer that incorporates what we believe to be honest and just parameters. Within this domain we still have to decide upon the uses and abuses of technologies such as sterilization, artificial insemination, fetal monitoring, therapeutic abortions, and carrier determinations as they counterbalance euphenic measures in genetic conservation.

If genetic conservation is not needed now, when we can still effectively treat only a handful of genetic diseases, when do we reach the critical point at which we should be concerned about the additive and interaction effects of euphenic measures? Do we have the responsibility to act before even small changes occur and thereby set a precedent for future euphenic developments, or should we treat the "euphenic fix" as a negligible societal problem fraught with academic dilemmas too far removed from the real problems of contemporary society to warrant premeditated actions? The task of incorporating euphenic measures into the medical practices of our society is clearly upon us. It would be wise to consider all costs and benefits judiciously and proceed with the utmost care. The gene pool is, after all, our own.

LEE EHRMAN AND JAMES J. NAGLE

[*Directly related are the entries* EUGENICS; *and* GENETIC CONSTITUTION AND ENVIRONMENTAL CONDITIONING. *For further discussion of topics mentioned in this article, see the entries:* GENE THERAPY; GENETIC DIAGNOSIS AND COUNSELING; GENETIC SCREENING; *and* RATIONING OF MEDICAL TREATMENT. *See also:* ABORTION; PRENATAL DIAGNOSIS; REPRODUCTIVE TECHNOLOGIES, *article on* ARTIFICIAL INSEMINATION; RIGHTS; *and* STERILIZATION.]

BIBLIOGRAPHY

AUGENSTEIN, LEROY. *Come, Let Us Play God.* New York: Harper & Row, 1969.

CALLAHAN, DANIEL. "Science: Limits and Prohibitions." *Hastings Center Report* 3, no. 5 (1973), pp. 5–7.

CROW, JAMES F. "The Quality of People: Human Evolutionary Changes." *BioScience* 16 (1966): 863–867.

GHENT, J. F. "Tort Liability for Wrongfully Causing One to Be Born: Annotation." *American Law Reports* 3d ser. 22 (1974): 1441–1448.

GOLDING, MARTIN P. "Ethical Issues in Biological Engineering." *UCLA Law Review* 15 (1968): 443–479. Symposium: Reflections on the New Biology.

HOLLOWAY, SUSAN M., and SMITH, CHARLES. "Effects of Various Medical and Social Practices on the Frequency of Genetic Disorders." *American Journal of Human Genetics* 27 (1975): 614–627.

HOWELL, R. RODNEY. "Genetic Disease: The Present Status of Treatment." *Medical Genetics.* Edited by Victor A. McKusick and Robert Claiborne. New York: Hospital Practice Publishing Co., 1973, pp. 271–280.

KUSHNICK, THEODORE. "When to Refer to the Geneticist." *Journal of the American Medical Association* 235 (1976): 623–625.

LAPPÉ, MARC. "Moral Obligations and the Fallacies of 'Genetic Control'." *Theological Studies* 33 (1972): 411–427.

LEDERBERG, JOSHUA. "Experimental Genetics and Human Evolution." *American Naturalist* 100 (1966): 519–531.

MEDAWAR, PETER BRIAN. "Do Advances in Medicine Lead to Genetic Deterioration?" *Mayo Clinic Proceedings* 40 (1965): 23–33.

MOTULSKY, ARNO G. "Brave New World?" *Science* 185 (1974): 653–663.

OMENN, GILBERT S. "Genetic Engineering: Present and Future." *To Live and to Die: When, Why, and How.* Edited by Robert H. Williams. New York: Springer-Verlag, 1973, pp. 48–63.

OUTKA, GENE. "Social Justice and Equal Access to Health Care." *Journal of Religious Ethics* 2, no. 1 (1974), pp. 11–32.

STERN, CURT. "The Place of Genetics in Medicine." *Annals of Internal Medicine* 75 (1971): 623–629.

TURNER, JOHN R. G. "How Does Treating Congenital Diseases Affect the Genetic Load?" *Eugenics Quarterly* 15 (1968): 191–197.

United States, National Institutes of Health, National Institute of General Medical Sciences. *What Are The Facts about Genetic Disease? Most Ubiquitous of All Human Maladies.* DHEW Publication no. (NIH) 76–370. Bethesda, Md.: Department of Health, Education, and Welfare, 1976.

WALLACE, BRUCE. "Genetic Engineering: The Promise of Things to Come." *Essays in Social Biology.* Edited by Bruce Wallace. Vol. 2: *Genetics, Evolution, Race, Radiation Biology.* Englewood Cliffs, N.J.: Prentice-Hall, 1972, pp. 41–44.

EUROPE

See MEDICAL ETHICS, HISTORY OF, *section on* EUROPE AND THE AMERICAS.

EUTHANASIA

See DEATH AND DYING: EUTHANASIA AND SUSTAINING LIFE; INFANTS; ACTING AND REFRAINING; LIFE-SUPPORT SYSTEMS.

EVOLUTION

Essentials of Darwin's theory

Although Charles Darwin (1809–1882) did, of course, have both precursors and partial anticipators, and although there have been considerable rival accounts, the public is quite right to link the idea of biological evolution indissolubly with his name. The epoch-making landmark is, therefore, the publication in 1859 of *The Origin of Species by Means of Natural Selection.* This, the full title, is significant and apt. There was also a subtitle, which has since acquired a sinister ring: *or the Preservation of Favoured Races in the Struggle for Life.* Darwin's theory is evolutionary inasmuch as it asserts, and provides an account of, the origin of species. Evolution is thus contrasted with the idea of the fixity of species, all of which were presumably specially created; as is assumed, for instance, in the picturesque creation stories of Genesis. Natural selection is here the key term in an account of how evolution, in this sense, has occurred and still is occurring.

None of these various notions was by itself new. For instance, the general hypothesis of the derivation of all present species from a small number, or perhaps even a single pair, of original ancestors was propounded by Maupertuis, as the President of the Berlin Academy of Sciences, in 1745 and 1751, and by Diderot, the organizer of the great French *Encyclopédie*, in 1749 and 1754. Again, there is a garish account of struggles for existence and of natural selection—combined with a notion of natural kinds, or fixed species, emphatically detached from any idea of divine creation—in the philosophical epic *Concerning the Nature of Things* by the Epicurean Roman poet Lucretius in the first century B.C. The actual phrases "a struggle for existence" and "the survival of the fittest" occurred in relevant contexts in, respectively, *An Essay on the Principle of Population* (1798)— the *First Essay*—by T. R. Malthus, and in an article by Herbert Spencer for the *Westminster Review* of 1852. So Darwin's claims to theoretical originality must rest upon the matter and the manner of his putting it all together.

He himself in his *Autobiography* described *The Origin* as "one long argument from the beginning to the end" (Darwin, 1958, p. 140), massively illustrated and supported by his vast knowledge of natural history. It runs:

If . . . organic beings present individual differences in almost every part of their structure, and this cannot be disputed; if there be, owing to their geometrical rate of increase, a severe struggle for existence at some age, season, or year, and this cannot be disputed; then . . . it would be an extraordinary fact if no variations had ever occurred useful to each being's own welfare, in the same manner as variations have occurred useful to man. But if variations useful to any organic being do occur, assuredly individuals thus characterized will have the best chance of being preserved in the struggle for life; and from the strong principle of inheritance they will tend to produce offspring similarly characterized. This principle of preservation, or the survival of the fittest, I have called natural selection [Darwin, 1859, pp. 169–170].

Certainly this core argument is valid, and the premises from which it proceeds can scarcely be contested. The Malthusian power to multiply and the tendency of like to produce like are two of the most familiar and fundamental facts of both the animal and the plant worlds. But this core argument is very far from proving what Darwin never thought it did prove: that all known species are descended, like varieties, from other species. Big questions remain. Has there, for one thing, been enough time for the often enormously elaborate and subtly arranged sorts of known life to have evolved in this way; or do we have to postulate some further, faster, much more directed mechanism? How, for a second thing, do hereditable differences or—for that matter—hereditable similarities appear, and are there sufficient of these, and of the right kinds?

In 1865 William Thomson (Lord Kelvin) argued that the physics of the cooling of the earth could not admit the vast ages which the geologists thought that the record of the rocks had revealed; and it was only well after Darwin's death that Kelvin could be shown to have been in fact mistaken. Darwin himself was convinced that natural selection has been the most important, but not the exclusive, means of modification. In a later work on *The Descent of Man* he protested that, whereas "my critics frequently assume that I attribute all changes of corporeal structure and mental power exclusively to the natural selection of such variations as are often called spontaneous," in fact he had from the beginning always "stated that great weight must be attributed to the inherited effects of use and disuse, with respect both to the body and the mind" (1874, p. viii). This was in fact Darwin's view, although such passages must come as a shock to those familiar with the ferocity of the neo-Darwinian rejection of any such Lamarckian suggestion of the inheritance of acquired characteristics.

On the second count Darwin was fully aware that he just did not know: "Our ignorance of the laws of variation is profound" (Darwin, 1859, p. 202). The work done in the early 1860s by Gregor Mendel—digging to lay the foundations of genetics—became known to his successors only after it had been independently repeated at the turn of the century by Hugo de Vries.

Darwinism and religion

The impact of Darwin's work has been wide-ranging and profound: It was altogether fitting that his compatriots buried him in Westminster Abbey, hard by the tomb of Sir Isaac Newton. It was Darwin and not any of his evolutionist predecessors who persuaded the scientific world that all the variety of life today has been the outcome of a gradual process of descent with modifications from a few original very simple forms —perhaps only one. Darwin succeeded where others had failed because he indicated a mechanism that he could prove must be operating, and because he deployed a mass of detailed evidence and argument to show how the development could have occurred.

Outside of science the first upset was to established religious ideas. For, although Darwinism was no more incompatible with a literal reading of Genesis than earlier evolutionary accounts of the origin of the solar system, or of the present condition of the earth's crust, it was nevertheless felt to be far more obnoxious. It seriously threatened, as they did not, the assumed special status of man. The epitome of this unease was the scandalized and scandalous question put by Bishop Wilberforce to the physiologist and publicist T. H. Huxley at an extraordinary meeting of the British Association for the Advancement of Science: "Is it on your father's or your mother's side that you are descended from a monkey?"

At least equally important was the threat to what should be known as the Argument or Arguments to Design. The most powerful expression of these in popular form was found in William Paley's *Natural Theology: or Evidences of the Existence and Attributes of the Deity Collected from the Appearances of Nature* (1802).

How could things so complex and so subtly integrated as organisms, and organs such as the human eye, come about, save by divine design? To this the Darwinian now replied that they could be, and were, the products of natural selection operating on spontaneous variation. His reply leaves the more sophisticated Argument to Design, which some find in the "Fifth Way" of St. Thomas Aquinas, untouched. The popular version appeals to divine design to fill lacunae in the scientific account of nature: "the God of the gaps." The more sophisticated alternative appeals first to whatever may be found to be the most fundamental regularities in the universe, including perhaps those from which evolution follows as a consequence. It then urges that this order cannot be intrinsic, but must be imposed by a divine orderer. The classical response to this is to be found in the posthumous masterpiece of the Scottish philosopher David Hume, *Dialogues concerning Natural Religion* (1779).

Social Darwinism

As the prestige of Darwin's theory grew, people began to see in it an endorsement for very diverse social and political policies. In America, William Graham Sumner (1840–1910) and, in Britain, Herbert Spencer (1820–1903) saw it as authorizing economic laissez-faire and no-holds-barred competition. J. D. Rockefeller declared in one of his Sunday school addresses:

The growth of a large business is merely a survival of the fittest. . . . The American Beauty rose can be produced in the splendour and the fragrance which bring cheer to its beholder only by sacrificing the early buds which grow up around it. This is not an evil tendency in business. It is merely the working out of a law of nature and a law of God [Hofstadter, p. 31].

At the opposite end of the spectrum of political economy Karl Marx wanted to dedicate the first volume of *Capital* to Darwin (Darwin declined), and in a speech at Marx's graveside Friedrich Engels claimed, "Just as Darwin discovered the law of development of organic nature, so Marx discovered the law of development of human history." Later socialists contrived to see Darwin's ideas as positively endorsing their own panacea, state monopoly. Thus in 1905 the future British Labour Prime Minister Ramsay MacDonald wrote that

. . . the Conservative and aristocratic interests . . . have armed themselves . . . with the law of the struggle for existence, and its corollary, the survival of the fittest. . . . Darwinism is not only not in intellectual opposition to Socialism, but is its scientific foundation. . . . Socialism is naught but Darwinism economized, made definite, become an intellectual policy, applied to the conditions of human society [Ferri, p. v].

A little later still, in the pre–World War I Vienna of his youth, the future Führer of German National Socialism wrote:

By means of the struggle the élites are continually renewed. The law of selection justifies this incessant struggle by allowing the survival of the fittest. Christianity is a rebellion against natural law, a protest against nature. Taken to its logical extreme Christianity would mean the systematic cult of human failure [Bullock, p. 693].

All such attempts to derive social, political, or bioethical norms directly from the findings of natural science must be unsound. Insofar as the survival of the fittest, and the so-called law of selection, really are laws of nature there cannot be any question of choosing either to obey or to disobey them. For where any descriptive law of nature holds it follows necessarily, by definition, that any occurrence incompatible with that law must be physically impossible. If there is to be room for a prescriptive law that lays down not what is but what ought to be, then it has to be physically possible either to do or to refrain from doing what the prescriptive law says ought to be done.

Many are inclined to believe that what is natural is by the same token good. Given this assumption it is almost impossible not to infer that a process of selection which is both natural and guaranteed to ensure the survival of the fittest must be for the best. The inference is, nevertheless, fallacious. The crux is the different criteria for what is fittest and what is best. Darwin's theory guarantees the survival of the fittest only and precisely insofar as actual survival is the criterion of fitness to survive. If some alternative and independent criterion is introduced, then Darwin's core argument ceases to be valid. The actual conclusion of Darwin's argument is entirely consistent with the familiar facts: that, for instance, men who are in every way wretched specimens exterminate superb species of animals; or that genius has often been laid low by the activities of unicellular creatures having no wits at all. The survivors, simply by surviving, show that they had what it took to survive. But those who seek in Darwinism an assurance that

the good will in the end prevail surely measure merit by some quite other standard. For to accept what the theory actually has to offer as if this were necessarily good would be to make time-serving your supreme principle: Whatever in fact wins will be as such in your eyes best.

Darwinism and progress

Darwin himself never misconstrued the expressions "struggle for existence" or "natural selection" in his theory as normative. Yet he was perhaps a little inclined to see in his own picture of biological evolution some promise of what he could value as progress. Thus in the penultimate paragraph of *The Origin* he wrote:

As all the living forms of life are the lineal descendents of those which lived long before the Cambrian epoch, we may feel certain that . . . no cataclysm has desolated the whole world. Hence we may look with some confidence to a secure future of great length. And as natural selection works solely by and for the good of each being, all corporeal and mental endowments will tend to progress towards perfection.

Before Hiroshima the second of these statements was reasonable enough. But the third was not warranted by what went before: No reason had been given for assuming that it is all, for the losers also, for the best; and it is perfectly possible for a species with great "corporeal and mental endowments" to be extinguished as a result of some competitive weakness elsewhere. Many of Darwin's successors, including several most distinguished biologists, have tried to develop his characteristically cautious hint of a promise of progress. After all, it certainly is the case that those animals which all would rate as, by other standards, higher, first appear in the most recent and, in that quite different sense, higher geological strata. (Darwin pinned into his copy of that once hugely popular book, Chambers' *Vestiges of the Natural History of Creation*, the memorandum slip: "Never use the words 'higher' and 'lower.'")

In our century Julian Huxley, one of the grandsons of T. H. Huxley, made several attempts to find in "the facts of evolutionary biology . . . a verifiable doctrine of progress" (1923, p. 19). It is, he said, a fundamental need "to discover something, some being or power, some force or tendency . . . moulding the destinies of the world—something not himself, greater than himself, with which [he can] harmonize his nature . . . achieve confidence and hope" (ibid., p. 17). Joseph Needham, another contemporary biological Fellow of the Royal Society, who maintains both a Christian and a Marxist–Leninist allegiance, reviews the same materials to find that "the new world-order . . . is no wild idealistic dream, but a logical extrapolation from the whole course of evolution, having no less authority than that behind it, and therefore of all faiths the most rational" (1943, p. 41). Later, in *History Is on Our Side*, he concluded: "Whatever force hinders the coming of the world cooperative commonwealth . . . is ultimately doomed. Against the world-process no force can in the end succeed" (1946, pp. 209–210).

The basic fault of every kind of social Darwinism is in logic. Albert Einstein expressed the heart of the matter with memorable clarity: "As long as we remain within the realm of science proper, we can never meet with a sentence of the type 'Thou shalt not kill.' . . . Scientific statements of facts and relations . . . cannot produce ethical directives." On the other hand, the trouble with the present sort of appeal to evolution as a guarantee of progress is that it ignores the decisive matter that members of our species already possess, or very soon will possess, the capacity to destroy all life on this planet. The point is made with salutary brutality by A. M. Quinton, writing on "Ethics and the Theory of Evolution." Man, he insists, "has certainly won the contest between animal species in that it is only on his sufferance that any other species exist at all, amongst species large enough to be seen at any rate" (p. 120).

Evolutionary biology cannot, therefore, provide either social and political norms or a promise of future progress. But what it can offer is a perspective. Huxley and Needham both wanted more, and sometimes believed that they had found it. What are available are possibilities of seeing our human activities in an evolutionary perspective. Thus, thirty years after he began his quest in *Essays of a Biologist*, Julian Huxley wrote:

In the light of evolutionary biology man can now see himself as the sole agent for further evolutionary advance on this planet, and one of the few possible instruments of progress in the universe at large. He finds himself in the unexpected position of business manager for the cosmic process of evolution [1953, p. 132].

Darwin, Lamarck, and the social engineers

Suppose that we do think of the life of mankind in this way, and suppose too that we are by temperament or conviction social engineers, eager to remake other people and human society nearer to our heart's desires. Then we are likely to be depressed by the implications, or the apparent implications, of Darwinism, especially when this is supplemented and reinforced by the findings of the geneticists. For this system of ideas defines certain limits to our ambitions. It suggests that our basic raw material—people, and especially the youngest—is in various genetically determined ways intractable; and that whatever shaping and molding we contrive to effect will have to be redone to all members of all succeeding generations.

Suppose again that we believe, conformably to our role as members of a quasi-Platonic elite of social engineers, that a very small group of ruthless and determined men can by seizing or creating a mighty state machine utterly transform a people and a society. Then we may well think that the neo-Darwinians present too passive a picture of the mechanisms of biological change. Surely there must be something we can do, other than just wait for natural (or artificial) selection to operate on spontaneously occurring variations?

These suppositions describe a ready market for Lamarckian notions of the inheritance of acquired characteristics. The Chevalier de Lamarck (1744–1829) developed a theory of evolution well before Darwin. Among the supposed laws of this theory are: (1) The production of a new organ in an animal body results from a new need which continues to make itself felt; (2) the development and effectiveness of organs are proportional to the use of these organs; and (3) everything acquired or changed during an individual's lifetime is preserved by heredity and transmitted to that individual's progeny. Almost all contemporary biologists believe that the vital third of these Lamarckian laws has been definitely refuted by experiment.

During the 1930s and 1940s similar ideas were put forward in the USSR by T. D. Lysenko. He succeeded in persuading the Soviet authorities both that his own researches were leading to results that would make possible a great leap forward in agricultural production and that orthodox Mendelian genetic theory was un-Marxist, and therefore to be eradicated in and by the party and the state. No such great leap forward in fact resulted. But it is indeed the case—though this has, of course, no bearing on the scientific question of which is the more true and tested—that Darwin's theory is more passive and less voluntaristic than that of Lamarck;

that it is, in Marxist terminology, metaphysical rather than dialectical. In the persecutions consequent upon the rise of Lysenko Russia's most distinguished geneticist, academician N. I. Vavilov, died, a martyr for science, in a concentration camp.

A less obscurantist response to the scientific picture of biological evolution is to make proposals for improving the human gene pool by encouraging the multiplication of approved genes and discouraging that of the disfavored. It was Darwin's cousin Francis Galton who introduced the label "eugenic" to describe such proposals, though the idea of policies for improving the human breed is at least as old as Plato's *Republic*. Eugenicists are, typically, concerned because modern medicine has enabled the victims of many formerly destructive genetic defects to survive to reproduce; and because those who rise or who stay at the top in socially mobile societies—and who are, therefore, presumed to have some of the best genes—tend to have fewer children than those who stay at or fall to the bottom.

More or less modest eugenic proposals, and attempts to draw moral and political conclusions from evolutionary biology, still are being made and will surely continue to be made; although it may sometimes seem that today we have rather more violent denunciation of putative proposals and alleged attempts than actual proposals and actual attempts. Consider, for instance, the controversies touched off in the last few years by the publication of Arthur Jensen's "How Much Can We Boost IQ and Scholastic Achievement?" and of Edward Wilson's *Sociobiology*.

Conclusion

Certainly evolutionary biology can provide a perspective for our thinking about human life, and certainly our policies must never fail to take account of stubborn biological and genetic facts. But policies are about possible choices; and no facts can by themselves determine in what sense choices ought to be made. Which is one, although only one, of the reasons why it must be wrong, for instance, to assume that admitting that any genetically determined average differences in talent or temperament between different racial and social groups would be to concede the propriety of advantaging or disadvantaging individuals for no other or better reason than that they happen to belong to one such group or another. The facts will remain whatever they are, whether we choose to face them or not,

whether we like them or not. But it is always for us to decide what we ought to do.

ANTONY G. N. FLEW

[*Directly related are the entries* BIOLOGY, PHILOSOPHY OF; MEDICINE, PHILOSOPHY OF; NATURAL LAW; PURPOSE IN THE UNIVERSE; *and* SCIENCE: ETHICAL IMPLICATIONS. *For discussion of related ideas, see the entries:* EUGENICS, *article on* ETHICAL ISSUES; GENETIC ASPECTS OF HUMAN BEHAVIOR, *article on* PHILOSOPHICAL AND ETHICAL ISSUES; *and* RACISM.]

BIBLIOGRAPHY

BARNETT, SAMUEL ANTHONY, ed. *A Century of Darwin*. Cambridge: Harvard University Press; London: Heinemann, 1958. Essays on the impact of Darwin in various areas.

BULLOCK, ALAN LOUIS CHARLES. *Hitler: A Study in Tyranny*. Completely rev. ed. Pelican Books, A564. Harmondsworth, England: Penguin Books, 1962.

CANNON, HERBERT GRAHAM. *Lamarck and Modern Genetics*. Manchester: Manchester University, 1959. A short polemical study by one of the few modern biologists with any time for Lamarckian ideas.

CHAMBERS, ROBERT. *Vestiges of the Natural History of Creation*. London: J. Churchill, 1844; New York: Wiley & Putnam, 1845. A dozen editions, 1844–1860.

DARWIN, CHARLES ROBERT. *The Autobiography of Charles Darwin*. Edited, with original omissions restored, by Nora Barlow. London: Collins, 1958. The first complete edition; all earlier, and some later, versions omit Darwin's various remarks about religion.

———. *The Descent of Man, And Selection in Relation to Sex*. 2 vols. London: John Murray, 1871. 2d ed. 1874.

———. *The Origin of Species by Means of Natural Selection, Or the Preservation of Favoured Races in the Struggle for Life*. London: John Murray, 1859. There is a modern edition of the first version by J. W. Burrow in the Pelican Classics series, Harmondsworth, England, and Baltimore: Penguin, 1968. A variorum text for the successive editions of Darwin's lifetime is edited by Morse Peckham, Philadelphia: University of Pennsylvania Press, 1959. References are to the modern edition.

DEWEY, JOHN. "The Influence of Darwinism on Philosophy." *The Influence of Darwinism in Philosophy and Other Essays in Contemporary Thought*. New York: Henry Holt & Co., 1910. Dewey always claimed that Darwinism was one of the continuing and formative influences on his own thought.

EISELEY, LOREN. *Darwin's Century: Evolution and the Men Who Discovered It*. Garden City, N.Y.: Doubleday Anchor Books, 1958. An exhilarating account of evolution and the men who discovered it.

FERRI, ENRICO. *Socialism and Positive Science: (Darwin-Spencer-Marx)*. Translated by Edith C. Harvey from the French ed. of 1896. 4th ed. The Socialist Library, no. 1. London: Independent Labour Party, 1906.

FLEW, ANTONY GARRARD NEWTON. *Evolutionary Ethics*. New Studies in Ethics. London: Macmillan; New York: St. Martin's Press, 1967. Reprint. *New Studies in Ethics*. 2 vols. Edited by William Donald

Hudson. London: Macmillan & Co.; New York: St. Martin's Press, 1974, vol. 2, pp. 217–268. A short philosophical study, aspiring to be definitive.

HOFSTADTER, RICHARD. *Social Darwinism in American Thought, 1860–1915*. Philadelphia: University of Pennsylvania Press; London: Oxford University Press, 1944. Hofstadter achieves what he undertakes admirably.

HUXLEY, JULIAN SORELL. *Essays of a Biologist* (1923). Pelican Books A51. Harmondsworth, England: Penguin Books, 1939.

————. *Essays of a Humanist*. London: Chatto & Windus; New York: Harper & Row, 1964.

————. *Evolution in Action*. London: Chatto & Windus; New York: Harper & Row, 1953. The Huxley works are landmarks in the search described in this article.

HUXLEY, THOMAS HENRY, and HUXLEY, JULIAN SORELL. *Evolution and Ethics: 1893–1943*. London: Pilot Press, 1947. A piquant confrontation between mighty grandfather and rather weaker grandson, hosted by the latter.

JENSEN, ARTHUR R. "How Much Can We Boost IQ and Scholastic Achievement?" *Harvard Educational Review* 39 (1969): 1–123.

KROPOTKIN, PETER ALEKSEEVICH. *Mutual Aid: A Factor of Evolution*. Rev. and cheaper ed. London: Heinemann, 1907. A counterblast to the traditional emphasis on competition, written with an eye to human applications.

NEEDHAM, JOSEPH. *History Is on Our Side: A Contribution to Political Religion and Scientific Faith*. London: G. Allen & Unwin, 1946.

————. *Time, The Refreshing River: Essays and Addresses, 1932–1942*. London: G. Allen & Unwin, 1943. Needham has an unusual width of interest, and a quite extraordinary combination of commitments.

QUINTON, ANTHONY M. "Ethics and the Theory of Evolution." *Biology and Personality: Frontier Problems in Science, Philosophy, and Religion*. Edited by Ian T. Ramsey. Oxford: Blackwell; New York: Barnes & Noble, 1965, pp. 107–131.

SPENCER, HERBERT. *The Principles of Ethics*. 2 vols. A System of Synthetic Philosophy, vols. 9, 10. London: Williams & Norgate, 1892, 1893. Very weary stuff, by a producer of evolutionary ethics more highly regarded by his contemporaries than by successors.

WADDINGTON, CONRAD HAL, ed. *Science and Ethics*. London: G. Allen & Unwin, 1942. A wartime discussion perhaps of antiquarian interest only.

WIENER, PHILIP PAUL. *Evolution and the Founders of Pragmatism*. Foreword by John Dewey. Cambridge: Harvard University Press, 1949. A serviceable study of a subject that may be of somewhat similar antiquarian interest.

WILSON, EDWARD OSBORNE. *Sociobiology: The New Synthesis*. Cambridge: Harvard University Press, Belknap Press, 1975.

EXPERIMENTATION, ANIMAL

See ANIMAL EXPERIMENTATION.

EXPERIMENTATION WITH HUMAN SUBJECTS

See HUMAN EXPERIMENTATION; PRISONERS, *article on* PRISONER EXPERIMENTATION; INFORMED CONSENT IN HUMAN RESEARCH; FETAL RESEARCH; CHILDREN AND BIOMEDICINE; AGING AND THE AGED, *article on* HEALTH CARE AND RESEARCH IN THE AGED; WOMEN AND BIOMEDICINE, *article on* WOMEN AS PATIENTS AND EXPERIMENTAL SUBJECTS.

EXTRAORDINARY TREATMENT

See DEATH AND DYING: EUTHANASIA AND SUSTAINING LIFE, *articles on* ETHICAL VIEWS *and* HISTORICAL PERSPECTIVES; INFANTS, *article on* ETHICAL PERSPECTIVES ON THE CARE OF INFANTS; LIFE-SUPPORT SYSTEMS; RIGHT TO REFUSE MEDICAL CARE.

DEMCO